Manual of
Oral Surgery

Matteo Chiapasco

Manual of Oral Surgery

THIRD EDITION

In collaboration with
M. Zaniboni

T. Anello, P. Casentini, A. Coggiola, E. Corsi, A. Flora, P. Fusari, G. Garattini, F. Gatti, L. Maccarini, R. Micolani, A. Montinari, A. Rossi, L. Serioli

Original title
Manuale illustrato di Chirurgia Orale – Terza edizione

ISBN 978-88-214-3469-3
eISBN 978-88-214-3725-0
Translation from Italian language, on behalf of Edra S.p.A., by: Marco Zaniboni

Publishing Manager
Costanza Smeraldi

Editor
Paola Sammaritano

Production Manager
Matteo Brambilla

Books Project Manager
Chiara Cucinella

Paper, Printing and Binding Manager
Michele Ribatti

Cover Design
Laura Barzacca

ISBN: 978-88-214-4756-3
eISBN: 978-88-214-4052-6

Edra S.p.A.
Via G. Spadolini 7, 20141 Milano
Tel. 02 881841
www.edizioniedra.it
Printed in Italy
Printed in August 2018 by "Printer Trento" S.r.l., Trento
(*) Edra S.p.A. is part of LSWR GROUP

Contributors

Tommaso Anello
Odontologist, Specialising in Oral Surgery, University of Milan
Tutor in Advanced Courses in Oral Surgery and Implantology, c/o Oral Surgery Unit of the Dental Clinic, Department of Health Sciences, University of Milan

Paolo Casentini
Odontologist, Private Practice
Lecturer in Advanced Courses in Oral Surgery and Implantology, c/o Oral Surgery Unit of the Dental Clinic, Department of Health Sciences, University of Milan

Alberto Coggiola
Surgeon, Odontologist, Specialising in Oral Surgery, University of Milan
Tutor and Lecturer in Advanced Courses in Oral Surgery and Implantology, c/o Oral Surgery Unit of the Dental Clinic, Department of Health Sciences, University of Milan

Elena Corsi
Odontologist, Specialising in Oral Surgery, University of Milan
Tutor in Advanced Courses in Oral Surgery and Implantology, c/o Oral Surgery Unit of the Dental Clinic, Department of Health Sciences, University of Milan

Andrea Flora
Odontologist, Specialising in Oral Surgery, University of Milan
Tutor in Advanced Courses in Oral Surgery and Implantology, c/o Oral Surgery Unit of the Dental Clinic, Department of Health Sciences, University of Milan

Pietro Fusari
Odontologist, Specialising in Oral Surgery, University of Milan
Tutor and Lecturer in Advanced Courses in Oral Surgery and Implantology, c/o Oral Surgery Unit of the Dental Clinic, Department of Health Sciences, University of Milan

Giovanna Garattini
Associate Professor of Orthodontics, Dental Clinic, Department of Health Sciences, University of Milan

Fulvio Gatti
Odontologist, Specialising in Oral Surgery, University of Milan
Tutor and Lecturer in Advanced Courses in Oral Surgery and Implantology, c/o Oral Surgery Unit of the Dental Clinic, Department of Health Sciences, University of Milan

Luca Maccarini
Odontologist, Specialising in Oral Surgery, University of Milan
Tutor and Lecturer in Advanced Courses in Oral Surgery and Implantology, c/o Oral Surgery Unit of the Dental Clinic, Department of Health Sciences, University of Milan

Roberto Micolani
Odontologist, Specialising in Oral Surgery, University of Milan
Tutor and Lecturer in Advanced Courses in Oral Surgery and Implantology, c/o Oral Surgery Unit of the Dental Clinic, Department of Health Sciences, University of Milan

Andrea Montinari
Odontologist, Specialising in Oral Surgery, University of Milan
Tutor and Lecturer in Advanced Courses in Oral Surgery and Implantology, c/o Oral Surgery Unit of the Dental Clinic, Department of Health Sciences, University of Milan

Alessandro Rossi
Odontologist, Specialising in Oral Surgery, University of Milan
Tutor and Lecturer in Advanced Courses in Oral Surgery and Implantology, c/o Oral Surgery Unit of the Dental Clinic, Department of Health Sciences, University of Milan

Laura Serioli
Odontologist, Specialising in Oral Surgery, University of Milan
Tutor in Advanced Courses in Oral Surgery and Implantology, c/o Oral Surgery Unit of the Dental Clinic, Department of Health Sciences, University of Milan

Marco Zaniboni
Odontologist, Private Practice, Milan, Bassano del Grappa

Preface

The *Manual of Oral Surgery* was first published in 2001. More than 15 years of life for a scientific textbook is quite a remarkable accomplishment, and a great source of satisfaction for its author and its publisher. Over the years, the manual has enjoyed a considerable diffusion among both professionals/specialists and academic students in Italy and abroad, thanks to a number of international editions. These significant results confirm its vitality and effectiveness. On the other hand, it is worth considering that the evolution of the diagnostic and therapeutic procedures and, particularly in the field of oral surgery, the evolution of the materials and surgical techniques, has been so significant as to render a comprehensive revision of the book necessary.

While the basic structure has remained unchanged to preserve the principles of clarity and effectiveness demonstrated by the first and second editions, the artwork and the clinical images have been significantly updated, and the text has been largely rewritten. Moreover, the most relevant innovations regarding the diagnostic possibilities and the surgical armamentarium, as well as the most recent minimally invasive surgical techniques, have been included. Furthermore, due to the considerable developments in the field of implant dentistry in recent years, a specific section of the text has been dedicated to a detailed description of the foundations of this fascinating discipline.

This revision has requested a significant effort and a great deal of work, something which would not have been feasible in a reasonable time frame all by myself. Therefore, I wish to thank all the colleagues that have contributed to the preparation of the new text, and who have helped me to select and organise the clinical pictures from the surgical interventions that I have performed over the years.

It is for me a great source of satisfaction to see that these colleagues, after graduating and specialising under my guidance, have maintained such a strong bond and still constitute a competent and close-knit group. Among them, I especially wish to thank Dr. Marco Zaniboni, who dedicated an enormous quantity of his time and intelligent energy in supporting me in the whole writing and revision processes.

Matteo Chiapasco

Contents

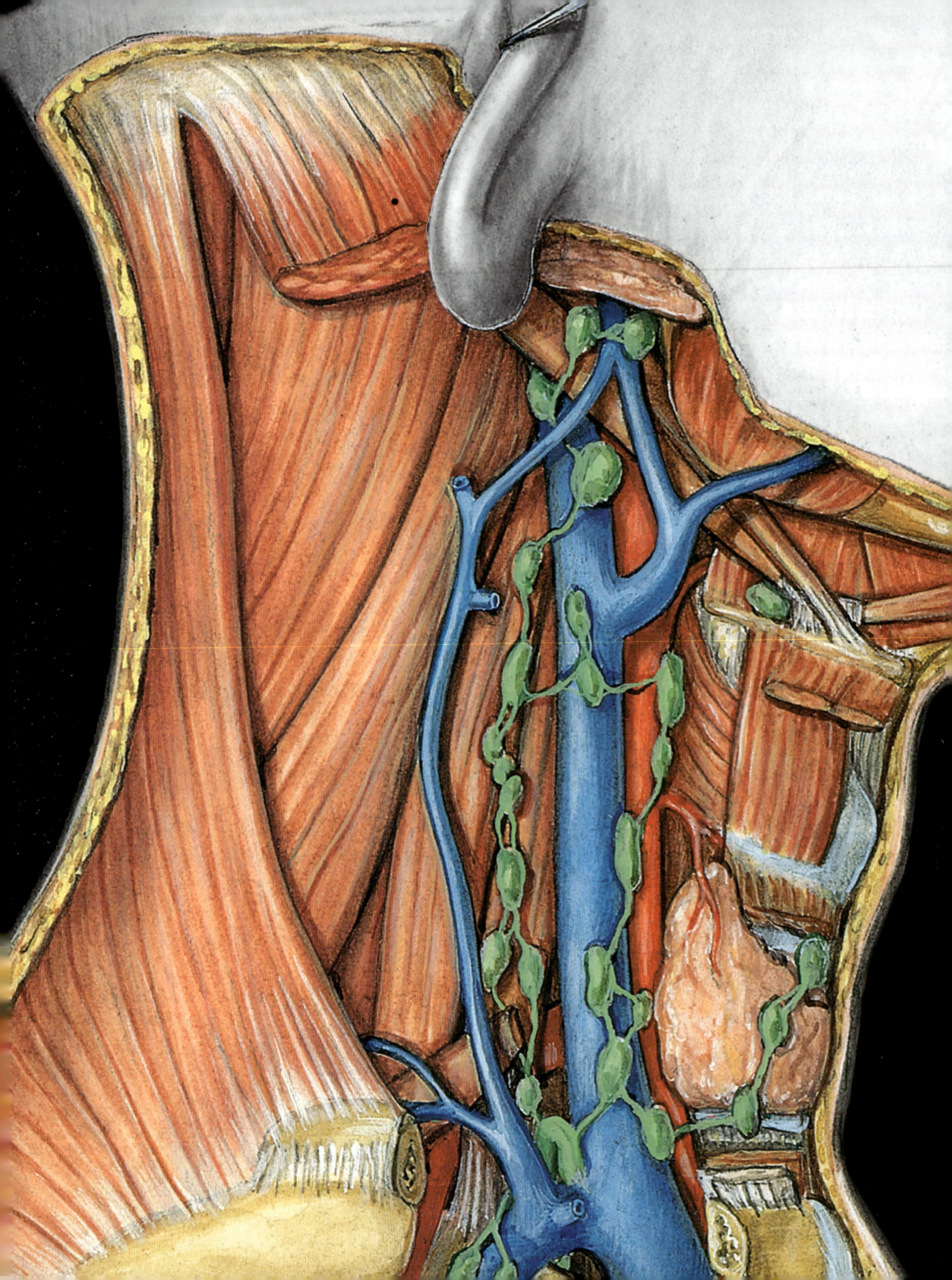

Basic principles

M. Chiapasco ▪ M. Zaniboni

Introduction

The domain of oral surgery, as with any other specialist surgery, is certainly not limited to surgical operation. In fact, the most important aspects of any surgical treatment are the preoperative evaluation and planning: if correctly performed, they can significantly reduce the risk of intraoperative and postoperative complications, and improve the outcome of the surgical intervention even when complications do arise. The sole application of a correct surgical technique never represents sufficient protection against complications or failures if surgery has not been properly planned.

Correct preoperative planning is founded on three pillars:

- Correct preoperative evaluation;
- In-depth study of the case;
- Knowledge of the local anatomy.

Adequate preoperative evaluation

Performing surgery is only the final stage of a thorough diagnostic workup, and entails not only gathering all the important information about the disease to be treated, but also assessing the patient's overall health. In addition, since oral surgery is largely elective and performed as an outpatient procedure, correct preoperative evaluation is essential in order to avoid complications during surgery (some of which can be quite severe), and complications in the postoperative period.

Given the practical nature of this text, it will not always follow the classic, semiological approach to the patient, but will instead adopt the approach that is used in daily practice in an outpatient setting.

To carry out a correct preoperative evaluation, it is necessary to follow a precise plan divided into several stages, each of which is a prerequisite of the following:

- Interview the patient about the reason for their visit, and a description of the main symptoms (recent medical history);
- Thorough clinical examination and recording of any signs;
- Prescription and subsequent analysis of X-ray examinations;
- Diagnostic hypothesis formulation;

- Assessment of the patient's general health (medical history) and request for additional examinations if necessary;
- Treatment plan decision and choice of the type of anaesthesia;
- Assessment of the risk-benefit ratio.

Chief complaint and description of the main symptoms (history of the present illness, HPI)

Any disease that falls within the scope of oral surgery presents its own peculiarities, and the latter will be analysed, in turn, in the dedicated chapters. Therefore, only the general aspects concerning the first visit will be described in this section.

The questions posed to the patient must be formulated in such a way that the most important information for identifying the active disease is gathered.

- What symptoms has the patient experienced, and how did he/she notice the onset of these symptoms?
- When did the symptoms appear?
- Is there any pain? What type of pain is it? (Continuous pain, intermittent, recurrent; is it associated with eating, or with the temperature of drink and food, etc.)
- Has the patient had a temperature? For how long?
- Has the patient noticed any swelling in the mouth or a change in facial profile? How long ago did this develop?
- Has the patient used any medications recently? For how long? What effects did they have?

For example, signs and symptoms such as the sudden appearance of an intra- or extraoral swelling associated with fever may be indicative of an acute infectious process, while they are very rarely associated with the presence of a neoplasm (📷 1.1). The concomitant ingestion of medications such as antibiotics can mask the clinical profile of an infection by reducing symptoms and clinical signs, thus making the diagnosis more difficult.

Clinical examination

The patient's description of his/her symptoms often provides a considerable amount of information about the active disease. However, this must be complemented by an in-depth analysis of clinical signs collected by means of a thorough physical examination. In addition, it is worth noting that frequently patients do not report any symptoms, so that clinical profiles are diagnosed by chance, after clinical or radiographic examinations have been performed to investigate other conditions.

Clinical examination is based on the manoeuvres of classic medical semiotics: inspection, palpation, and percussion (auscultation is rarely indicated in oral surgery, except for the diagnosis of temporomandibular joint disorders). Such manoeuvres are used to identify and assess the typical signs of pathology, such as swelling, redness, increased temperature of the skin and/or mucosa, pain, and functional impairment (*tumor*, *rubor*, *calor*, *dolor*, *functio laesa*); basic manoeuvres are summarised in this section. For a detailed description of the methodology, please refer to a specialty textbook on clinical semiology.

Intraoral inspection should not be limited to the area where the patient identifies the symptoms, but should be extended to the entire oral cavity (dental arches, floor of the mouth, tongue, palate, buccal mucosa and oropharynx). In this way, the presence of dental crown lesions, morphological alterations of the oral cavity, swelling and/or redness of the oral mucosa, fistulas, etc. can be detected (1.1). It is worth remembering that, apart from the symptoms reported by the patient, signs of different pathological conditions may be present (lesions such as periapical cysts, tumours, etc. may be completely asymptomatic) and should be identified.

Extraoral inspection can reveal anomalies such as asymmetry of the facial profile and areas of skin redness. These signs, associated with intraoral evidence, may lead to a presumptive diagnosis that will eventually be confirmed by the results of other semiological manoeuvres, and by the results of instrumental examinations (1.2).

Intraoral palpation provides useful information to assess the extent of a lesion, tissue consistency, tooth mobility, the presence of pain on compression, the degree of mobility of a lesion, the presence of drainage from a fistula, etc. Palpation can be performed with one or two hands: bimanual palpation is typically indicated to examine the soft tissues of the cheeks and the floor of the mouth (1.3). A single hand, in fact, can cause dislocation of the tissues and may fail to identify lesions developing between the intraoral mucosa and the skin.

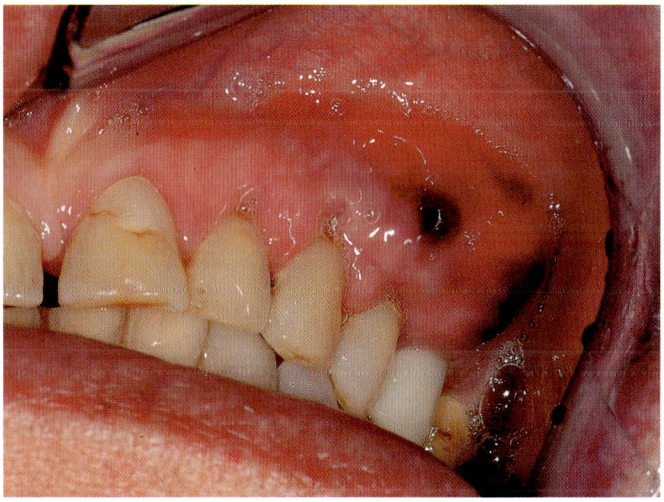

1.1 Localised swelling of the buccal mucosa in the left hemimaxilla (premolar region) caused by an odontogenic infection.

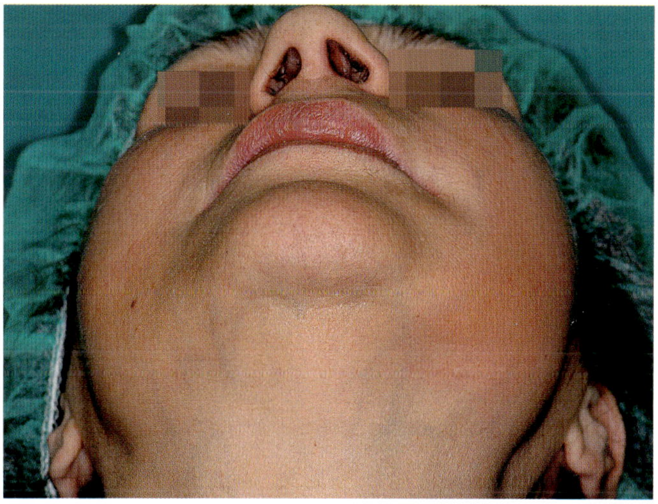

1.2 The same patient exhibiting swelling of the left cheek, redness of the skin and an altered facial profile.

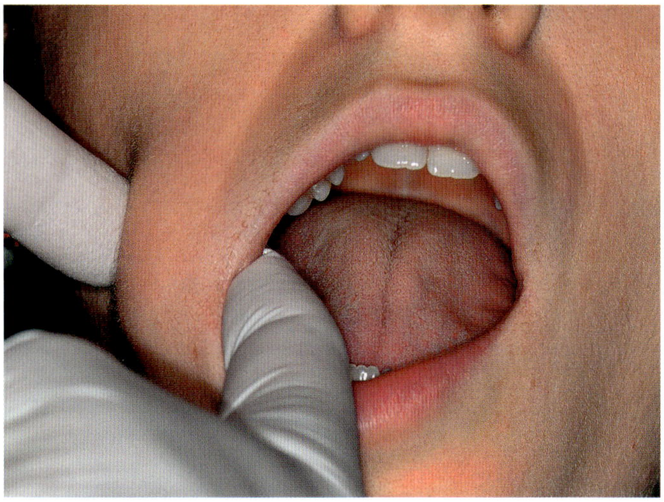

1.3 Bimanual palpation of the cheek.

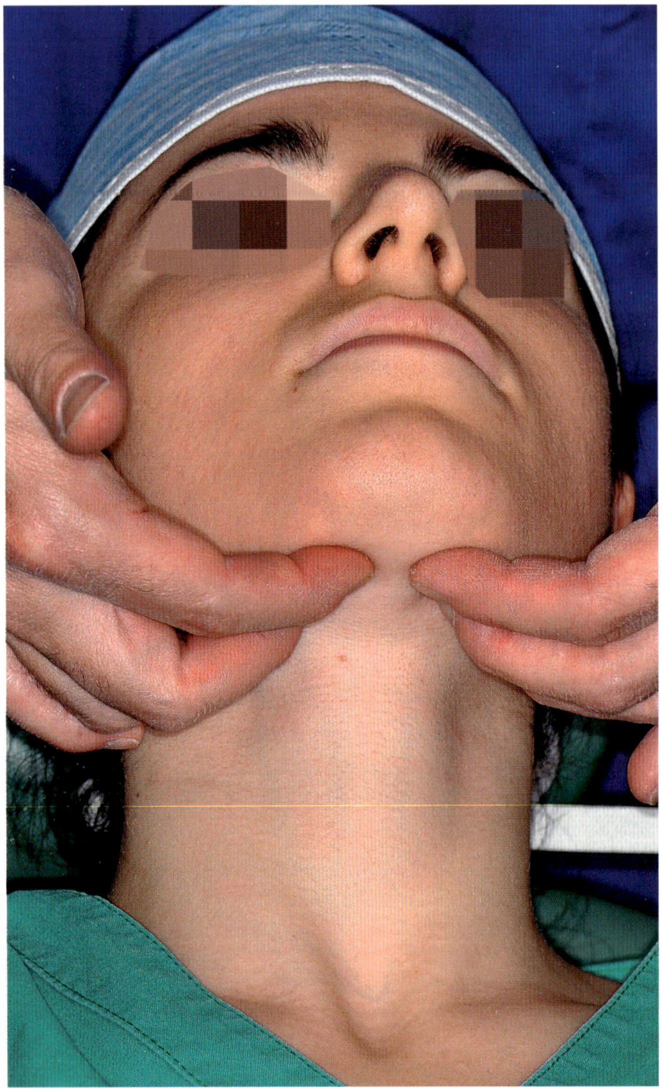

1.4 Palpation of the submandibular region.

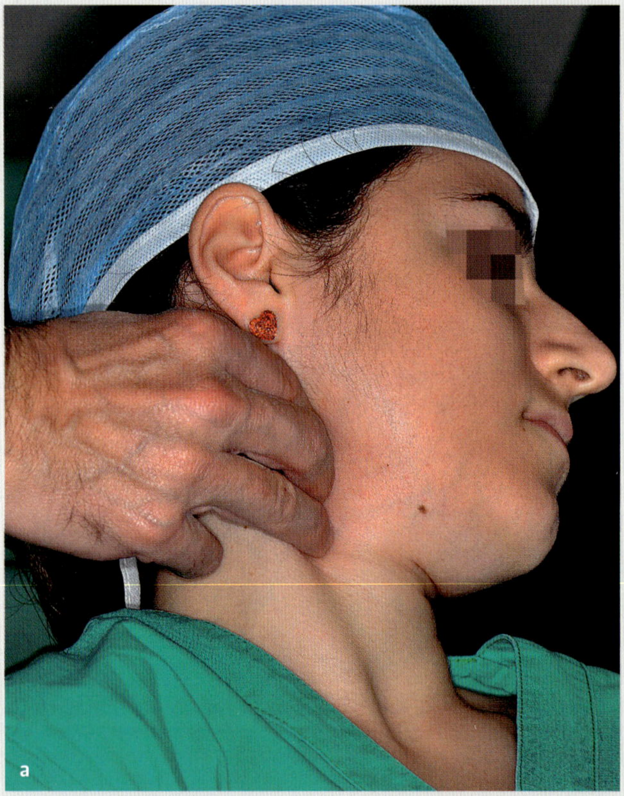

1.5 **a)** Palpation of the cervical lymph nodes. **b)** Anatomical drawing of the neck region highlighting the main cervical lymph node stations (from *Sobotta Atlante di Anatomia Umana*. Elsevier, Milano 2012).

Extraoral palpation is useful for evaluating signs of lesions that develop towards the cutaneous plane and for assessing cervicofacial lymph node stations (1.4, 1.5a-b).

Percussion is particularly useful for assessing pathologic conditions related to dental elements (periapical endodontic lesions, periodontal lesions, etc.).

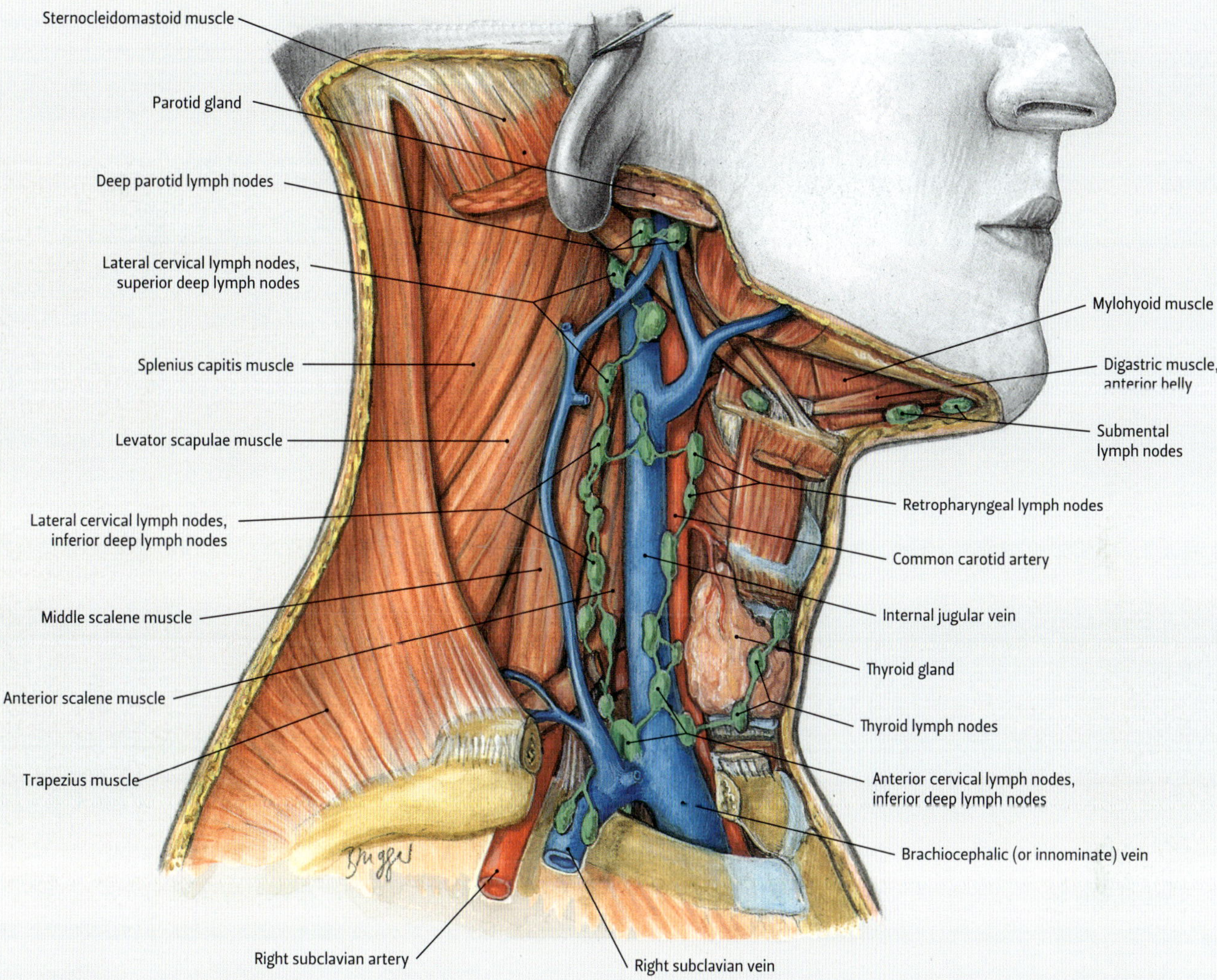

b

Radiographic examinations

Radiographic examinations alone are not sufficient to formulate a definitive diagnosis or decide every detail of the treatment plan. Nonetheless, they play a fundamental role in the diagnostic process and in the planning of every surgical intervention.

ANALOGUE AND DIGITAL MEDICAL IMAGING

Radiographic images are produced when an X-ray beam passes through a solid (human body) and then meets a support (a plate or a sensor) which is designed to be exposed. With regard to the first phase, i.e. the production and emission of an X-ray beam, little has changed over the years. Developments have instead been remarkable with regard to the second phase, namely the capture of radiographic images on a suitable support. Traditionally, the workflow in medical imaging was entirely analogue, as the support was represented by an X-ray film (plate) which was exposed and then developed. Increasing the sensitivity of X-ray films to radiation allows for a decrease in the radiation dose needed to obtain a good radiographic image. For this reason, even during the "analogue era" of radiology, developments in materials (plates/films) led to a marked reduction in radiation doses compared with those used at the dawn of the technique. The advantages of analogue images reside mainly in their high level of detail, while their limitations are due to the need for a development process by means of a darkroom and toxic developing/fixing agents, special procedures for the disposal of these fluids, storage space for the developed images, and the impossibility of applying post-processing techniques to the resulting images.

To overcome, as much as possible, the limitations of analogue media, alternative solutions using technological developments in detectors/sensors were subsequently explored. The first step was taken with the introduction of phosphor plate imaging systems, which represented the bridge between analogue and digital radiology. **Phosphor plates** are physically similar to analogue plates, but they present two *main advantages* over the traditional medium:

- each phosphor plate can be used several times, because the image can be deleted and the support can be exposed again;
- phosphor plates are not developed like traditional plates: instead, they are placed in a special scanner that captures the image in digital format.

This method eliminates the need to use a darkroom and developing/fixing agents, as well as the need for space to store the plates, because the exams are digitised by the scanner and stored directly on a computer. In addition, with this method of acquisition and digital storage, the resulting images can be edited with appropriate image processing software. However, this method also presents some *disadvantages*:

- media plates cannot be used indefinitely: after several exposures they retain traces of previously exposed images and must therefore eventually be replaced at costs which are not negligible;
- a scanner is required to acquire the images exposed on the phosphor plates.

The limits of analogue radiology and phosphor plate imaging systems were finally overcome with the advent of **digital sensors**, which enable the acquisition of radiographic images without the need for any external acquisition system. The image is captured by a CCD (*Charge Coupled Device*) sensor and directly transferred to a computer, eliminating the scanning and acquisition procedures, as well as the respective waiting times. The image obtained is directly stored and accessible from a computer connected to the X-ray sensor or, if a network is created, from any other computer on that network. The image can also be treated with post-processing techniques using suitable software, which can create ad hoc elaborations that are useful for investigating different anatomical and/or pathological situations. As far as this latter possibility is concerned, there are two categories of software capable of treating images, by acting at two different levels:

- the first level is a simple modification of the basic parameters of the scanned image, i.e. variation of brightness, contrast, sharpness, exposure, etc.;
- the second level is represented by the possibility of modifying the images by applying filters or (in the case of a series of images, e.g. CT scans) by creating alternative projections, three-dimensional elaborations of the acquired areas, etc.

The most important *advantage* of digital radiology is represented by the significant reduction in exposure times needed to obtain a good radiographic image, thanks to the enhanced sensitivity of CCD sensors over traditional films. The only *disadvantage* of digital radiology is the lower definition of the resulting image when compared to the analogue method. However, considerable technological developments in the field of digital sensors have occurred in recent years, suggesting that in a relatively short time sensors will become available that can acquire images with the same level of definition as analogue and phosphor plates.

Nevertheless, two possible issues related to the digital acquisition and processing of radiographic images remain:

- the possibility of modifying radiographic exams at will involves great medico-legal responsibilities, and it is therefore appropriate to limit the modifications to the correction of possible defects that may render the images difficult to read (incorrect exposure, inadequate contrast, etc.), while retaining a copy of the original image;
- not all post-processing software for digital images available on the market is officially approved for use on medical images for diagnostic purposes. It is therefore essential to use only certified applications. It would be incorrect and dangerous to base a diagnosis on calculations made with software not specifically designed to be used for medical purposes.

RADIOGRAPHIC EXAMINATIONS COMMONLY USED IN ORAL SURGERY

Regardless of the type of radiographic exam chosen to investigate a condition, it is fundamental that not only the entire area of the lesion, but also a portion of the surrounding healthy tissues, is visible. Secondly, when prescribing a radiographic exam, the relationship between biological costs and diagnostic benefits should be carefully evaluated, with the aim of limiting the amount of radiation to which the patient is exposed. For this reason, clinical evidence and diagnostic requirements must be thoroughly assessed in order to select the most appropriate radiographic procedure for each clinical situation.

The most frequently used radiographic exam in a private practice environment is the **periapical radiograph**, which is particularly suited to evaluate dental elements and lesions of limited extension that develop in the alveolar ridge (📷 1.6). Despite the disadvantages represented by the limited visible area and the two-dimensional nature of the image, periapical radiographs provide high definition images that, if the appropriate receptor instrument with X-ray beam ring guide is used, are immune to artefacts such as foreshortening or elongation of the captured anatomical structures, thus allowing accurate measurements to be performed.

Occlusal radiographs of the upper arch are indicated to evaluate the position (buccal or palatal) of impacted teeth, while occlusal radiographs of the mandible may be indicated to assess the buccal or lingual position of impacted teeth, to assess radiopaque mandibular formations on the lingual or buccal bone plates, and to investigate the presence of salivary stones inside the sublingual glands or the submandibular ducts (📷 1.7). Advantages and disadvantages of occlusal radiographs are similar to those described for periapical radiographs; however, occlusal radiographs are rarely used due to their limited indications.

When the limited dimension of intraoral radiographs precludes the possibility of capturing the entire area under investigation (📷 1.8a), the recourse to a **panoramic radiograph** is indicated. The panoramic radiograph (pantomogram, orthopantomography) provides an overview of the maxillary-mandibular complex, making it possible to evaluate the morphology of the maxilla and mandible, as well as of several other anatomic structures of the middle and lower third of the face such as the inferior alveolar nerve, the maxillary sinuses, the nasal cavities, the mandibular condyles, the glenoid fossae and articular eminences, the maxillary and mandibular dentition. It also makes it possible to verify the

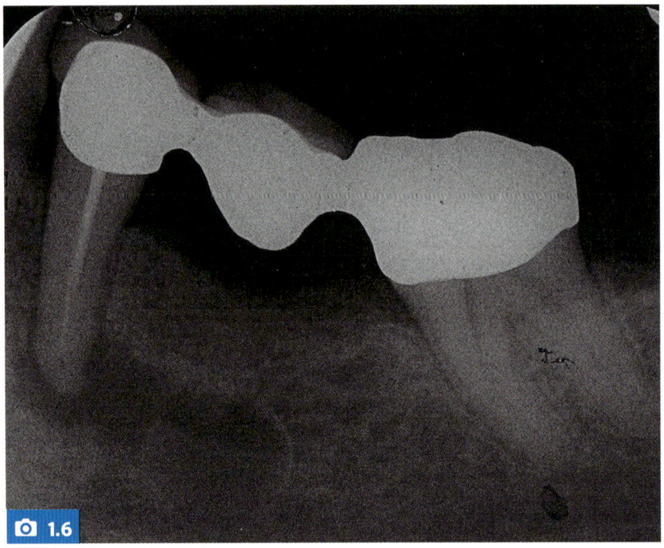

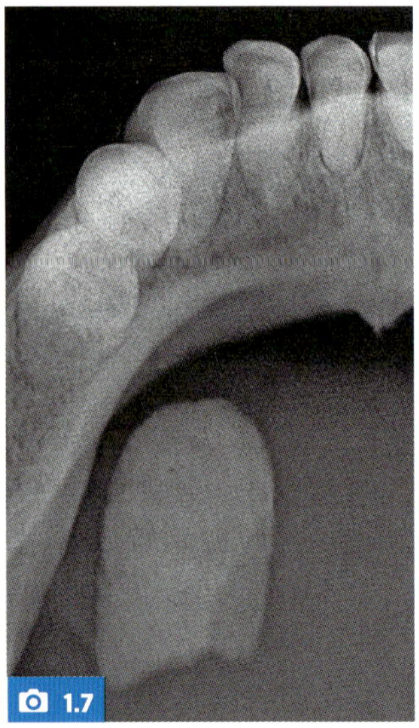

1.6 Periapical radiograph showing a radiolucent lesion around the apex of 35.

1.7 Occlusal radiograph showing a salivary stone in the left submandibular duct.

presence of possible radiolucent or radiopaque lesions of the jaws, such as cysts or odontogenic tumours (1.8b). The main limitations of panoramic radiographs are related to the non-negligible (and often non-measurable) dimensional distortion of the image, which is caused by the discrepancies between the curvatures of the jawbones and the path followed by the X-ray generator around the patient's head. Moreover, due to the bidimensional nature of the image, the superimposition of anatomical structures that are on different planes may lead to the generation of artefacts and, in general, may render the interpretation of the image difficult, particularly for the untrained eye.

If more information is required, or if a three-dimensional view of the area under examination is necessary, the radiographic exam of choice is **the X-ray computed tomography** (CT scan), which has long supplanted other imaging techniques, such as stratigraphy (1.8c). According to the method used for the acquisition of the images, three types of CT scan are in use: axial CT, spiral CT, and volumetric CT. Regardless of the method with which images are acquired, the most important factor to evaluate in the choice of a suitable 3D imaging system is the data processing software: in fact, the software should be expressly developed to work in combination with the coupled CT machine and specifically designed for use in dentistry and oral surgery. For many years, axial CT scans were processed with specific software (e.g. DentaScan) to obtain coronal and cross-sectional images that could be useful for oral surgery. Currently, **cone beam volumetric tomography** or **CBVT** (also known as **cone beam computed tomography** or **CBCT**), which was actually created to be used specifically for dental and maxillofacial purposes, allows the acquisition of selected volumes of the maxillofacial complex, the reslicing of the acquired volume according to different planes or curves, the tridimensional rendering of the anatomical structures (hard and soft tissues), the application of colour filters, the tridimensional navigation through pneumatic spaces, and more.

The world of applications for the management of medical images, however, has undergone a remarkable evolution in recent years, and today a considerable variety of software capable of advanced processing is available. The decreasing cost of such software, once exclusively found in hospitals and large private medical centres, has also made them available to dentists who require the greatest amount of diagnostic information from computed tomography. These applications permit the reformatting of acquired images to display axi-

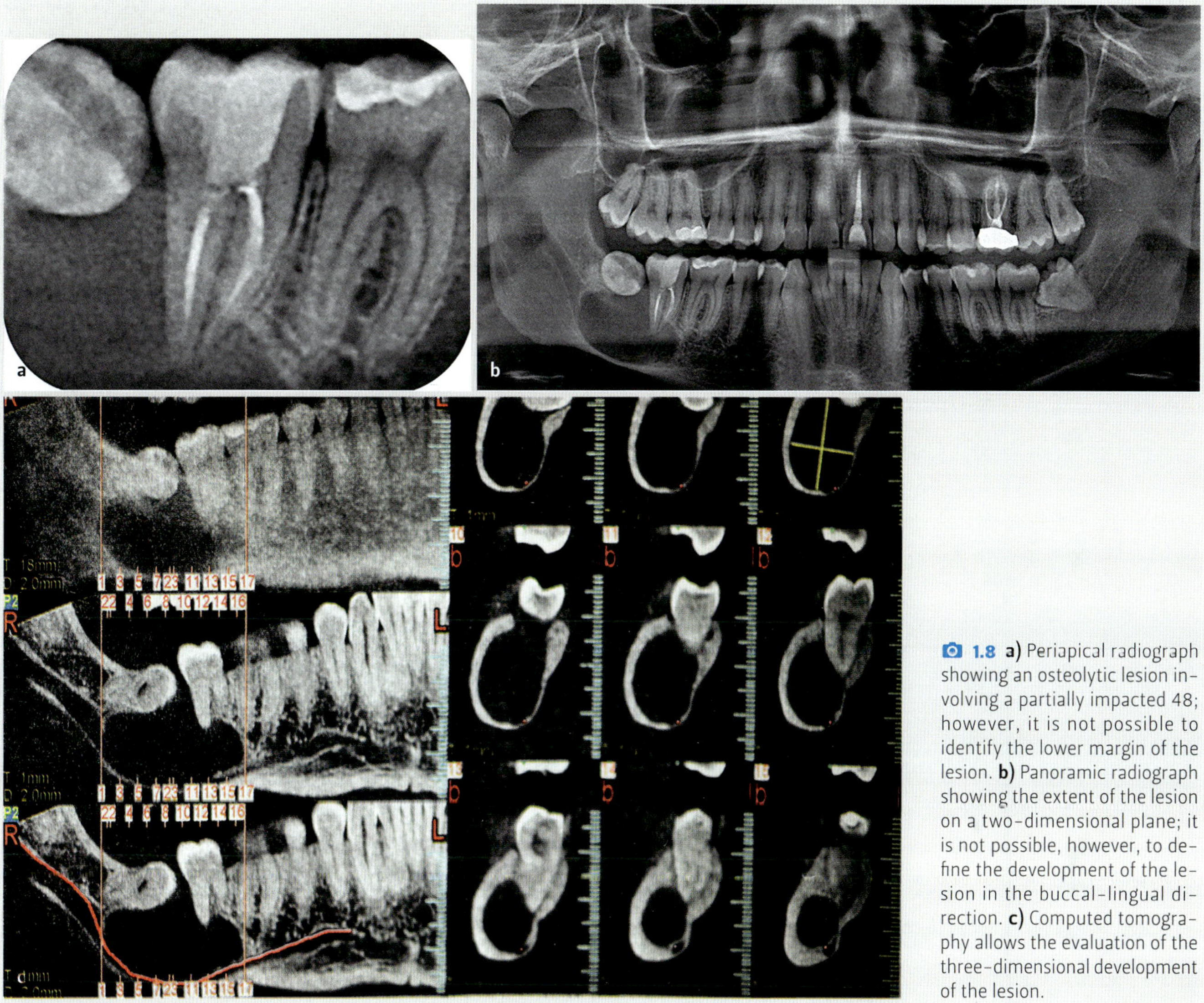

1.8 **a)** Periapical radiograph showing an osteolytic lesion involving a partially impacted 48; however, it is not possible to identify the lower margin of the lesion. **b)** Panoramic radiograph showing the extent of the lesion on a two-dimensional plane; it is not possible, however, to define the development of the lesion in the buccal-lingual direction. **c)** Computed tomography allows the evaluation of the three-dimensional development of the lesion.

al, sagittal or coronal sections, as well as sections that are referred to as **panorex**, which allow for the obtaining of panoramic images by reslicing the acquired volume along the curve of the jawbones (1.9a). A three-dimensional model of the facial skeleton (1.9b) and the soft tissues (1.9c) can also be created using special functions. The three-dimensional model may be treated with filters to change colours, to apply photorealistic rendering, or colour spectrums designed to highlight specific anatomical parts or characteristics (filters to highlight bone density, blood vessels, soft tissues, paranasal sinuses, etc.) (1.10a-b).

Additional functions create transparency effects that accurately display the size and orientation of radiopaque or radiolucent intraosseous structures (impacted teeth, cysts, etc.) (1.11), while others allow for navigation through three-dimensionally reconstructed hollow structures (nasal cavity, paranasal sinuses, large blood vessels, bony channels) in a virtual endoscopic view (1.12a-b). Finally, developments in technology and computer sciences have led to the creation of software that exploit tomographic images and their corresponding three-dimensional reconstructions to plan virtual surgical interventions such as implant placement (1.13), bone reconstruction, and orthognatic procedures. Moreover, these ap-

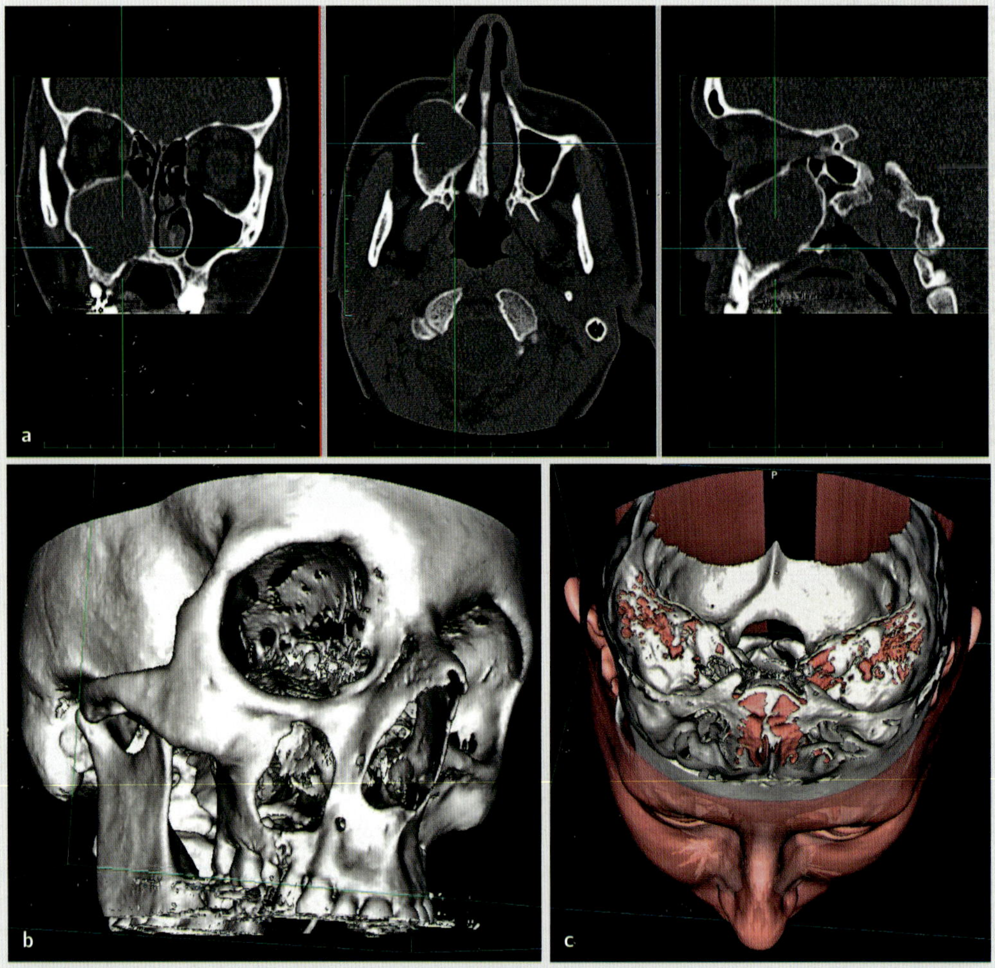

1.9 **a)** Computed tomography. Coronal, axial and sagittal sections of the maxilla, showing a large cystic lesion that occupies the entire maxillary sinus, has eroded the lateral wall of the nose and leans against the inferior orbital floor. **b)** Three-dimensional reconstruction of the same CT scan, which shows the erosion of the buccal cortical plate. **c)** Three-dimensional reconstruction of the same CT scan, including the soft tissues: swelling of the right cheek is evident.

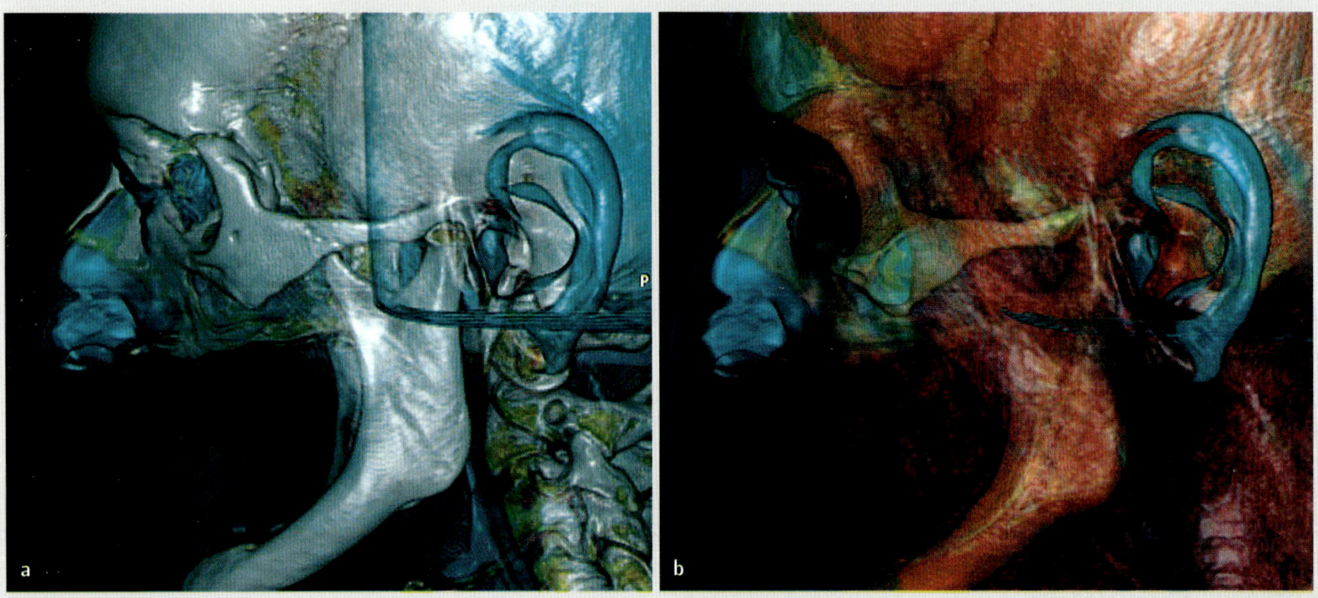

1.10 **a–b)** Three-dimensional reconstruction of the face: specific software allows the photorealistic rendering of the hard and soft tissues.

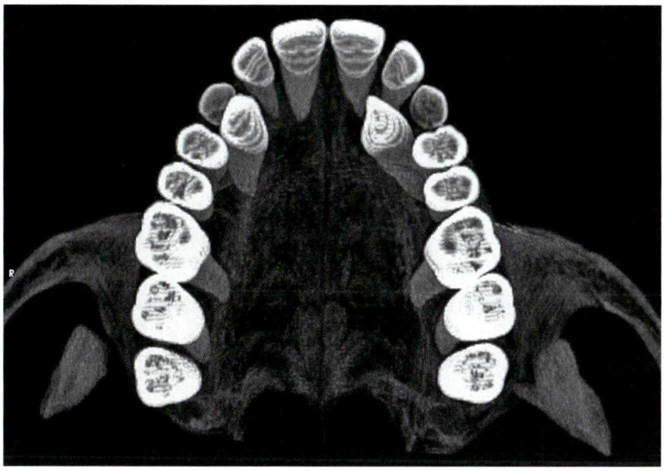

1.11 Three-dimensional MIP (maximum intensity projection) of the upper maxilla showing the position and orientation of impacted maxillary canines.

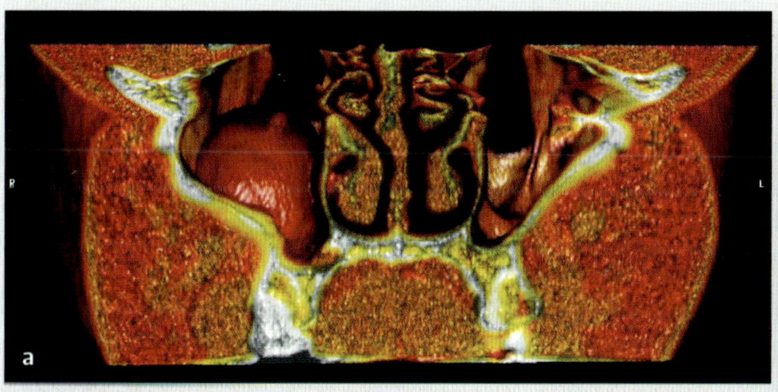

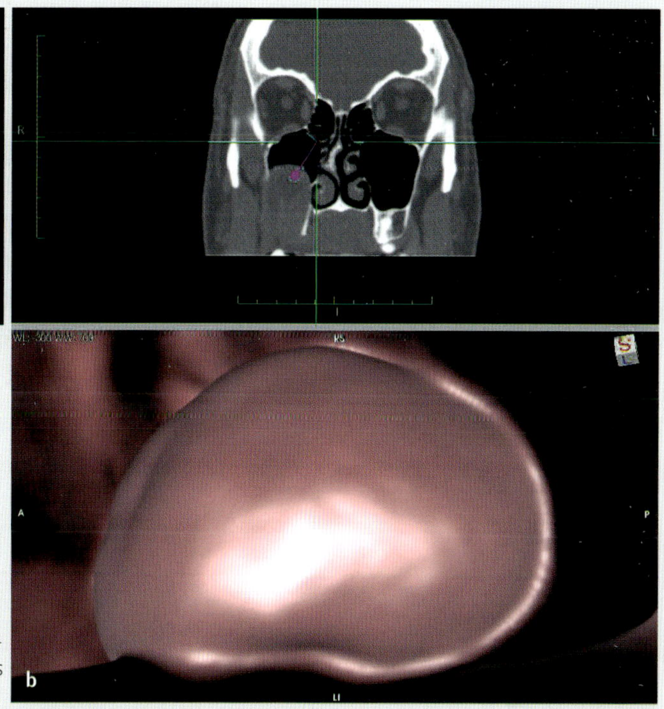

1.12 a–b) Three-dimensional reconstruction of a CT scan: specific functions allow navigating inside the maxillary sinus, where a radiopaque mass occupies the lower two-thirds of the antrum.

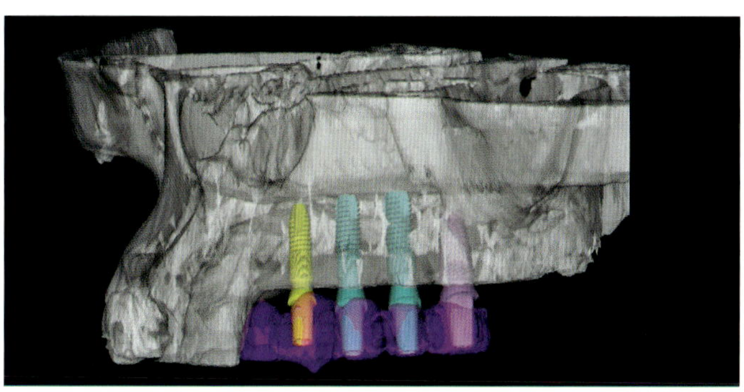

1.13 Dedicated software makes possible the creation not only of a three-dimensional reconstruction of the jaws, but also of a virtual plan for the position of implants. A surgical stent is then produced by stereolithography according to the virtual plan, thus allowing computer-guided placement of implants to be performed.

plications can export all data on skull anatomy and the virtual plan to a stereolithographic 3D printer, in order to create accurate resin reproductions of the jawbones and surgical guides that allow an exact reproduction of the planned implant positions during surgery.

Finally, even though indications are still limited, it is worth remembering that methods have been developed (particularly in the field of implantology) to facilitate intraoperative navigation and provide the ability to see anatomical structures of interest during surgery. A typical example is the ability to check, in real-time, the preparation of an implant site, with the huge advantage of being better able to prevent damage to important anatomical structures such as the inferior alveolar nerve or the maxillary sinus.

IMAGING TECHNIQUES RARELY USED IN ORAL SURGERY

In addition to those described, other imaging techniques may be used for diagnostic purposes in oral surgery, such as lateral cephalometric radiograph, ultrasonography and magnetic resonance imaging (MRI).

The **lateral cephalometric radiograph (lateral cephalogram)** is a radiographic exam generally used for orthodontic purposes, while it is rarely of help in oral surgery mostly due to the superimposition of anatomic structures caused by lateral projection. Exceptions may be represented by the study of fully edentulous jaws presenting severe bone atrophy and requiring pre-implant reconstructive surgery, or the planning of orthognatic surgery to correct maxillomandibular dysmorphisms. Nonetheless, it is worth noting that this imaging technique, although not a first choice, can occasionally provide useful information for the evaluation of specific aspects, such as the position of maxillary and mandibular impacted canines or incisors (1.14). Therefore, in the event that this exam has already been prescribed for other purposes, its analysis may supply enough information in specific cases to avoid further unnecessary radiation exposure for the patient.

Ultrasonography and **MRI** permit the evaluation of soft tissue lesions and alterations that radiographic examinations are not able to display. These examinations do not involve the use of X-rays or other forms of radiation. Therefore, while being burdened by non-negligible economic costs, they present no biological risk. Ultrasonography of the head and neck area may be indicated for the identification of salivary stones, the dynamic analysis of temporomandibular joints, the evaluation of tumours developing in the soft tissues of the floor of the mouth or inside the parenchyma of a major salivary gland, etc. (1.15).

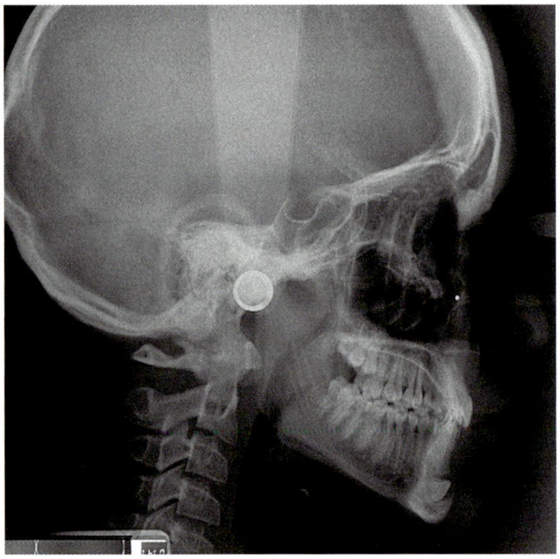

1.14 Lateral cephalometric radiograph showing an impacted mandibular canine.

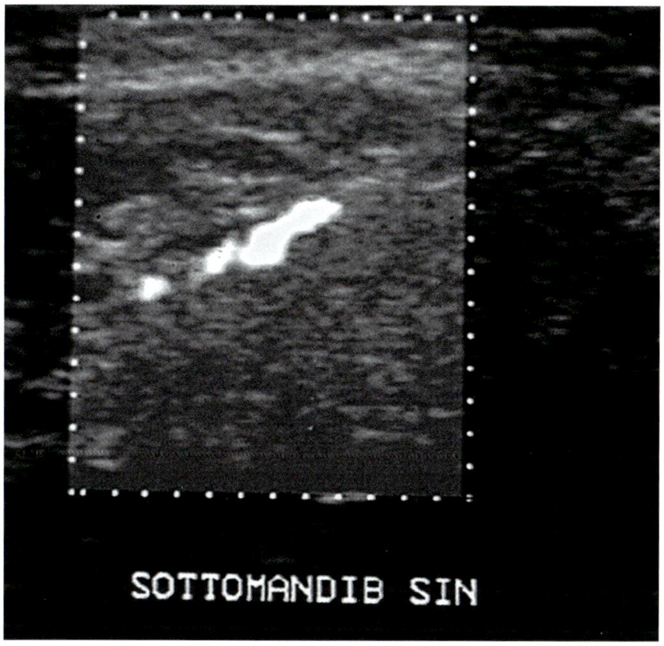

1.15 Ultrasonography of the floor of mouth showing the presence of a hyperechoic structure: this type of image is indicative of a salivary stone.

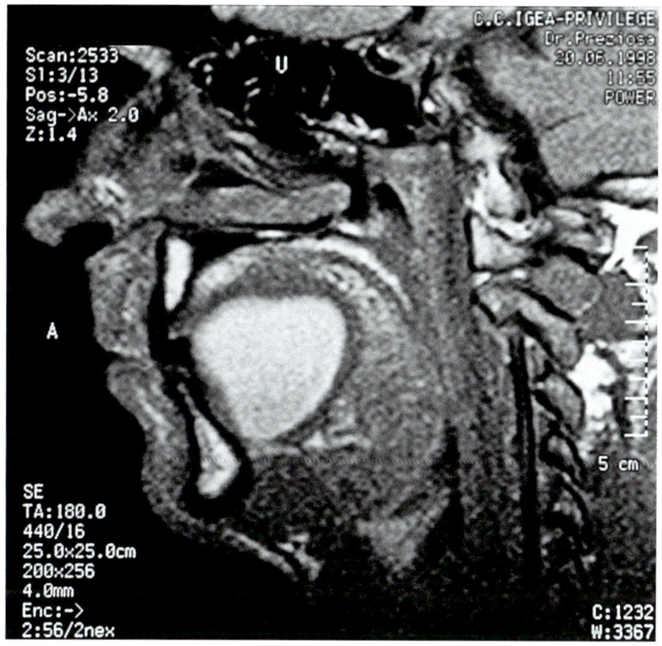

1.16 Magnetic resonance imaging of the face showing a large disembryogenic cyst of the oral floor.

MRI is particularly suitable for the tridimensional evaluation of lesions, malformations and tumours of the soft tissues of the oral cavity and cervicocephalic region, and for the analysis of the temporomandibular joints and articular disc (1.16). The only limitation to the use of MRI is represented by the presence of metallic objects in the oral cavity: those made of non-ferromagnetic alloys (such as titanium implants, amalgam fillings, etc.) seem to have negligible interactions with the magnetic field produced during the MRI scan, while those made with alloys containing a significant quantity of ferromagnetic metals (such as some orthodontic appliances and some fixed prosthetic restorations) may pose serious problems ranging from detachment, deformation, overheating, and dislodgement.

RADIODIAGNOSTIC PROCEDURE

The correct radiodiagnostic procedure should provide an adequate balance between the necessity to evaluate every aspect that can be useful to diagnose a condition and the biological and economic costs of the prescribed exams. In order to reduce the radiation dose the patient is exposed to, a simple set of rules can be followed:

- check whether the patient has recently undergone a similar examination (or one that could provide similar information);
- carefully estimate the extent of the area to be investigated: if it is small and in a favourable position, taking a periapical radiograph may be sufficient to provide the information required, thus eliminating the need for a panoramic radiograph; conversely, if the area is larger than the dimension of a periapical radiograph or is in a position that cannot be reached using this method, a panoramic radiograph should be the first choice. The recourse to periapical radiographs is often unnecessary: for example, in the evaluation of impacted third molars, or periapical cysts, or maxillary sinuses prior to sinus lifting procedures, etc., the images acquired are not able to display the entire area to be investigated, thus determining the need to perform additional radiographic exams;

- when the vestibular-palatal or buccal-lingual position of an impacted tooth that is not in close proximity to important anatomical structures is to be assessed, it is preferable to avoid the recourse to a CT scan in favour of an occlusal radiograph; the same information can be obtained without further exams if the patient has recently had a lateral cephalometric radiograph taken for orthodontic reasons;
- the recourse to computed tomography should be restricted to situations where it is necessary to know the exact tridimensional relationships between possible lesions and important anatomical structures. However, it is worth noting that, since oral surgery interventions are mainly elective, only computed tomography can provide complete information and precise measurements of the area to be treated: for this reason, whenever there is the slightest chance this information could result in a difference in the course and outcome of a surgical procedure, it is essential to use a CT scan.

The ultimate aim of these simple rules is to have access to all the diagnostic information required for every clinical situation, while exposing the patient to the lowest possible radiation dose. It is indeed incorrect to prescribe more radiographic examinations than necessary, or to prescribe a certain radiographic exam if a lower-radiation alternative can provide the same information. On the other hand, it is also incorrect to plan surgical treatment without the necessary information, as this increases the probability of committing errors and therefore the risk of complications.

Interpretation of radiographic exams

After selecting and prescribing the appropriate radiographic exams, the second fundamental step is to interpret the results correctly. The difficulty in the interpretation is inversely proportional to the sharpness of the image and directly proportional to the extent of the area under investigation. For instance, a periapical radiograph shows a small area (often limited to two or three contiguous teeth) and, as previously mentioned, provides a very clear image. As such, periapical radiographs are the easiest radiographic exams to interpret. Conversely, a panoramic radiograph shows a large area (both jawbones, teeth, nasal cavity, maxillary sinuses, temporomandibular joints, base of the skull, cervical vertebrae, and hyoid bone) and, because the image is captured by a sensor/plate that rotates around the patient's head, it is less sharp, particularly due to the superposition of all the bony structures of the facial skeleton. Consequently, interpretation of panoramic radiographs is more difficult, especially as regards the areas with the most significant superposition of anatomic structures (📷 1.17).

Theoretically, computed tomography is the most accurate examination, although the interpretation of a CT scan can be difficult particularly for those clinicians who rarely request it, or when anatomic structures with which the clinician is unfamiliar are present in the area under investigation. Specialised training in interpreting such exams is necessary, as it is not advisable to rely completely on the radiologist's report to plan a surgical intervention.

In addition to the unique characteristics of each radiographic investigation, an element that causes further difficulty for interpretation can be caused by mistakes or artefacts. Errors may be represented by incorrect positioning of the plate/sensors or patient, or incorrect parameter settings on the device (exposure times, angle of incidence of the X-ray beam, etc.), by failure to remove metallic objects from the area under examination and (only in the case of radiographic exams performed with analogue methods) errors in the development and/or fixation process.

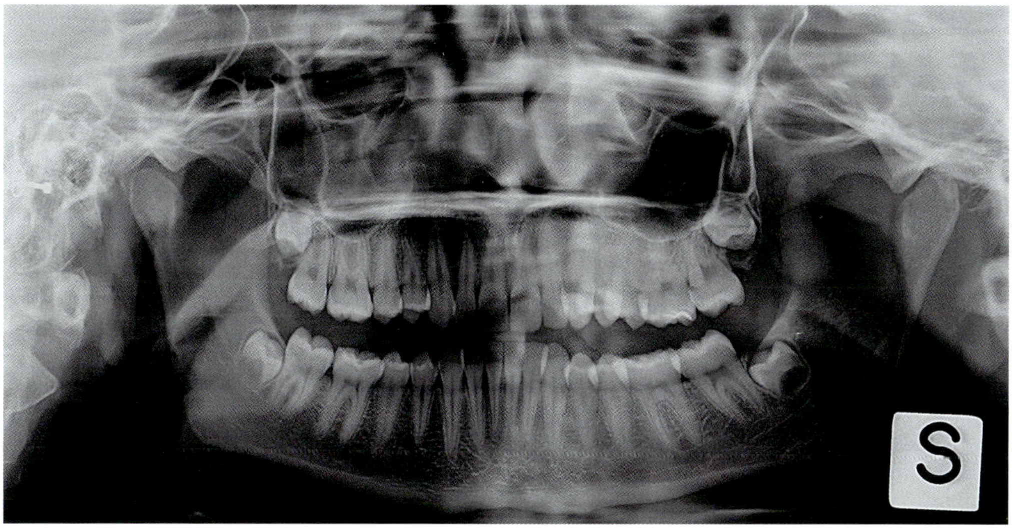

1.17 Panoramic radiograph demonstrating the presence of four impacted third molars.

The incorrect positioning of the sensors/plates leads to distortion of the final image: alterations can involve the dimension, the morphology, and the position of the structures under examination. Incorrect positioning of the patient can cause similar problems. Furthermore, it can lead to artefacts that make it difficult or impossible to interpret the radiographic image or some parts of it. For instance, in a panoramic radiograph, incorrect positioning of the patient's tongue may create a black arch that could completely hide the maxillary dentition and alveolar ridge. Such an artefact is caused by the air trapped between the tongue and palate when the patient's tongue lies against the floor of the mouth instead of the correct position, which is against the palate. Errors in setting the device parameters may cause overexposure or underexposure of the images, resulting in a variable loss of detail depending on the magnitude of the error, or (especially with computed tomography) can lead to image distortion that is amplified if the images are post-processed with dedicated software. Failure to remove metallic objects from the oral cavity (removable partial dentures, tongue piercings), the neck, lips, nose or ears (necklaces, nose jewellery, earrings) can result, as previously mentioned, in movement shadows (panoramic radiographs) or scattering phenomena (emission of secondary radiation in CT scans). Such errors can render some areas of the image partially or wholly unreadable. Finally, errors in the development and/or fixation of the radiographic film can lead to partial or complete discolouration of the image, varying degrees of underexposure, or stains on the surface of the film.

Diagnostic hypothesis

The clinical and radiographic information collected is, in most cases, sufficient to formulate an initial diagnostic hypothesis. It should be remembered that signs and symptoms are not always specific for each type of pathology (pathognomonic signs). It is therefore always necessary to include all the observed signs and symptoms in a differential diagnostic procedure. In the case of neoplasms, such as cysts or odontogenic and non-odontogenic tumours, a definitive diagnosis can only be obtained after histological examination of a tissue sample excised from the lesion.

Evaluation of the patient's general health (review of systems, ROS), past medical history (PMH) and possible request for additional exams

After a presumptive diagnosis is made, and before the surgical intervention is planned, the patient's general health should be thoroughly assessed.

This review of systems (ROS) and the recording of the patient's past medical history (PMH) are fundamental because the patient, regardless of the nature of the present illness, will undergo elective surgery and he/she must be in good general health. In fact, an undiagnosed systemic condition can expose the patient to intraoperative and/or postoperative complications. The patient must therefore be questioned in detail to exclude pre-existing or current conditions, which they may not declare spontaneously. To simplify the collection of information, and as a precaution from a medico-legal perspective, it is advisable to have the patient fill out a medical history form prior to the first examination. The form should contain a complete review of systems and a list of all the conditions that could represent a contraindication to a surgical intervention. A detailed description of all the systemic conditions that might expose patients to a higher risk of intraoperative and postoperative complications, and so contraindicate the surgical treatment, lies beyond the scope of this book. However, a summary of these conditions has been reported to serve as a quick reference guide for the reader (tab. 1.1), while a comprehensive treatise can be found in internal medicine manuals.

If the medical history of the patient contains evidence of any condition that might have a negative influence on the outcome of a surgical treatment, consultation with the general practitioner and/or consultant treating the patient for that condition is mandatory. In some cases, it may be necessary to carry out further examinations (instrumental screenings, blood tests, etc.).

Treatment plan and anaesthesia selection

Once the patient's health status has been thoroughly evaluated, the surgical intervention to treat the diagnosed condition can be adequately planned. This phase involves the analysis of additional factors that must be evaluated preoperatively in order to optimise the final result and minimise the risks. In particular, these factors determine the choice of the type of anaesthesia between:

- local anaesthesia;
- local anaesthesia associated with premedication (oral administration of sedatives);
- local anaesthesia in association with nitrous oxide/oxygen sedation;
- local anaesthesia in association with procedural sedation and analgesia (previously referred to as conscious sedation);
- general anaesthesia.

Factors determining the choice of the type of anaesthesia can be summarised as follows:

- patient's age;
- patient's level of cooperation and duration of the surgical intervention;
- type of pathology;
- localisation of the pathology and accessibility of the operating field;
- surgeon's experience.

Clinical record for surgery under local anaesthesia

Date ______________________________

First name ______________ Last name ______________

Place of birth ______________ Date of birth ______________

City ______________ County/State ______________ Postcode/ZIP Code ______________

Street ______________________________

Home phone ______________ Mobile phone ______________

Surgeon ______________________________

Diagnosis ______________________________

Do you have, or have you ever had, any of the following diseases or problems?

			Please specify
1) Respiratory diseases	no ❑	yes ❑	....
2) Heart disease	no ❑	yes ❑	....
3) Digestive disorders	no ❑	yes ❑	....
4) Genitourinary diseases	no ❑	yes ❑	....
5) Diabetes	no ❑	yes ❑	....
6) Haemorrhages	no ❑	yes ❑	....
7) Allergies	no ❑	yes ❑	....
8) Hepatitis	no ❑	yes ❑	....
9) Nervous system disorders	no ❑	yes ❑	....
10) Psychological disorders (nervous breakdown, etc.)	no ❑	yes ❑	....
11) Complications associated with anaesthesia	no ❑	yes ❑	....
12) Blood pressure values...			
13) What medications are you taking?.........................			
14) Are you pregnant?	no ❑	yes ❑	....
15) Do you smoke?	no ❑	yes ❑	....
16) Do you drink alcohol?	no ❑	yes ❑	....

Place and date ______________ Patient's signature ______________

Tab. 1.1 Clinical situations that contraindicate surgery

Cardiovascular diseases

Congestive heart failure

Issues related to surgery

- Intraoperative heart failure
- Myocardial infarction
- Cardiac arrest
- Cerebrovascular accidents
- Major bleeding

Precautions

- If the patient is well compensated:
  - minimally invasive and brief surgical procedures should only be scheduled after consultation with the treating doctor
- If the patient is in treatment with digitalis:
  - avoid prescribing macrolides or tetracyclines (these would enhance the toxic effect)
  - avoid administration of adrenalin, which can trigger arrhythmias
- If the patient is following an anticoagulation therapy:
  - assess the prothrombin time and, should it be necessary, modify anticoagulation therapy (replace with calciparin)
- If the patient is taking diuretics:
  - limit the use of adrenalin or acetylcholinesterase inhibitors
- If the patient is non-compensated:
  - refer the patient to a specialist, and avoid any elective procedures until compensation is obtained
  - urgent surgical procedures should be performed in a safe environment (e.g. hospital)

Heart failure

Issues related to surgery

Congestive heart failure

Precautions

- Postpone all elective surgeries until correction of the condition has been achieved
- Schedule only short, non-invasive surgeries
- Keep the patient as upright in the chair as possible
- If the patient is taking digitalis or anticoagulants, see Congestive Heart Failure

Myocardial infarction

Issues related to surgery

- Angina pectoris
- Recurrent infarction
- Cardiac arrest

Precautions

- In the first six months after the heart attack, undertake only emergency surgical procedures in a safe environment (e.g. hospital)
- All elective procedures should be postponed to at least six months after the heart attack and only performed if good functional recovery of myocardial activity is achieved (contact the treating physician)
- Schedule the procedure in the late morning or early afternoon
- Monitor vital signs (blood pressure, heart rate, saturation, etc.) before, during, and after surgery
- Reduce perioperative stress with anxiolytics
- Limit the use of vasoconstrictors. However, this aspect remains controversial, because a reduced use of vasoconstrictors limits the effects of the anaesthetic and the duration of its effect. The onset of pain can trigger the secretion of adrenalin, with paradoxical endogenous effects that are more dangerous than exogenous adrenalin administration
- If the patient is taking anticoagulants, antiarrhythmics, or digitalis, see Congestive Heart Failure

Angina pectoris

Issues related to surgery

- Angina episode
- Arrhythmias
- Acute myocardial infarction

Precautions

- In cases of stable angina:
  - schedule short appointments if possible
  - reduce perioperative stress with anxiolytics
  - limit the use of vasoconstrictors
- In cases of unstable angina:
  - postpone elective operations until stabilisation
  - perform urgent surgeries in a safe environment (e.g. hospital)
  - consult with the treating doctor

Arterial hypertension

Issues related to surgery

- Angina episode
- Excessive intraoperative bleeding
- Hypertensive crisis

Precautions

Diastolic blood pressure $>$ 105 mmHg and systolic blood pressure $>$ 200 mmHg lead to high risks.

- In cases of diastolic and systolic blood pressure values of $>$ 105 mmHg and 200, respectively:
  - refer the patient to hospital for urgent surgery
  - postpone elective surgery until blood pressure is under control
- In cases of diastolic and systolic values of $<$ 105 and 200 mmHg, respectively:
  - limit the use of vasoconstrictors
  - avoid long sessions
  - administer anxiolytics if possible
  - at the end of the session, raise the patient slowly to avoid postural hypotension

Congenital cardiac abnormalities and acquired valvular diseases

Issues related to surgery

- Risk of bacterial endocarditis

Precautions

- Antibiotic prophylaxis (2 grams of amoxicillin orally 1 hour before the surgery or 2 grams IV or IM 30 minutes before the surgery)
- In allergic patients: 600 mg of clindamycin orally 1 hour before surgery

Congenital coagulopathies

Issues related to surgery

- Prolonged bleeding

Precautions

- Perform coagulation tests preoperatively
- Consult with the treating doctor
- Avoid all drugs that delay platelet aggregation (salicylates, NSAIDs, etc.)
- Refer to the hospital if necessary
- Compensate for the missing coagulation factors

Diabetes

Issues related to surgery

- Delayed healing of the surgical wound
- Increased risk of infection
- Hypoglycaemic crisis

Precautions

- In the case of uncontrolled diabetes:
  - refer to the hospital for emergency treatment and postpone elective procedures until after compensation is achieved
- In the case of controlled diabetes:
  - Administer antibiotic prophylaxis preoperatively
  - Keep glucose solutions at hand, to be administered in the event of a hypoglycaemic crisis

(continued)

Tab. 1.1 Clinical situations that contraindicate surgery (*continued*)

Pregnancy

Issues related to surgery
- Drugs can interfere with embryogenesis
- The use of adrenaline in anaesthesia can cause placental ischaemia and foetal hypoxia

Precautions
- Simple surgical procedures under local anaesthesia without vasoconstrictor can be performed without restrictions, especially if urgent
- Elective surgical procedures should be postponed

Liver diseases

Cirrhosis

Issues related to surgery
- Altered drug metabolism
- Prolonged bleeding due to impaired synthesis of coagulation factors

Precautions
- Prescribe preoperative coagulation tests
- Compensate possible deficits with vitamin K, platelets, plasma
- Avoid medications that have a liver metabolism
- Refer to the hospital if necessary

Hepatitis

Issues related to surgery
- Altered drug metabolism
- Prolonged bleeding due to impaired synthesis of coagulation factors

Precautions
- Prescribe coagulation tests
- Protect operators and assistants from infection
- Compensate possible deficits with vitamin K, platelets, plasma
- Avoid medications that have a liver metabolism
- Refer to the hospital if necessary

Nephropathy

Issues related to surgery
- Anaemia, prolonged bleeding, hypertensive crisis, bacterial endarteritis

Precautions
- Preoperative assessment of blood pressure and coagulation factors
- Antibiotic prophylaxis (erythromycin or clindamycin)
- Plan only simple surgeries for the uncontrolled types
- Avoid medications that have a kidney metabolism
- Refer the patient to hospital in case complex surgical procedures are necessary

Hypothyroidism

Issues related to surgery
- Hypothyroid coma in uncontrolled forms (bradycardia, hypothermia, hypotension, convulsive crises)

Precautions
- Perform thyroid function tests and request an endocrinology consultation
- Avoid the use of anxiolytics
- Plan only simple surgeries
- Refer the patient to hospital in case complex surgical procedures are necessary
- Administer hydrocortisone 100300 mg for symptoms of acute hypothyroidism

Hyperthyroidism

Issues related to surgery
- Thyroid storm (thyrotoxic crisis) in noncompensated hyperthyroidism (abdominal pain, dulling of the sensorium, tachycardia, hyperthermia)

Precautions
- Perform thyroid function tests and request an endocrinology consultation
- Do not use adrenalin
- In noncompensated forms, refer the patient to hospital
- Administer an antibiotic prophylaxis

Allergy

Issues related to surgery

Anaphylactic crises (itching and hives, nausea and vomiting, oedema of the soft palate and pharynxlarynx, tachycardia and/or arrhythmia, hypotension, tachypnoea, bronchospasm, coma)

Precautions
- Identification of allergic patients and risk factors
- Consult with the treating doctor
- Refer to hospital if an accident occurs:
  - Supine patient
  - 0.5 ml adrenalin solution 1:1,000 IM or subcutaneously
  - Respiratory support

Immune system disorders

AIDS (HIV antigen positivity in the absence of symptoms)

Issues related to surgery
- Possibility of infection transmission to health professionals, and crossinfection between patients

Precautions

All the precautions available to prevent crossinfections

AIDS (AIDS related complex, ARC)

Issues related to surgery
- Possibility of infection transmission to health professionals, and crossinfection between patients
- Patients in the advanced stages of ARC may be thrombocytopenic and/or have severe immunodepression

Precautions
- All the precautions available to prevent crossinfections

AIDS (fullblown phase)

Issues related to surgery
- Increased susceptibility to secondary infections after surgical procedures
- Increased tendency towards prolonged bleeding due to thrombocytopenia and abnormalities in the coagulation process
- Possibility of infection transmission to health professionals, and crossinfection between patients

Precautions
- Assess the platelet count and bleeding time
- Administer an adequate postoperative antibiotic therapy (the need for prophylaxis in severely immunocompromised patients is not documented)
- Patients in the advanced or terminal stages, more conservative therapies should be preferred whenever possible
- All the precautions available to prevent crossinfections
- Refer the patient to hospital

Leukaemia

Issues related to surgery
- Increased susceptibility to postoperative infections
- Tendency towards increased and prolonged bleeding
- Delayed healing process

(continued)

Tab. 1.1 Clinical situations that contraindicate surgery (*continued*)

Precautions

- Do not treat patients in the acute phase of the disease
- Assess the platelet count before any invasive treatment
- Consider the recourse to an appropriate preoperative antibiotic prophylaxis
- Patients in remission can undergo routine treatments; it is important to motivate the patient to maintain good hygiene
- Referral to hospital for surgical treatment is advised

Multiple myeloma

Issues related to surgery

- Increased susceptibility to postoperative infections as well as immune alterations which are secondary to both the pathology and the radio and/or chemotherapy
- Tendency towards increased and prolonged bleeding caused by thrombocytopenia and/or alterations in clot formation

Precautions

- Careful evaluation of platelet count and bleeding time; in invasive treatments, consider the increased risk of secondary infectious complications
- In patients with stable clinical profiles, elective treatments can be performed
- In terminal patients, only supportive care should be implemented
- Treatment in a safe environment (e.g. hospital) is suggested

Lymphomas

Issues related to surgery

- Increased susceptibility to postoperative infections
- Patients receiving radiation therapy of the head and neck are likely to develop osteoradionecrosis

Precautions

- In patients with stable clinical profiles, elective therapies should always be performed depending on the prognosis of the systemic disease
- Platelet count and bleeding time must be assessed preoperatively
- In terminal patients, implement only supportive care
- Treatment in a safe environment (e.g. hospital) is suggested

Adrenal insufficiency

Issues related to surgery

- Increased susceptibility to infections
- Tissue healing problems
- Blood pressure imbalances
- Poor stress tolerance

Precautions

- When invasive and/or stressful surgeries are necessary, the need for an increase in the usual corticosteroid therapy should be assessed
- In noncompensated forms, surgical treatment in a safe environment (e.g. hospital) is indicated

Irradiated patients

Issues related to surgery

- For doses > 48 Grey:
  - delayed healing of the surgical wounds
  - increased risk of infection
  - risk of osteoradionecrosis

Precautions

- Perform only urgent procedures in a safe environment (e.g. hospital)
- Administer adequate antibiotic therapy
- Follow a chlorhexidine mouthwash protocol
- The recourse to hyperbaric oxygen therapy is suggested

Patient's age

The patient's age is a very important parameter, but it is frequently overlooked in the preoperative evaluation. This factor can be less significant when surgery is performed under general anaesthesia, but when surgery is performed under local anaesthesia, it is crucial to consider this variable. While generalisations are impossible due to interindividual variability, it is advisable to avoid prolonged and bloody surgery in patients under the age of 8-9 for three reasons:

- the tolerance threshold of a child is lower than that of an adult;
- young patients, unlike adults, are generally cooperative for short time spans;
- invasive or painful treatments may represent negative experiences that can result in odontophobic sequelae, which are then difficult to resolve.

Patient's cooperation and duration of the surgical procedure

Patients should be questioned about their previous experiences with dentists, to assess their psychological approach to an oral surgery intervention. In fact, such procedures, however simple, are perceived by patients to be "more dramatic" (preparation of the surgical field, surgical incision of the soft tissues, sutures, etc.) when compared to common dental procedures. While taking into account considerable interindividual variability in behaviour, it is possible to give some general indications derived from clinical experience. With normally compliant subjects, surgeries lasting between 60-90 minutes can be performed under local anaesthesia without any particular problem. Some patients are able to tolerate longer sessions, but it is important to bear in mind that surgery, unlike other dental treatments (root canal treatments, restorations, prosthetic treatments) must be completed in the same session and cannot be postponed to a later date. Therefore, it is fundamental to overestimate surgery duration as often as possible, and this can only be assessed by the surgeon on the basis of personal experience. Surgical procedures requiring more than 90 minutes to complete should always be planned considering the recourse to other types of anaesthesia (conscious sedation, general anaesthesia).

When performing surgery on uncooperative patients (due to conditions such as odontophobia, belonephobia, claustrophobia, psychological or physical disabilities, etc.), it is advisable to do so in a safe environment (hospital or clinic with adequate facilities), under conscious sedation or general anaesthesia to shorten the operating time and to reduce the risk of intraoperative complications that may arise due to the lack of cooperation of the patient if treated under local anaesthesia.

Type of pathology

The type of pathology may influence the choice of the operating environment, the type of anaesthesia and the duration of the surgery, irrespective of the localisation of the pathology. For example, the removal of an angioma of the cheek, even if located in a favourable position, can cause profuse bleeding that is difficult to manage. In such cases, surgery under local anaesthesia is contraindicated.

Localisation of the pathology and accessibility of the operating field

The localisation of the pathology must be evaluated with great care. Surgeries in the rearmost portion of the oral cavity, or in areas that are difficult to access, may not be easily performed under local anaesthesia. As such, accessibility of the operating field and/or maximum mouth opening must be assessed preoperatively. Moreover, a significant number of patients have hypersensitive pharyngeal reflex: any stimulus exerted in proximity to the soft palate or the posterior two-thirds of the tongue and floor of the mouth can cause gagging, rendering surgery impossible under local anaesthesia.

A thorough evaluation of possible functional alterations of the temporomandibular joints should always be performed. These conditions may cause the patient to be unable to maintain an adequate opening of the mouth for more than a few minutes. In addition, after the onset of pain, the patient may no longer be able to open the mouth sufficiently, making it very difficult to complete the surgery. In these cases, it is advisable to choose local anaesthesia only for short procedures that do not require the patient to maintain the mouth in the maximum opening position.

Surgeon's experience

Where the surgeon has extensive experience, this usually translates into reduced operating times and reduced trauma to hard and soft tissues. Less experienced surgeons may require more time to complete the same procedure, which, in some cases, can be difficult for the patient to bear. A correct general indication is therefore always to overestimate the difficulties that may be encountered during surgery if local anaesthesia is used, and to consider the recourse to conscious sedation or general anaesthesia when complex surgeries are necessary.

Relationship between biological risks and benefits obtained

Any surgery results in some degree of trauma to the hard and/or soft tissues of the oral cavity. This requires a healing period that may not always lead to a complete *restitutio ad integrum*. Therefore, every surgical intervention carries a biological cost that must always be preoperatively compared to the benefits that may be obtained. This concept - *primum non nocere* - is particularly true for elective surgery, which represents a significant share of all oral surgery interventions. In the absence of symptoms or a valid indication for surgery, the opportunity to perform such procedures must be carefully weighed. As an illustration, the removal of an asymptomatic, deeply impacted inferior third molar in close proximity to the inferior alveolar canal may result in sensory alterations to the teeth of the corresponding hemiarch, and to the ipsilateral half of the lower lip and of the mental region. The biological cost, in this case, is too high compared to the benefits obtained, and the patient may not tolerate the impairment suffered, with possible medico-legal sequelae. On the contrary, a case presenting strong indications would be the removal of an impacted inferior third molar associated with an infected odontogenic cyst that has eroded part of the corpus and mandibular ramus and caused the patient intense pain. Therefore, even if the surgical removal of the tooth causes the same sensory alterations occurring in the first example, the indications (removal of a cyst that would continue to grow, elimination of infection and its associated symptoms) determine the necessity for surgery and lead to the consideration that the biological cost, in this case, is inferior to the benefits achieved.

Informed consent for surgical procedures

Before any surgical procedure is performed, it is necessary to communicate to the patient, in a clear and complete way, the results of clinical and radiographic/instrumental examinations, the diagnosis obtained and the proposed treatment plan (or alternative plans) to solve the clinical problem. It is worth remembering that, regardless of the medico-legal value of the informed consent document (which is intrinsic in a courtroom), it is mandatory for every doctor to inform patients about their conditions and different treatment options, avoiding the use of technical expressions in favour of terms that are easy to understand. Thus, the informed consent document is not only a form of protection for the patient and the treating doctor from a legal perspective, but also, and most importantly, the formalisation of a pact of mutual trust between doctor and patient that should always be the basis of any treatment plan.

In any case, there is in fact no clear regulation that defines the technical details about how to prepare and compile an informed consent form. Nonetheless, a few rules can be followed to serve as valuable guidelines to compile a document that is as clear and complete as possible:

- To be considered "informed", the consent must be expressed by an explanation that the patient can easily understand. For this reason, technical expressions used to define all aspects of the proposed treatment plan should be backed up, where necessary, by an explanation in common terms so that the patient can independently read the document to assess its contents and their clinical implications;
- It is preferable that the patients complete the registry section of the document in their own handwriting, rather than entering their personal data by computer or in the doctor's handwriting. This represents an element of patient empowerment, and provides

proof that patients have had the document in their hands, and had the opportunity to read it and personally fill in the section regarding their personal data;

- The document must not omit information about the imaging studies performed to assess the clinical situation because, as mentioned earlier (see section about radiographic examinations), they have specific indications and are not free of biological costs, in addition to being one of the pillars underpinning the diagnosis and the choice of the treatment plan;
- It is fundamental that the diagnosis be very clearly indicated, as it represents the patient's clinical situation at the time of the visit and, as a result, the starting point for the entire treatment;
- It is necessary to report in full, and in terms that the patient can easily understand: a) the description of the proposed treatment to achieve resolution of the condition or to improve the prognosis; and b) the reasons that led to the selection of the proposed treatment plan, and the possible alternatives that may have equal efficacy (if any);
- Any medical, pharmacological or surgical therapies that are to be performed before the proposed treatment should be clearly listed, in order to ensure the completeness of the information given to the patients about all the treatments required;
- It is of the utmost importance that any inevitable consequences of the proposed surgical procedure and possible specific complications be reported in a way that is in a clear and understandable. The inevitable consequences are the common postoperative sequelae of all surgical procedures (such as pain, swelling, bleeding from the surgical wound) that do not necessarily always occur, but are a normal consequence of surgery. The possible complications must also be included: occasional intra or postoperative events that may arise for a specific procedure or site (infection, haematomas, visible morphological changes of hard and/or soft tissues, transient or permanent paraesthesia/anaesthesia, bone fractures, partial or total failure of the surgical treatment, etc.). Every possible complication should be explained in detail to the patient when the diagnosis and the proposed treatment plan are discussed, so that the patient is aware of the possible benefits as well as all potential risks related to the treatment of their condition;
- The patient must be adequately informed about possible variations in the proposed treatment plan that may become necessary at any stage, and these variations must be explained in a comprehensive manner;
- It is necessary to inform the patient about the possible consequences of leaving the condition untreated. In particular, patients must be warned about the degeneration or aggravation of the pathological profile, or the possibility of aesthetic, functional or anatomical changes resulting from non-treatment;
- Finally, it is advisable that the informed consent document, once completely compiled with the information listed above, is delivered to the patient before the set surgery date. In this way, the patient has the opportunity to reread the document several times independently, to express any doubts or uncertainties to the doctor, and to obtain further explanations.

Informed consent for surgical procedures

I, the undersigned, Born on / /

Nationality Spoken language

Declare that I was informed by Doctor

in an understandable and appropriate way about:

- my current clinical situation
- any investigations recommended for diagnosis
- medical or surgical treatment recommended for healing or to improve prognosis of the disease
- alternative treatment options, of substantially equal effectiveness, and the reasons motivating the proposed surgical treatment
- medical/pharmacological treatment to be performed before the recommended surgery
- expected benefits of the surgical treatment
- discomfort, side effects and inevitable consequences of the recommended surgery
- possible risks and complications or limitations connected with the recommended surgery
- possible modifications to the proposed treatment, as already planned and authorised, that may become necessary to deal with any unforeseen situations that are difficult to predict at present
- foreseeable consequences of non-treatment
- I have understood the situation as illustrated and asked for further explanations about

I, the undersigned, confirm that I have had full and complete answers from Dr

to all of my questions, and that I am fully conscious, aware and free to make choices that affect my person.

I have understood the situation illustrated here and declare that I [ACCEPT] – [REJECT] with a current and spontaneous choice, the procedure that has been proposed to me.

The signature below confirms that my [REJECTION OF] – [CONSENT TO] the medical or surgical procedure proposed has been expressed by myself in a present, free and informed manner, and that this documentation is compliant with the interview/discussions that I had with

Doctor

Patient's signature

Parent's signature

Guardian's signature

Interpreter's signature

Doctor's signature:

Signature of any witnesses

NOTE: PATIENTS WHO HAVE EXPRESSED THEIR CONSENT ARE FREE TO REJECT THE PROCEDURE AT ANY TIME

REFERENCES

Chiapasco M. Manuale illustrato di Chirurgia Orale. 2a ed. Elsevier Masson, Milano 2007.

DuBrul EL. Anatomia Orale di Sicher. Edi-Ermes, Milano 1988.

Escoda CG, Aytés LB. Cirugía Bucal. In: Escoda CG, Micas MM, Tost AE, Albiol JG. Otras inclusiones dentarias. Mesiodens y otros supernumerarios. Ergon, Madrid 1999; 511-50.

Kassab MM, Radmer TW, Glore JW, Visotcky A, Robertson J, Degroot B. A retrospective review of clinical international normalized ratio results and their implications. *J Am Dent Assoc* 2011 Nov; 142(11):1252-7.

Paulsen F., Waschke J. Sobotta Atlante di Anatomia Umana. Elsevier, Milano 2012.

Peterson LJ, Indresano AT, Marciani RD, Roser SM. Principles of oral and maxillofacial surgery. JB Lippincott Company, Philadelphia 1992.

Sailer HF, Pajarola GF. Chirurgia Orale. Masson, Milano 1996.

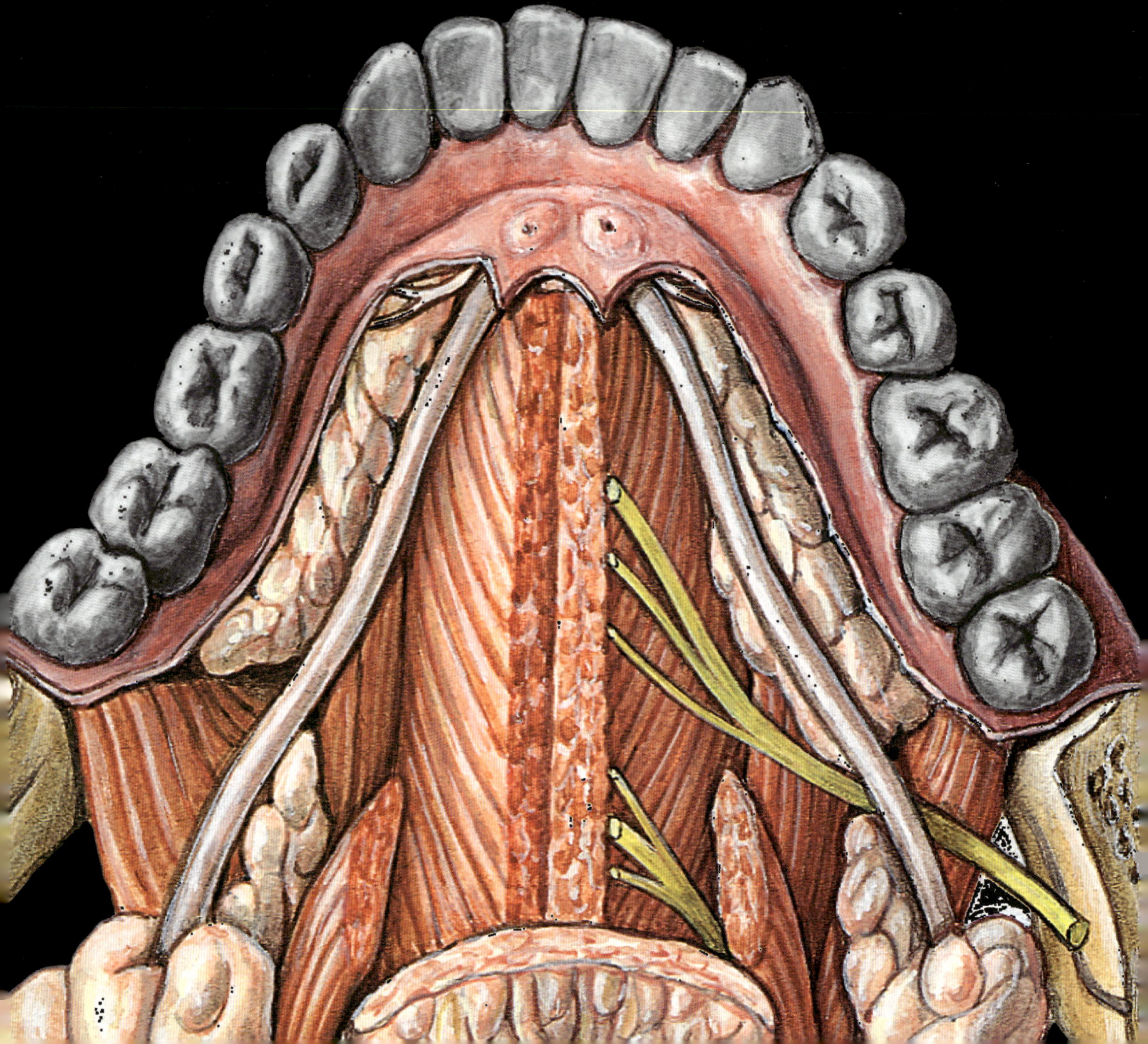

Surgical anatomy of the jaws

M. Chiapasco ▪ M. Zaniboni

Introduction

Thorough knowledge of maxillofacial anatomy, including the oral cavity, is fundamental to performing correct surgical procedures that respect the integrity of anatomical structures, both in the operating field and adjacent areas. Although it is beyond the scope of the current project to describe the topographical anatomy of this area in detail, the reader may refer to specialised textbooks for more information. Thus, the present chapter briefly describes key anatomical structures (muscles, nerves, blood vessels, pneumatic cavities, etc.), with particular attention given to those that should be respected during the most common oral surgery interventions. To facilitate understanding and to make learning more effective, these anatomical structures will be described in the context of the topographical area in which they lie. Therefore, the anatomy of the oral cavity will be divided into different areas of intervention and described accordingly.

These areas can be divided as follows:

- posterior mandible;
- anterior mandible;
- floor of the mouth;
- tongue;
- anterior maxilla;
- posterior maxilla;
- palate;
- cheek (malar region);
- upper and lower lip.

Posterior mandible

This is the portion of the jaw located posterior to the mental foramen. It is formed by the posterior part of the mandibular body and by the ramus.

From a surgical perspective, the following anatomical planes can be distinguished: mucosa, submucosa, muscles (only in the basal part of the mandible), periosteum, and bone (2.1a-e). Each anatomical plane is a potential cleavage plane during surgical dissection, and it is essential to know which structures are found in the different planes. While it is not possible to generalise, it can be assumed that the vascular and nervous structures all lie within the submucosal or muscular planes, except in the areas of the foramina (mental foramen, infraorbital foramen, etc.) or in the case of perforating vessels. Therefore, the cleavage conducted between the bony plane and the periosteal plane makes it possible to keep the periosteum intact (subperiosteal dissection) and corresponds to the creation of a so-called full-thickness flap, which normally prevents copious bleeding and nerve injuries (2.1e). Cleavage above the periosteum (which may be indicated under certain circumstances) can still be performed, but it must be done bearing in mind that there are vessels and nerves running within the muscular and submucosal plane (2.1f). This principle is obviously applicable to all of the other maxillary and mandibular areas. Consequently, further analysis of this aspect will be avoided to avoid unnecessary redundancy.

BONY PLANE – MANDIBULAR BODY AND RAMUS

The dominant structure is represented by the inferior alveolar neurovascular bundle, which consists of the inferior alveolar nerve, accompanied by the homonymous artery and vein.

Inferior alveolar nerve

Origin: it arises from the posterior trunk of the mandibular nerve, third branch of the trigeminal nerve (cranial nerve V) (2.2).

Function: it is a mixed nerve, but with a high prevalence of sensory fibres. The sensory component innervates the dental alveoli, teeth, and gums distal to the first premolar, while the motor component consists of fibres innervating the mylohyoid muscle.

Course: it arises, along with the lingual nerve, from the posterior-medial branch of the mandibular nerve a few millimetres below the oval foramen, and, like the lingual nerve, it describes an arch with an upper anterior concavity. It then continues between the in-

Posterior mandible

Surgical procedures

- Impacted or erupted molars
- Cysts of the ramus and body of the mandible
- Bone harvesting from the mandibular ramus
- Implant placement

Notable anatomic structures

- Lingual nerve
- Inferior alveolar neurovascular bundle and facial artery
- Buccal nerve
- Mylohyoid artery

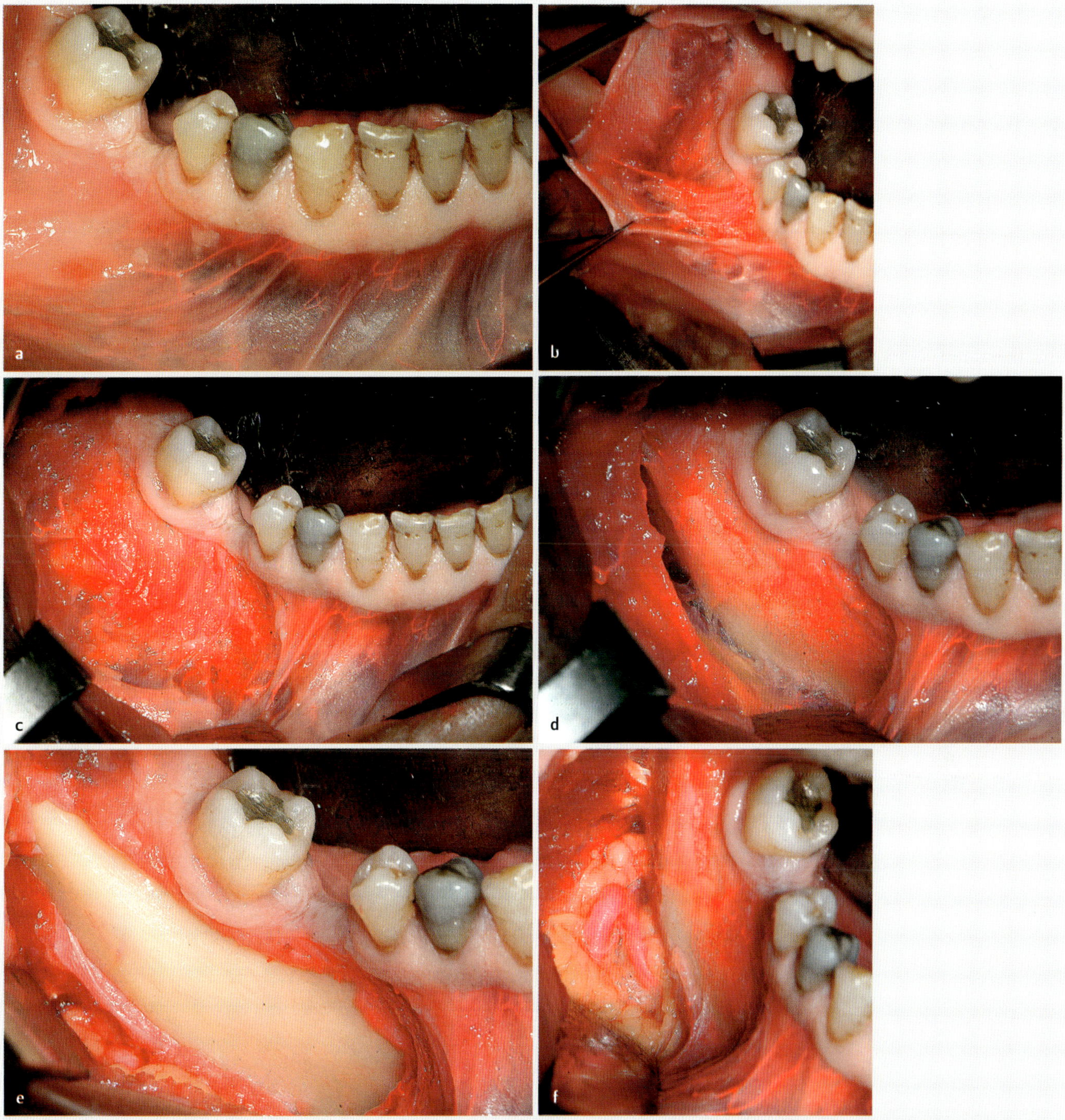

2.1 Anatomical dissection of the mandible: **a)** mucosa; **b)** submucosa; **c)** muscles; **d)** periosteum; **e)** bone plate (neurovascular structures are normally present within the soft tissues in the intermediate layers); **f)** the facial artery is visible below and towards the vestibule, at the inferior margin of the mandible between the periosteum and the muscles.

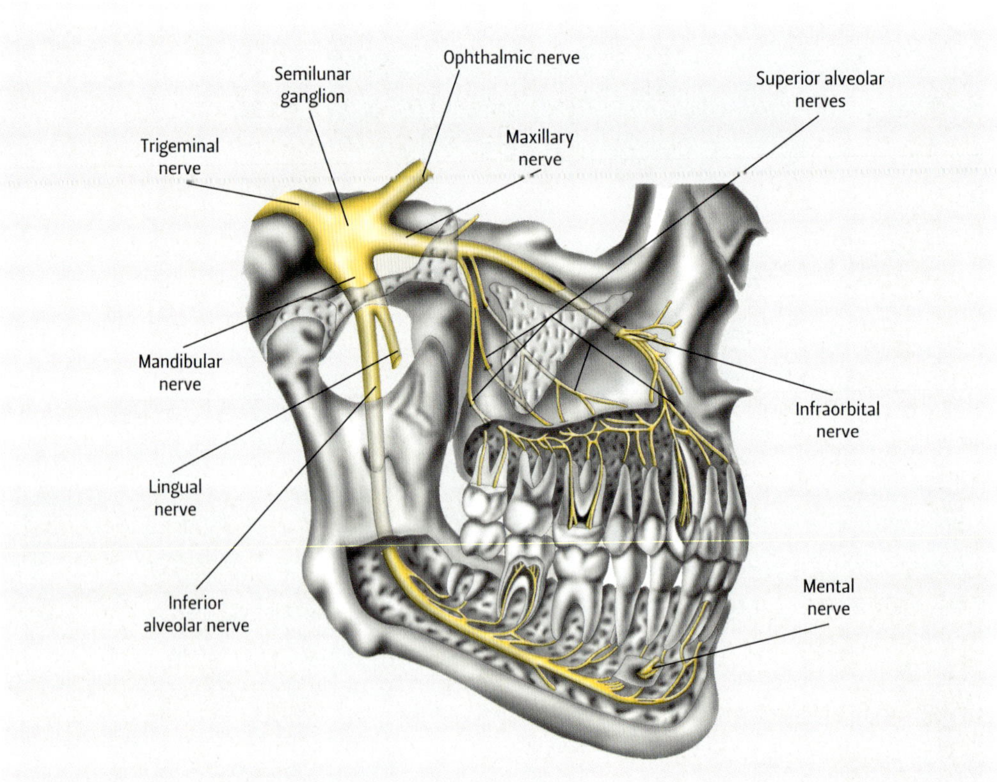

2.2 Anatomic illustration showing the course of the mandibular nerve (third branch of the fifth cranial nerve) from its origin in the trigeminal ganglion (or Gasser's ganglion or semilunar ganglion) to its peripheral branches.

ternal pterygoid muscle and the medial side of the mandibular ramus until it reaches the opening of the mandibular canal. Before entering it at the Spix's spine, it gives off a collateral branch, the mylohyoid nerve, which supplies motor fibres to the mylohyoid muscle.

The position of the Spix's spine, where the inferior alveolar nerve enters the mandibular canal, shows considerable interindividual variability, in both the vertical and anterior-posterior aspects; this must be considered, particularly when locoregional anaesthesia manoeuvres are performed. On average, the foramen can be clinically located slightly above the level of the occlusal plane, and 2 centimetres distally to the anterior margin of the mandibular ramus (2.3a-b) (see the Anaesthesia section for further details). Once it has entered the mandible, the inferior alveolar nerve runs the entire length of the mandibular canal below the teeth apexes until it reaches the premolars, where it divides into its two terminal branches: the mental nerve (which runs through the homonymous foramen) and the incisive nerve (which runs along the mandibular canal until it anastomoses with the contralateral at the midline) (2.3c-d).

The course of the nerve shows a great interindividual variability with respect to its coronal-apical and vestibular-lingual position. Special attention must be paid to the end of its course in the mandibular canal. Before engaging the mental foramen, the nerve describes a knee (or *loop*) of variable size pointing mesially: after this anterior angle, the nerve bends distally and engages the foramen to emerge on the vestibular side of the mandibular body. Therefore, it is of paramount importance to assess the entire course of the nerve carefully, in order to avoid damaging it during surgical procedures performed in the area of the mandibular molars and premolars (removal of erupted and impacted teeth, surgical endodontics, cyst enucleations, placement of implants, etc.) (2.3e).

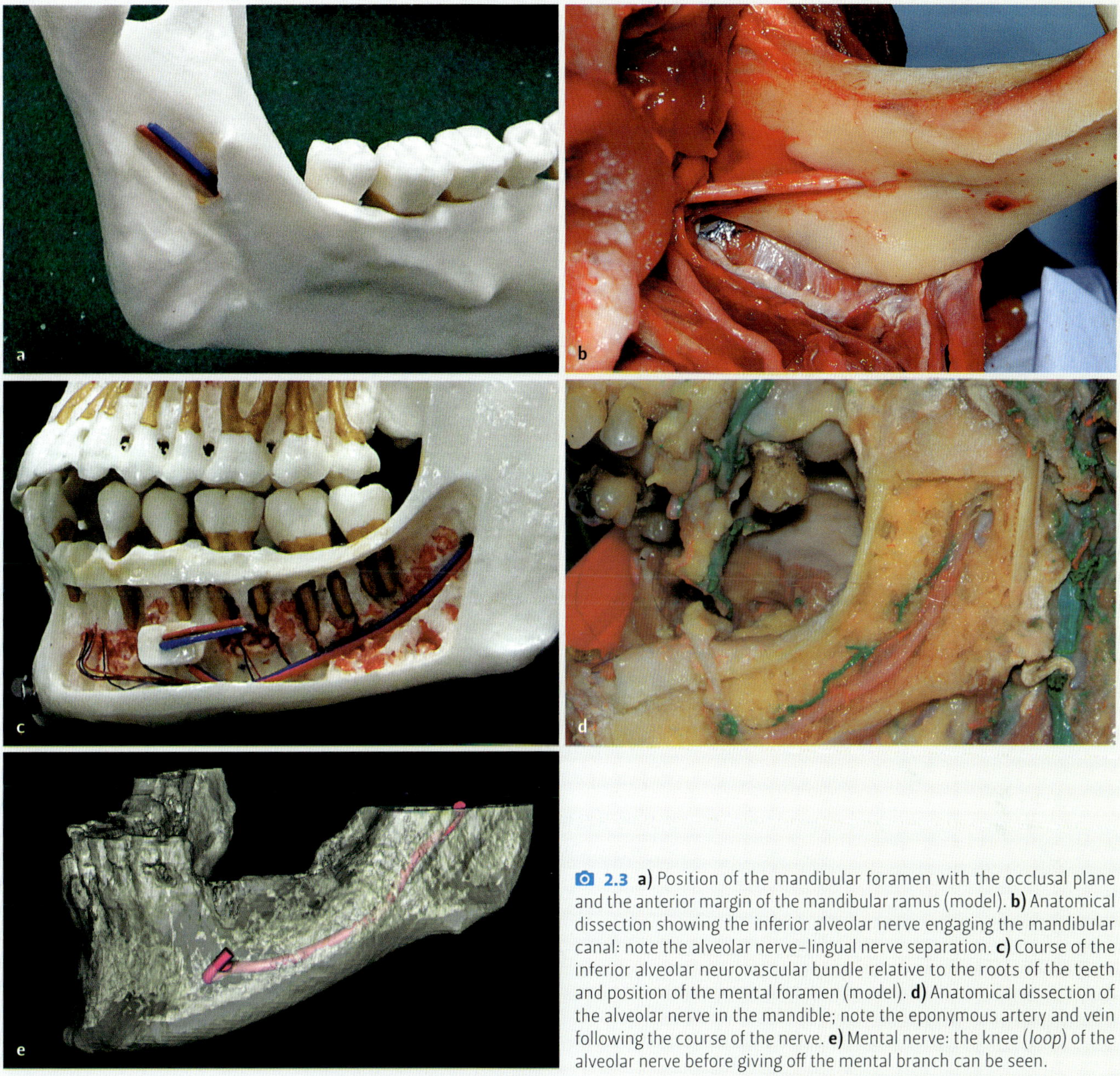

2.3 **a)** Position of the mandibular foramen with the occlusal plane and the anterior margin of the mandibular ramus (model). **b)** Anatomical dissection showing the inferior alveolar nerve engaging the mandibular canal: note the alveolar nerve-lingual nerve separation. **c)** Course of the inferior alveolar neurovascular bundle relative to the roots of the teeth and position of the mental foramen (model). **d)** Anatomical dissection of the alveolar nerve in the mandible; note the eponymous artery and vein following the course of the nerve. **e)** Mental nerve: the knee (*loop*) of the alveolar nerve before giving off the mental branch can be seen.

Inferior alveolar artery

Origin: arises from the first tract (mandibular portion) of the internal maxillary artery that runs between the neck of the mandible and the sphenomandibular ligament.

Function: it is responsible for the endosteal blood supply to the mandibular body distal to the first premolar.

Course: from its point of origin, it descends along the medial side of the mandibular ramus. Just above the mandibular foramen, it gives off a mylohyoid branch to vascularise the homonymous muscle, and then penetrates inside the mandibular canal, along with the inferior alveolar nerve. It then follows the same course as the nerve, finally dividing into its two terminal branches (the mental and incisive arteries).

To protect the integrity of the inferior alveolar artery, the same precautions described for the inferior alveolar nerve apply: being aware of the position of the mandibular canal is the best way to avoid damaging the neurovascular bundle. Today it is possible, thanks to the new techniques of digital radiographic imaging, to identify the mandibular canal and its relationship to adjacent anatomical structures (teeth, cysts, etc.) with dedicated three-dimensional image processing techniques, thus reducing the risk of complications (2.3e).

Inferior alveolar vein

Origin: it is a tributary of the internal maxillary vein, which is in turn a tributary of the posterior facial vein.

Course: its course is similar to that of the homonymous artery; it is a vessel with a negligible diameter, and damaging it does not create any significant risks.

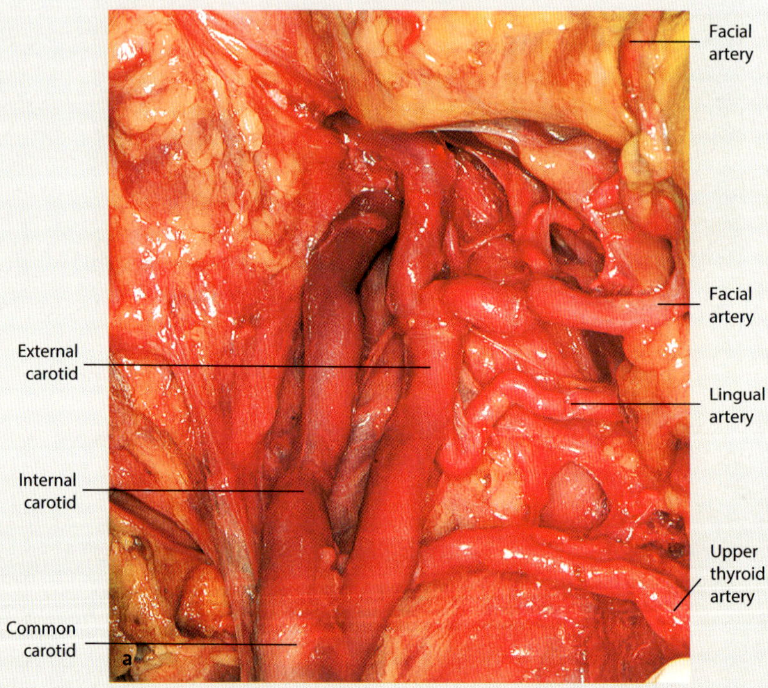

2.5 a) Anatomical dissection of the great vessels of the neck (common carotid artery, external carotid artery, and internal carotid artery): the last branch (top) is the facial artery. **b)** The dissection shows the proximity of the facial artery and vein to the buccal bone plate of the mandibular body. **c)** Anatomical dissection showing the proximity of the facial artery and vein to the vestibular bone plate of the mandibular body.

BUCCAL SIDE

Facial artery

Origin: arises from the external carotid artery just above the point of origin of the lingual artery, at the level of the great horn of the hyoid bone (2.4, 2.5a–c).

Function: provides the vascularisation of the soft palate, the palatine tonsil, the submandibular gland, the skin and muscles of the chin and lips, the mucosa and skin of the cheeks, and the skin of the nasal pyramid.

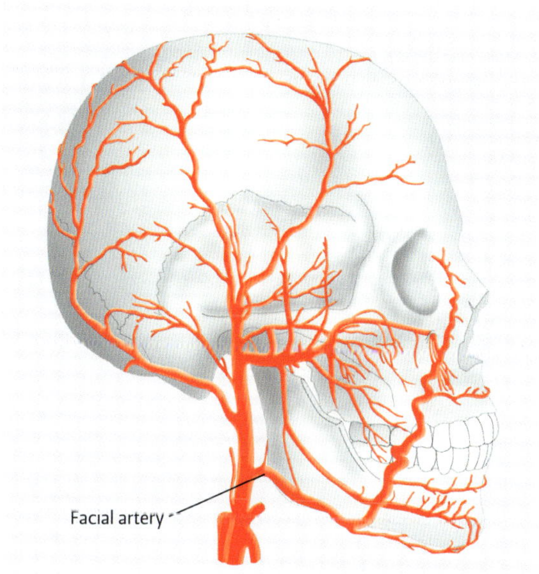

2.4 Anatomic illustration highlighting the course of the facial artery.

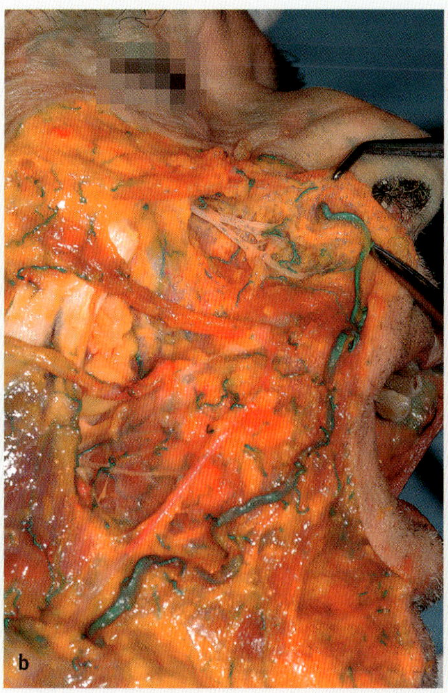

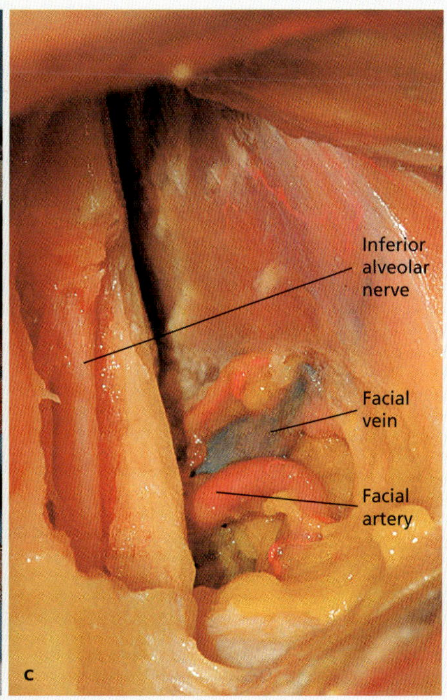

Course: it ascends along the lateral wall of the pharynx, until it crosses the posterior pole of the submandibular gland. The collateral branches that the facial artery gives off in the neck are as follows: the ascending palatine artery, the tonsillar branch, the glandular branches (submaxillary branches) for the submandibular gland, and the submental artery.

It then ascends anteriorly, skirting the inferior border of the mandible just in front of the anterior insertions of the masseter muscle, where it is only covered by the superficial cervical fascia, the platysma muscle, and the skin. From there, taking a sinuous course, it crosses the face towards the oral commissure, running below the muscles of the cheek, to become superficial at the level of the buccal mucosa. The collateral branches it gives off in the face are the inferior and superior labial arteries.

Finally, it ascends to the wing of the nose where it ends in its terminal branch, the lateral nasal artery (or the artery of the wing of the nose); often, after giving off this branch, the facial artery continues into a thinner branch called the angular artery (📷 2.5c).

The facial artery can be accidentally damaged in all surgical procedures performed on the buccal side of the mandible in the premolar and molar area (extraction of impacted third molars, bone harvesting from the mandibular ramus, vestibuloplasty, etc.), or on the buccal mucosa. To prevent bleeding from the facial artery it is advisable to perform, whenever possible, a subperiosteal dissection when raising flaps on this area (📷 2.6), and a blunt dissection with adequate surgical instruments when working on the intra- and extraoral malar soft tissues (📷 2.7). In cases where it is necessary to perform the drainage of an abscess in the buccal region with an extraoral approach, it is essential to identify the course of the facial artery to prevent possible damages.

For more details, please refer to the section regarding the malar region.

Buccal nerve

Origin: it arises from the anterior trunk of the mandibular nerve.

Function: it is responsible for the sensitivity of the skin and mucosa of the cheek, of the gingiva/buccal mucosa in the area of the molars, but it also supplies secretory fibres for the buccal and labial glands.

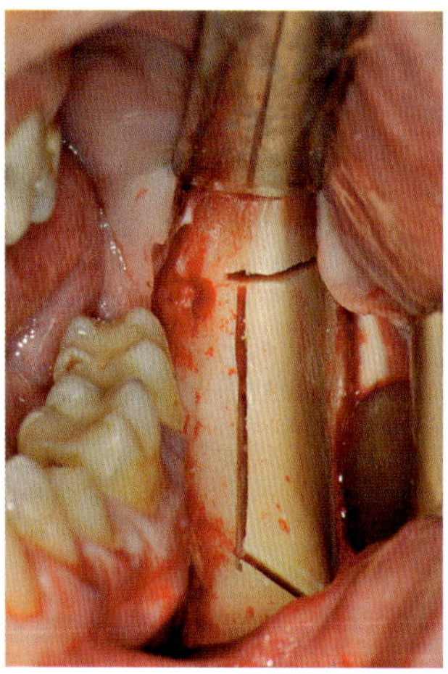

📷 **2.6** Protection of the facial artery during bone harvesting from the mandibular ramus.

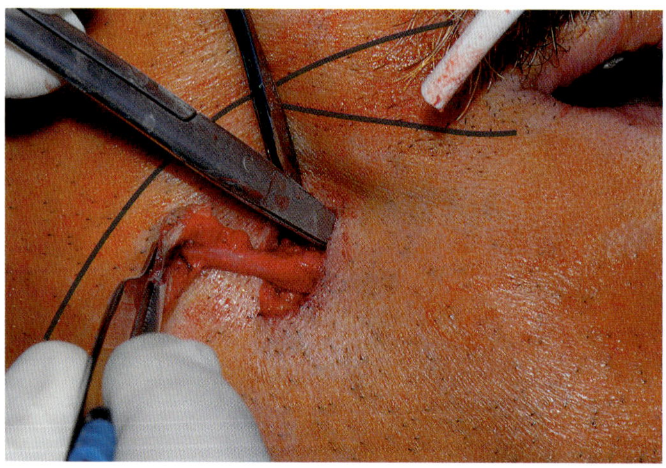

📷 **2.7** Presence of a cutaneous fistula near the facial artery (the course of the artery is represented on the patient's skin): dissection must take into account the relationship between the fistula and the artery.

Course: from its point of origin, it descends laterally, crossing the anterior margin of the mandibular ramus, and reaches the lateral side of the buccinator muscle. From here, some fibres are distributed to the skin of the cheek, while others penetrate the muscle, emerging on its medial side to innervate the buccal mucosa and minor salivary glands in the area.

The nerve can be clinically located approximately 1-2 centimetres buccally to the third molar, at the level of the occlusal plane, along the external oblique line (2.8a). The buccal nerve can be damaged by full-thickness releasing incisions extending distally to the retromolar trigon. To prevent such injuries, the full-thickness incision must not extend more than two centimetres distally to the retromolar trigon: if a longer incision is necessary to allow a wider retraction, the further extent of the incision must be performed split-thickness (involving only the superficial mucosa and submucosa). The buccal nerve can be retracted without being dissected, thus allowing adequate access to the mandibular ramus (2.8b).

Arterial ramusculi

They follow the course of the buccal nerve. Bleeding resulting from their accidental section is not complicated to manage.

When describing cleavage planes in the posterior mandible it is worth remembering the retromolar papilla, which is located at the base of the mandibular ramus and is connected to the inferior part of its anterior margin, just behind the third molar.

Immediately behind the papilla, the malar mucosa contains minor salivary glands, which are referred to as the *retromolar glands*. While this glandular aggregate has rather loose connections and is therefore easily elevated, the retromolar papilla is characterised by a rather tenacious attachment to the deeper planes.

These structural features are particularly important, especially in the surgery of third molars, for which an adequate dissection is essential to achieving correct intraoperative vision.

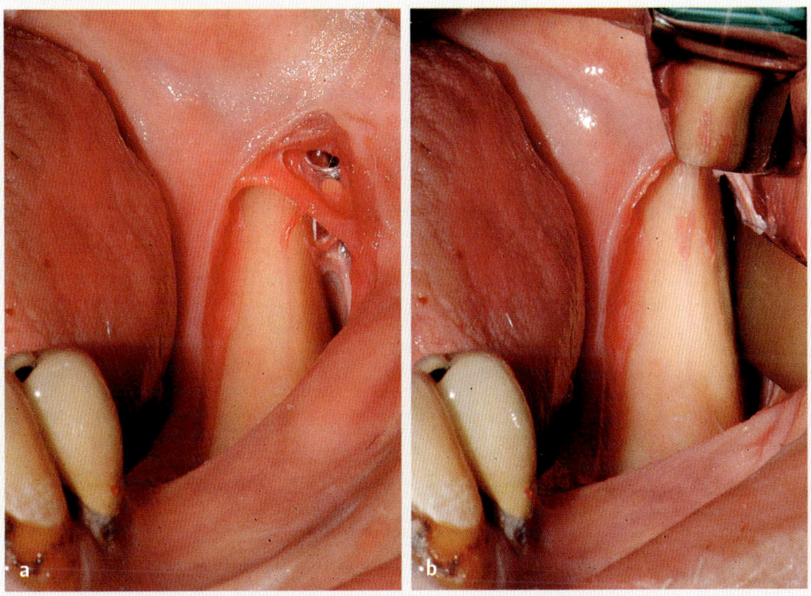

2.8 **a)** Anatomical dissection of the buccal nerve. **b)** Protection of the buccal nerve.

LINGUAL SIDE

The anatomical planes are similar to those described earlier, and the anatomical structures to consider are the lingual nerve, the mylohyoid nerve, and the mylohyoid artery.

Lingual nerve

Origin: it arises from the posterior trunk of the mandibular nerve, along with the inferior alveolar nerve.

Function: it is a sensory nerve, and it innervates the mucosa of the anterior two-thirds of the tongue, the mucosa of the floor of mouth, and the gingiva/alveolar mucosa on the lingual side of the mandible. It also carries two contingents of fibres from the chorda tympani, which it receives from an anastomotic branch. One contains fibres destined to the submandibular and sublingual secretory glands, while the other contains visceral sensory fibres gathering the sense of taste from the tongue.

Course: from its point of origin, similar to the inferior alveolar nerve, it maintains an anterior-medial position to it; it then runs down, describing an arch with an upper and anterior concavity. Next, it passes between the two pterygoid muscles and from there between the internal pterygoid muscle and the mandibular ramus, thus extending to the outer side of the tongue. In this area, the nerve is found in the alveolo-lingual sulcus, covered only by the mucosa of the oral floor. Its path begins between the hyoglossus and genioglossus muscles medial to the sublingual gland, and finally crosses beneath the submandibular duct, where it ends in giving off its terminal branches for the innervation of the apex of the tongue (📷 2.9a-c).

In the retromolar and third/second molar area, the nerve can be extremely superficial (2-3 mm medially to the gingival margin) (📷 2.9b).

It is important to remember that the mandibular ramus develops from the body of the mandible towards the condyle fossa, with an axis oriented more towards the vestibule compared to the line connecting the central fossae of the molars. This has significant surgical implications, because an incision made in the retromolar area following this line exposes the lingual nerve to a high risk of section. Therefore, incisions in this area must be performed at an angle towards the vestibule, to avoid damaging the nerve (📷 2.9d). The dissection must be strictly subperiosteal, and the soft tissues on the lingual side of the flap must be adequately protected using appropriate instruments (📷 2.9e). Surgical removal of impacted third molars, bone harvesting from the mandibular ramus, and enucleation of cysts in this region (particularly when they develop towards the lingual side of the mandible) are the most frequent surgical procedures that require adequate protection of the soft tissues on the lingual side to avoid any damage to the lingual nerve.

In this area, the insertions of the mylohyoid muscle are also found: the two mylohyoid muscles merge on the median raphe along the midline, and represent the inferior limit of the floor of the mouth (📷 2.10). Resting on the muscle, the mylohyoid nerve and artery run along the homonymous line.

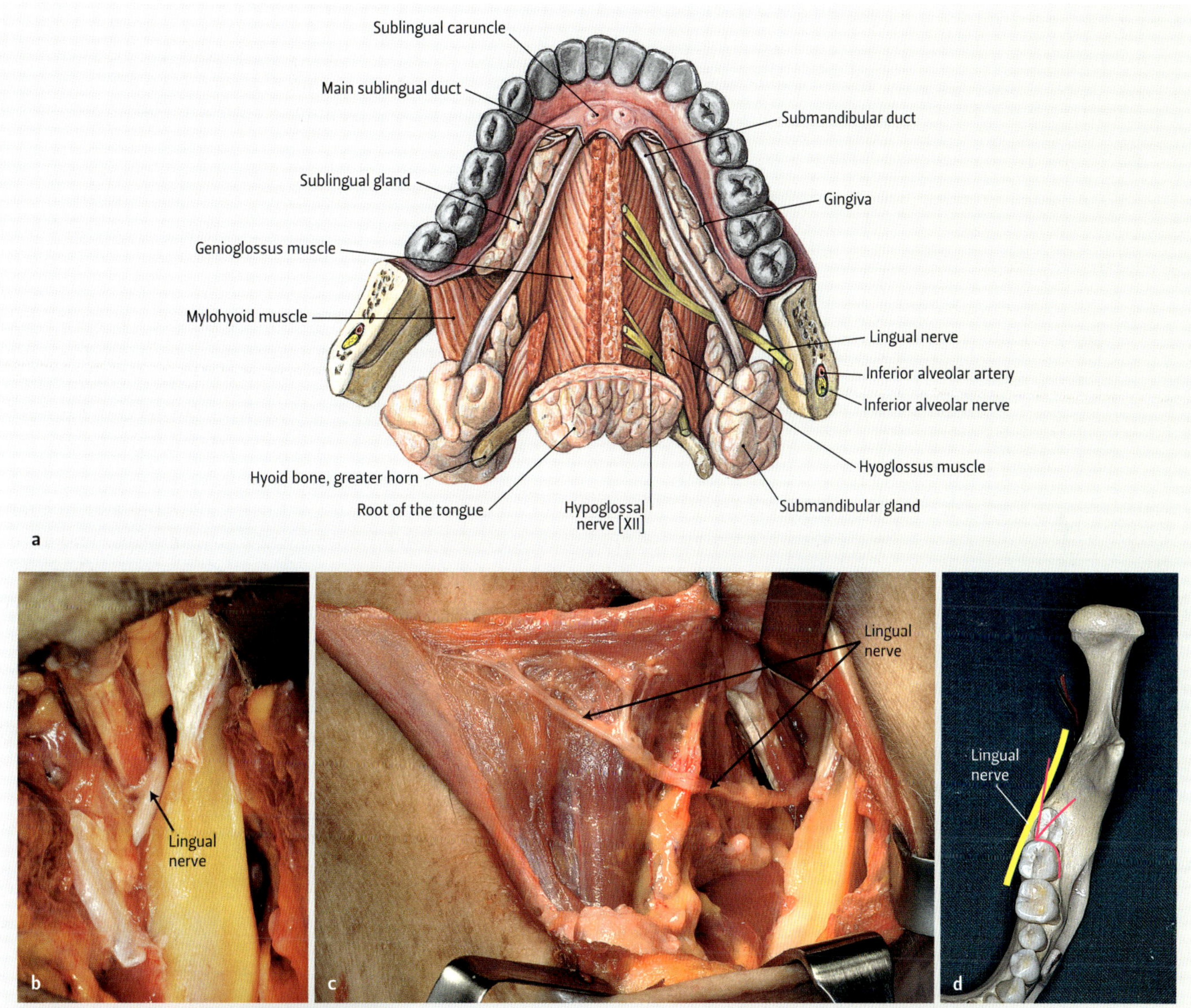

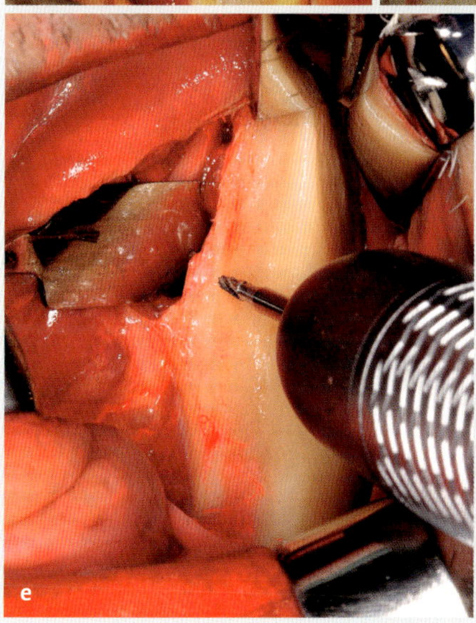

2.9 a) Anatomic illustration highlighting the course of the lingual nerve on the lingual side of the mandible (from *Sobotta Atlante di Anatomia Umana*. Elsevier, Milano 2012). **b)** Anatomical dissection of the lingual nerve near the mandibular body. **c)** Anatomical dissection of the lingual nerve within the tongue. **d)** At its root, the mandibular ramus abruptly changes direction, heading upwards towards the vestibule. Therefore, incisions in the area of the retromolar trigone should be directed buccally. **e)** Protection of the lingual nerve with a retractor.

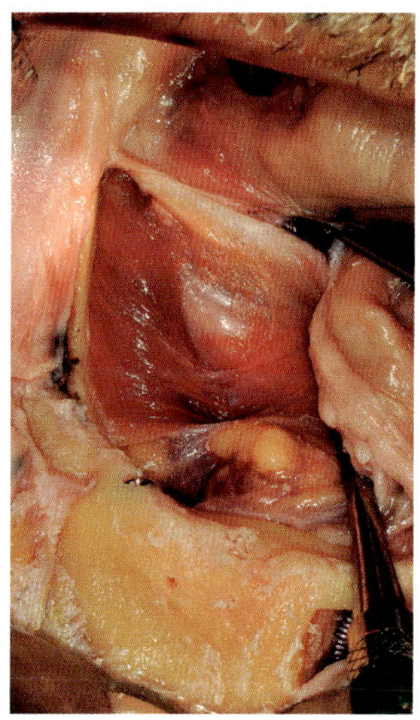

2.10 Anatomical dissection of the mylohyoid muscle.

Mylohyoid artery

Origin: it arises from the inferior alveolar artery, just above the mandibular foramen.

Function: it is responsible for the vascularisation of the homonymous muscle.

Course: from its point of origin, it runs down along the medial side of the mandibular ramus and then bends anteriorly to rest on the homonymous muscle, running along the mylohyoid line. Along its path, it provides branches to the muscle itself, some of which pass through it and create anastomoses with branches of the submental artery.

The accidental lesion of the mylohyoid artery can induce considerable bleeding. Therefore, it is important that elevation of the soft tissues in this area be performed subperiosteally in order to avoid major bleeding, which can be difficult to control in the course of surgeries performed under local anaesthesia (2.11a-b). It is thus appropriate, in order to limit this risk, to perform radiographic evaluations which permit a three-dimensional analysis of local anatomy when planning surgical procedures in this region, because the mandibular body in the molar and premolar area can present significant undercuts that implicate an increased risk of penetrating the oral floor during surgery (2.12). In these cases, the

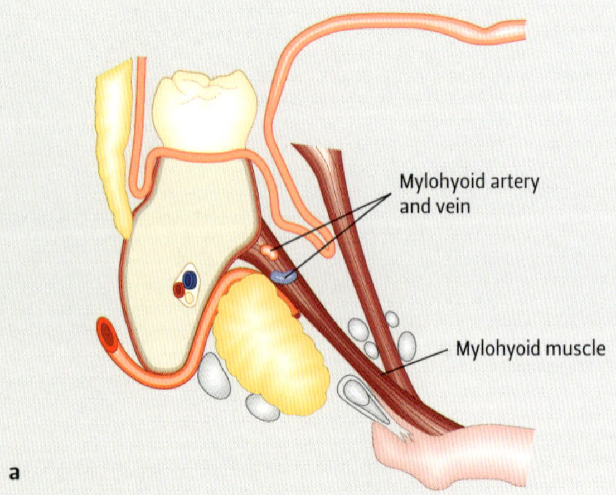

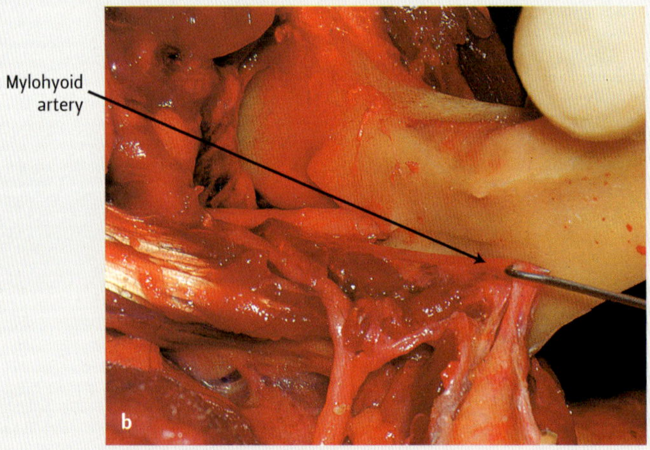

2.11 **a)** Cross-section of the jaw showing insertions of the mylohyoid muscle and the course of the homonymous artery and vein. **b)** Cadaveric dissection of the mylohyoid artery.

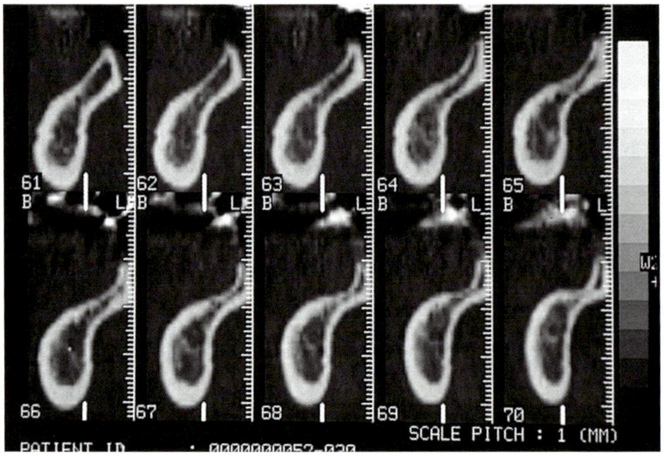

2.12 Computed tomography of the mandible (cross-section) showing a considerable undercut that would not be visible on panoramic and periapical radiographs: the mylohyoid artery might be injured, for example, while preparing an implant site.

mylohyoid artery can be damaged while preparing implant sites if the bur tip perforates the lingual cortical plate of the mandible, during tooth sectioning manoeuvres of impacted molars, or during manoeuvres to enucleate mandibular cysts that have eroded the lingual cortical plate.

Mylohyoid nerve

Origin: it arises from the inferior alveolar nerve just above the mandibular foramen.

Function: it is a motor nerve that innervates the mylohyoid muscle and the anterior belly of the digastric muscle. However, in a variable percentage of patients, it can also have sensitive fibres that, passing through the mandibular cortex, contribute to innervation of the premolars, canines and incisors, as well as the skin overlying the inferior border of the mandible. This anatomical variation must be considered when performing local anaesthesia on these teeth. In fact, despite adequate nerve block anaesthesia of the inferior alveolar nerve, the patient may still report pain, for example during molar tooth extraction.

Course: it follows the course of the homonymous artery.

To protect the nerve during surgical manoeuvres, the same recommendations described for the protection of the mylohyoid artery apply.

Anterior mandible

It is the portion of the lower jaw found between the two mental foramina.

The anatomical planes are the same described previously for the posterior mandible.

BONY PLANE – MANDIBULAR BODY

Running inside the incisive canal, the incisive neurovascular bundle is formed by the incisive artery and vein and the incisive nerve, one of the two terminal branches of the inferior alveolar nerve. The nerve gives off branches to the anterior teeth and the corresponding gingiva (📷 2.13a). Even with an adequate knowledge of the course of this nerve, it is often difficult to identify it during surgery because of its frequently small diameter, and as it runs deep within the cancellous bone (📷 2.13b). Damages to this nerve (e.g. as a result of tooth extraction, removal of cysts, implant placement, bone harvesting from the chin, etc.) may cause paraesthesia-anaesthesia of the corresponding teeth. This event may lead to functional and medico-legal implications that are in any case not comparable in severity to those resulting from damage to the main trunk of the inferior alveolar nerve. The only serious complication that may occur involving the incisive nerve is the indirect (retrograde) damage of the inferior alveolar nerve/mental nerve. This can happen in cases in which the diameter of incisive nerve is larger than usual: when using rotary instruments in close proximity to the incisive nerve (e.g. creation of implant sites, removal of intraosseous lesions, etc.), the nerve may be caught by the bur and be pulled by the rotation. This results in its stretching, therefore involving the fibres of the main trunk of the mental nerve and inferior alveolar nerve. In such a case, all or part of the area innervated by the latter can be affected by paraesthesia/anaesthesia, with much more relevant sequelae (📷 2.13c). In the specific case of implant placement in the interforaminal area of the mandible, keeping a "safety distance" of 4-5 millimetres from the mental foramen is recommended to prevent this complication.

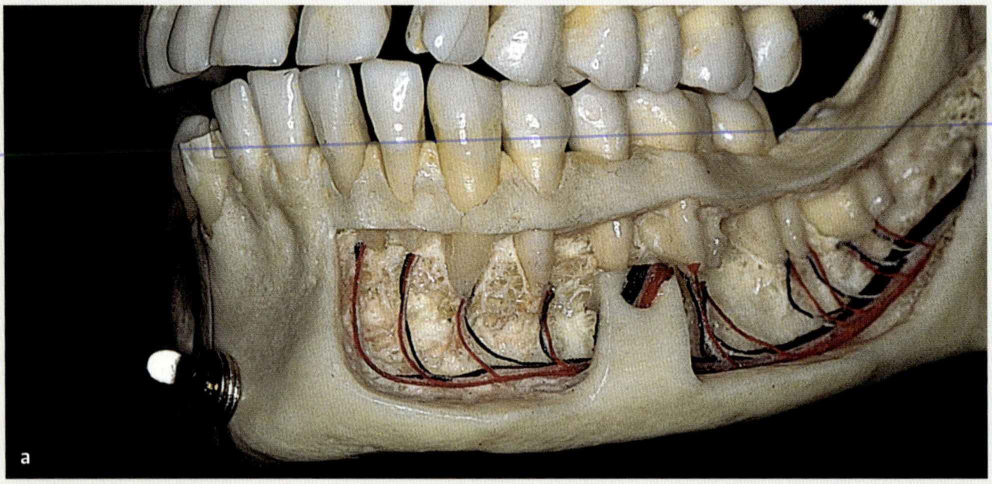

2.13 **a)** Course of the incisive nerve within the mandibular body, and position of the mental foramen relative to the premolars (model). **b)** Anatomical dissection showing the course of the incisive nerve within the mandibular body and the position of the mental foramen. **c)** Anatomical dissection of the inferior alveolar nerve including its terminal branches: the incisive nerve and the mental nerve.

Anterior mandible

Surgical procedures

- Impacted or erupted premolars
- Cysts and soft tissue lesions
- Bone harvesting from the mandibular symphysis
- Vestibuloplasty
- Implant placement in the interforaminal region
- Biopsy

Notable anatomic structures

- Branches of the submental artery
- Secondary branches of the deep lingual and sublingual arteries
- Mental neurovascular bundle

BUCCAL SIDE

The dominant structure is represented by the inferior alveolar neurovascular bundle, which consists of the inferior alveolar nerve, accompanied by the homonymous artery and vein.

Mental nerve

Origin: it arises from the inferior alveolar nerve, of which it is the bigger terminal branch, given off at the mental foramen.

Function: it is a sensory nerve that innervates the skin of the chin and lower lip.

Course: it leaves the mandible through the homonymous foramen, which is generally located below the apexes of the first and second mandibular premolars. The distinctive feature of the mental nerve is its course in the area of the foramen, as it often forms a mesially oriented loop inside the mandibular canal, then bends distally and engages the mental foramen. The presence of this anatomical characteristic is significant, because identification of the mental foramen on periapical or panoramic radiographs alone is not sufficient, and can be deceptive as far as the actual course of the nerve (particularly, its mesial loop) is concerned.

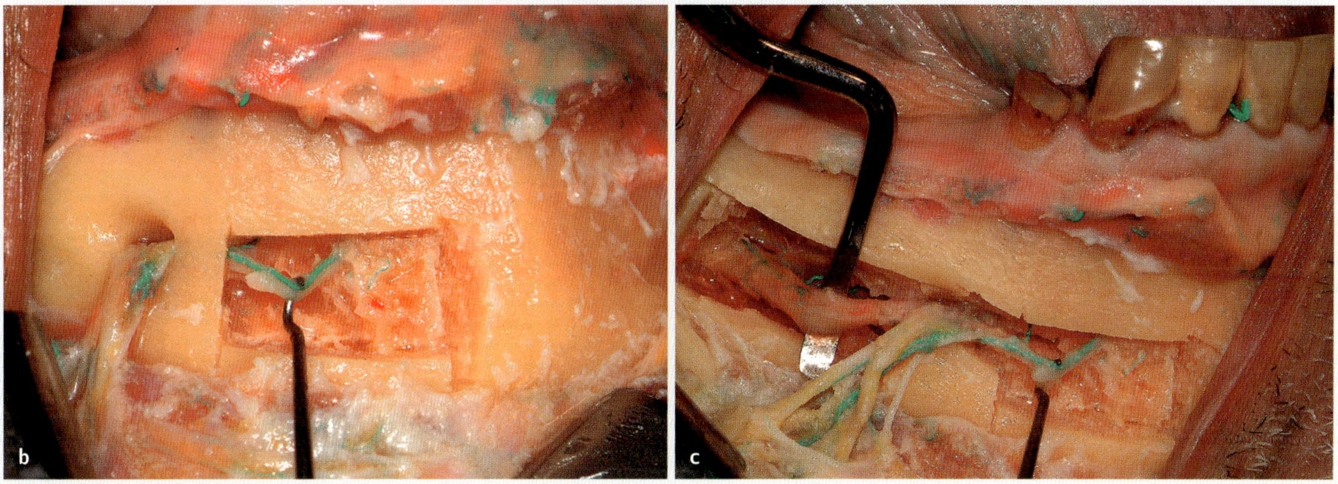

After emerging from the foramen, the nerve divides into three main branches, which take different directions (mesial, middle and distal) supplying somatic sensory innervation to the skin of the chin and lower lip (2.14a-b).

For surgeries in the inferior premolar region, it is always indicated to perform a full-thickness dissection (except when it is necessary to remain above the periosteum, e.g. removal of soft tissue lesions, vestibuloplasty), which makes it possible to locate the mental foramen and the nerve exit. Identifying and protecting the nerve prevents any intraoperative damage, particularly during surgical manoeuvres involving the use of sharp or rotating surgical instruments. The same applies to the mental artery: a subperiosteal dissection prevents profuse bleeding.

Thorough knowledge of the mental nerve and artery course is particularly important in the case of surgical procedures on edentulous patients with significant resorption of the alveolar ridge. In such situations, the mental foramen can be very superficial. In cases of extreme atrophy, the mental nerve, as well as the inferior alveolar nerve, may be found on top of the ridge, just below the mucosa, because the roof of the mandibular canal has been lost due to bone atrophy (2.14c).

Surgeries requiring partial-thickness flaps (deepening of the vestibular sulcus/vestibuloplasty, removal of fibromas, biopsies, etc.) carry a higher risk of damaging the mental neurovascular bundle or its terminal branches if not performed with due care and attention. The identification and careful isolation of the mental bundle by blunt dissection will prevent this possibility.

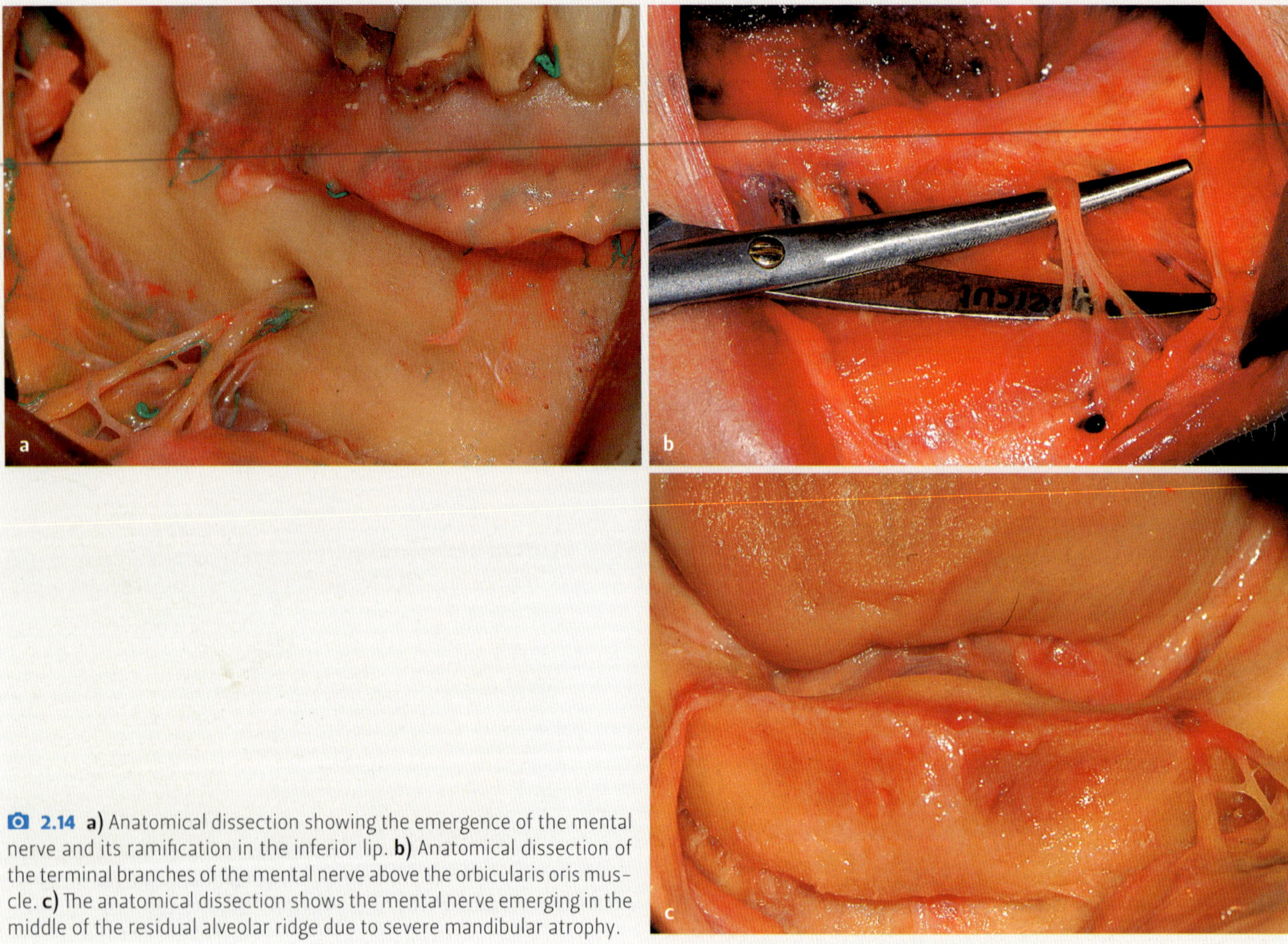

2.14 **a)** Anatomical dissection showing the emergence of the mental nerve and its ramification in the inferior lip. **b)** Anatomical dissection of the terminal branches of the mental nerve above the orbicularis oris muscle. **c)** The anatomical dissection shows the mental nerve emerging in the middle of the residual alveolar ridge due to severe mandibular atrophy.

LINGUAL SIDE

No anatomical structures that, if damaged, would cause a severe risk are present, as long as a subperiosteal elevation of the soft tissues is performed. Lateral to the midline are the mental spines, which receive the insertions of the two genioglossus muscles (2.15a-d). This muscle extends distally and then upwards to become a part of the tongue body by opening like a fan. It contributes to the backward, forwards, and lowering movements of the tongue.

The anatomical structures located superficially to the periosteum will be described in the section dedicated to the anterior portion of the floor of the mouth. There are also intramuscular perforating arteries that anastomose with the incisor vessels and penetrate the mandible laterally to the midline. These originate from secondary branches of the deep lingual artery and from the sublingual artery. Their identification may be useful during dissection in order to prevent bleeding.

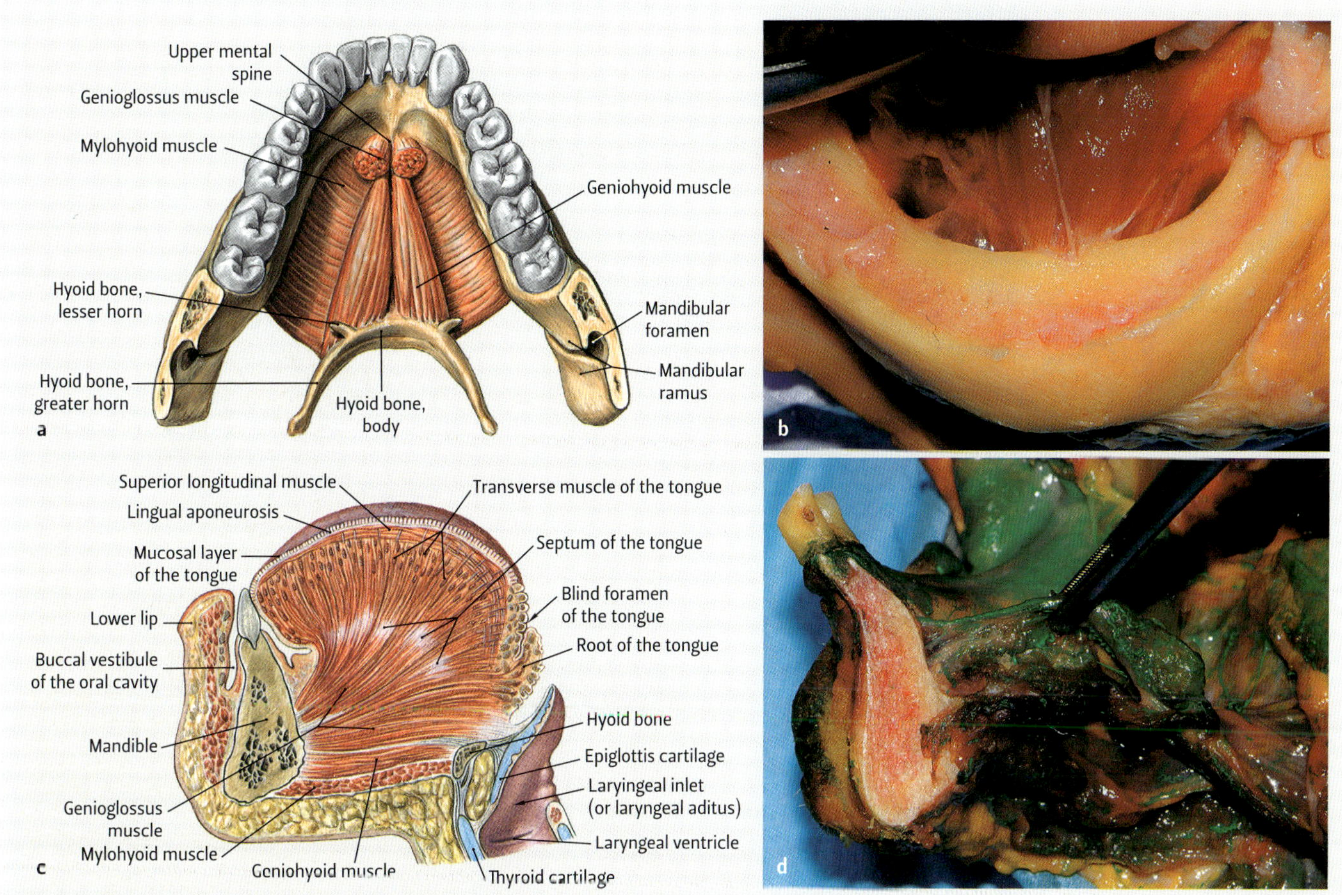

2.15 a–b) Anatomic illustration (modified from *Sobotta Atlante di Anatomia Umana*. Elsevier, Milano 2012) and dissection showing the insertion of the genioglossus muscles immediately lateral to the midline of the mandible. **c–d)** Anatomic illustration (modified from *Sobotta Atlante di Anatomia Umana*. Elsevier, Milano 2012) and sagittal dissection showing the insertions of the genioglossus, geniohyoid and mylohyoid muscles on the mandible.

INFERIOR BORDER

The inferior border of the mandible is not usually involved in basic oral surgery procedures. However, it may be involved in the case of enucleation of large cysts, of deeply impacted teeth, or during the preparation of implant sites. The only notable structures are the branches of the submental artery (a branch of the facial artery), which runs just over the periosteal plane: a subperiosteal dissection avoids intraoperative complications (2.16).

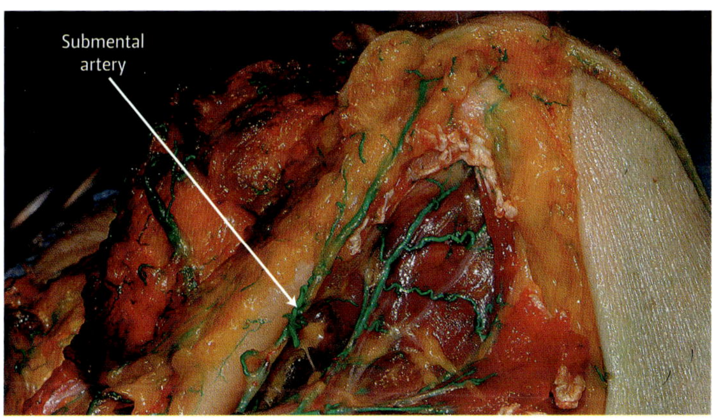

2.16 Anatomical dissection showing the course of the submental artery along the inferior border of the mandible.

Submental artery

Origin: it arises from the facial artery at the inferior edge of the mandible, just behind the mesial insertions of the masseter on the mandibular border.

Function: it is responsible for the vascularisation of the skin and muscles of the chin and lower lip.

Course: from its point of origin, it runs forwards and close to the mylohyoid muscle, along the inferior border of the mandible, medially to the submandibular gland; on its path, it gives off branches to the aforementioned anatomical structures. In addition, it gives off several perforating branches, which cross the mylohyoid muscle and create anastomoses with branches of the mylohyoid and sublingual arteries (2.16).

Floor of the mouth

From a surgical point of view, the floor of the mouth is one of the most delicate regions of the oral cavity, because it is composed entirely of soft tissues and, thus, no bony reference planes are present. Therefore, the anatomical planes are more difficult to identify. For this reason, a very precise knowledge of local anatomy is essential to correct performance of surgical procedures in this area. The area is highly vascularised: incautious surgical manoeuvres can cause diffuse bleeding which is difficult to manage, especially if the procedure is performed under local anaesthesia. In the anterior portion of the floor of the mouth and on the ventral surface of the tongue, the mucosal layer is thin, and it is possible to see through it the ranine arteries and veins, and the terminal branches of the sublingual artery and vein (2.17). A dissection in this area (e.g. to remove a ranula) must take into account the presence of these vessels, with the aim to preserving their integrity whenever possible (2.18a-b). Laterally, at the base of the lingual frenulum, the sublingual caruncle is found, which hosts the outlet of the submandibular (Wharton's) duct, the excretory duct of the submandibular gland (2.19a-b). The position of the submandibular duct outlet should always be located when performing surgeries in this area, in order to avoid any damage to it, or its ligation when suturing (for example, following a lingual frenulectomy). Laterally and behind the two caruncles, numerous small orifices can be seen; these are the outlets of the excretory ducts of the sublingual gland. Between these orifices and the dental arches, the floor of the mouth is raised from beneath by the sublingual gland to form the sublingual folds (2.17).

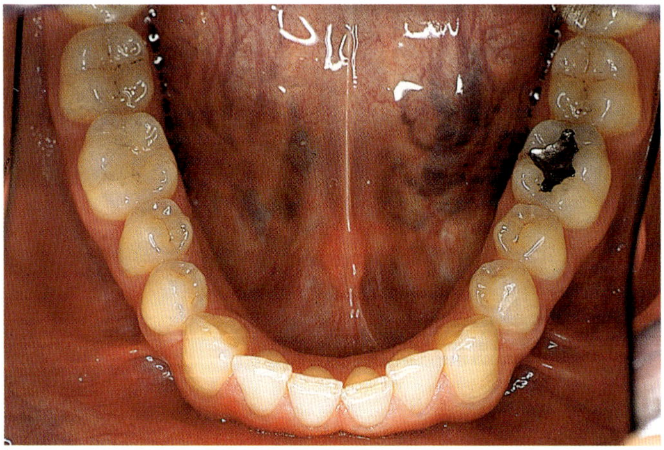

2.17 Clinical appearance of the floor of the mouth: the rich submucosal vascular structure is evident.

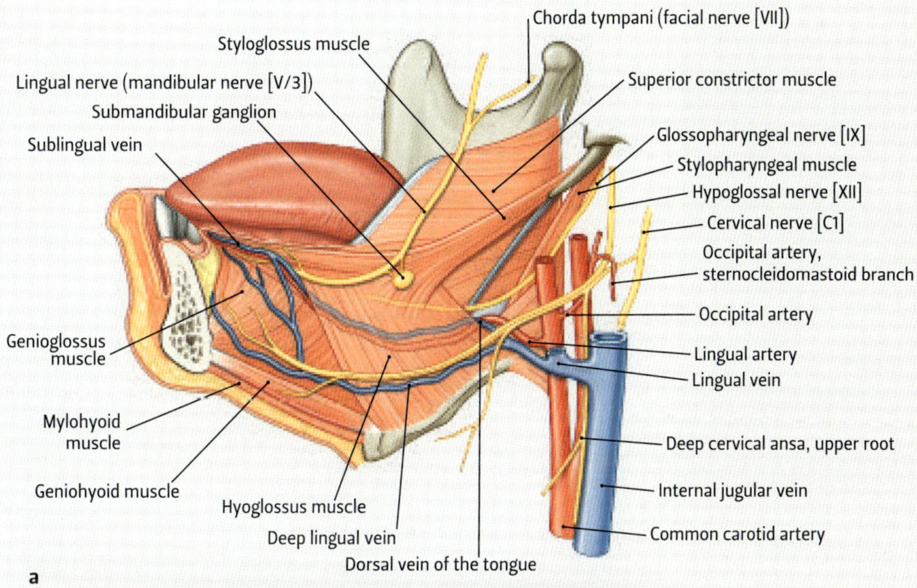

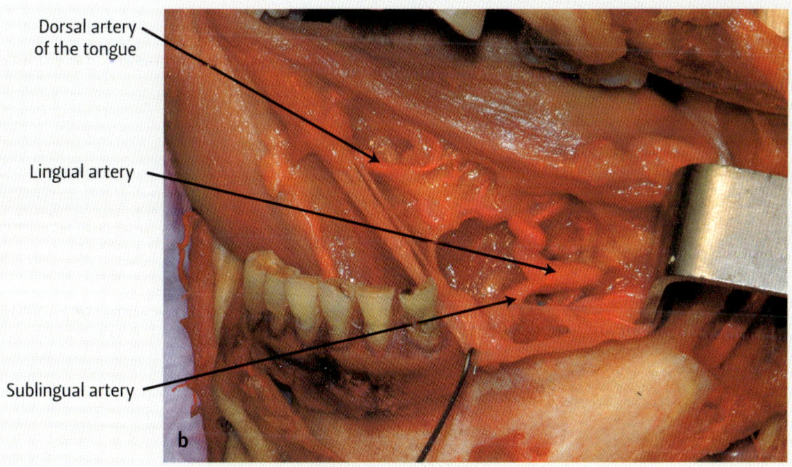

2.18 a) Anatomic illustration showing the course of the sublingual vessels within the floor of the mouth (modified from Drake R, A. Wayne Vogl, Mitchell A. *Gray's Anatomy for Students*. Churchill Livingstone, Philadelphia (PA) 2009). **b)** Anatomical dissection of the lingual artery dividing into the dorsal and sublingual arteries.

Underneath the mucosa of the sublingual sulcuslies lies a cavity separating the base of the tongue from the inner side of the mandible: the sublingual space. In the anterior portion, the walls of this sublingual space are:

- superiorly, the oral mucosa;
- on the anterior-lateral side, the portion of the inner side of the mandibular body that is above the mylohyoid line;
- on the posterior-medial side, the hyoglossus muscle;
- on the inferior part, the mylohyoid muscle, which separates the floor of the mouth from the suprahyoid region.

The sublingual space communicates extensively, in the area behind the posterior margin of the mylohyoid muscle, with the submandibular space. Notable anatomical structures are as follows: the sublingual gland, submandibular gland, submandibular duct, lingual nerve, mylohyoid artery, branches of the deep artery of the tongue, and sublingual artery.

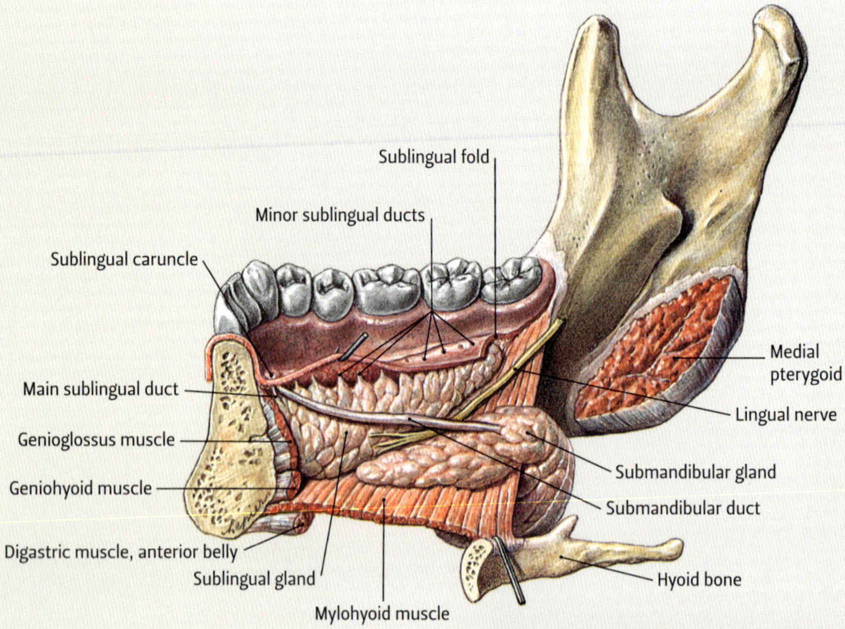

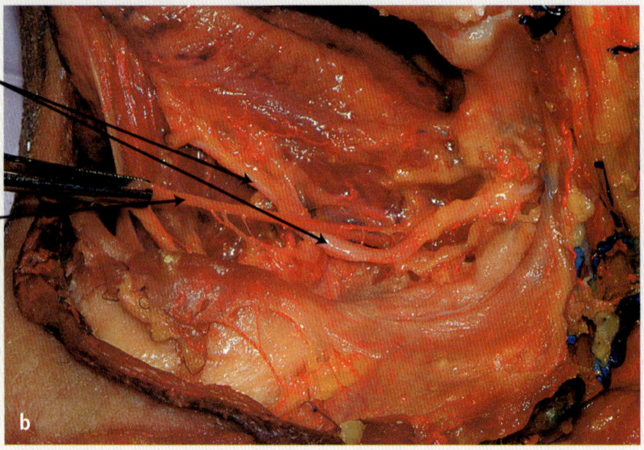

2.19 **a)** Anatomic illustration showing the intraoral course of the submandibular duct, its outlet in the oral cavity, and the excretory ducts of the sublingual gland (modified from *Sobotta Atlante di Anatomia Umana*. Elsevier, Milano 2012). **b)** Anatomical dissection showing the submandibular duct crossing the lingual nerve.

SUBLINGUAL GLAND

It is located immediately below the mucosa of the anterior portion of the floor of the mouth. It is almond-shaped, with a lateral face corresponding to the sublingual fossa of the mandibular body, a medial side that leans against the tongue muscles, a superior margin that lifts the mucosa of the floor of the mouth creating the sublingual fold, and a posterior end that corresponds to the anterior extension of the submandibular gland (2.20).

The sublingual gland may be involved in surgical manoeuvres during procedures to remove lesions of the mucosa overlying the floor of the mouth, or when the interruption of the periosteum on the lingual side of the mandible is necessary (e.g. after bone reconstructive procedures, to allow a tension-free suture). In such cases, the gland may herniate and invade the operating field: it is important to protect it to prevent any involvement or injury, especially when suturing.

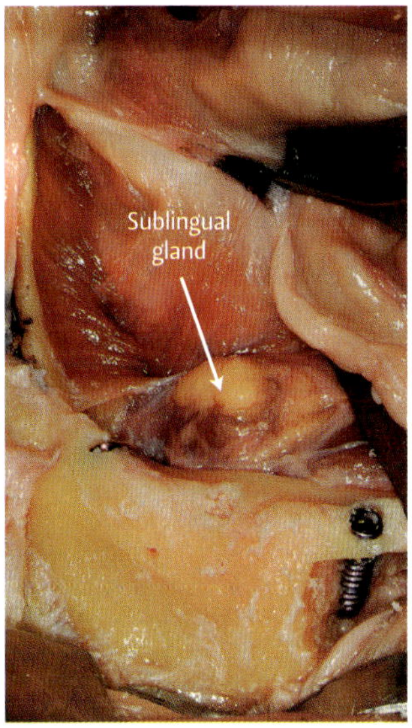

2.20 Anatomical dissection highlighting the sublingual gland, just below the mucosal layer of the anterior portion of the floor of the mouth.

Floor of the mouth

Surgical procedures

- Salivary pseudocysts
- Submandibular salivary stones
- Neoplasms of the mucosa

Notable anatomic structures

- Sublingual and submandibular glands
- Submandibular duct
- Lingual nerve
- Mylohyoid artery
- Secondary branches of the deep lingual and sublingual arteries

SUBMANDIBULAR GLAND

As the gland is deep-seated, it is almost never involved in oral surgery procedures. While it is not necessary to detail its anatomical relationships, it is nonetheless important to know the exact location of its anterior extension and the course of the submandibular duct. The gland has a roughly conical shape and, once it has passed into the gap between the hyoglossus muscle and the posterior margin of mylohyoid muscle, it penetrates into the floor of the mouth and in certain cases can make contact with the posterior pole of the sublingual gland.

The submandibular duct emerges from the medial part of the submandibular gland and runs forwards and medially, accompanying the extension of the gland; it then crosses above the lingual nerve in the area of the 1st-2nd molar, and then penetrates the sublingual space. Here, it runs along the medial aspect of the sublingual gland, very close to the sublingual artery, and finally emerges at the lingual caruncle (2.19b).

It is essential to know the path of the duct and its position relative to the other anatomical structures, for surgeries on the mucosa of the anterior portion of the floor of the mouth, or for removal of submandibular salivary stones, which are often located inside the duct (see Chapter 10 for more details).

Sublingual artery

Origin: it arises from the lingual artery at the point where it passes between the genioglossus muscle and the anterior margin of the hyoglossus muscle.

Function: it supplies the vascularisation for the sublingual gland, the surrounding muscles, the mucosa of the floor of the mouth and the lingual gingiva of the incisors.

Course: from its point of origin, it moves forwards, between the mylohyoid muscle and the genioglossus muscle below the submandibular duct, and it gives off several branches to vascularise the aforementioned anatomical structures, terminating in the soft tissues on the anterior lingual side of the mandible (in the area of the lateral incisors/canines) (2.21).

This vessel can be damaged when working on the lingual aspect of the anterior portion of the jaw, causing severe bleeding, as the artery sometimes has a significant diameter. Therefore, surgeries in this area must be conducted with great care: when performing a subperiosteal dissection, when working on the lingual side of the anterior mandible, or when performing a blunt tissue dissection, avoiding any damage to the artery is paramount. The section or tearing of the artery wall can induce severe bleeding during preparation of the implant site, if the drills being used perforate the lingual cortex in the region of the canine and lateral incisor. This is particularly true if relevant undercuts are present, or if the thickness of the alveolar ridge is reduced. Surgical procedures in this area must therefore be conducted with caution, after careful clinical inspection and evaluation of mandibular morphology, possibly with the aid of a CT scan. Bleeding that results from an injury to the vessel can spread among the soft tissues causing extensive swelling of the floor of the mouth and of the lingual pelvis, with risk of obstructing the upper aero-digestive tract. Cases have been described in the literature where a patient's life was at risk, had there not been the possibility of prompt hospitalisation and emergency surgeries under general anaesthesia to ligate the vessel; in some of these cases, emergency tracheostomy had to be performed create an airway and save the patient's life.

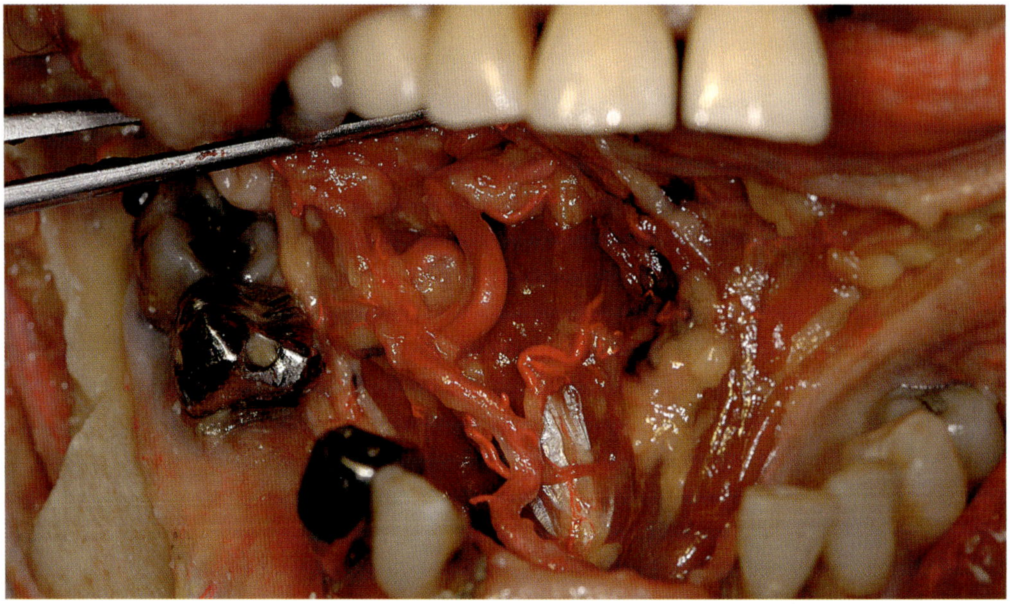

2.21 Anatomical dissection of the sublingual artery in the anterior portion of the floor of the mouth.

The lingual nerve, previously described with regard to its relationship with the posterior mandible (particularly the region of the third molar), may also be encountered during surgeries on the floor of the mouth. In this region, the nerve is in close contact with the posterior pole of the sublingual gland and crosses the submandibular duct at the level of the first-second molar, which passes underneath. This reference point is particularly important when working on the duct (e.g. when removing a salivary stone). The nerve then runs forwards, dividing into its terminal branches.

Tongue

The tongue can be involved in oral surgery procedures, in particular when removing small benign neoplasms that have developed in its superficial layers. In the case of lesions located deep inside the body or root of the tongue, the patient should instead be referred to a maxillofacial surgery unit for treatment since, given the rich vascularisation and the consequent risk of profuse intraoperative bleeding, surgery must be conducted under general anaesthesia and by adequately trained specialists.

The tongue presents two anatomical planes, which are easily distinguishable when adequate haemostasis is obtained: the mucosal plane and the muscular plane (2.22). Surgeries on the mucosal plane do not present particular risks, because the anatomical structures whose damage could create serious complications (lingual artery, dorsal and sublingual arteries of the tongue, previously described) all run within the confines of the muscular layer. For a detailed description of the lingual musculature, refer to systematic human anatomy textbooks.

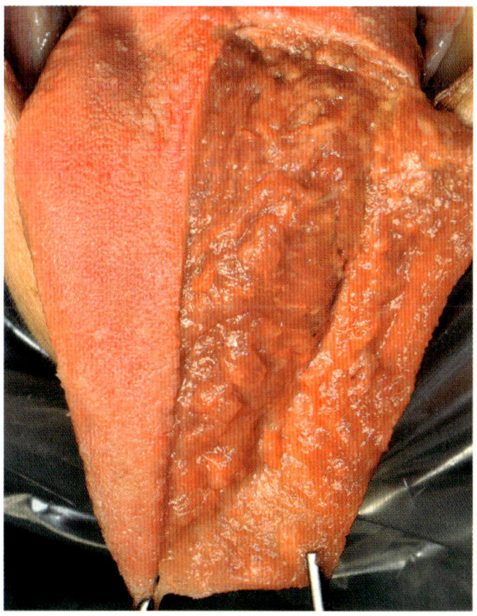

2.22 Anatomical dissection of the tongue: the mucosa is reversed, showing the submucosal and muscular layers.

Tongue

Surgical procedures
- Benign neoplasms

Notable anatomic structures
- Lingual artery
- Dorsal lingual and sublingual artery

Lingual artery

Origin: it arises from the external carotid artery near the great horn of the hyoid bone.

Function: it vascularises the suprahyoid muscles, the palatine tonsil, the sublingual gland, and the tongue.

Course: from its point of origin, it runs upwards in the neck close to the middle pharyngeal constrictor, medially to the posterior belly of the digastric muscle and to the stylohyoid muscle, crossing the hypoglossal nerve. It then runs forwards, medially to the hyoglossus muscle, which separates it from the submandibular gland, and then runs upwards between the genioglossus muscle and the anterior margin of the hyoglossus muscle (where it gives off the sublingual artery), ending as a deep artery of the tongue. Its location is somewhat deeper at the root of the tongue, while it tends to become superficial towards the tongue apex (2.23a-b; see also 2.21).

A lesion of the lingual artery causes severe bleeding, which is difficult to control and can put the patient's life at risk. Therefore, surgeries on the body of the tongue should be performed by trained maxillofacial surgeons under general anaesthesia in a safe environment (hospital).

Dorsal artery of the tongue

Origin: arises from the lingual artery, deep within the hyoglossus muscle.

Function: it is responsible for the vascularisation of the posterior portion of the dorsum of the tongue, the palatine tonsil, and the epiglottis.

Course: from its point of origin, it passes through the muscles of the tongue to the back of the tongue, where it divides into its terminal branches.

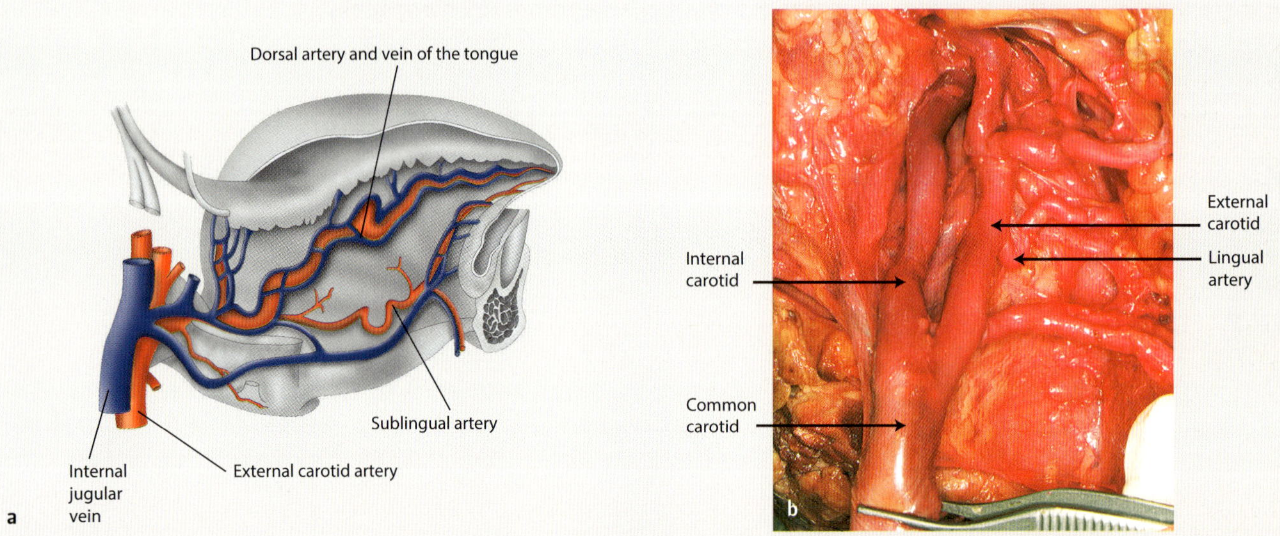

2.23 a) Anatomic illustration showing the course of the lingual, sublingual and dorsal arteries of the tongue. **b)** Anatomical dissection of the great vessels of the neck (common carotid, external carotid, and internal carotid): the penultimate branch (top) is the lingual artery.

As a rule, it is recommended that surgeries on the body of the tongue be performed by experienced maxillofacial surgeons in a safe environment (hospital), under general anaesthesia. These measures make it possible to manage any intraoperative complications using adequate instruments (bipolar coagulation systems), or by recourse to emergency manoeuvres (extraoral access for the ligation of arteries, etc.).

Anterior maxilla

This corresponds to the embryological premaxilla, the portion of the maxilla located mesially to the intercanine line.

BONY PLANE

From a surgical perspective, the most important structure to consider is the nasopalatine neurovascular bundle. This structure, often described as single, is actually formed by two symmetrical nerves (with their accompanying arteries and veins) that converge on the median line and engage the incisive canals. The right and left canals are also symmetrical, but they are so close together that they almost constitute a single channel, divided by a thin bone lamina which may nevertheless be absent in certain cases.

Nasopalatine nerve

Origin: it is part of a nerve group called the posterior-superior nasal nerves, which arise from the sphenopalatine ganglion (located in the pterygopalatine fossa).

Function: it supplies the anterior portion of the palatine mucosa, mesially to the intercanine line.

Course: from the point of origin in the pterygopalatine fossa, it descends obliquely along the wall of the nasal septum to reach the incisive canal. It emerges from the nasopalatine foramen, located posteriorly to the central incisors (📷 2.24a).

As previously mentioned, the right and left nasopalatine nerves (and the accompanying vessels) converge on the midline in the opening of the incisive foramen. In some cases, the incisive canal may be undivided; the neurovascular bundles of the two sides are thus united, and emerge as a single structure from the incisive foramen (📷 2.24b-c).

The presence of the canal must be considered in the case of surgeries performed on the palatal side of the anterior maxilla (removal of impacted or supernumerary teeth, enucleation of cysts, placement of implants, etc.). The accidental section of the bundle does not cause significant functional sequelae, but causes intraoperative bleeding and may cause paraesthesia/anaesthesia of the innervated area.

In cases of severe atrophy of the upper maxilla, the position of the incisive foramen relative to the usual anatomical landmarks may vary considerably. Centripetal bone resorption of the upper maxilla results in bone loss from the buccal side towards the palatal side, which causes a shift of the centre of the residual alveolar ridge in the palatal direction; this results in the possibility of finding the bundle on the centre of the residual alveolar ridge, particularly in cases of extreme bone resorption. This must be considered when the position of surgical access is planned and during incision and elevation of the soft tissues.

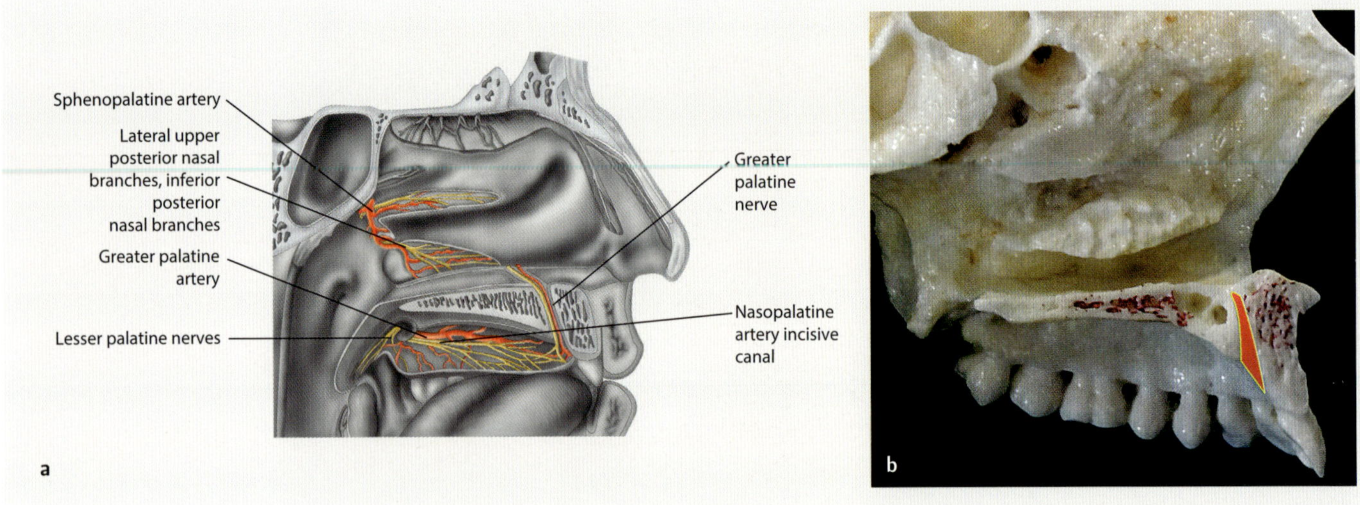

Anterior maxilla

Surgical procedures
- Impacted teeth
- Cysts

Notable anatomic structures
- Nasopalatine neurovascular bundle
- Infraorbital neurovascular bundle
- Nasal floor

The nasopalatine artery and vein follow the course of the nerve: to avoid any damage during the surgical manoeuvres, the same suggestions described for the nerve apply.

Both the nasopalatine vessels and nerves have numerous anastomoses with branches of the major neurovascular palatine bundles (📷 2.24d).

The upper anatomical limit of the anterior maxilla on the midline is represented by the floor of the nose. When working in its proximity (impacted/supernumerary teeth, cysts, implants, etc.), it is fundamentally necessary to identify the margins of the nasal fossae and, if necessary, dissect and protect the nasal mucosa with adequate retractors (📷 2.25). If damaged, the nasal mucosa may bleed profusely, and blood may invade both the surgical field and the nasal cavities: this can render the management of such complications difficult when carrying out the procedure under local anaesthesia.

BUCCAL SIDE

On the buccal side of the anterior maxilla, several anatomical planes can be distinguished that correspond to an equal number of cleavage planes: the mucosal, submucosal, muscular, periosteal and bony planes (📷 2.26a-c). As mentioned earlier, subperiosteal cleavage reduces intraoperative bleeding and the risk of damage to the neurovascular structures, except in the areas where foramina or perforating vessels are present.

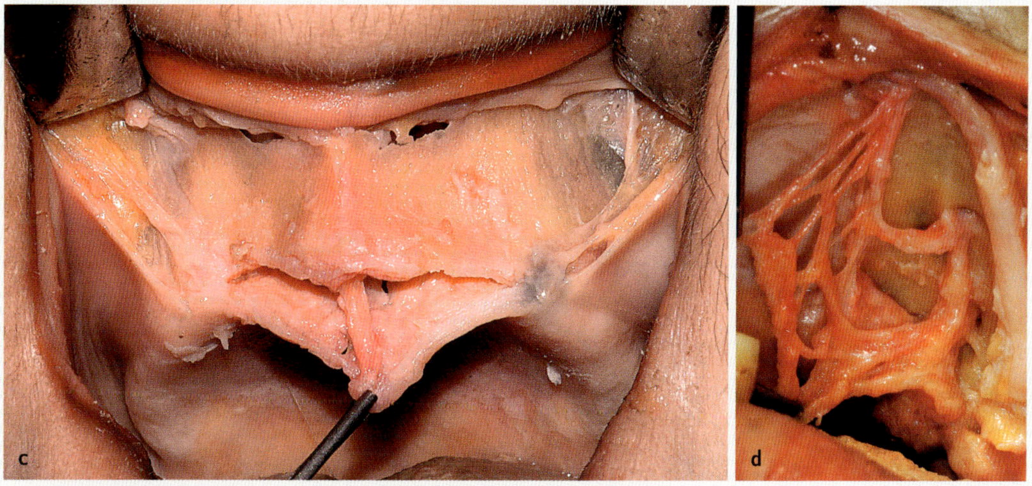

2.24 **a)** Anatomic illustration of the arterial blood supply and innervation of the palate. **b)** Course of the nasopalatine canal (model). **c)** Anatomical dissection showing the exit of the nasopalatine nerves at the incisor foramen. **d)** Anatomical dissection showing the neurovascular nasopalatine bundle and anastomotic circuits with the palatine bundle.

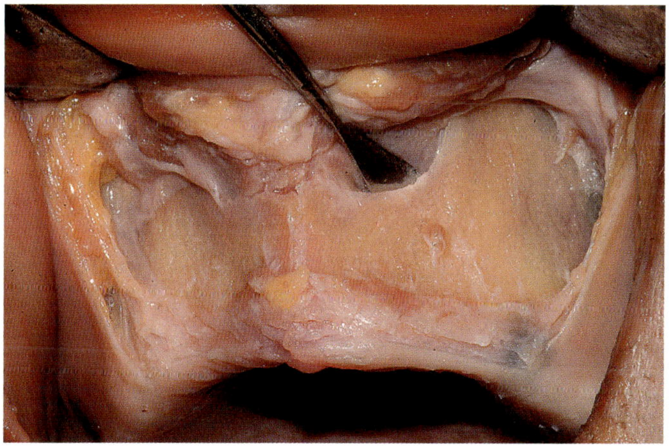

2.25 Anatomical dissection of the nasal floor.

In the intercanine region and below the nasal floor, no relevant anatomical structures are present. However, it is worth remembering that the soft tissues in this area are highly vascularised and innervated. For this reason, a subperiosteal dissection significantly reduces the risk of copious bleeding and prevents significant damage to the anterior terminal branches of the infraorbital nerve (2.26a-c).

On the border between the anterior and posterior regions of the maxilla, the most notable anatomical structure is the infraorbital neurovascular bundle, which emerges from the eponymous foramen.

Infraorbital nerve

Origin: it arises from of the maxillary nerve, the second branch of the trigeminal nerve (cranial nerve V), (2.27a), and is one of its terminal branches.

Function: it is responsible for the sensory somatic innervation of the skin of the middle third of the face (malar and cheek regions, lower eyelid, and nasal pyramid), the conjunctiva of the lower eyelid, the nasal vestibule, the skin and mucosa of the upper lip and the corresponding portion of the gingiva.

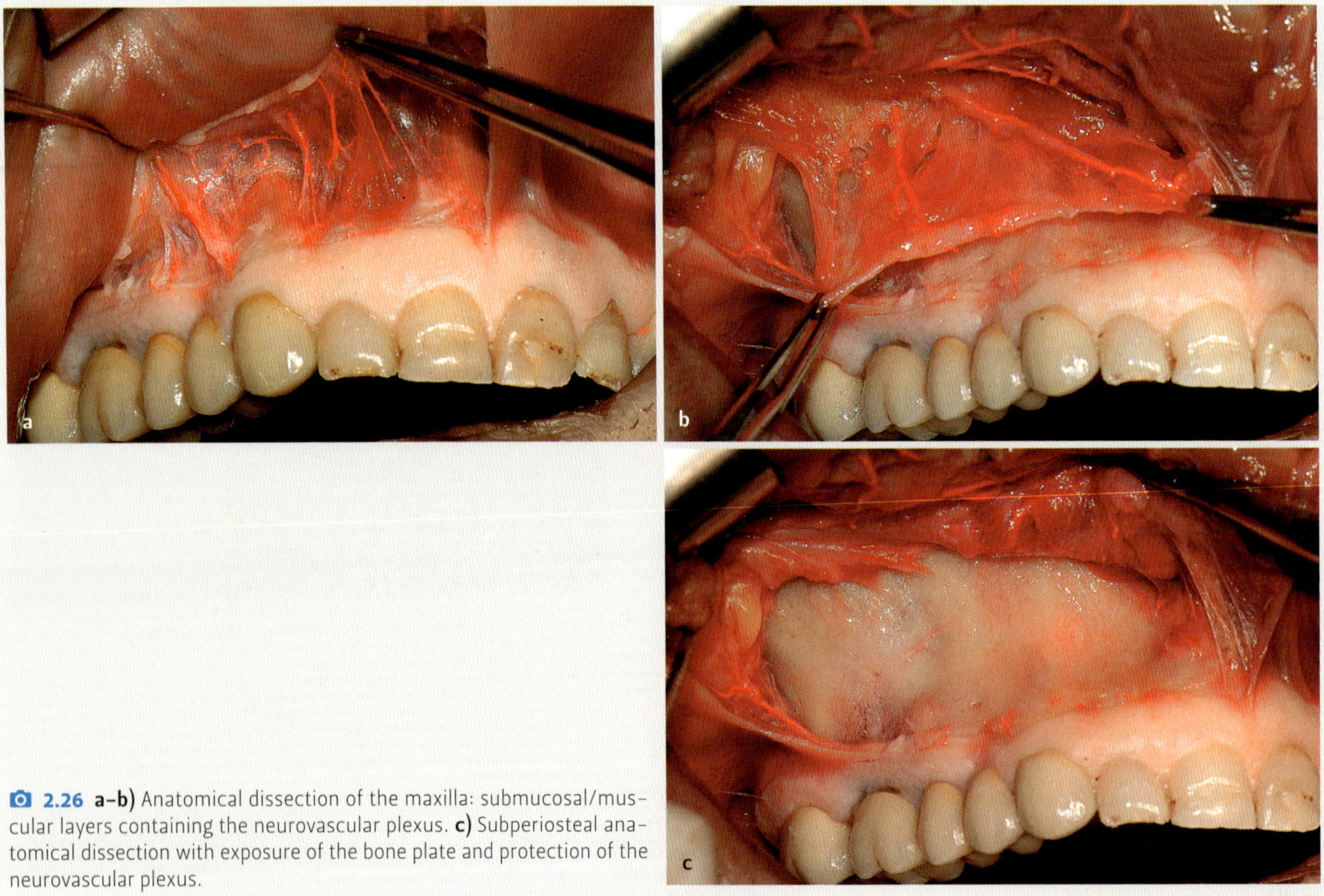

2.26 **a–b)** Anatomical dissection of the maxilla: submucosal/muscular layers containing the neurovascular plexus. **c)** Subperiosteal anatomical dissection with exposure of the bone plate and protection of the neurovascular plexus.

Course: from its point of origin at the inferior orbital fissure, it runs forwards along the floor of the orbit to engage the infraorbital canal. It then runs along the canal to emerge at the infraorbital foramen, located below the inferior orbital margin above the maxillary canine fossa. Here, the nerve divides into its terminal branches (2.27b–c).

The area of the infraorbital foramen is not generally involved in oral surgery procedures. However, in cases of severe atrophy of the maxilla (typical of longstanding total maxillary edentulism) or in cases where nerve block anaesthesia is needed (see Chapter 3), its position must be identified. Because the nerve distributes to the skin of the cheek and the nasal pyramid, a subperiosteal dissection prevents accidental damage to most of its branches, as well as to the homonymous intramuscular arteries. As in the case of the mental nerve, when surgery is needed near the infraorbital foramen, it may be useful to identify it by careful subperiosteal dissection of the soft tissues and adequate protection of the nerve (to read more about identifying the infraorbital nerve for performing anaesthesia, see the dedicated section of this book).

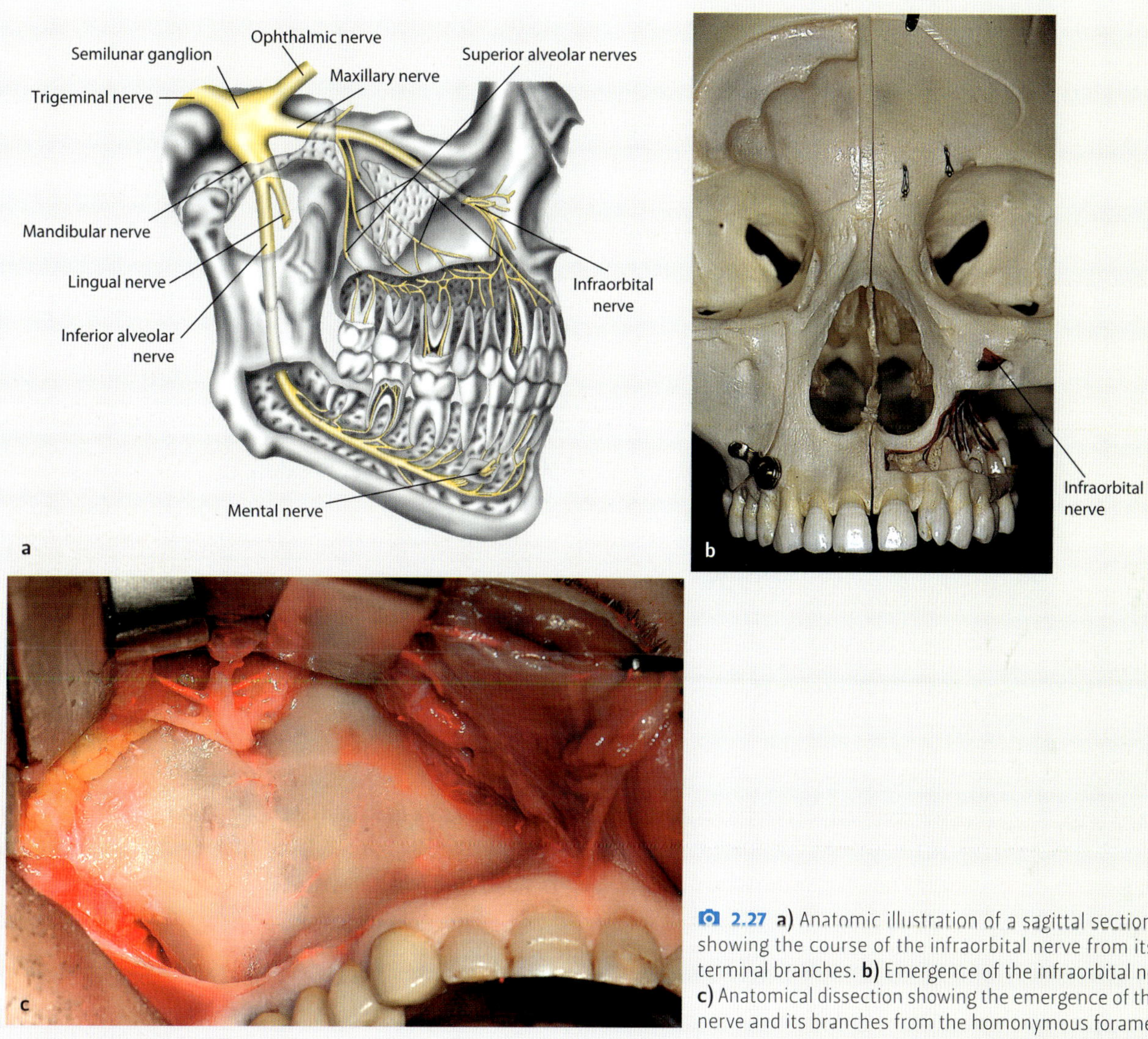

2.27 **a)** Anatomic illustration of a sagittal section of the skull, showing the course of the infraorbital nerve from its origin to its terminal branches. **b)** Emergence of the infraorbital nerve (model). **c)** Anatomical dissection showing the emergence of the infraorbital nerve and its branches from the homonymous foramen.

Posterior maxilla

This corresponds to the portion of the maxilla that develops distally to the intercanine line. The distinction in planes is similar to that previously described for the anterior maxilla.

BONY PLANE

The predominant anatomical structure is the maxillary sinus. It is the largest of the paranasal sinuses and shows wide interindividual variability in its development. Its size and relationships with adjacent anatomical structures are also linked to age and the presence or absence of premolars and molars. Its lumen is lined by the Schneider's membrane, which is often misidentified as simple respiratory mucosa. It is actually a mucoperiosteum, a structure composed of a thin layer of the respiratory mucosa (facing the sinus lumen) and a layer of periosteum (facing the walls of the sinus), with the interposition of a loose connective tissue layer. This anatomical peculiarity evidently results when action is taken to enucleate antral pseudocysts, also referred to as "rising sun cysts". It consequently develops in the obstruction of the excretory duct of a secretory cell in the mucosal layer, and its expansion separates this layer from the periosteal layer below. It is therefore possible to eliminate these cysts without completely interrupting the continuity of the sinusal lining.

The maxillary sinus is very small at birth, its appearance being that of a pneumatised "cell" below the orbit floor and lateral to the nasal cavity. It then undergoes a process of progressive expansion across the entire lifespan. In cases where one or more posterior teeth are lost, the maxillary sinus tends to expand downwards, in the direction of the alveolar ridge (2.28a-b). An accurate preoperative radiographic study is therefore crucial when surgical procedures are performed in this area (complex extractions of erupted or impacted teeth, surgical endodontics, implant placement, etc.), to minimise the risk of accidentally damaging the integrity of the maxillary sinus.

The alveolar-antral artery runs along the anterior-lateral wall of the maxillary sinus (2.29a). It originates from the internal maxillary artery and is part of an anastomotic circuit with branches of the infraorbital artery, which is responsible for the vascularisation of the maxillary sinus. It has a variable diameter (usually under one millimetre, but in rare cases up to two millimetres), and it is often possible to verify its presence in the coronal slices of a CT scan (2.29b), since in most cases it runs inside a small channel in the anterior-lateral wall of the maxillary sinus. More rarely, it runs between the inner side of the anterior-lateral wall of the sinus and the Schneider's membrane. In most cases, damages or section of this artery do not cause significant sequelae, but bleeding may complicate some procedures (particularly, maxillary sinus lifting with a lateral approach) by reducing the visibility in the surgical field and thus increasing the risk of intraoperative complications.

The last notable anatomical structure in the region, although rarely responsible for severe complications if damaged, is the superior-posterior alveolar artery. The artery enters the maxilla above the apex of the third molar, originating directly from the internal maxillary artery, and supplies branches for the maxillary endosteum and the molar apices. It may be involved in the surgical manoeuvres for the removal of deeply impacted third molars: the resulting bleeding does not give rise to particular risks, but reduces visibility, already scarce, in the operating field.

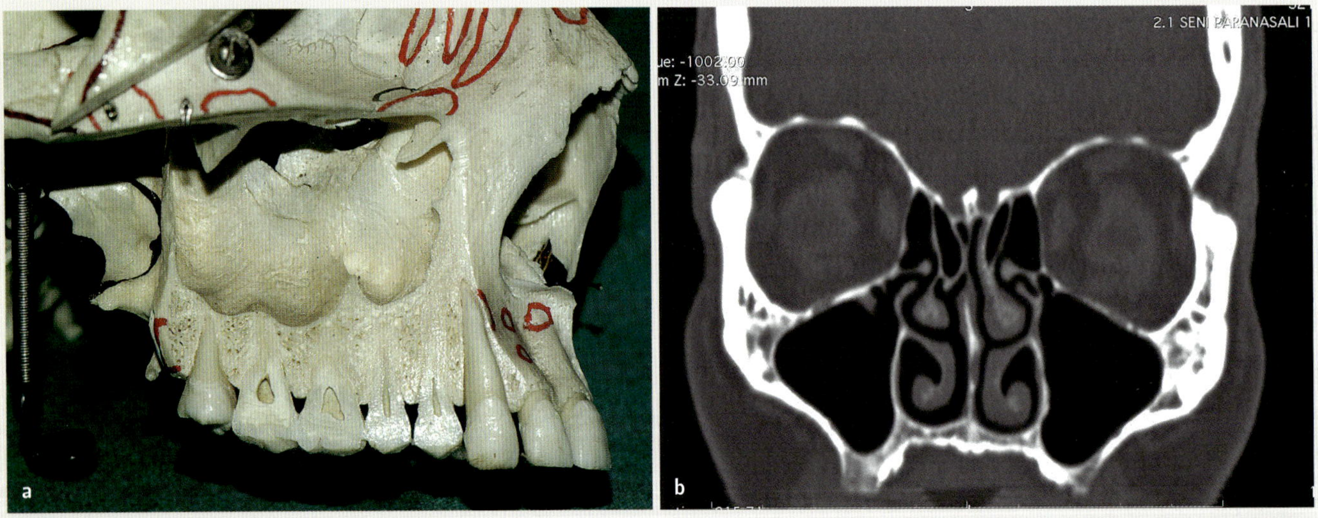

2.28 a) The lumen of the maxillary sinus after removal of the anterior wall (model). **b)** CT of the facial skeleton (coronal section), highlighting the maxillary sinuses.

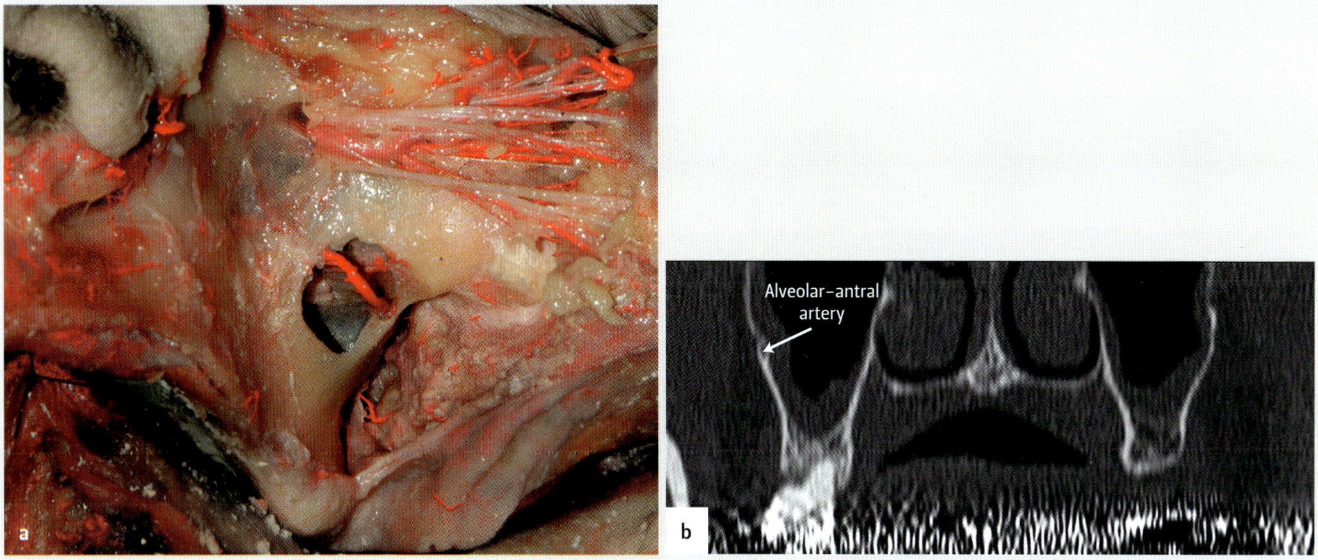

2.29 **a)** Anatomical dissection showing the course of the alveolar-antral artery inside the anterior wall of the maxillary sinus. **b)** CT scan showing the intraosseous course of the alveolar-antral artery in the anterior wall of the maxillary sinus.

Posterior maxilla

Surgical procedures

- Erupted or impacted teeth
- Endodontic surgery
- Sinus lifting procedures
- Sinusal cysts
- Fibromas, biopsies, angiomas
- Implant placement
- Impacted third molars, endosseous cysts, neoformations

Notable anatomic structures

- Alveolar antral artery
- Maxillary sinus
- Parotid duct, buccal fat pad
- Pterygopalatine fossa

BUCCAL SIDE

On the buccal side of the maxilla, inside the soft tissues, numerous arterial branches and nerve fibres supplied by the infraorbital neurovascular bundle are present, as previously described.

In addition, three further anatomical structures must be taken into consideration: the parotid duct (or Stensen), the buccal fat pad (also known as Bichat's fat) and the pterygopalatine fossa.

Parotid duct

The parotid duct, after emerging from the glandular parenchyma, runs across the masseter muscle to reach its anterior border. Here, the duct turns sharply inwards, passing through the buccal fat pad and piercing the buccinator muscle. Then, it runs obliquely forwards for a short distance just under the buccal mucosa to reach its orifice located at the salivary papilla, opposite the second upper molar (2.30a-c).

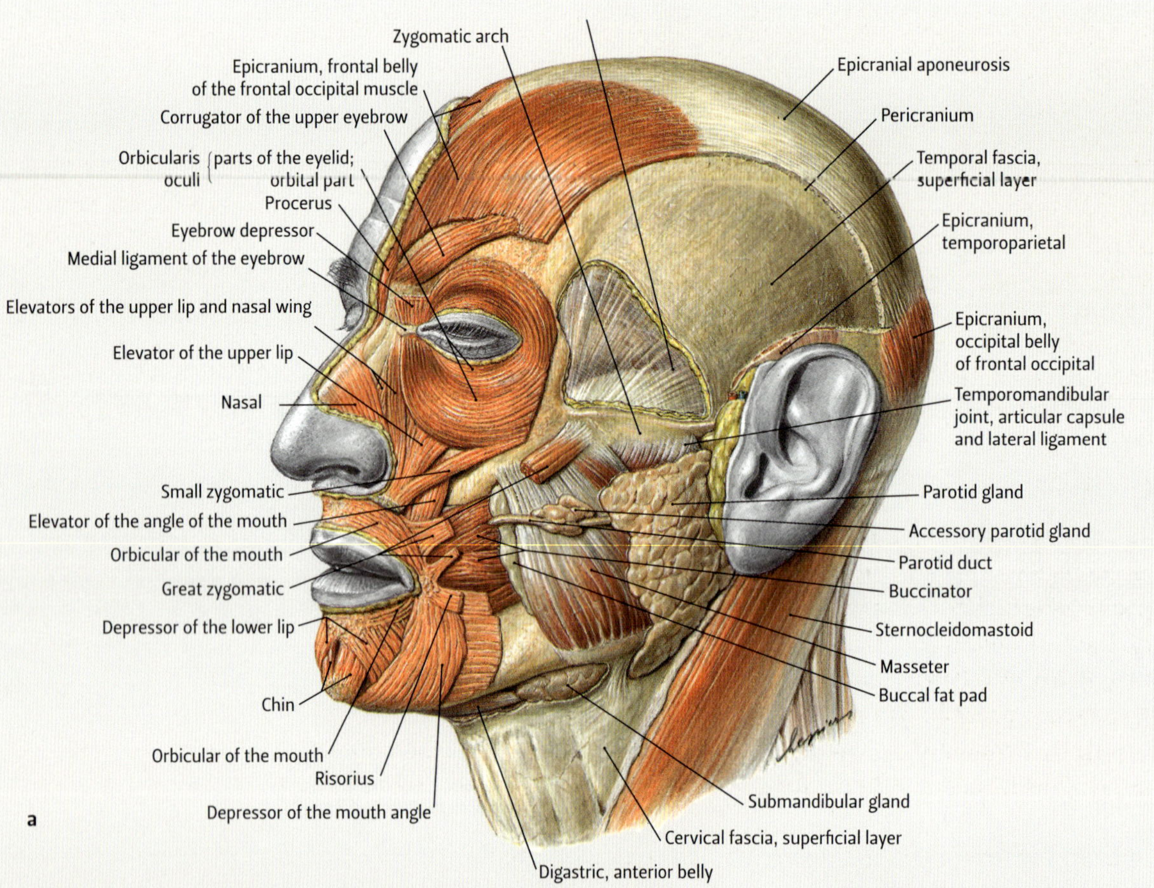

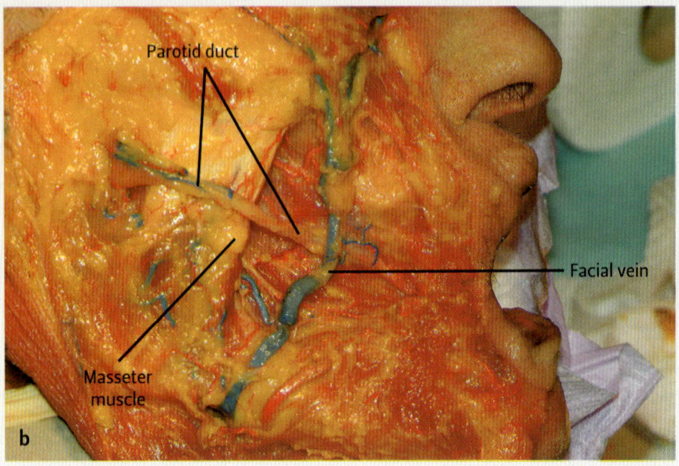

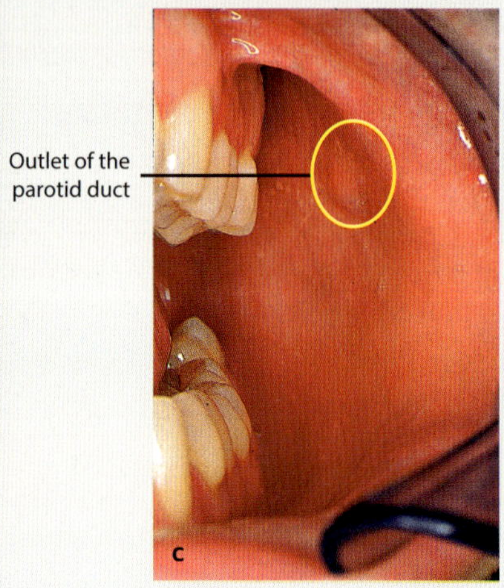

2.30 **a)** Anatomic drawing of the parotid region and the gallery that contains the buccal fat pad (modified from *Sobotta Atlante di Anatomia Umana*. Elsevier, Milano 2012). **b)** Anatomical dissection showing the course of the parotid duct above the masseter muscle: note the relationship with the facial vein. **c)** Intraoral view of the upper buccal vestibule indicating the outlet of the parotid duct.

Subperiosteal dissection in this area prevents any damage to the duct. However, the duct must be identified whenever vertical releasing incisions or dissection of the buccal soft tissues is to be performed (biopsies, excision of neoplasms, removal of intraductal salivary stones, etc.). Moreover, it is worth considering that any surgical procedure performed in close proximity to the duct can cause its obliteration from scarring, with subsequent retrograde damage to the parotid gland (see Chapter 10).

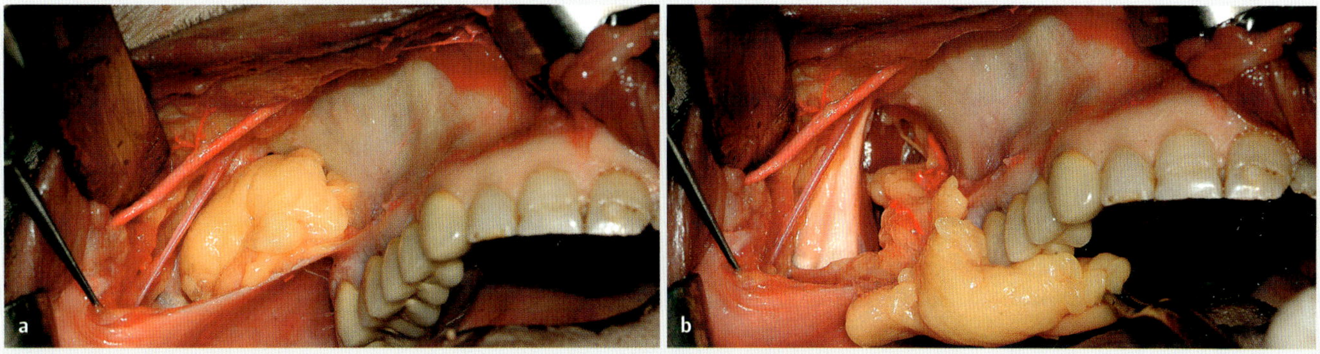

2.31 **a)** Anatomical dissection of the buccal fat pad. **b)** The buccal fat pad can be used for the closure of oroantral communications after its capsule is opened.

Buccal fat pad

It is a mass of adipose tissue contained in a space between the buccinator and masseter muscles in the buccal region, opposite the upper molars (2.31a). Subperiosteal dissection and elevation of a full-thickness flap in this area prevent the herniation of the fat pad. If, on the contrary, the periosteum is interrupted either accidentally or as a part of the surgical procedure (e.g. Rehrmann flap, periosteal incision to allow a tension-free suture after bone grafting, etc.) the buccal fat pad may partially invade the operating field.

Opening the capsule that contains the buccal fat pad has no serious consequences, but accidental herniation of the fat pad in the operating field can cause a reduction in intraoperative visibility.

Knowledge of the local anatomy is useful not only in preventing this problem, but also because in opening the capsule carefully so as not to damage the vascular pedicle feeding it, the fat pad may then be used for the closure of oroantral communications (see Chapter 15 for details) (2.31b).

Pterygopalatine fossa

The pterygopalatine fossa is a small triangular space between the maxillary tuberosity (anteriorly) and the anterior face of the pterygoid process (posteriorly) (2.32a):

- the anterior wall is formed by the maxillary tuberosity, which corresponds to the posterior wall of the maxillary sinus; on this surface is the posterior-superior alveolar foramen, which acts as a pathway for the homonymous nerves and arteries;
- the posterior wall is formed by the anterior face of the pterygoid process; from this wall, the maxillary nerve (the second branch of the trigeminal nerve, cranial nerve V) enters the fossa through the round foramen;
- the lateral wall is formed by the pterygomaxillary fissure, which connects this fossa to the infratemporal fossa.

The anatomical structures found inside the pterygopalatine fossa are as follows: the maxillary nerve, the maxillary artery and its branches, and the venous pterygoid plexus (2.32b).

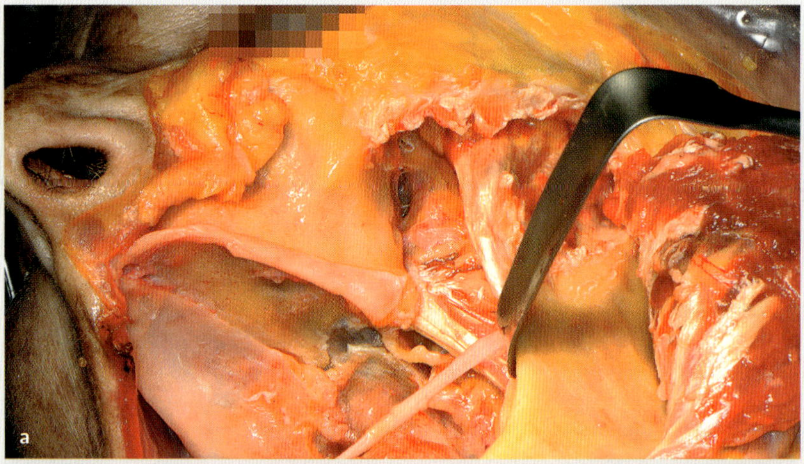

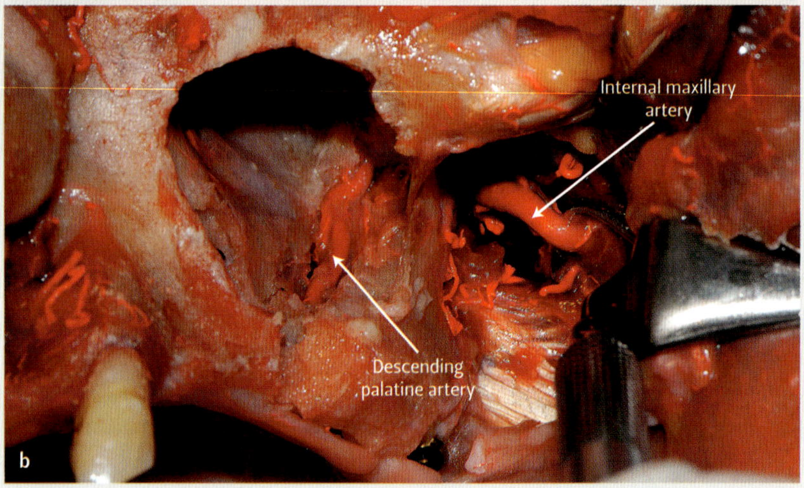

2.32 **a)** Anatomical dissection of the pterygopalatine fossa emptied of its contents (pterygoid plexus, internal maxillary artery, maxillary nerve, etc.). **b)** Anatomical dissection of the pterygopalatine fossa, in which the internal maxillary artery and the descending palatine artery are highlighted.

The maxillary nerve (somatic sensory) crosses the fossa in a horizontal direction, in proximity to the vault and above the maxillary artery, and then penetrates the orbital cavity through the inferior orbital fissure. It subsequently runs along the orbital floor until it enters the infraorbital canal: from this point on it takes the name of its terminal branch, the infraorbital nerve. The maxillary nerve gives off several branches along its course: the middle meningeal nerve, the zygomatic nerve, the sphenopalatine nerves and the superior alveolar nerves. The only ones among these that can be affected during oral surgery are the superior alveolar nerves.

Superior posterior, median, and anterior alveolar nerves

Origin: they arise from the maxillary nerve in the stretch that runs within the infraorbital groove on the orbital floor.

Function: they are responsible for the innervation of the dental alveoli, the teeth, and the gingiva of the corresponding hemimaxilla.

Course: from their points of origin, these nerves run inside small bone canals until they reach the alveolar ridge, where they form a plexus from which branches are distributed to the aforementioned structures.

These are nerve branches with a very small diameter and are therefore difficult to identify; due to their small size and complex distribution, accidental sectioning of one or more branches may cause changes in the sensitivity of the innervated teeth that nonetheless bear a high probability of spontaneous recovery, with little or no risk of permanent clinical and medico-legal sequelae.

The internal maxillary artery (one of the terminal branches of the external carotid artery), after crossing the infratemporal fossa, ends in the pterygopalatine fossa. This artery and its branches (the infraorbital artery, descending palatine artery, pterygoid channel artery, sphenopalatine artery) supply blood to the upper jaw, the mandible, teeth, palate, jaw muscles and portions of the nasal cavity (2.33). Given the significant diameter of this vessel and its location inside a bone cavity that is difficult to access, it is crucial that, during the course of any surgery in the posterior region of the maxilla (removal of third molars, placement of implants, etc.), any damage to the content of the pterygopalatine fossa be avoided. If the internal maxillary artery is injured the resulting bleeding is copious and impossible to control under local anaesthesia. Due to the difficulty of isolating the damaged maxillary artery inside the pterygopalatine fossa with an intraoral approach, ligation of the external carotid artery via an extraoral access is necessary, because failure to interrupt the bleeding can be fatal for the patient.

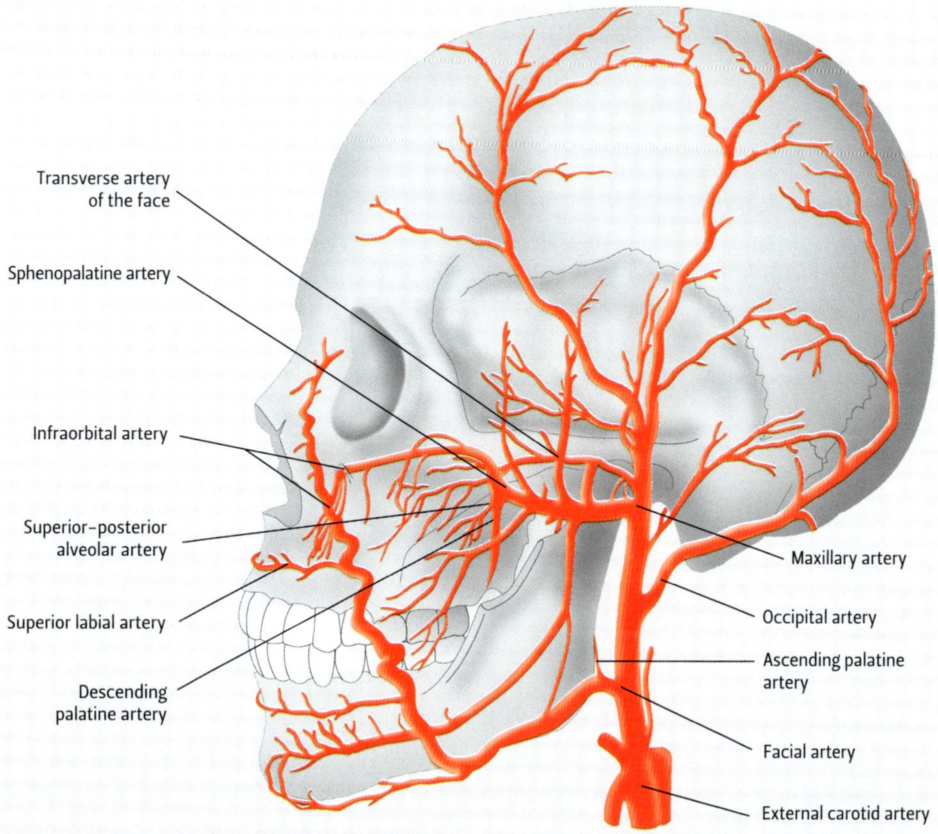

2.33 Anatomic illustration highlighting the course of the superior-posterior alveolar artery.

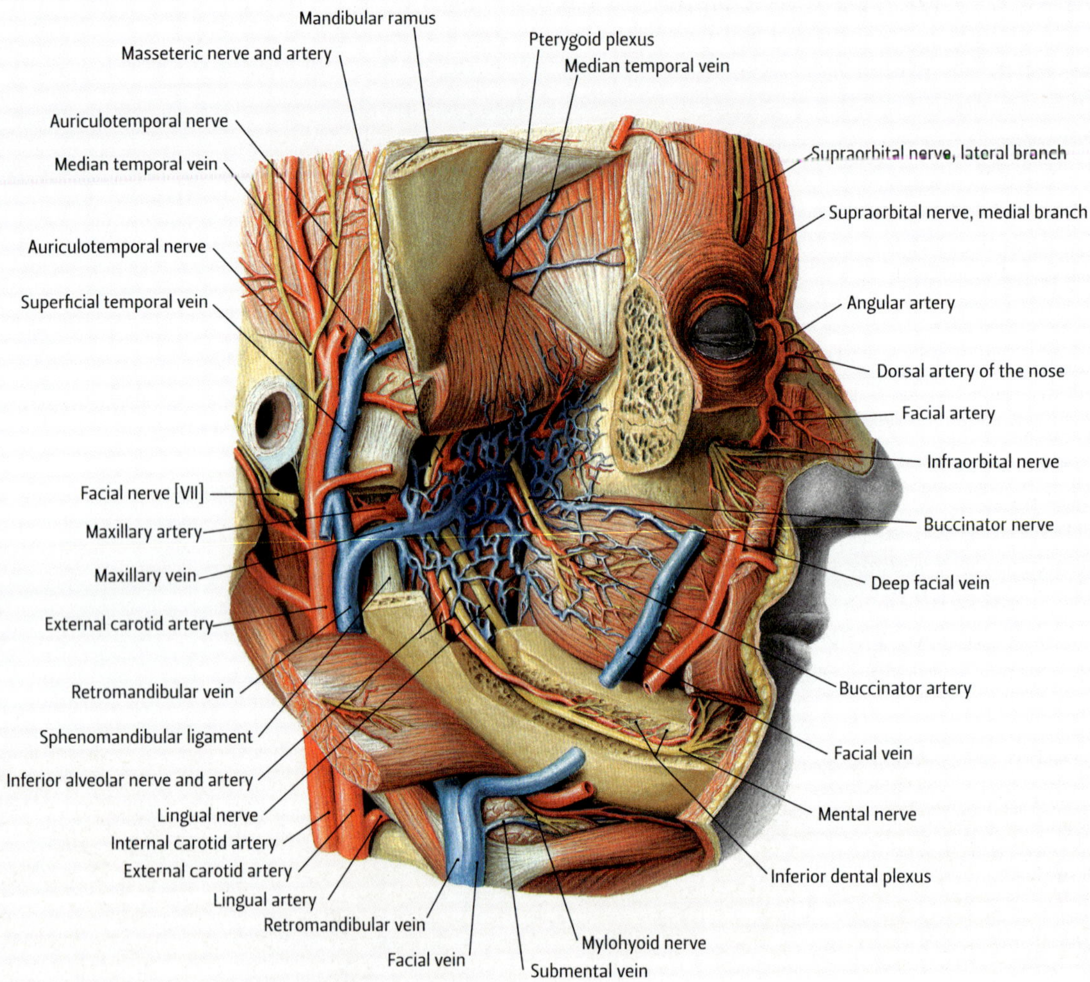

2.34 Anatomic illustration showing the pterygoid plexus (adapted from *Sobotta Atlante di Anatomia Umana*. Elsevier, Milano 2012).

The pterygoid plexus is a dense venous plexus that extends from the neck of the mandible to the pterygopalatine fossa: its tributaries are the inferior alveolar vein, the masseterine veins, the deep temporalis veins, the middle meningeal veins, the sphenopalatine vein and the venous plexus of the foramen ovale. The pterygoid plexus drains mainly into the internal maxillary vein, which is itself a tributary of the posterior facial vein (2.34). During surgeries in this area, it is important to avoid damaging the branches of the pterygoid plexus. Although a venous bleeding is not as risky as an arterial one (considering a vessel of the same diameter), the bleeding caused by damages to this plexus is often diffuse and may be significant, making surgical manoeuvres difficult due to reduced visibility in the operating field, in addition to causing extensive postoperative haematomas.

Palate

Two different areas can be identified in the palatine region: the hard palate and the soft palate. The anatomical planes in the hard palate are as follows: mucosa, submucosa, periosteum, and the horizontal plate of the palatine bone. The soft palate presents the following anatomical planes: mucosa, submucosa, muscles and palatine aponeurosis, and pharyngeal mucosa.

Generally speaking, surgical procedures on the soft palate are not performed by oral surgeons. However, on the other hand, it is essential that the oral surgeon have precise knowledge of details regarding the anatomical structures that are present in the area of the hard palate.

The mucosa in the area shows no peculiar features, except for the fact that it is entirely keratinised. For this reason, when a mucosal graft is needed to treat a keratinised mucosa defect around teeth or implants, the hard palate is always the donor site of choice.

Within the submucosa, numerous minor salivary glands are present; neurovascular structures are also contained in a loose connective tissue between the periosteum and the submucosa (2.35a-c).

As previously pointed out in the previous description of other anatomical regions, a full-thickness elevation of the soft tissues in the hard palate avoids the risk of damaging the anatomical structures (vessels and nerves) which are present in this area, with the exception of the areas of the foramina at which neurovascular bundles (greater palatine and nasopalatine) emerge from bone canals. Therefore, the exact position of these foramina must be well known and, if surgery is to be performed in the area, it is essential that the emerging neurovascular bundles be identified and adequately protected.

Notable anatomical structures in the hard palate are the greater palatine neurovascular bundle and the nasopalatine neurovascular bundle; the latter and the surgical implications of its course have already been described (for details, see section on the Anterior maxilla).

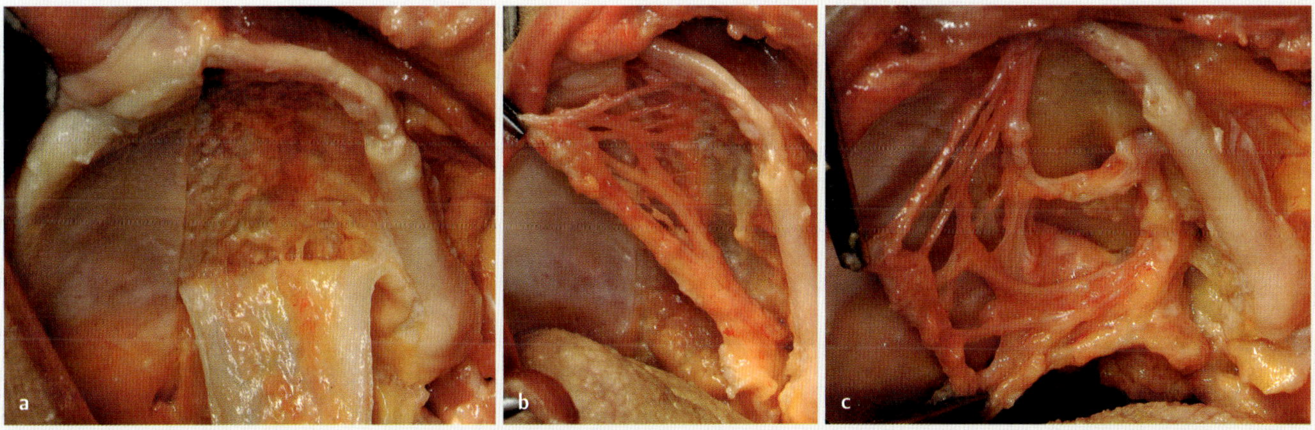

2.35 **a)** Anatomical dissection of the palate after removal of the mucous layer: numerous minor salivary glands are visible. **b)** Anatomical dissection: in the connective layer, the neurovascular structures of the palate are visible. **c)** Anatomical dissection of the greater palatine bundle and its anastomotic circuit with the nasopalatine bundle.

Palate

Surgical procedures

- Harvesting of the palatine mucosa and/or the underlying connective tissue
- Apicoectomy of the palatal roots of molars
- Incisional or excisional biopsy of lesions developing on the palatine mucosa

Notable anatomic structures

- Greater palatine neurovascular bundle
- Lesser palatine neurovascular bundle

Greater palatine nerve (or anterior palatine nerve)

Origin: it arises from the sphenopalatine ganglion, located near the roof of the pterygopalatine fossa.

Function: it supplies somatic sensory innervation to the mucosa of the corresponding hemipalate; it also contains parasympathetic fibres to control the secretion of minor salivary glands in the same area.

Course: from its point of origin, it descends to enter the greater palatine canal, and emerges onto the palatal vault from the homonymous foramen, located about 1 cm medially to the second molar. From this point, the nerve runs forwards, close to the horizontal plate of the palatine bone, in the curve formed by the base of the alveolar ridge; along its course, it gives off branches for the innervation of the aforementioned anatomical structures (2.36; see also 2.35b). It is worth noting that in cases of severe atrophy of the alveolar ridge (particularly in totally edentulous patients), the relative position of the palatine foramen with respect to the centre of the residual alveolar ridge can be much closer. This must be considered during surgeries in this area (palatal mucosa harvesting, biopsy, removal of benign tumours of the palatal mucosa, bone reconstruction, etc.).

Greater palatine artery

Origin: it arises from the maxillary artery within the pterygopalatine fossa.

Function: it supplies vascularisation to the bone, mucosa, minor salivary glands, and gingiva of the corresponding hemipalate.

Course: from its point of origin, it follows the same course as the greater palatine nerve (2.37; see also 2.32b).

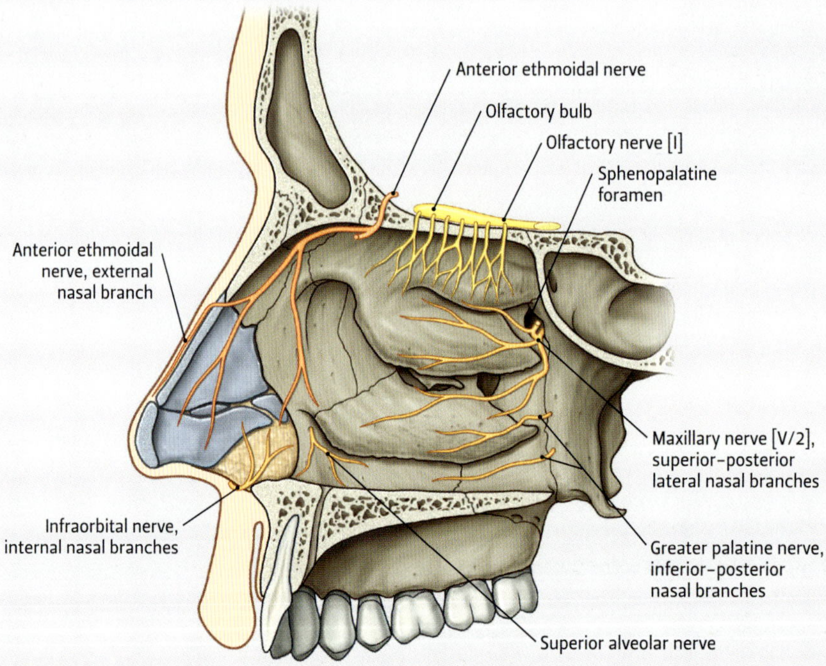

2.36 Anatomic illustration showing the course of the greater palatine nerve (modified from *Sobotta Atlante di Anatomia Umana*. Elsevier, Milano 2012).

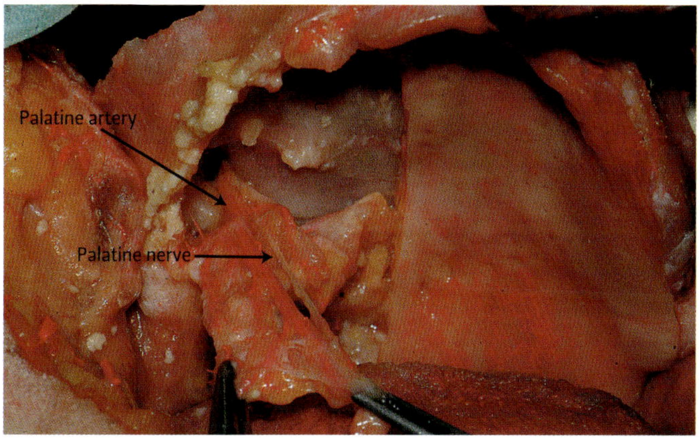

2.37 Anatomical dissection showing the emergence of the greater palatine artery and nerve on the horizontal plate of the palatine bone.

To preserve the integrity of the artery, subperiosteal dissection is indicated. Where this is not possible (mucosal and palatal biopsies, harvesting of connective tissue from the palate for muco-gingival surgeries, etc.), identifying the course of the artery to prevent or control the bleeding caused by dissection of its branches or main trunk is essential. In cases of significant bleeding, an adequate haemostasis can be achieved either with bipolar coagulation systems, or by ligature of the vessel. However, the latter solution can prove more complicated if the lesion occurs near the palatine foramen, due to the possible retraction of the artery inside the palatine canal.

Cheek

Within the soft tissues of the cheek, from the oral to the facial side, it is possible to identify the following anatomical planes: mucosa, buccinator muscle, subcutaneous tissues, and skin. As previously mentioned regarding the oral floor, a detailed knowledge of local anatomy is crucial since there are no bone plates to act as reference points. It is thus more difficult to identify the various cleavage planes where the most significant anatomical structures are present. The oral surgeon is rarely involved in surgical procedures on the skin of the cheek (except, for example, when removing orocutaneous fistulas or abscesses of the cheek). On the other hand, surgery on the mucosal side may be necessary in the presence of lesions of the buccal mucosa and underlying tissues (traumatic pseudofibromas, cysts or pseudocysts of the minor salivary glands, angiomas, salivary stones inside the parotid duct, etc.).

Notable anatomical structures in this region are as follows: the buccal fat pad (also known as Bichat's fat pad), the parotid duct, the facial artery, and the facial nerve.

Descriptions of the buccal fat pad and parotid duct were previously given (see dedicated section).

Cheek

Surgical procedures

- Intraoral procedures and drainage of odontogenic abscesses
- Removal of lesions

Notable anatomic structures

- Facial artery
- Facial nerve

As for the aforementioned facial artery, it is worth noting that it may be involved not only during surgical procedures using an intraoral approach, but also when odontogenic abscesses are drained through a cutaneous incision. It is therefore necessary to perform a careful dissection to avoid any damage to the artery (please refer to Chapter 6 for more details).

The facial nerve and its branches run between the subcutaneous tissues and the mimic muscles, and so are almost never involved in surgical manoeuvres on the buccal side of the cheek. The branches of the nerve must instead be identified and protected during the removal of lesions/tumours that develop deep within the subcutaneous tissues. However, it is advisable that these surgical procedures only be performed by experienced surgeons.

Upper and lower lip

The surgical anatomical planes of the lips are represented by the mucosa, the submucosal layer, the muscles, the subcutaneous layer, and the skin (2.38).

The cutaneous and subcutaneous layers do not present any peculiar features.

The orbicularis oris muscle extends from the margin of the lips to the base of the nose and to the mentolabial fold. It is divided into two loops: an inner loop, near the free margin of the lips, and an outer loop, in which its fibres intersect with fibres from the mimic muscles.

For surgical procedures in this area (removal of benign tumours, minor salivary gland cysts, etc.), it is essential to consider the course of the upper and inferior labial arteries and facial nerve branches (2.39a-b). Cutting the vessels may result in significant bleeding; therefore, they should be identified and isolated to preserve their integrity whenever pos-

Upper and lower lip

Surgical procedures

- Removal of lesions developing under the mucosal layer

Notable anatomic structures

- Labial arteries

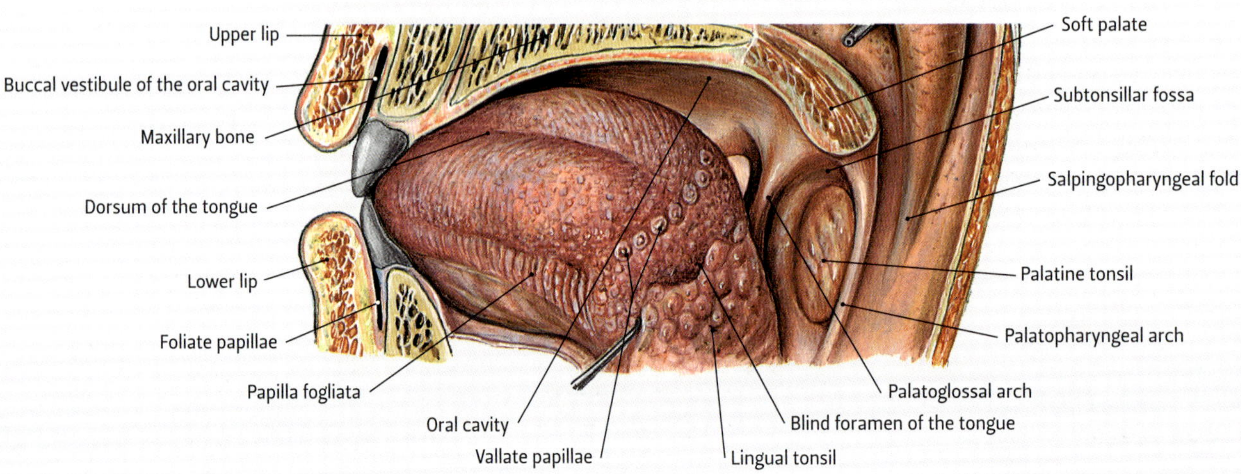

2.38 Anatomic illustration of the upper lip (cross-section) showing the labial vessels (modified from *Sobotta Atlante di Anatomia Umana*. Elsevier, Milano 2012).

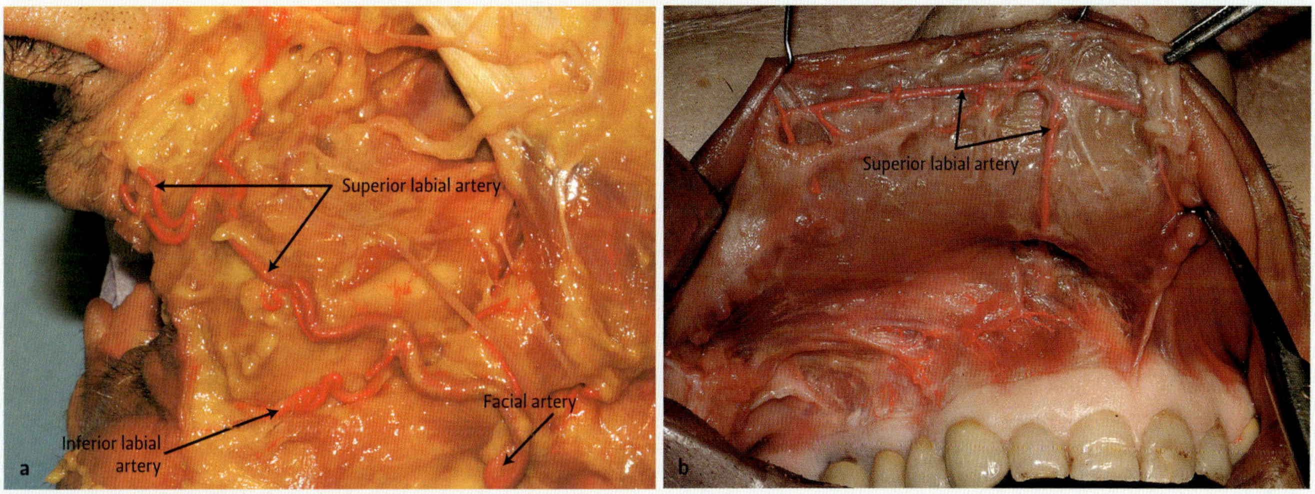

2.39 **a)** Anatomical dissection showing the origin of the upper and lower labial artery from the facial artery. **b)** Anatomical dissection showing the course of the upper labial artery and its branches.

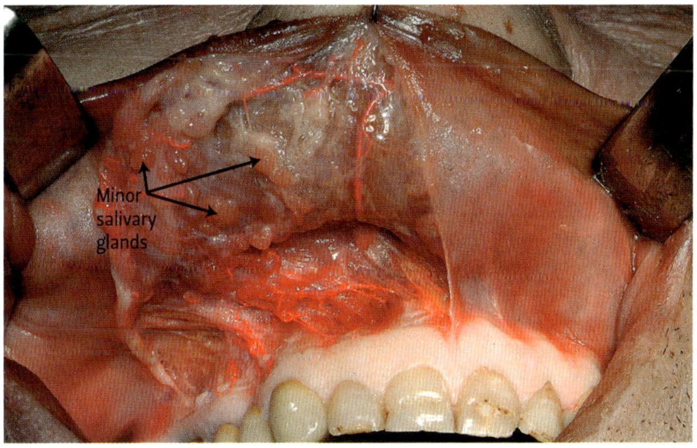

2.40 Anatomical dissection: after removal of the mucosa, numerous minor salivary glands and the terminal branches of the labial artery are revealed.

sible. If this is not possible, then it is recommended that a bipolar coagulation system or ligature of the vessel be used prior to its section (see Chapter 15). Coagulation or ligation of the labial artery carries no risk of lip ischaemia due to the presence of several anastomotic circuits that can guarantee adequate vascularisation to the lips.

The submucosal tissues contain numerous minor salivary glands, as well as the terminal branches of the mentalis nerve and infraorbital nerve, in the upper and lower lip respectively (2.40). For surgical procedures extending in the submucosal layer, the salivary glands are easily detectable and the surgeon must be careful to avoid involving the glands when suturing the surgical access, as this may cause an obstruction of the excretory ducts with the formation of retention cysts.

REFERENCES

CHIAPASCO M. Manuale illustrato di Chirurgia Orale. 2ª ed. Elsevier Masson, Milano 2007.

CHIAPASCO M. Procedure di chirurgia orale nel rispetto dell'anatomia. Utet, Torino 2007.

DUBRUL EL. Anatomia Orale di Sicher. Edi-Ermes, Milano 1988.

PAULSEN F, WASCHKE J. Sobotta Atlante di Anatomia Umana. Elsevier, Milano 2012.

PETERSON LJ, INDRESANO AT, MARCIANI RD, ROSER SM. Principles of oral and maxillofacial surgery. JB Lippincott Company, Philadelphia 1992.

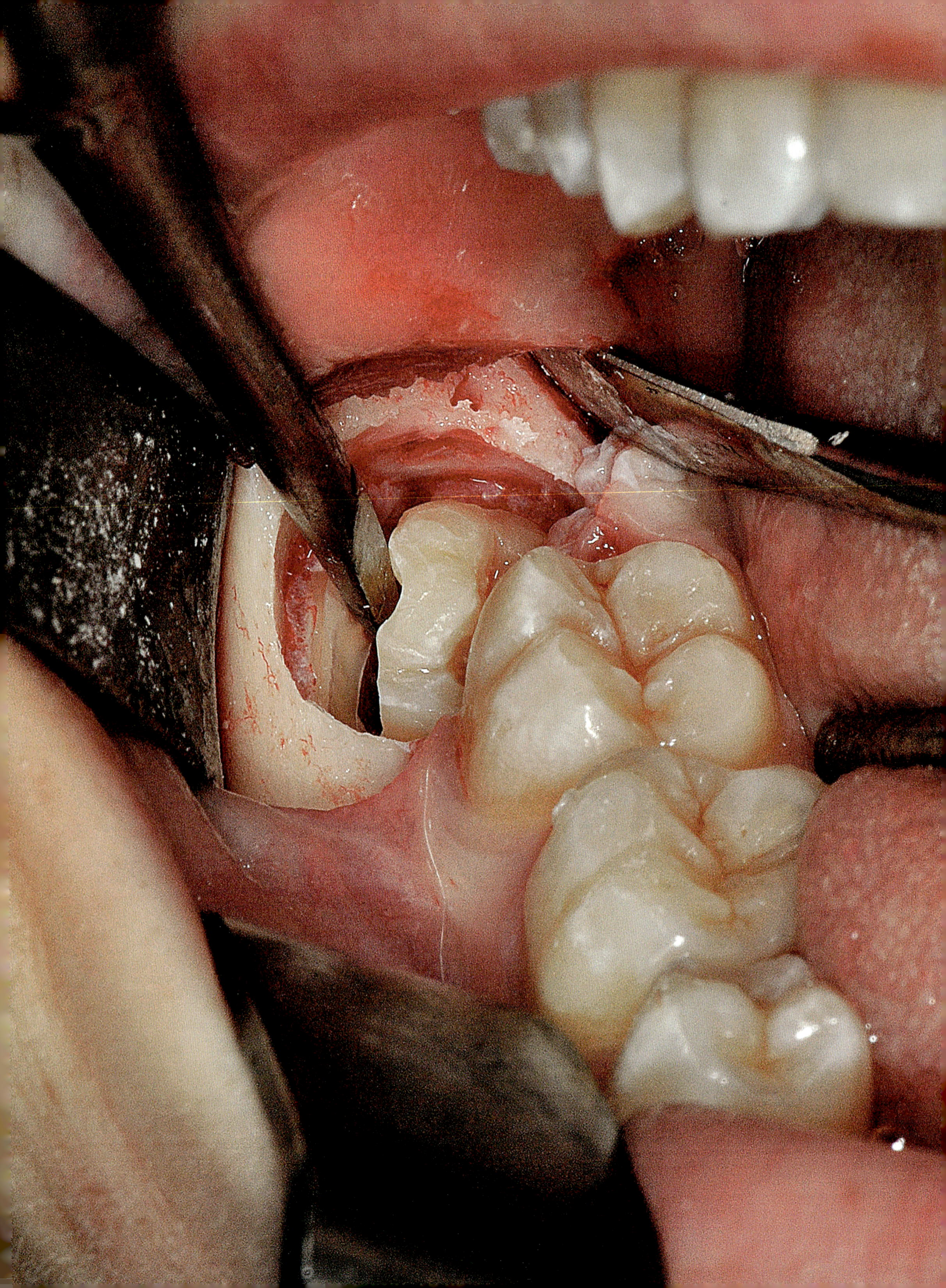

The surgical intervention

M. Chiapasco · M. Zaniboni · L. Serioli
A. Flora · T. Anello · E. Corsi

Preparation: environment, operators, surgical armamentarium, patient

Performing an oral surgery procedure involves the interruption of the mucosal barrier and exposing deeper tissues to the oral environment, which is permanently colonised by a specific kind of bacterial flora. Bacterial contamination can result in a higher risk of local or systemic infection.

The objective of correct preparation is to minimise the risk of infection by following basic principles aimed at:

- reducing the number of bacteria in the patient's oral cavity and perioral region;
- preventing bacteria in the external environment from contaminating the surgical field.

Preoperative preparation being equal, the risk of infection is caused by the type of surgical procedure. Generally, this risk is very low for short procedures involving only the superficial tissues, while it is higher in the case of more invasive and prolonged procedures. Moreover, when autogenous and heterologous grafting materials are used, the risk of infection increases.

The incidence of postoperative complication caused by bacterial contamination may be rather low, if the correct protocols are followed when preparing the operating environment, the operators, the surgical armamentarium, and the patient.

The four crucial passages to eliminate all contaminants are as follows: decontamination, cleaning, disinfection, and sterilisation.

Decontamination and cleaning: a set of procedures aimed at the removal of biologic materials from any surface (operating room, surgical instruments, etc.) together with part of the bacterial contaminants. Decontamination and cleaning may be sufficient for non-invasive procedures where no interruption of the soft tissues is necessary; when invasive procedures are involved, they represent mandatory steps to complete prior to disinfection and sterilisation.

Tab. 3.1 Activity level

Activity level	Action	Disinfectant	Concentration	Action time	Inactivation by biological material
High	Also active on the spores, even if it does not guarantee complete elimination of all spores	Glutaraldehyde	>2%	20'	+/–
		Chlorine derivatives	>1000 ppm Cl available	20'	++*
Medium	Active on the vegetative cells, but not on the spores (a process that eliminates a resistant microorganism such as *Mycobacterium tuberculosis* is sufficient to eliminate also weaker microorganisms such as HIV and HBV viruses)	Glutaraldehyde	<2 %	10'	+/–
		Chlorine derivatives	>500 ppm	10'	++*
		Alcohols	70%	10'	+
		Phenol derivatives	s.s.p.**	10'	–
		Iodophors	s.s.p.	10'	+
Low	Not active on the spores and vegetative cells	Chlorine derivatives	>100 ppm		++*
		Chlorhexidine in water	s.s.p.		+/–
		Quaternary ammonium compounds in water	s.s.p.		++

*When biological material is present, keeping above 5000 ppm is recommended.

**According to the manufacturer's specifications.

Disinfection: a set of procedures aimed at reducing the microbial load to a safe level. Disinfection causes the elimination of the majority of pathogenic microorganisms; however, some pathogens may survive after disinfection is completed.

Chemical (antiseptics and disinfectants) and physical (heat, ultrasound) agents are the two commonly used means to reduce the microbial load in the environment and on surgical instruments. Three levels of disinfection – high, medium, and low – can be identified, depending on the activity of the chosen agents against *Mycobacterium tuberculosis var. bovis* according to specific tests (tab. 3.1):

- high-level disinfectants (glutaraldehyde solutions > 2%, and chlorine derivatives > 1000 ppm available Cl) can inactivate all microbial forms, including resistant bacteria and spores;
- mid-level disinfectants (glutaraldehyde solutions < 2%, alcohols, phenolic derivatives, iodophors) inhibit all microbial forms, including *Mycobacterium tuberculosis*, but they have no effect on the spores;
- low-level disinfectants (chlorine derivatives < 1,000 ppm available Cl, chlorhexidine digluconate solution, aqueous solutions of quaternary ammonium compounds) inactivate some viruses, bacteria and fungi.

The choice between the different levels should be based on the risk of contamination. Generally, low-level disinfection should be limited to the work surfaces, the operating table/dental chair, and to the operating room furniture.

Disinfectant: chemical agent designed to eliminate microbial contamination from work surfaces and surgical instruments.
Antiseptic: chemical solution designed to reduce microbial contamination from the living tissues (skin and mucosa).

Among oral antiseptics, the most commonly used is an aqueous solution containing 0.12% or 0.2% chlorhexidine digluconate as the antiseptic agent. Among skin antiseptics, the most commonly used are iodine and chlorine solutions (see the section dedicated to patient preparation for details).

Sterilisation: a set of procedures aimed at eliminating all microorganisms, including the spores. Either chemical or physical agents can be used: chemical sterilisation may be performed with glutaraldehyde and ethylene oxide, while physical sterilisation may be obtained using heat, saturated steam, and high pressures (autoclave), or radiations.

An expiry date accompanies every sterilised item: generally, sterilisation lasts from 30 to 90 days. After the reported date has passed, the absence of contaminants is not guaranteed.

As far as the preparation of the environment, the operators, and the patient is concerned, two different procedures can be described: clean preparation and sterile preparation.

Clean preparation

Clean preparation is indicated (for apparently healthy patients) for performing the majority of oral surgery interventions, namely short and less invasive procedures such as extraction of erupted or impacted teeth, minor dentoalveolar trauma, surgical endodontic treatments, minor preprosthetic surgery, biopsies, and the enucleation of small cystic lesions.

Preparing the environment: all surfaces are cleaned and disinfected, and sterile drapes are used to cover the surgical trays before arranging the surgical armamentarium. In cases of asymptomatic carriers (hepatitis, HIV, etc.), it is recommended that all surfaces and objects be covered with clean disposable plastic wraps that are removed at the end of the procedure. In fact, the use of rotary instruments and sterile saline sprays causes nebulisation that can carry contaminants up to 3 metres away from the operating field.

Preparing the surgical armamentarium: sterilised instruments should be placed on sterile drapes in a logical order (📷 3.1). To reduce the risk of contamination and improve ergonomics, it is recommended that prearranged sterile instrument kits be prepared in advance. Insufficient armamentarium means wasted time and the need for one more assistant to search for missing instruments; in fact, to avoid further contamination of the surrounding environment, members of the surgical team should never leave the operating field.

Preparing the patient: a one-minute chlorhexidine (0.2%) mouth rinse is used to lower the intraoral microbial load before surgery. The patient should enter the operating room wearing shoe covers and a clean surgical cap, and should be covered with clean drapes (not necessarily sterile) (📷 3.2).

Preparation of the operators: the operators should wear disposable shoe covers or dedicated footwear, dedicated scrubs, a clean surgical cap, and a clean surgical facemask. Hands should be cleaned with specific antiseptic soaps. Clean disposable gloves should be used (📷 3.3a-c). The use of protective glasses is indicated to guarantee the safety of the operators. Hands and forearms must be free from accessories such as rings, watches, and bracelets, which are difficult to clean and disinfect and, therefore, represent a possible source of contamination.

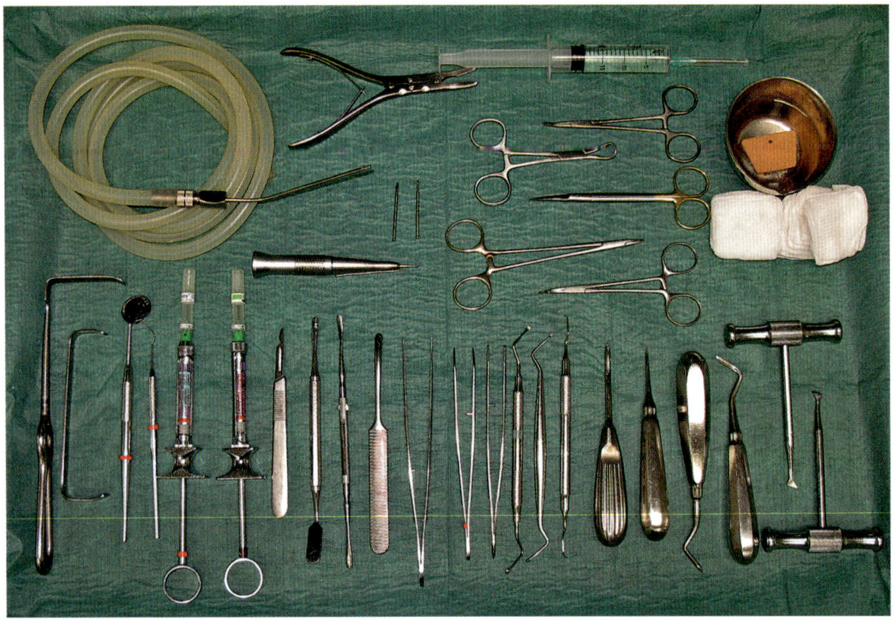

3.1 Surgical armamentarium is logically arranged on a sterile surface (e.g. Mayo stand covered with a sterile drape).

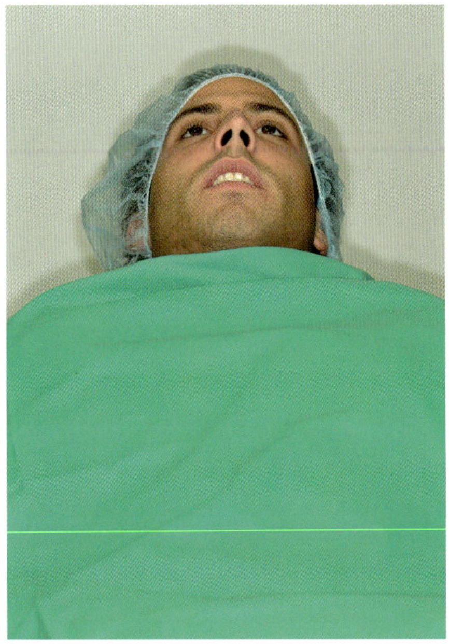

3.2 Patient preparation (clean surgery preparation): the patient wears a hair bonnet and is covered with a clean drape.

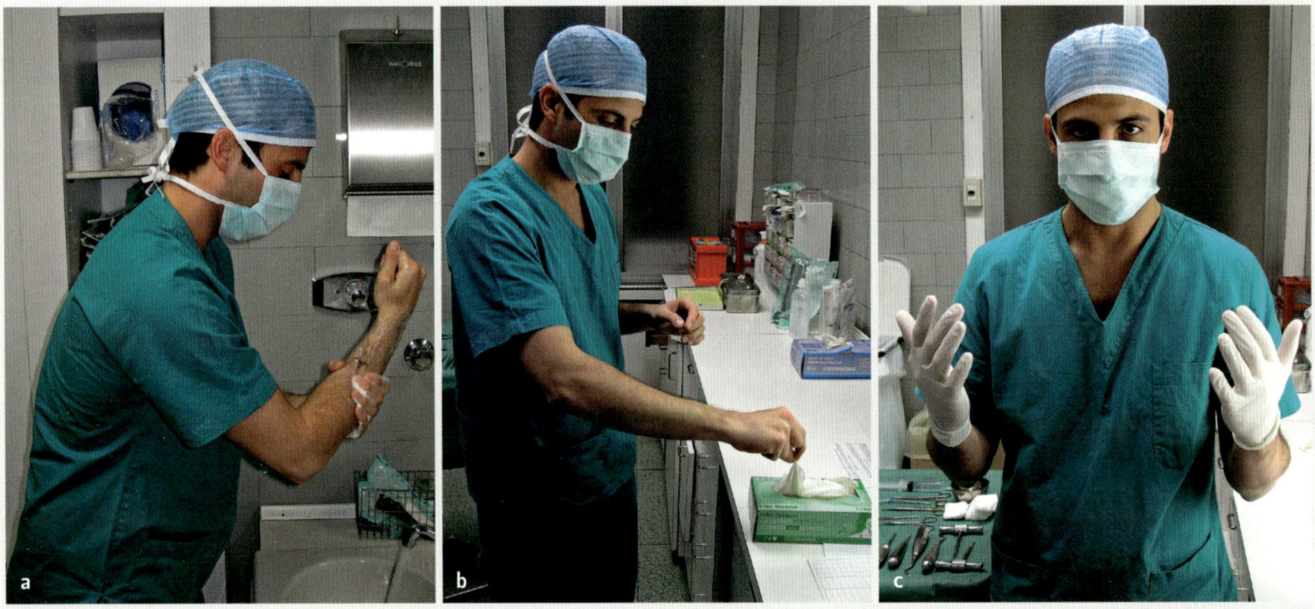

3.3 Operator preparation for clean surgery: **a)** after the surgical cap and mask are put on, hands and forearms are thoroughly washed (hands should be kept higher than elbows to avoid contamination); **b)** the operator picks up a disposable glove from its container, grabbing it by the edge; **c)** after the gloves are put on without touching their outer surface, the operator is ready.

Sterile preparation

A sterile preparation is indicated for the more invasive, prolonged surgeries, particularly when implants, grafting materials, and barrier membranes are used, or when the risk of postoperative infection is higher.

Preparing the environment and the surgical armamentarium: the same procedures described for the clean preparation apply. Complex surgeries performed under intravenous sedation or general anaesthesia should be performed in an adequately equipped operating theatre.

Preparing the patient: as with clean preparation, the patient must enter the operating room wearing shoe covers and a clean surgical cap: a one-minute chlorhexidine (0.2%) mouth rinse is used to lower the intraoral microbial load. In addition, to complete the sterile preparation of the patient:

- the perioral skin must be prepared with antiseptics such as iodophors (e.g. povidone iodine solutions) to reduce the risk of contamination of the surgical field;
- the patient must be covered with sterile drapes: only the perioral area, which is prepared with antiseptics, can be left uncovered to access the surgical field (3.4).

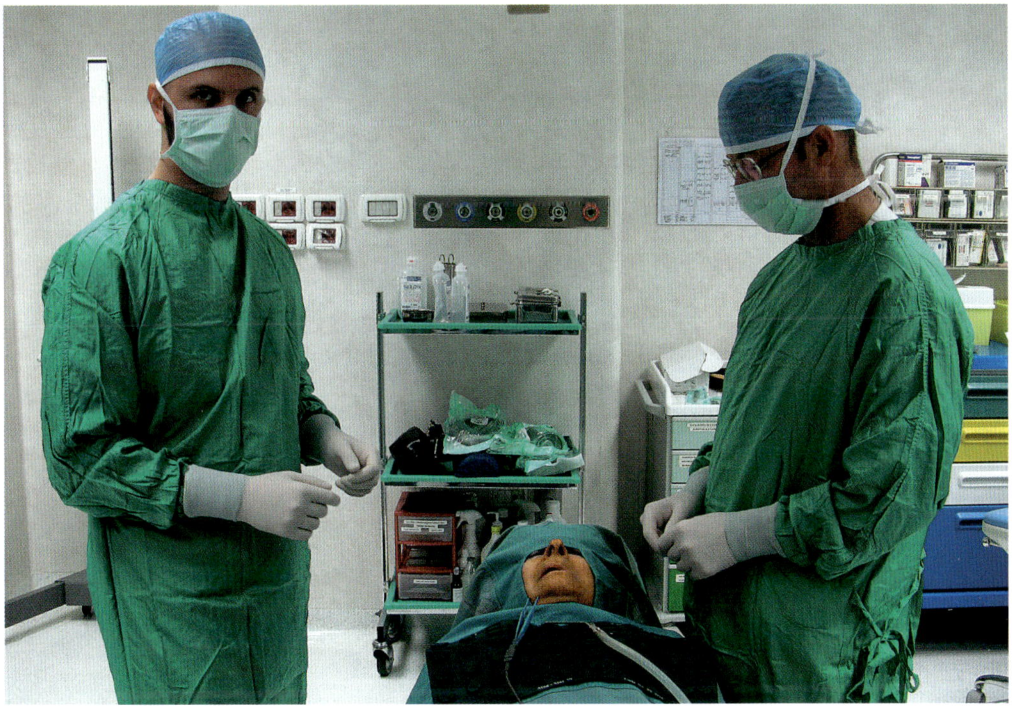

3.4 Preparation of the environment, the operators, and the patient for sterile surgery.

Preparation of the operators: operators must wear disposable shoe covers or dedicated (sterilised) footwear, clean surgical caps, clean surgical masks, sterile surgical gowns and sterile gloves. Protective glasses can be used to guarantee the safety of the operators.

The surgeon must first put on shoe covers, the surgical cap, and the surgical mask. Next, hands are thoroughly washed with antiseptic soaps, and sterile towels are used for hand drying (3.5a). The surgeon then puts on a sterile surgical gown with the aid of an assistant (3.5b). Sterile gloves can be put on with the aid of an assistant already dressed with sterile gown and sterile gloves (3.5c-d), or a specific procedure can be followed to put on the gloves without contaminating their outer surface (3.6a-d).

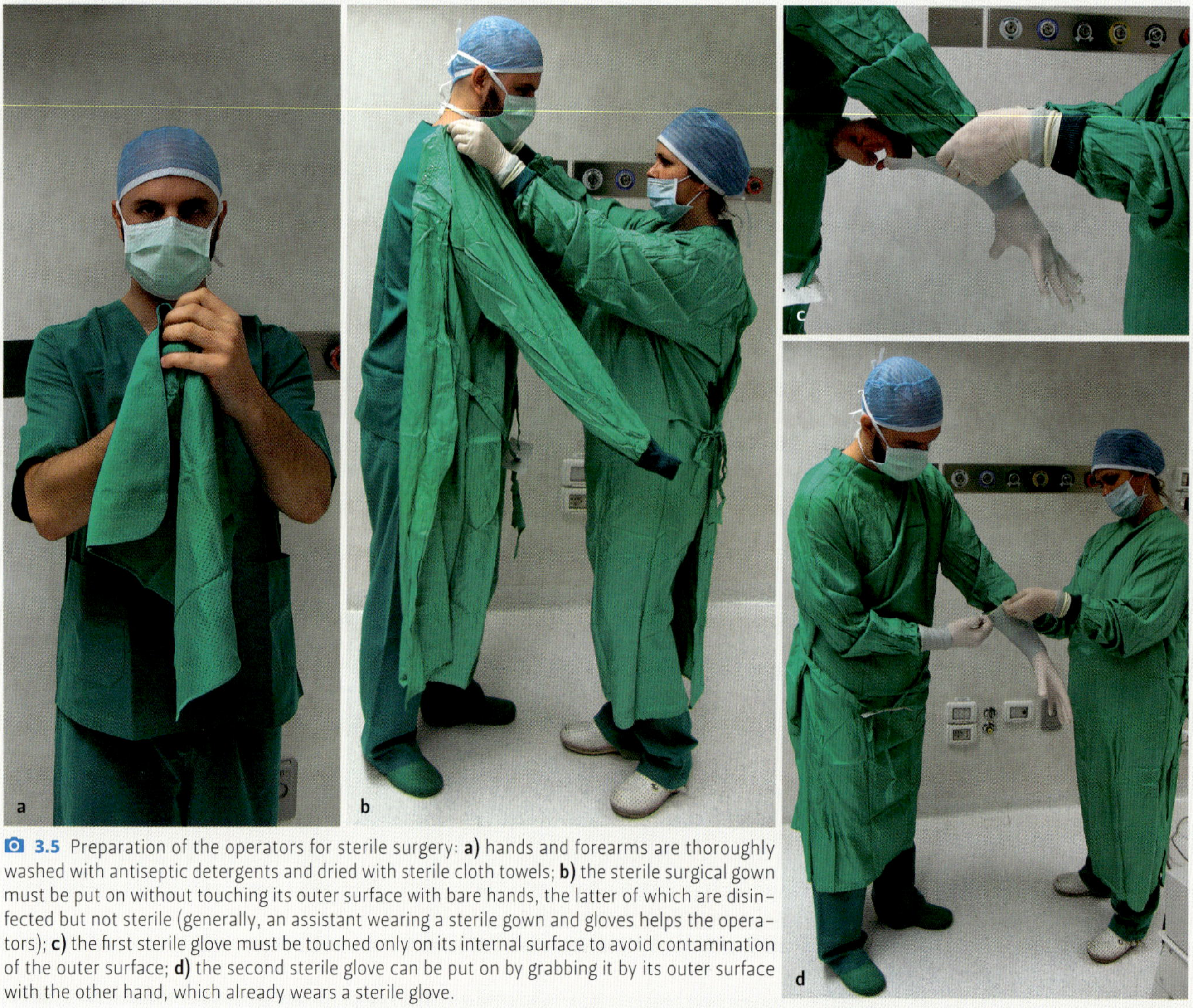

3.5 Preparation of the operators for sterile surgery: **a)** hands and forearms are thoroughly washed with antiseptic detergents and dried with sterile cloth towels; **b)** the sterile surgical gown must be put on without touching its outer surface with bare hands, the latter of which are disinfected but not sterile (generally, an assistant wearing a sterile gown and gloves helps the operators); **c)** the first sterile glove must be touched only on its internal surface to avoid contamination of the outer surface; **d)** the second sterile glove can be put on by grabbing it by its outer surface with the other hand, which already wears a sterile glove.

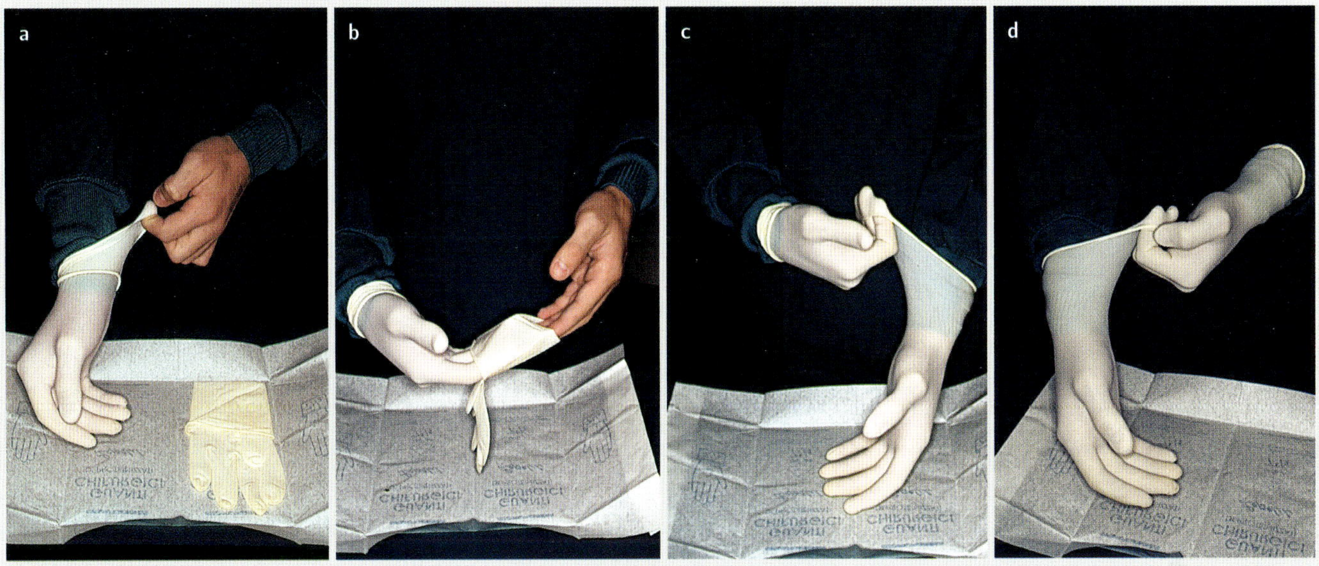

3.6 The operator may put on sterile gloves by himself/herself following a specific procedure: **a)** the first sterile glove must be grabbed only by its inner surface to avoid contamination of the outer surface: the glove is initially left folded into itself and it does not completely cover the cuff of the surgical gown; **b)** the second glove is grabbed by its outer surface with the hand already wearing the first glove; **c)** the second glove is completely unfolded to cover the cuff of the surgical gown; **d)** unfolding of the first glove is completed.

Local anaesthesia

The detailed description of the mechanism of action of local anaesthetics is beyond the scope of this manual. Therefore, only the practical aspects of their use are described.

Techniques to obtain local anaesthesia are:

1. topical anaesthesia, which is obtained by direct application of the anaesthetic (spray or cream) on the mucosa;
2. refrigeration anaesthesia, which is obtained by direct application of refrigerants (e.g. ethyl chloride or chloroethane sprays) on the mucosa;
3. infiltration anaesthesia, which is obtained by infiltration of the anaesthetic under the mucosa, is subdivided into:
   - intraligamentary anaesthesia (infiltration of the anaesthetic in the periodontal space);
   - supraperiosteal anaesthesia (infiltration of the anaesthetic around free nerve endings);
   - nerve block or conduction anaesthesia (infiltration of the anaesthetic near the main trunk of a nerve).

Topical and refrigeration anaesthesia may be used to desensitise the mucosa to reduce the discomfort caused by infiltration anaesthesia, or to obtain superficial numbing for short, atraumatic procedures such as the extraction of mobile deciduous teeth.

Infiltration anaesthesia allows effective interruption of the signal transmission of sensory fibres to be achieved.

Supraperiosteal infiltration is used when it is not possible, or it is not necessary, to reach the main trunk of a nerve but only its peripheral ramifications.

Conduction anaesthesia, on the other hand, is used to obtain a complete block of the sensory signals on the entire area innervated by the targeted nerve, with the same dose of anaesthetic.

In cases of tooth extraction, intraligamentary anaesthesia is typically used in conjunction with supraperiosteal infiltration.

Another important aspect to evaluate is the choice between anaesthetics containing vasoconstrictors and anaesthetics without vasoconstrictors. The role of the vasoconstrictor (generally, adrenaline/epinephrine) is to reduce intraoperative bleeding, and to prolong the effect of anaesthesia. Potential disadvantages are represented by a reduced diffusion of the anaesthetic, and by the systemic effects (e.g. tachycardia) that these vasoconstrictors may induce.

In particular, the use of adrenaline is generally advised against in patients presenting a risk of cardiac ischaemia, and in patients suffering from hyperthyroidism. However, it has been observed that the earlier onset of pain caused by the use of anaesthetics without vasoconstrictors, particularly in the case of prolonged surgical interventions, may trigger the secretion of quantities of endogenous catecholamines, which can be higher than those that are present in anaesthetics containing vasoconstrictors. Therefore, the resulting effect on the patient may be worse. According to recent research, the use of anaesthetics associated with vasoconstrictors is indicated in the majority of cases. In patients suffering from hyperthyroidism and patients presenting a risk of cardiac ischaemia, these anaesthetics can be used in lower doses, and in association with anxiolytics.

Standard cartridges used in dentistry contain 1.8 ml of anaesthetic, and the concentration of vasoconstrictor ranges between 1:50,000 to 1:200,000. As a rule, the limit of 10 cartridges should not be exceeded in a single surgical session to avoid the onset of toxic effects.

For the sake of clarity, the description of anaesthesia techniques follows the same principles applied to the description of local anatomy (see Chapter 2): specific techniques are described for every area of the oral cavity.

Posterior mandible

The main nerve trunks in the area are:
- inferior alveolar nerve;
- lingual nerve;
- buccal nerve.

INFERIOR ALVEOLAR NERVE BLOCK

Inferior alveolar nerve block causes anaesthesia of the ipsilateral hemimandible (bone and teeth), the ipsilateral half of the lower lip and chin, and the buccal mucosa (except in the molar area) (3.7a-b).

Indications

Surgical interventions involving the teeth, bone, or soft tissues of the corresponding hemimandible (e.g. extraction of erupted or impacted teeth, surgical endodontics procedures, enucleation of endosseous cysts, implant placement).

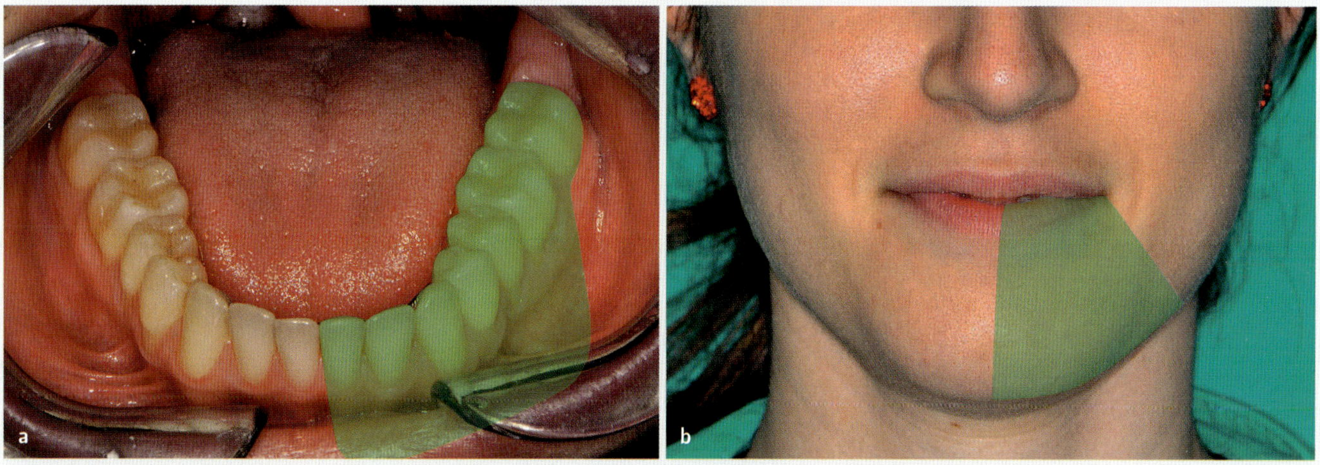

3.7 Area anaesthetised by an inferior alveolar nerve block: **a)** intraoral; **b)** extraoral.

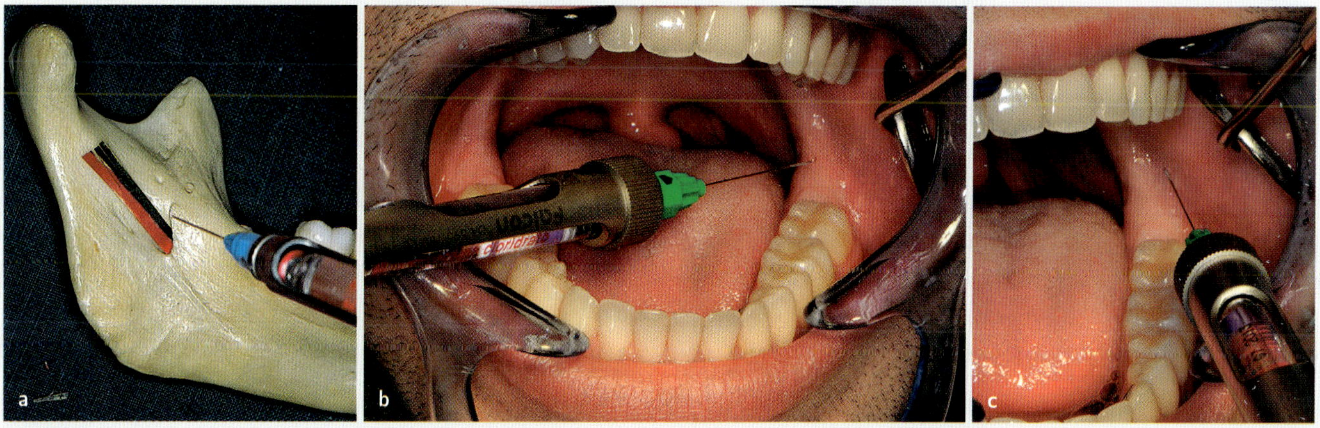

3.8 Inferior alveolar nerve block: **a)** the location of the Spix's spine and inferior alveolar neurovascular bundle with respect to the occlusal plane and anterior margin of the mandibular ramus can be seen; **b)** direct technique: the needle penetrates 1.5 cm above the occlusal plane, posteriorly to the anterior margin of the mandibular ramus, while the syringe is kept perpendicular to the contralateral premolars; **c)** indirect technique: the needle penetrates medially to the anterior margin of the mandibular ramus while the syringe is kept parallel to the mandibular body.

Technique

With the patient's mouth open, the anterior margin of the mandibular ramus is identified by palpation. The penetration point is located at the pterigomandibular depression (1-1.5 cm above the occlusal plane and 1-1.5 cm distally to the area of the third molar). If the "direct" technique is used, the needle is inserted while keeping the syringe inclined towards the contralateral premolars. Once the cortical plate in the area of the Spix's spine is encountered, the needle is slightly withdrawn (1 mm) and aspiration is attempted to exclude penetration of the needle inside a blood vessel; if no blood is visible inside the cartridge, then the anaesthetic can be slowly injected (3.8a-b). If the "indirect" technique is chosen, then the syringe is kept parallel to the medial face of the mandibular ramus. The needle is inserted to reach the area of the Spix's spine, and if the aspiration test is negative, the anaesthetic can be injected (3.8c).

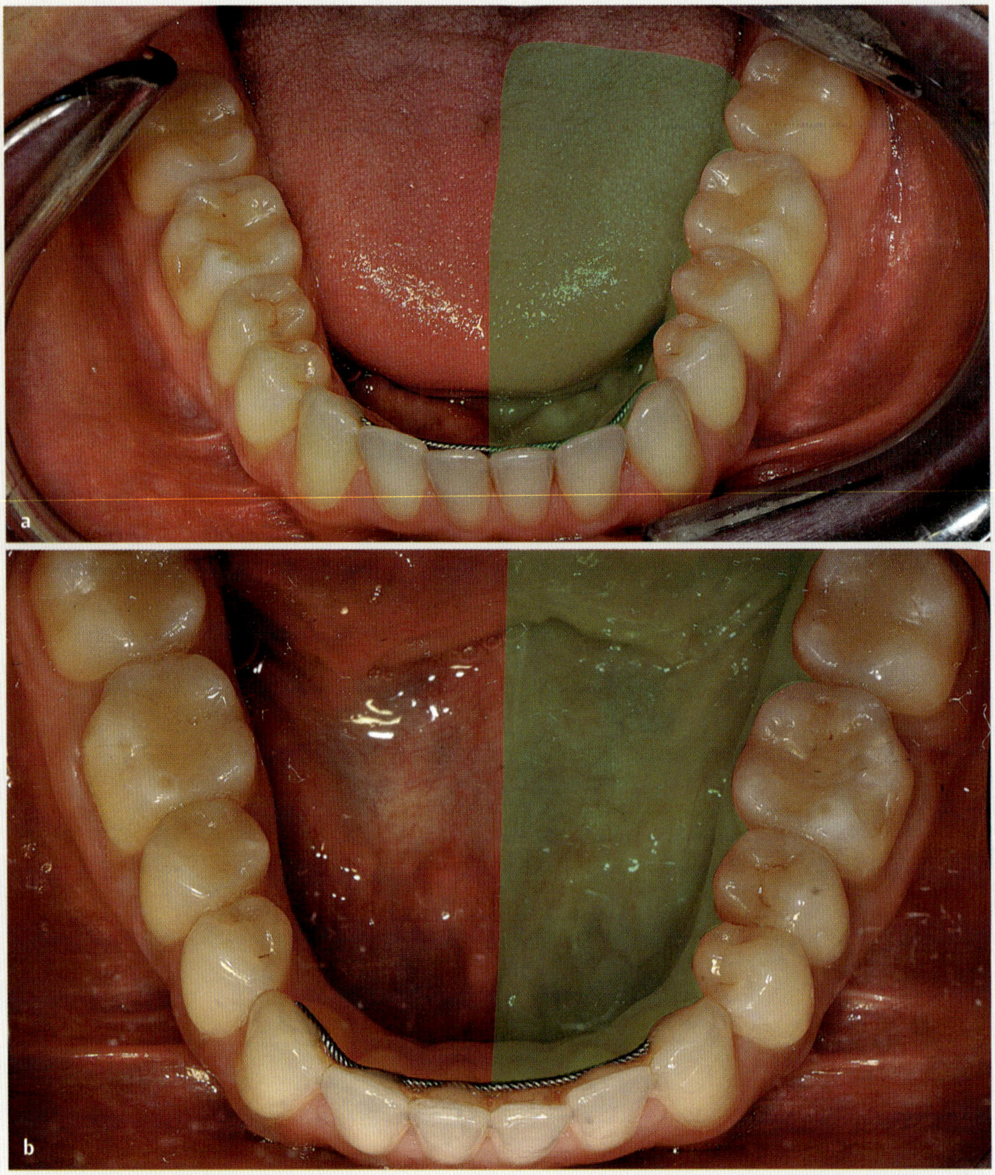

3.9 Area anaesthetised by a lingual nerve block: **a)** tongue; **b)** floor of the mouth.

LINGUAL NERVE BLOCK

Lingual nerve block causes anaesthesia of the anterior two thirds of the ipsilateral hemitongue, of the alveolar mucosa on the lingual side of the mandible, and of the ipsilateral half of the floor of the mouth (3.9a-b). Frequently, the lingual nerve block is obtained while performing the inferior alveolar nerve block, due to the proximity of the two nerves in the area of the Spix's spine.

Indications

Surgical interventions involving the floor of the oral cavity, the alveolar mucosa on the lingual side of the mandible, and the anterior two thirds of the corresponding hemitongue.

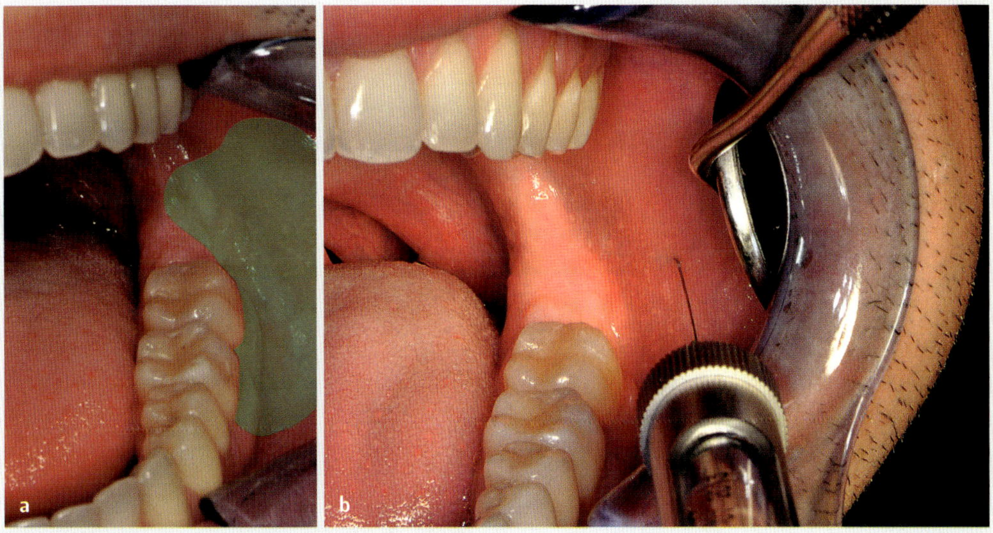

3.10 **a)** Area anaesthetised by a buccal nerve block. **b)** Technique for buccal nerve block.

Technique

The technique is similar to the one described for the inferior alveolar nerve block: the penetration point is 1 cm medially to the retromolar trigone, where the lingual nerve is covered only by the oral mucosa.

BUCCAL NERVE BLOCK

Buccal nerve block causes anaesthesia of the mucosa and buccal vestibule in the molar area (3.10a).

> ### *Indications*
>
> Extraction of erupted or impacted molars, surgical procedures involving the buccal mucosa in the molar region, bone harvesting from the mandibular body and ramus (in association with block anaesthesia of the inferior alveolar nerve).

Technique

The penetration point is located 1 cm buccally to the third molar area, where the external oblique line is (3.10b).

Anterior mandible

Anaesthesia in the anterior mandible can be obtained either via the inferior alveolar nerve block, the mental nerve block, or by supraperiosteal infiltration, due to the reduced thickness of the buccal cortical plate in the area.

MENTAL NERVE BLOCK

Mental nerve block causes anaesthesia of the buccal soft tissues of the ipsilateral hemimandible mesially to the second premolar, and of the corresponding half of the inferior lip and chin (3.11a).

Indications

Surgical interventions involving the buccal soft tissues of the corresponding hemimandible (enucleation of salivary cysts, excision of superficial lesions of the labial mucosa, etc.). It is worth emphasising that the mental nerve block alone causes anaesthesia of the soft tissues; indeed, it has no effects on the mandibular body and teeth until perfusion occurs, either through the mental foramen (where the injection can also be directed to improve the effect) or through the thin buccal cortical plate. Therefore, this type of anaesthesia should be associated with the inferior alveolar nerve block for surgical interventions involving the hard tissues (bone, teeth) in the anterior mandible.

Technique

Panoramic and periapical radiographs may facilitate identification of the mental foramen. The needle is inserted perpendicularly to the buccal cortical plate between the first and second premolar, below the level of the apex (3.11b-c). The anaesthetic can be injected just outside the mental foramen, or the needle can be inserted a few millimetres inside the foramen before injecting. This latter technique allows a better anaesthetic effect on the incisive nerve; however, it also increases the risk of damaging the mental nerve. Therefore, the association of this type of anaesthesia with the inferior alveolar nerve block should always be considered.

In edentulous patients, particularly when severe bone atrophy is present, palpation may help to identify the actual position of the mental foramen, which can be relatively superficial.

INCISIVE NERVE BLOCK

Incisive nerve block causes anaesthesia of the teeth and periodontal tissues in the anterior region of the corresponding hemimandible. However, the incisive nerve cannot be independently blocked, as it runs inside its canal in the anterior portion of the mandibular body. Therefore, incisive nerve block is obtained by means of supraperiosteal infiltration of anaesthetic on the buccal side of the mandible: the concomitant numbing obtained on the buccal soft tissue is due to the anaesthesia of the terminal branches of the mental nerve (3.12a).

Indications

Extraction or surgical endodontics procedures involving the first premolar, canine and incisors in the ipsilateral hemimandible. Surgical procedures involving the soft and hard tissues of the corresponding side of the mandible.

Technique

Anaesthesia, which cannot be considered a true block, is obtained by supraperiosteal infiltration of the anaesthetic in the buccal vestibule, between the mental foramen and the median line of the mandible (3.12b).

In some cases, it is necessary to associate infiltration of anaesthetic in the anterior third of the floor of the mouth to block the sensory branches of the mylohyoid nerve that may reach the incisives.

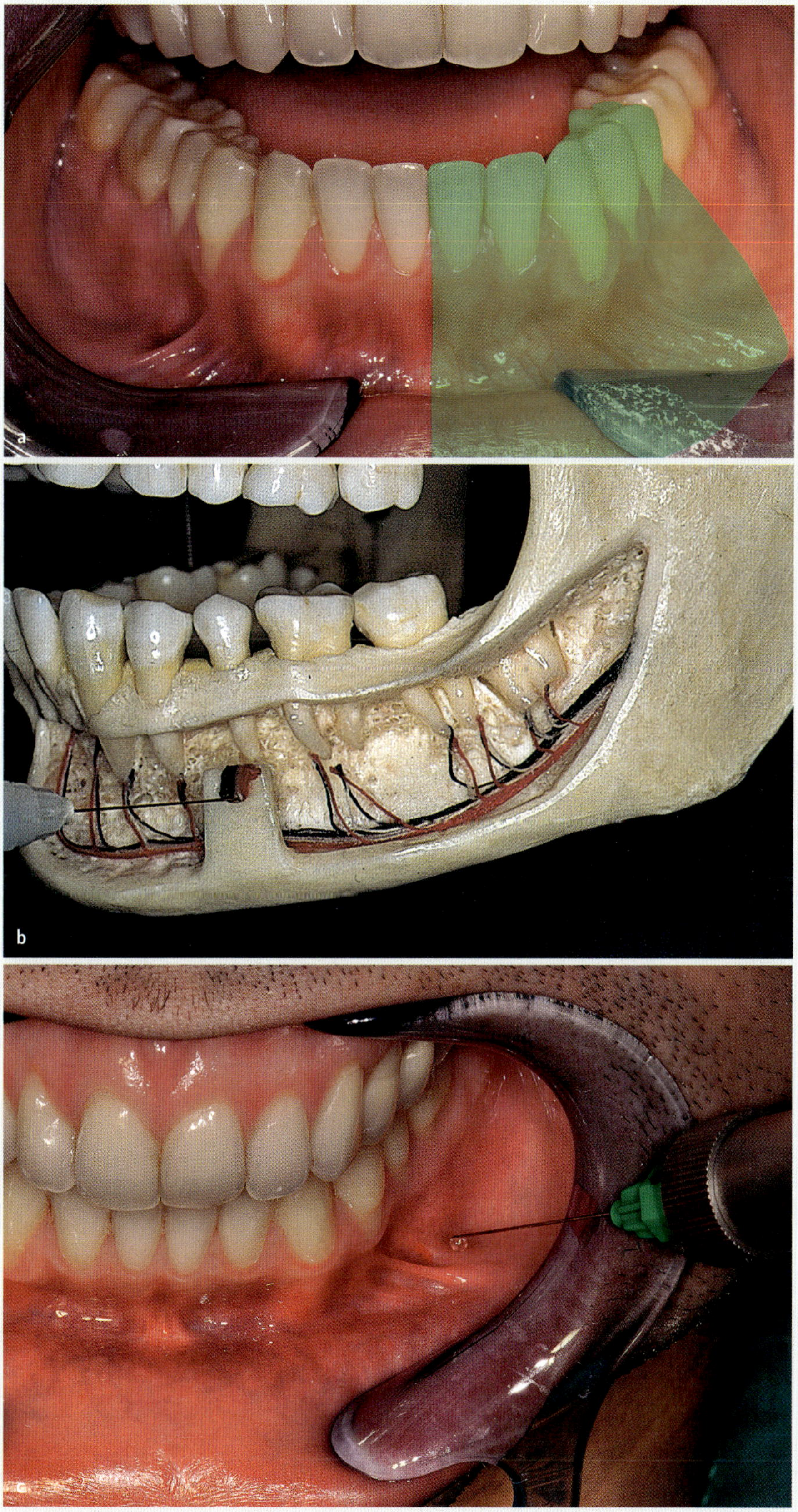

3.11 Mental nerve block: **a)** area anaesthetised by buccal nerve block; **b)** mental nerve block simulated on a skull model; **c)** point of penetration of the needle to obtain the mental nerve block.

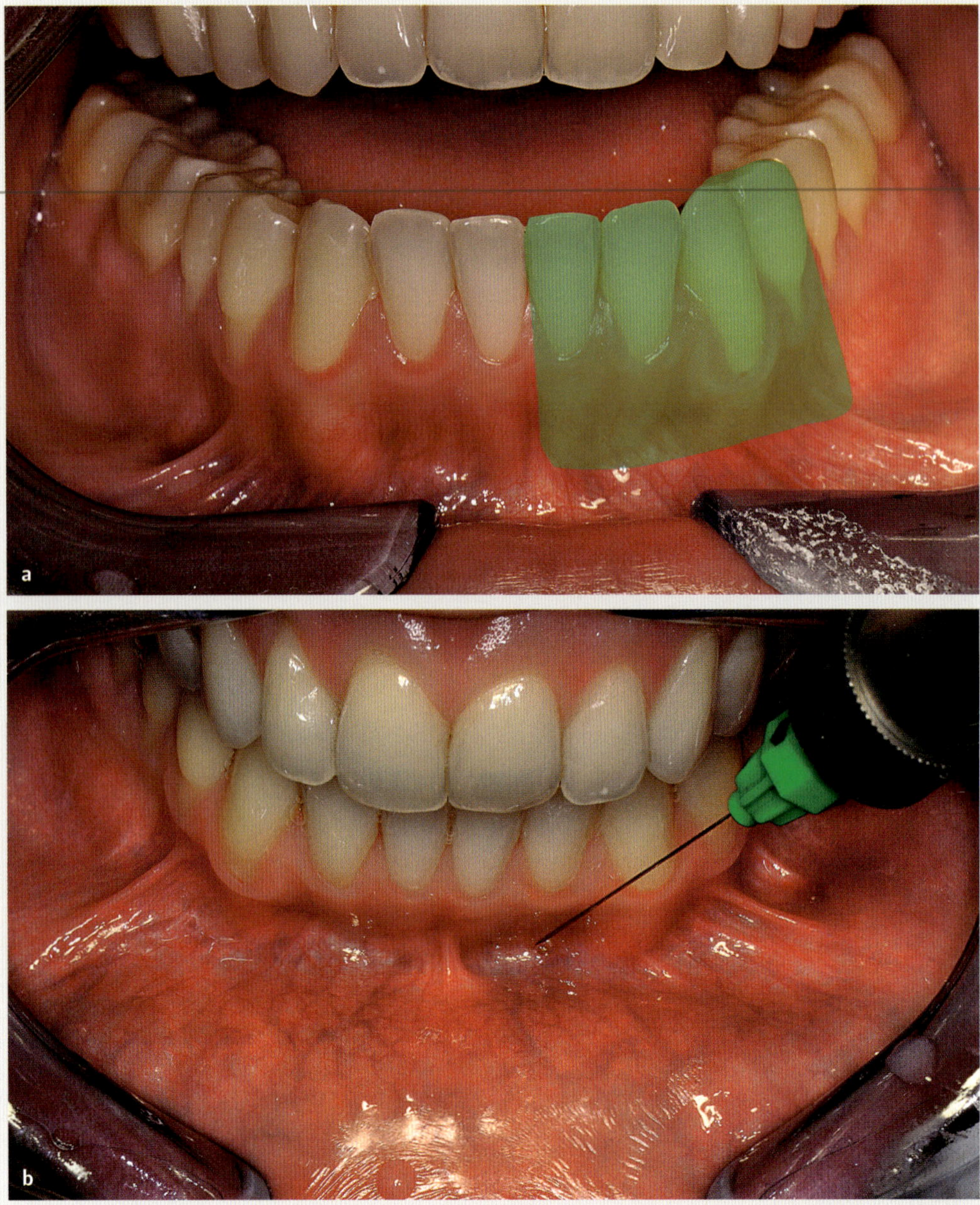

3.12 Incisive nerve block: **a)** area anaesthetised by an incisive nerve block; **b)** point of penetration of the needle to obtain the incisive nerve block.

Floor of the mouth

Innervation of the floor of the mouth is mainly provided by the lingual nerve and its branches. Lingual nerve block anaesthesia has already been described. Nevertheless, in cases of surgical procedures on the superficial tissues involving small areas, local submucosal infiltration (or perilesional injection) may be sufficient (3.13).

The floor of the mouth has a rich vascularisation. Therefore, the use of anaesthetics containing vasoconstrictors is indicated to reduce intraoperative bleeding, and to prolong the anaesthetic effect.

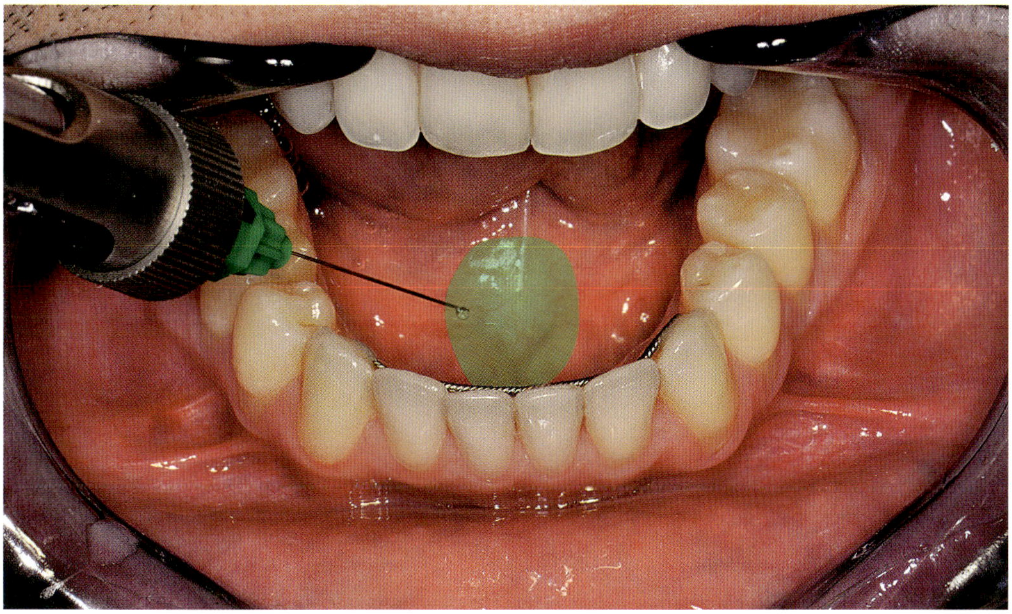

3.13 Point of penetration of the needle in the floor of the mouth to obtain anaesthesia of the terminal branches of the lingual nerve.

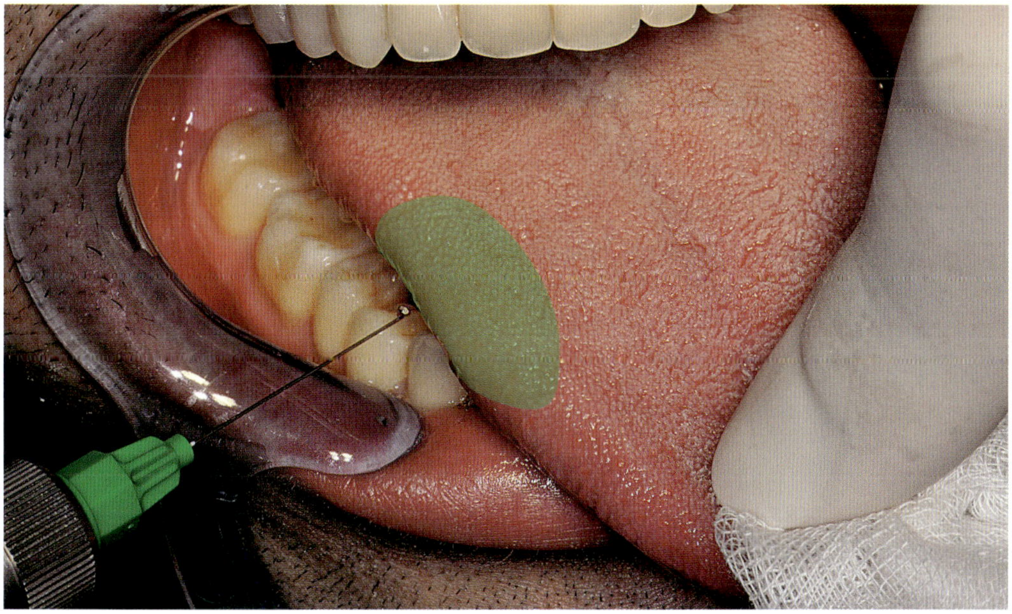

3.14 Local infiltration in the anterior portion of the tongue.

Tongue

Surgical interventions on the anterior two thirds of the tongue require block anaesthesia of the lingual nerve, which has already been described. Anaesthesia can also be obtained by submucosal infiltration in a specific area, or perilesional injection of anaesthetics (3.14).

Posterior maxilla

Innervation in this area is provided by the superior-posterior and middle alveolar branches (arising from the maxillary nerve), and by the infraorbital nerve: the first are blocked by supraperiosteal infiltration of anaesthetics in the buccal vestibule, while block anaesthesia of the latter can be obtained with either an intra- or extraoral approach.

ANAESTHESIA OF THE SUPERIOR-POSTERIOR ALVEOLAR BRANCHES

Superior-posterior alveolar nerve block causes anaesthesia of the alveolar ridge, molars, and alveolar mucosa of the corresponding area (3.15a).

Indications

Surgical procedures involving the alveolar ridge, molars, and alveolar mucosa of the posterior maxilla (extraction of erupted or impacted molars, surgical endodontics, enucleation of endosseous lesions, implant placement, etc.).

Technique

The needle penetrates in the buccal vestibule beside the third molar, and reaches the superior portion of the maxillary tuberosity (3.15b-c).

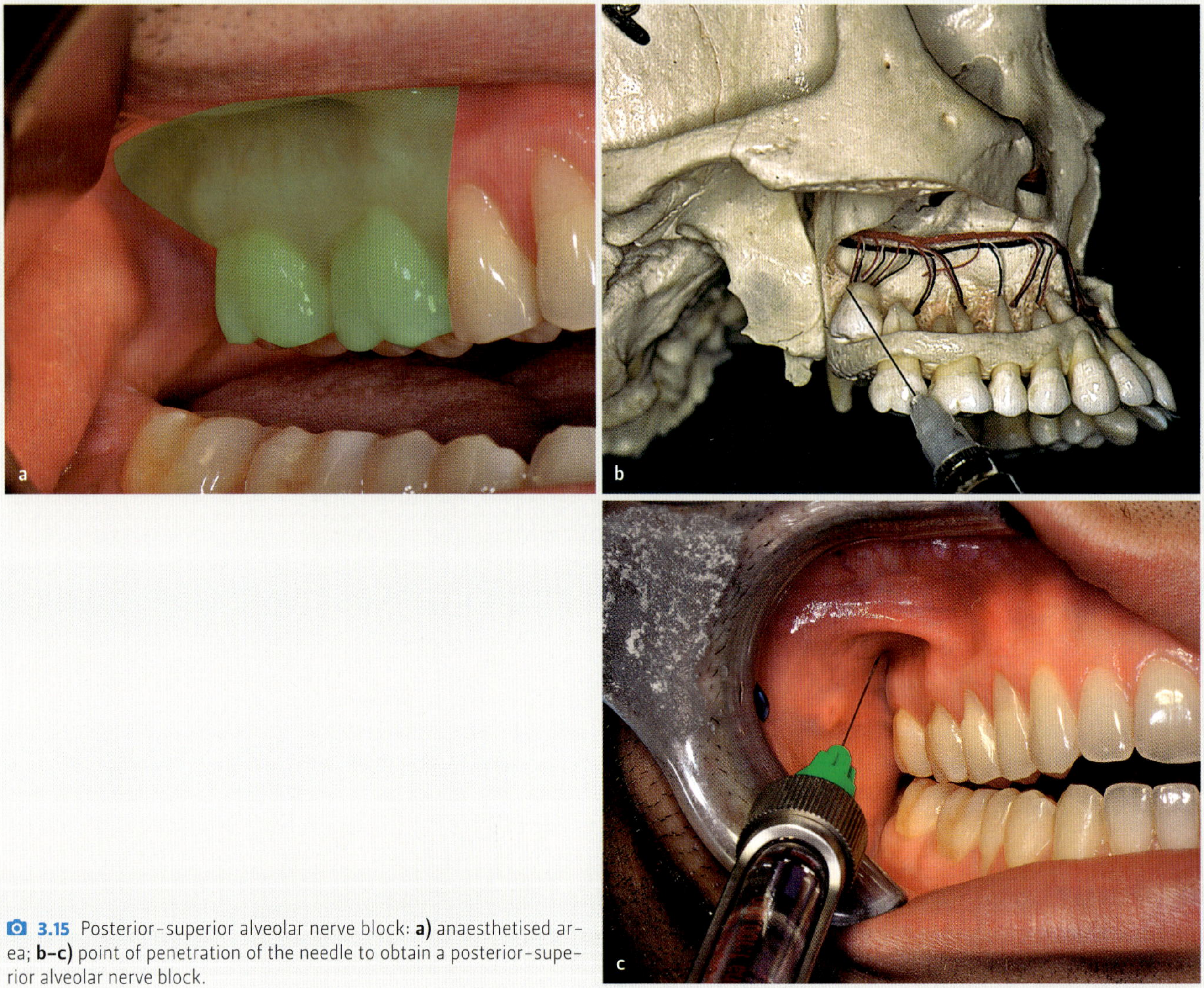

3.15 Posterior-superior alveolar nerve block: **a)** anaesthetised area; **b-c)** point of penetration of the needle to obtain a posterior-superior alveolar nerve block.

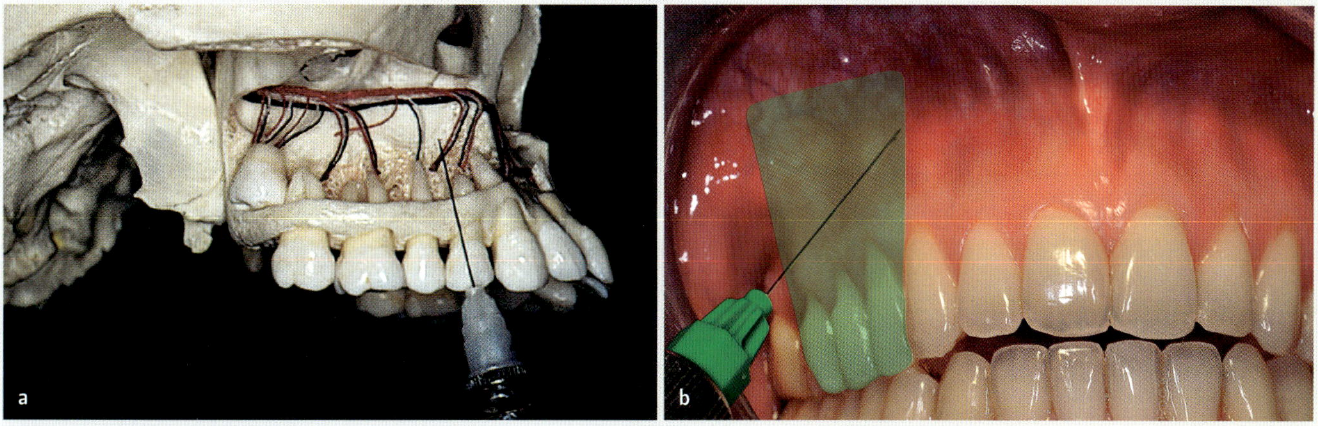

3.16 a–b) Middle-superior alveolar nerve block: point of penetration of the needle and anaesthetised area.

ANAESTHESIA OF THE SUPERIOR-MIDDLE ALVEOLAR BRANCHES

Superior-middle alveolar nerve block causes anaesthesia of the alveolar ridge, premolars, and alveolar mucosa of the corresponding area.

Indications

Surgical procedures involving the alveolar ridge, premolars, and alveolar mucosa of the lateral maxilla (extraction of erupted or impacted premolars, surgical endodontics, enucleation of endosseous lesions, implant placement, etc.).

Technique

The needle penetrates in the buccal vestibule beside the premolars and supraperiosteal injection of the anaesthetic is performed (3.16a-b).

INFRAORBITAL NERVE BLOCK

Infraorbital nerve block causes anaesthesia of the ipsilateral hemimaxilla, including teeth, the buccal mucosa, the mucosa and skin of the corresponding half of the upper lip, the skin of the corresponding half of the nose, the skin of the corresponding malar region, and the skin of the corresponding lower palpebral area (3.17a).

Indications

In the case of surgical procedures involving the alveolar ridge, teeth, and the alveolar mucosa, supraperiosteal infiltration to obtain anaesthesia of its terminal branches is sufficient. When the maxillary sinus, deeply impacted teeth (e.g. canines), and the skin in the malar region (e.g. abscess drainage) are involved, infraorbital nerve block anaesthesia is recommended.

Technique

Block anaesthesia of the infraorbital nerve can be performed via an intra- and extraoral approach.

Intraoral approach: the needle penetrates laterally to the canine fossa and follows the anterior wall of the maxillary sinus up to 1 cm below the inferior orbital rim, where the infraorbital foramen opening can be found (3.17b). Extraoral palpation helps to verify that the anaesthetic is injected in the correct area. The main disadvantage of this approach is represented by the fact that, due to the horizontal course of the infraorbital canal, it is not possible to obtain an effective block of the nerve branches coming from inside the canal itself, but only of the terminal branches coming from the nerve outside of the infraorbital foramen.

Extraoral approach: the needle penetrates perpendicularly to the anterior wall of the maxilla: the penetration point is located 1 cm laterally to the alar groove of the nose and 1 cm below the inferior orbital rim (3.17c). The percutaneous technique allows the needle to penetrate inside the infraorbital canal, causing a more effective block of the branches coming from the infraorbital nerve inside the canal.

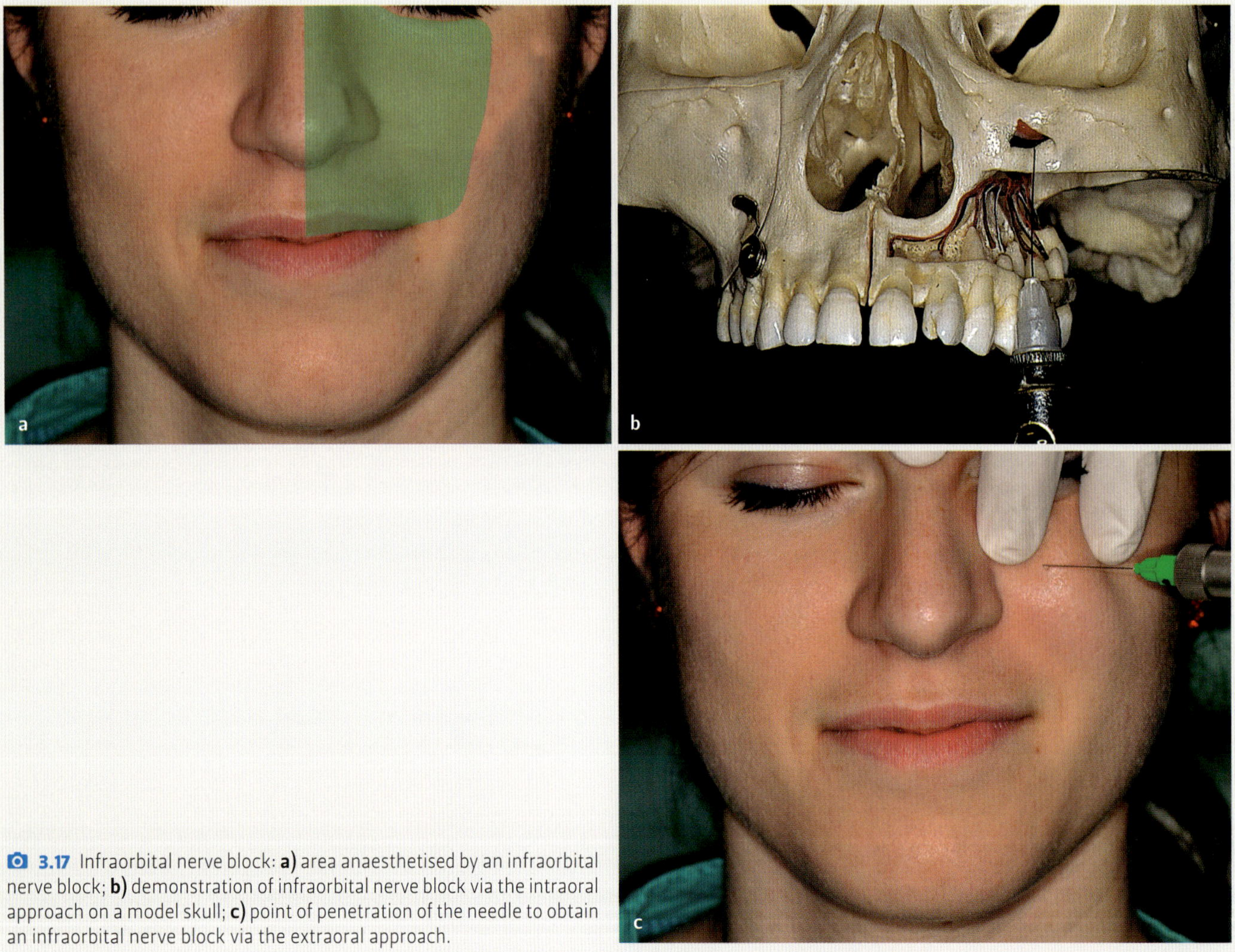

3.17 Infraorbital nerve block: **a)** area anaesthetised by an infraorbital nerve block; **b)** demonstration of infraorbital nerve block via the intraoral approach on a model skull; **c)** point of penetration of the needle to obtain an infraorbital nerve block via the extraoral approach.

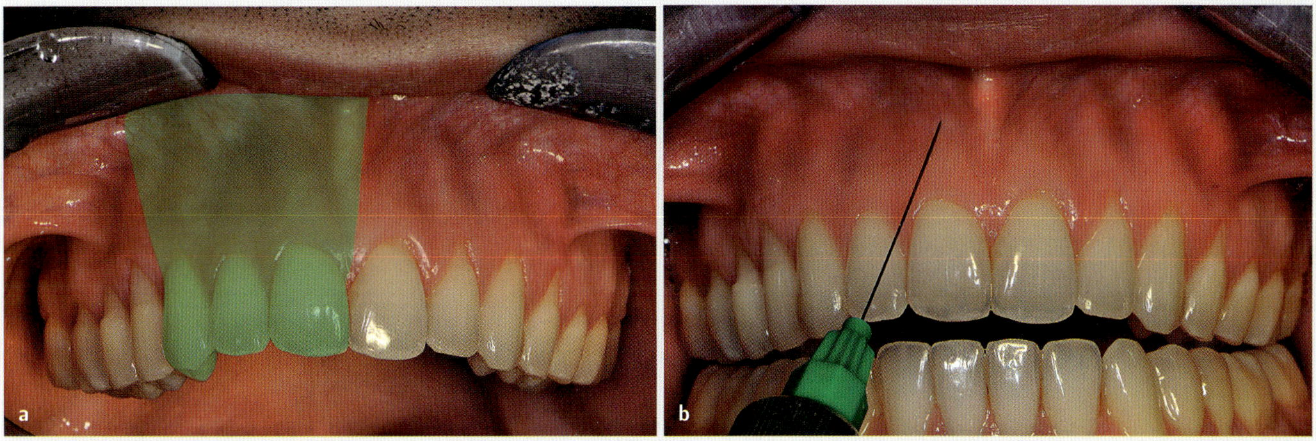

3.18 a-b) Area anaesthetised by an anterior-superior alveolar nerve block and point of penetration of the needle.

Anterior maxilla

Innervation in this area is provided by the superior-anterior alveolar nerves and by the terminal branches of the infraorbital nerve.

ANAESTHESIA OF THE SUPERIOR-ANTERIOR ALVEOLAR NERVES AND TERMINAL BRANCHES OF THE INFRAORBITAL NERVE

Anaesthesia of these nerves causes numbing of the alveolar ridge, alveolar mucosa and teeth in the canine-incisor area of the ipsilateral hemimaxilla.

Indications

Surgical procedures involving the canines and incisives, the alveolar ridge, and the alveolar mucosa on the buccal side of the anterior maxilla.

Technique

The area of penetration is the bottom of the buccal vestibule, above the apexes of the canines and incisors (3.18a-b). As previously mentioned, in cases of more invasive surgical procedures, the recourse to block anaesthesia of the infraorbital nerve via the extraoral approach is indicated.

Palate

As far as the hard palate is concerned, innervation is provided by the major palatine nerve and by the nasopalatine nerve, while innervation of the soft palate is provided by the lesser palatine nerve arising from the maxillary nerve.

NASOPALATINE NERVE BLOCK

Nasopalatine nerve block causes anaesthesia of the palatine mucosa in the intercanine region. The right and left nasopalatine nerves share the same canal; therefore, from a practical viewpoint they constitute a single functional unit.

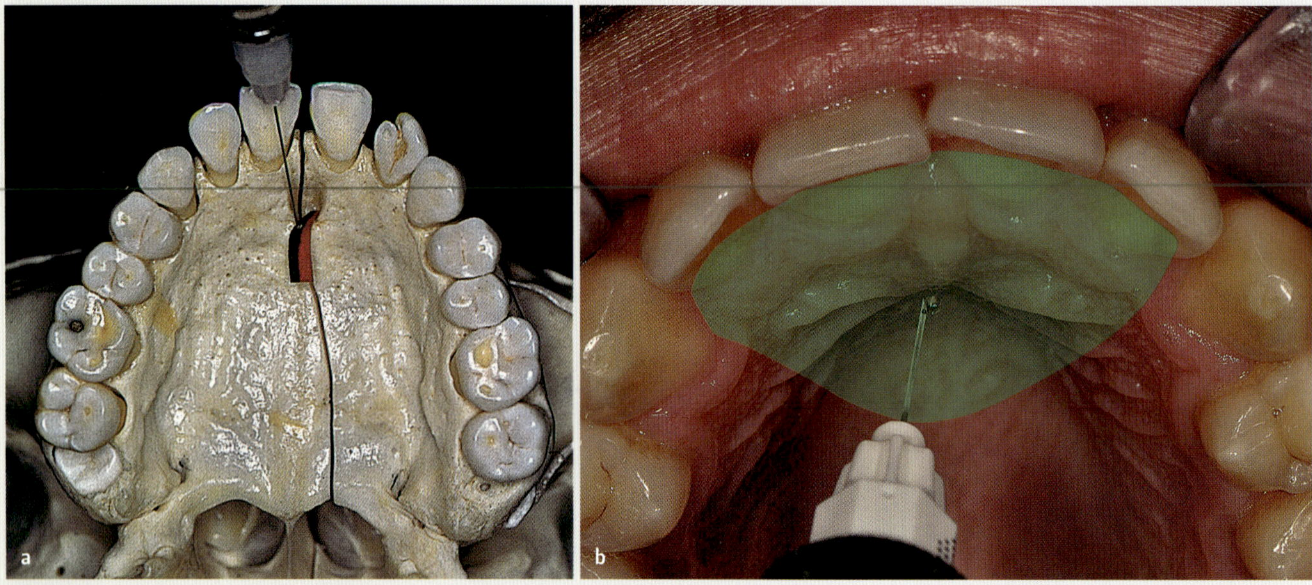

3.19 Nasopalatine nerve block: **a)** demonstration on a model skull; **b)** area anaesthetised.

Indications

Surgical interventions involving the incisors and canines, as well as the palatine mucosa and the alveolar ridge in the intercanine region (extraction of erupted or impacted teeth, surgical endodontics, endosseous lesions developing towards the palatal side of the alveolar ridge, etc.).

Technique

In dentate patients, the needle is kept parallel to the central incisors: the area of penetration corresponds to the retroincisive papilla (3.19a-b). The injection of anaesthetics in this area, particularly those containing vasoconstrictors, causes a visible ischaemia of the palatine mucosa, thus significantly reducing intraoperative bleeding. In edentulous patients, particularly in the case of severe bone atrophy, the nasopalatine foramen (and the overlying interincisive papilla) may be found on top of the residual alveolar ridge: care must be taken when choosing the area of injection, and when performing crestal incisions, to avoid any damage to the neurovascular bundle.

MAJOR PALATINE NERVE BLOCK

Major palatine nerve block causes anaesthesia of the palatine mucosa of the ipsilateral hemimaxilla from the area of the third molar to the area of the canine, where numerous anastomoses with branches of the nasopalatine nerve are present.

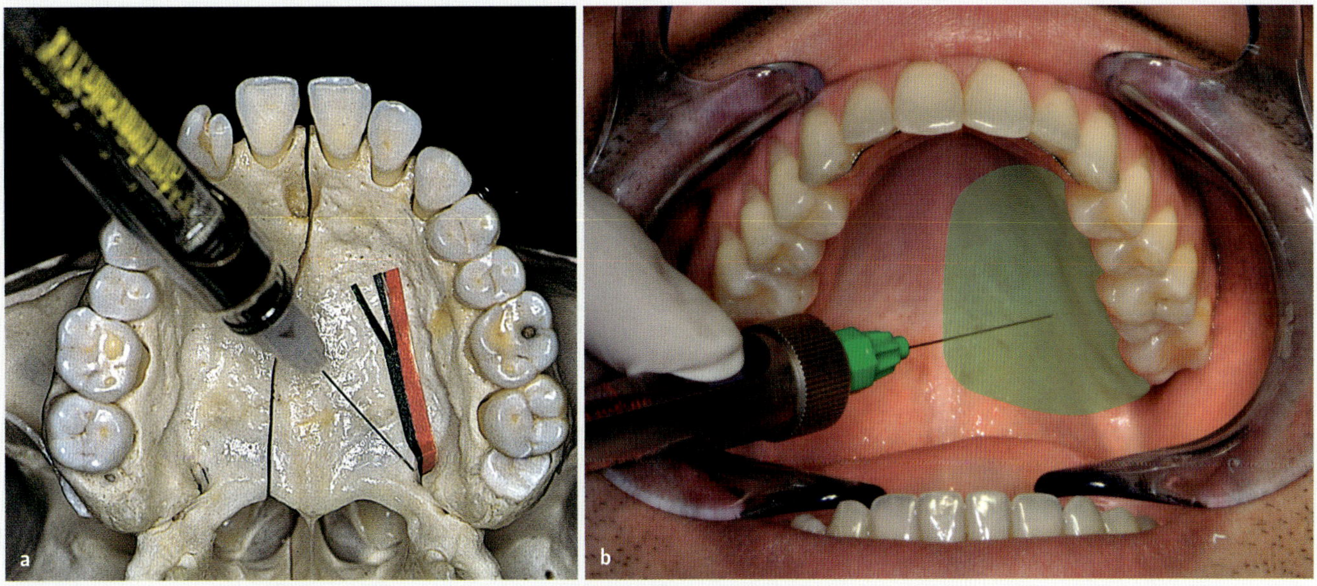

3.20 Major palatine nerve block: **a)** demonstration on a model skull; **b)** area anaesthetised.

Indications

Surgical interventions involving the palatine mucosa, the alveolar ridge, the palatal vault, the molars, and the premolars (extraction of erupted and impacted teeth, endosseous lesions developing towards the palate, harvesting of keratinised mucosa, etc.).

Technique

In dentate patients, the reference point is represented by the third molar, where the alveolar ridge meets the palatine process (3.20a-b). The injection of anaesthetics in this area, particularly those containing vasoconstrictors, causes a visible ischaemia of the palatine mucosa, thus significantly reducing intraoperative bleeding. In edentulous patients, particularly in the case of severe bone atrophy, the major palatine foramen may be found in relative proximity to the top of the residual alveolar ridge. Care must be taken when choosing the area of injection, and when performing crestal incisions to avoid any damage to the neurovascular bundle.

LESSER PALATINE NERVE BLOCK

Lesser palatine nerve block causes anaesthesia of the soft palate.

Indications

Surgical procedures involving the soft palate.

Infiltration anaesthesia

Type	Area	Indications
Inferior alveolar nerve block	Posterior mandible	Teeth of the corresponding hemimandible Endosseous neoformations
Lingual nerve block	Posterior mandible Posterior portion of the floor of the mouth	Floor of the mouth, lingual mucosa Anterior portion of the ipsilateral hemitongue
Buccal nerve block	Posterior mandible	Extraction of erupted or impacted molars Buccal soft tissues
Mental nerve block	Anterior mandible Lower lip	Anterior teeth Endosseous neoformations Buccal mucosa, ipsilateral hemimandible and ipsilateral half of the lower lip
Superior-posterior nerve block	Posterior maxilla	Molars, posterior alveolar ridge, buccal mucosa
Infraorbital nerve block	Posterior maxilla Upper lip	Maxillary teeth, maxillary sinus surgery
Nasopalatine nerve block	Anterior palate	Mucosa, alveolar ridge, palatine bone in the anterior maxilla
Major palatine nerve block	Posterior palate	Mucosa, alveolar ridge, palatine bone in the area of the premolars and molars
Middle and posterior palatine nerves block	Soft palate	Soft palate
Incisive nerve	Anterior mandible	Anterior mandibular teeth Endosseous neoformations Buccal mucosa, ipsilateral anterior hemimandible and ipsilateral half of the lower lip
Superior-middle alveolar nerve	Posterior maxilla	Premolars, alveolar ridge, corresponding buccal mucosa
Superior-anterior alveolar nerve and terminal branches of the infraorbital nerve	Anterior maxilla	Incisors and canines Alveolar ridge and corresponding buccal mucosa

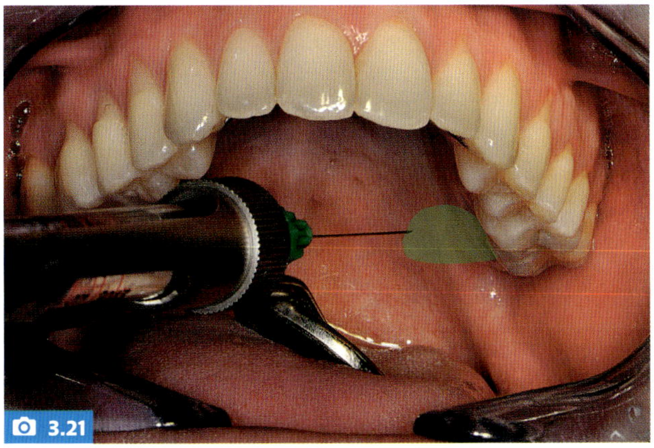

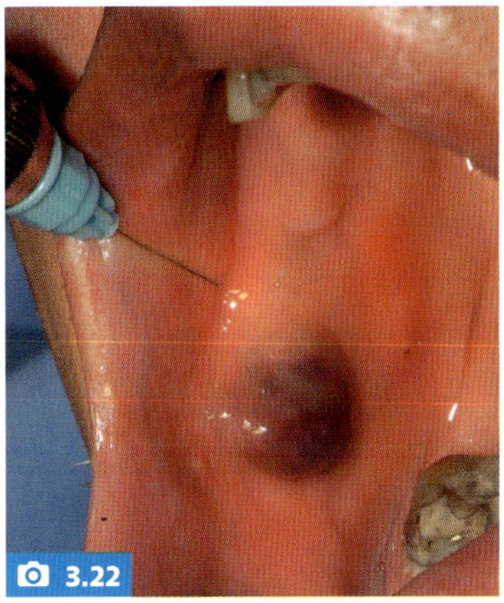

3.21 Lesser palatine nerve block: area anaesthetised.

3.22 Perilesional infiltration to remove a lesion on the malar mucosa.

Technique

The area of insertion is located posteriorly and medially with respect to the major palatine foramen, at the junction between the hard and soft palate (3.21). It is worth emphasising that, due to the absence of reference points, the rich vascularisation, and the functional implications, surgical procedures involving the soft palate should be performed only by specifically trained surgeons.

Malar region

Typically, anaesthesia of the malar mucosa is necessary for surgical removal of superficial lesions of the soft tissues in the area, which is obtained by means of perilesional infiltration of the anaesthetic (3.22). If necessary, buccal nerve block and infraorbital nerve block can be associated with the perilesional infiltration (see dedicated sections for details).

Lower lip

Anaesthesia of the inferior lip is obtained by mental nerve block (see dedicated section for details). To reduce intraoperative bleeding even further, perilesional anaesthesia can be used in conjunction with mental nerve block.

Upper lip

Anaesthesia of the upper lip is obtained by infraorbital nerve block (see dedicated section for details). To reduce intraoperative bleeding even further, perilesional anaesthesia can be used in conjunction with mental nerve block.

Techniques for soft tissue incision and flap preparation

Incision of the soft tissues is aimed at gaining access to the operating field by elevating one or more flaps that are retracted to perform a surgical procedure. The principles upon which the preparation of an access flap must always be based are as follows:

- preventing ischaemia;
- preventing flap lacerations;
- preventing damage to important anatomical structures;
- preventing wound dehiscence.

Oral surgery procedures are performed on both the soft and the hard tissues. With the provision that the aforementioned principles are respected, relevant differences concerning the armamentarium and techniques exists between surgical procedures performed on the hard (bone, teeth) and soft (mucosa) tissues. In particular, specific dissection/cleavage techniques are used to enucleate lesions from the soft tissues.

Preventing ischaemia

Every incision causes an interruption, albeit partial and temporary, of the blood supply of the flap, in which a free portion (delimited by the incisions) and a pedicle (the base, where no incisions are made to preserve blood supply for the entire flap) can be identified. Therefore, the principles underlying the blood supply of surgical flaps must always be respected to guarantee flap vitality.

Two types of flap can be identified according to blood supply: axial and random flaps.

Axial flaps receive their blood supply by a specific artery: the flap is designed around the artery so that this latter penetrates from the pedicle and gives off branches that can guarantee adequate blood supply even to extended flaps. An example of intraoral axial flap is the mucoperiosteal flap based on the major palatine artery (3.23a-b).

In random flaps, a main artery is not present, and they receive their blood supply from a network of smaller arterial branches; they represent the majority of flaps that can be prepared in the oral cavity, and the length of their pedicle (base) must be at least equal to that of the free portion, or greater, so that this latter can always receive adequate blood supply. A shorter pedicle may cause partial or total flap necrosis (3.24a-b).

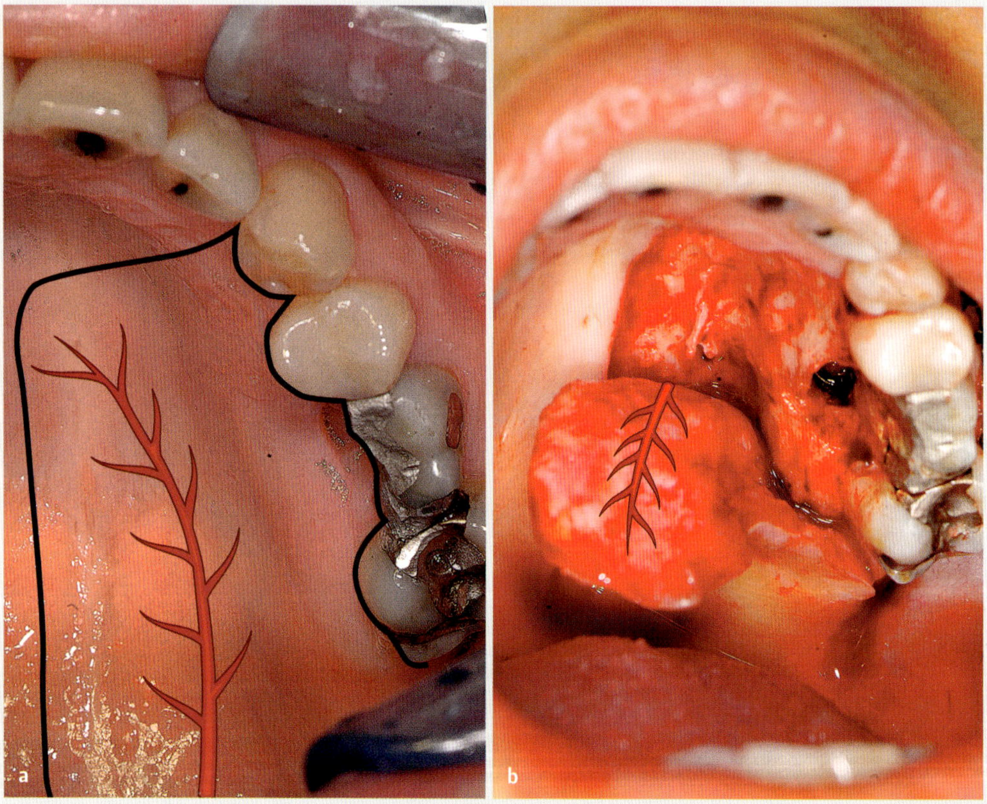

3.23 a) Design of an axial flap based on the major palatine artery. **b)** Full-thickness elevation of the axial flap.

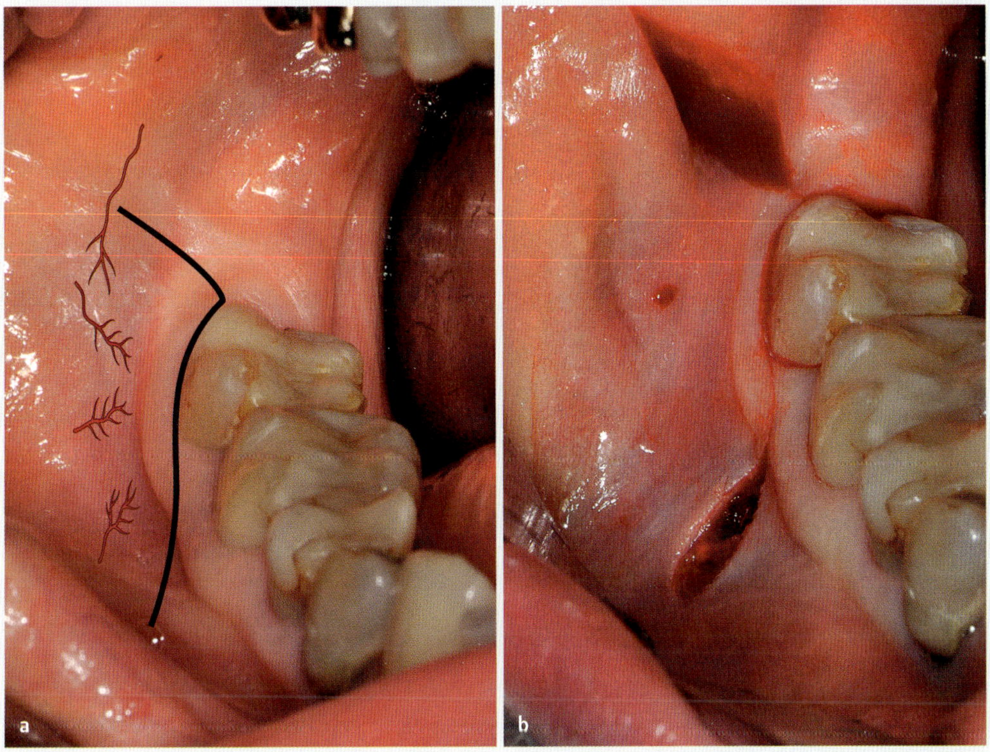

3.24 **a)** Design of a random flap on the buccal side of the posterior mandible. **b)** Incision of the random flap.

Preventing flap laceration

Soft tissue laceration typically occurs when the flap is undersized with respect to the extent of the area of intervention. Consequently, access to the surgical field and visibility are inadequate. If excessive retraction is attempted, then lacerations involving either the flap or the surrounding soft tissues may result.

Different types of flap can be identified according to their shape:

- flaps without releasing incisions (envelope flaps);
- flaps with one releasing incision (three-corner flaps);
- flaps with two releasing incisions (four-corner flaps);
- semilunar flap.

FLAPS WITHOUT RELEASING INCISIONS

These flaps are constituted by a single, linear incision. They offer the best blood supply, because the integrity of the soft tissues is interrupted on one side only. On the other hand, retracting these flaps during surgery is more difficult than retracting flaps with releasing incisions. Therefore, a longer incision is required to obtain the same exposure of the surgical field.

Envelope flaps are particularly indicated for concave surfaces, as for example the palatal side of the maxilla, or the lingual side of the mandible (3.25). The advantages are represented by easier suturing, and generally a reduced intraoperative bleeding.

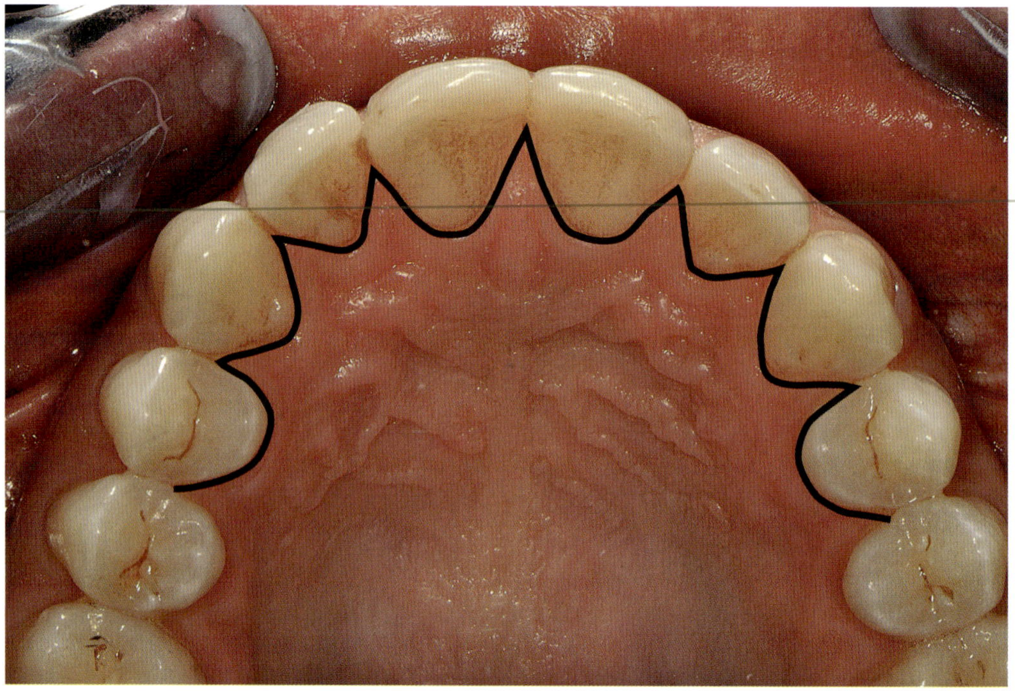

3.25 Marginal flap without releasing incisions.

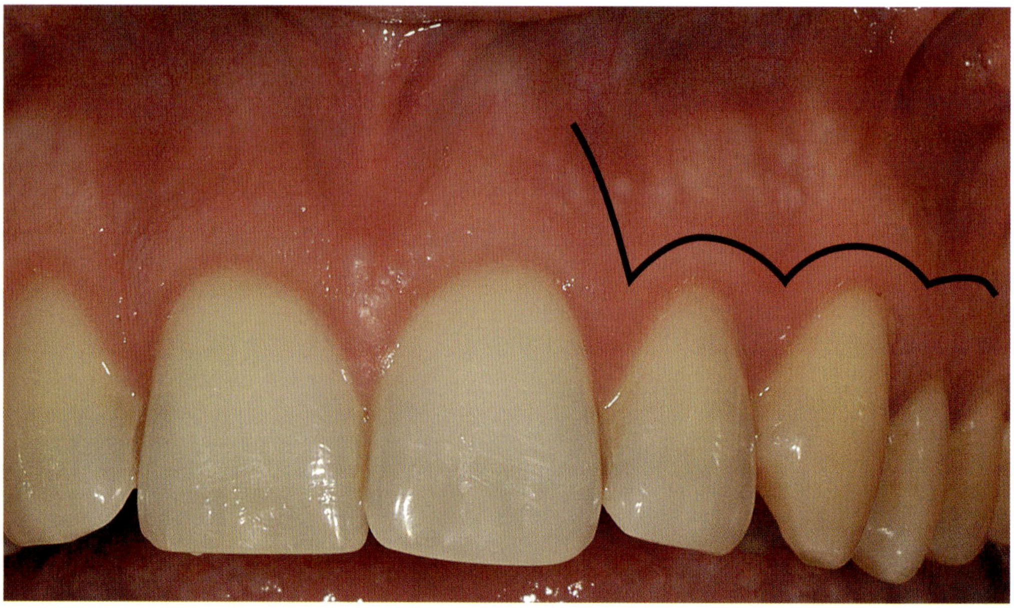

3.26 Three-corner submarginal flap (mesial releasing incision).

FLAPS WITH ONE RELEASING INCISION

These flaps are constituted by a linear incision associated with a single vertical releasing incision. The addition of the vertical releasing incision renders the retraction of these flaps easier, thus reducing the risk of soft tissue laceration. Since blood supply in the alveolar mucosa is guaranteed by arterial branches distributed in a mesial direction, the releasing incision should always be made mesially, and the angle between the main incision and the releasing incision should never be less than 90° to avoid ischaemia of the flap margin. In dentate patients, the releasing incision should never fall on the bisector of the interdental papillae, but rather mesially or distally (3.26).

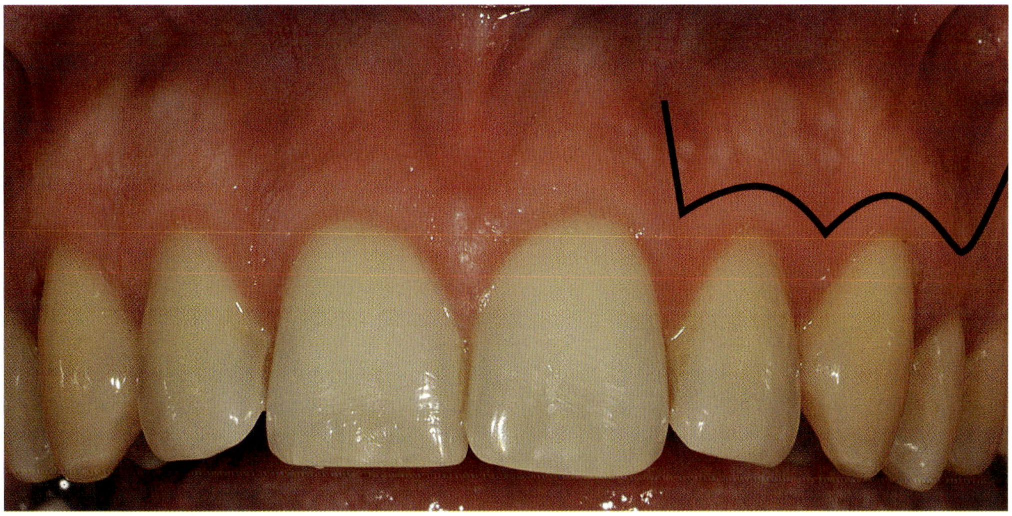

3.27 Four-corner submarginal flap.

The vertical releasing incision in the area of the mandibular premolars should never extend apically between the first and second premolar, to avoid damaging the mental nerve. The releasing incision can be made mesially to the first premolar or canine, with a mesial and apical inclination to obtain ample access to the surgical field. Moreover, releasing incisions must also be avoided on the palatal side of the maxilla, to avoid any damage to the major palatine neurovascular bundle.

FLAPS WITH TWO RELEASING INCISIONS

These flaps are constituted by a linear incision associated with mesial and distal releasing incisions, and offer the best view of the operating field and the easiest retraction. However, the blood supply is guaranteed only by the pedicle. As such, the principles described for flap preparation must always be respected to prevent partial or total flap necrosis. The angles between the main incision and the releasing incisions must measure no less than 90°, or must be obtuse (3.27).

SEMILUNAR FLAP

This flap is obtained with a single, arched incision with upper (in the maxilla) or lower (in the mandible) concavity. It is rarely used, but it may be indicated in treatment of a single tooth to remove a small periapical lesion and perform apicoectomy and retrograde endodontic treatment (3.28).

Preventing damages to important anatomic structures

Irrespective of the design of the access flap, it is mandatory that incisions be made each time at a safe distance from important anatomic structures. For example, a vertical releasing incision extending apically between the first and second mandibular premolar creates a high risk of damaging the mental nerve (3.29). As far as the maxilla is concerned, as mentioned earlier, palatal releasing incisions must be avoided to prevent damages to the major palatine neurovascular bundle.

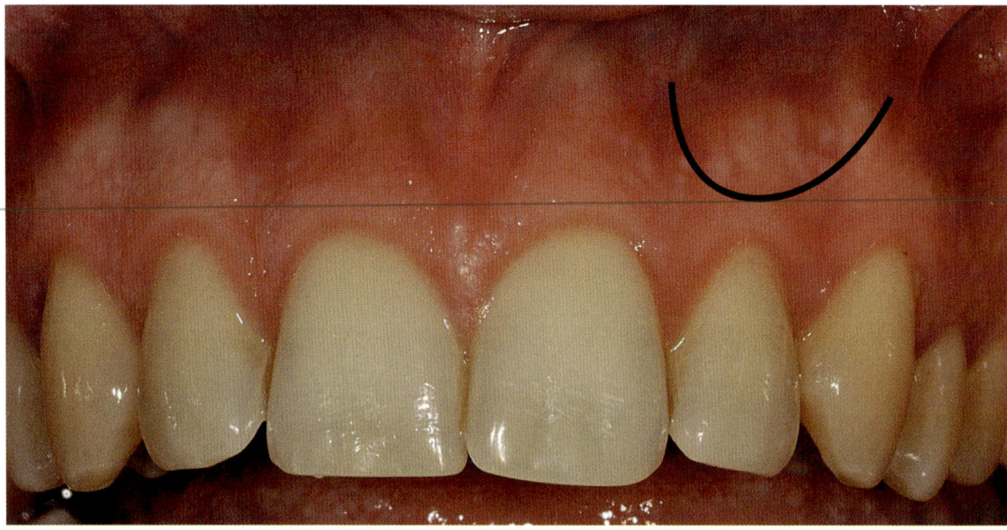

3.28 Semilunar flap.

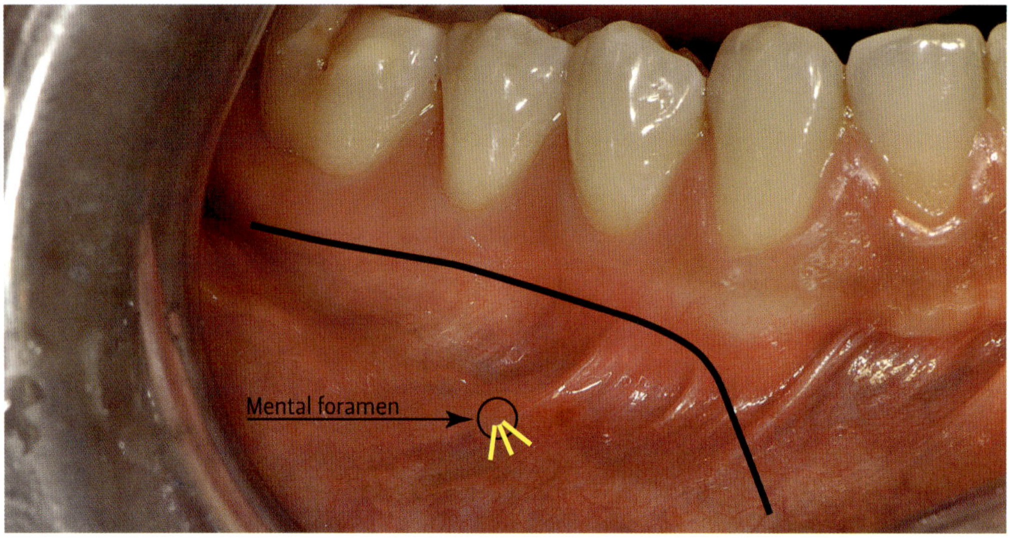

3.29 Correct positioning of the mesial releasing incision in the area of the mental foramen.

Preventing wound dehiscence

To prevent wound dehiscence (delayed spontaneous opening of the surgical wound) it is important to:

- suture the access flap over healthy and well vascularised tissues;
- perform a tension-free suture.

The first objective can be obtained by creating a flap wider than the underlying defect that is caused at the end of the surgical procedure (e.g. when endosseous lesions are enucleated, or an impacted tooth is extracted). An undersized flap may constrain to suture the access flap over a bony void, thus exposing to the risk of dehiscence due to the lack of flap support (3.30a-c).

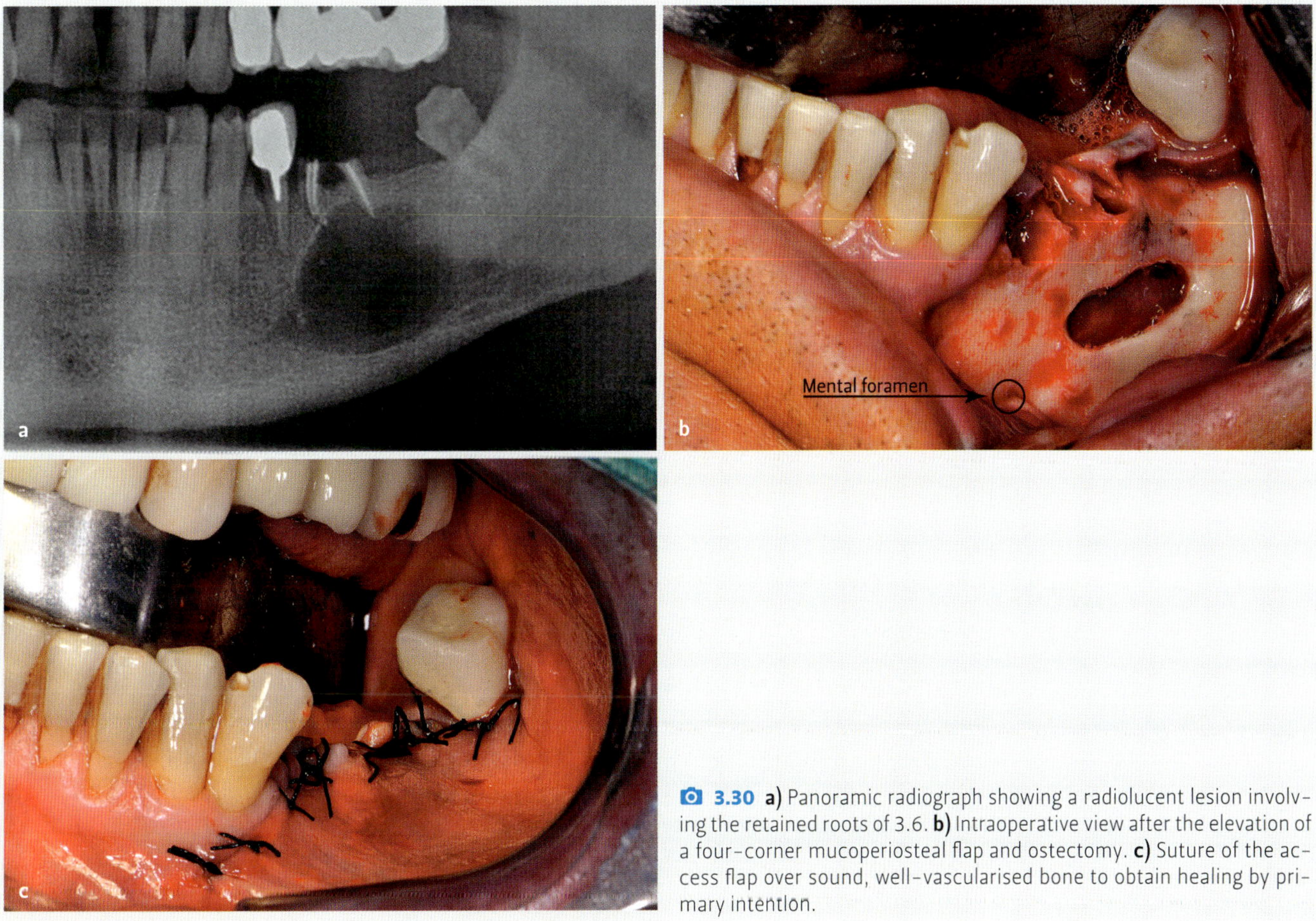

3.30 **a)** Panoramic radiograph showing a radiolucent lesion involving the retained roots of 3.6. **b)** Intraoperative view after the elevation of a four-corner mucoperiosteal flap and ostectomy. **c)** Suture of the access flap over sound, well-vascularised bone to obtain healing by primary intention.

The second objective is attained when the flaps are free to close without effort: this aspect is even more crucial when the volume of the underlying tissues is augmented (e.g. bone regeneration/reconstructions). The most effective method for obtaining a tension-free closure of the access flap is to perform periosteal releasing incisions. In fact, while the mucosal and submucosal tissues are stretchable, the periosteum is inextensible: a horizontal periosteal incision allows extension of the flap, to obtain a passive closure of the surgical access (3.31a-d).

Position of the incision relative to the gingival margin

Based on the position of the incision relative to the gingival crest, flaps can be classified into the following categories:

- marginal (intrasulcular) flaps, when the incision is made inside the gingival sulcus;
- submarginal flaps, when the incision is made at a variable distance from the gingival margin, either on the keratinised tissue or on the alveolar mucosa;
- crestal flap, when the incision is made on top of the alveolar ridge in edentulous areas.

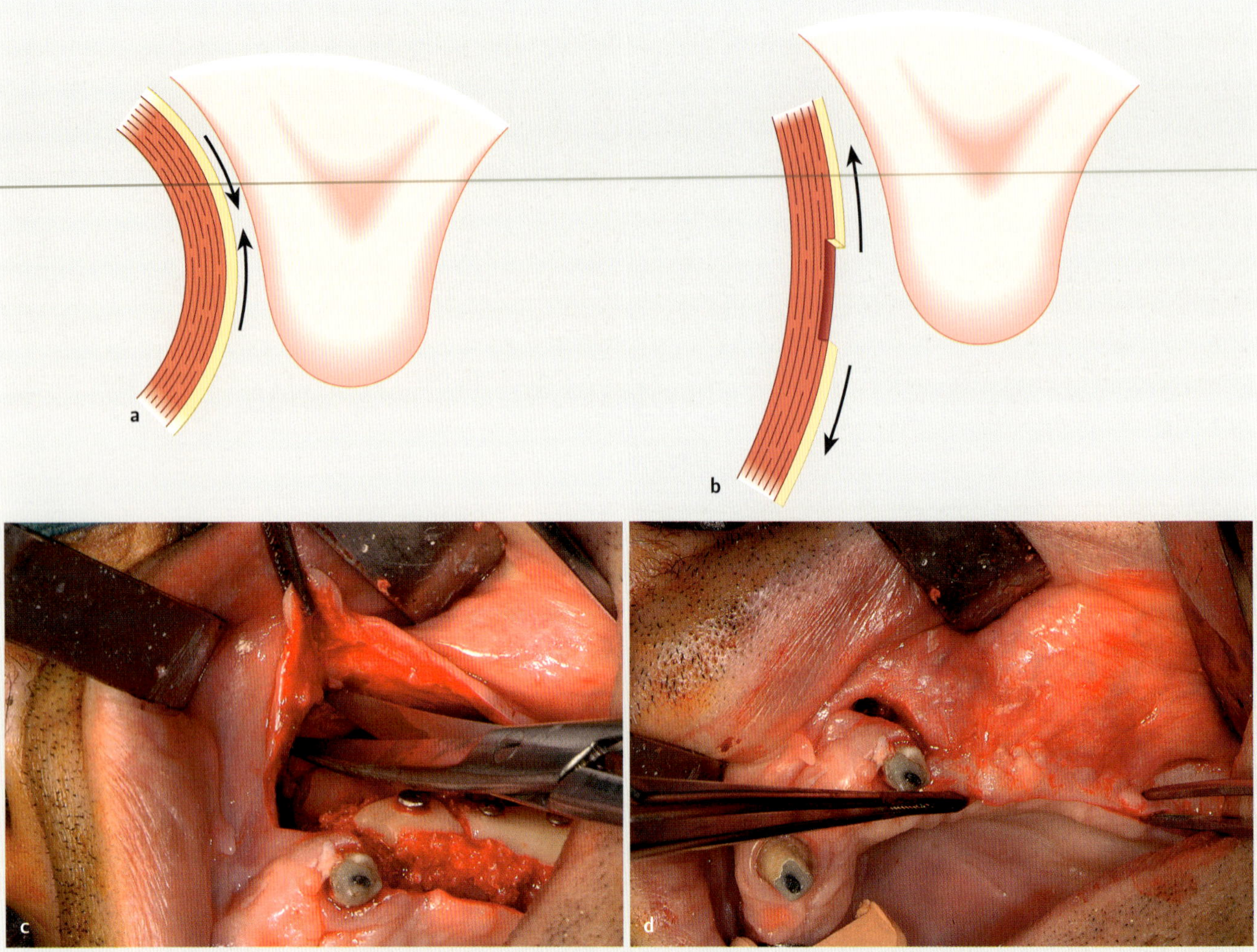

3.31 **a)** The flap, albeit adequately elevated, does not extend due to the inextensibility of the periosteum. **b)** Releasing incisions to interrupt the periosteum are made. **c)** Periosteal releasing incisions performed with dissecting scissors to obtain tension-free flap adaptation over a bone defect corrected by means of autogenous onlay grafts. **d)** Tension-free adaptation of the flap over the reconstructed alveolar ridge is verified.

MARGINAL FLAPS

In marginal flaps, the horizontal incision is made inside the gingival sulcus (3.32a). Therefore, the use of marginal flaps is indicated when exposure of the alveolar crest up to the neck of teeth is necessary. The main advantage is represented by the absence of visible scars, while the main disadvantage is represented by the interruption of the periodontal fibres around the teeth involved in the incision. This may cause, particularly in elderly patients and in teeth rehabilitated with fixed prostheses, gingival recession after wound healing.

SUBMARGINAL FLAPS

The horizontal incision is made outside of the gingival sulcus, either on the keratinised mucosa or on the alveolar mucosa (3.32b).

The distance of the incision from the gingival margin is dictated by different factors, such as the width of the keratinised tissue and the apico-coronal position of the underlying lesion.

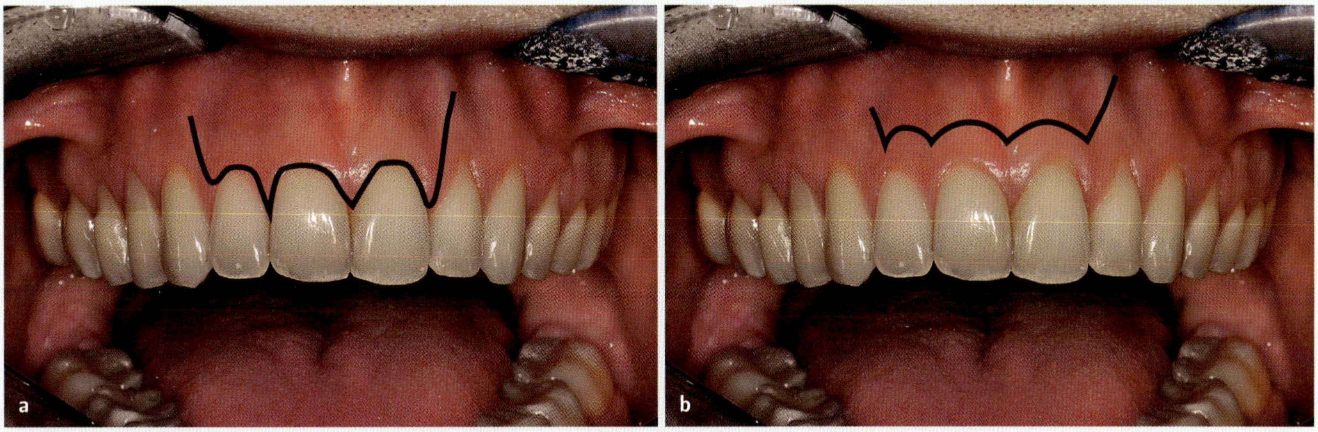

3.32 **a)** Marginal (intrasulcular) flap. **b)** Submarginal flap.

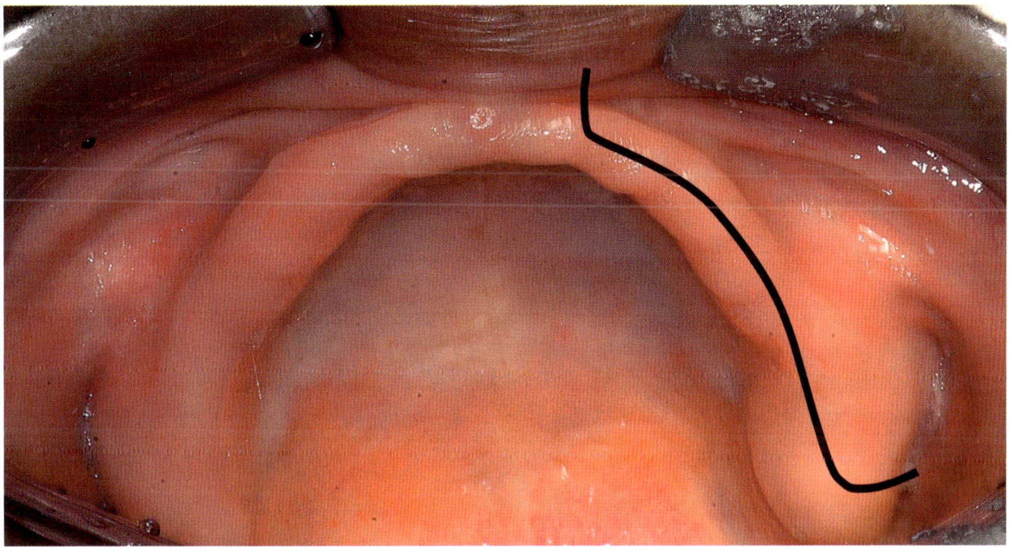

3.33 Crestal flap.

The advantages of making the incision on keratinised tissue are represented by the lower risk of visible scar formation and the higher resistance to traction compared to the alveolar mucosa, thus reducing the risk of wound dehiscence.

The recourse to incisions performed on the alveolar mucosa may be indicated for lesions developing far from the gingival margin in an apical direction.

CRESTAL FLAPS

In edentulous areas, the horizontal incision can be made on top of the alveolar ridge (3.33). This type of incision shares the same indications of intrasulcular incisions, and presents the advantage of simplifying the suture, which is generally performed on keratinised tissue that exhibits a higher resistance to traction and is therefore less prone to dehiscence.

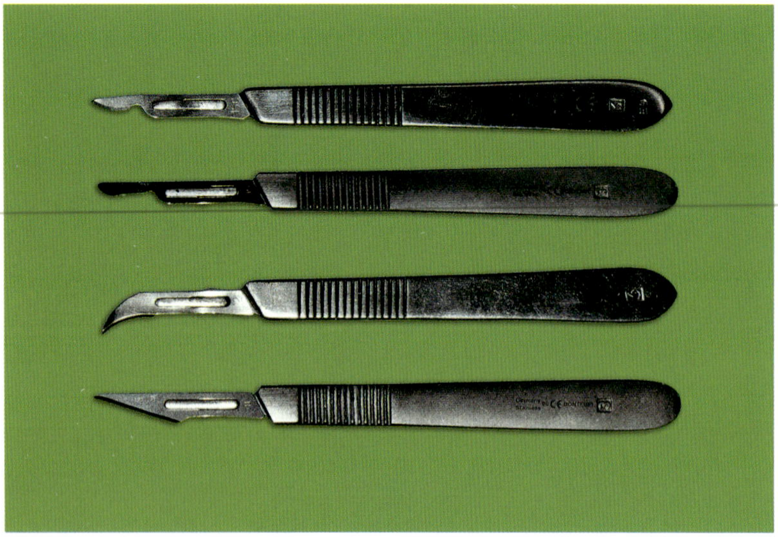

3.34 Scalpel handle and scalpel blades (top to bottom): No.15, No.15C, No.12, No.12.

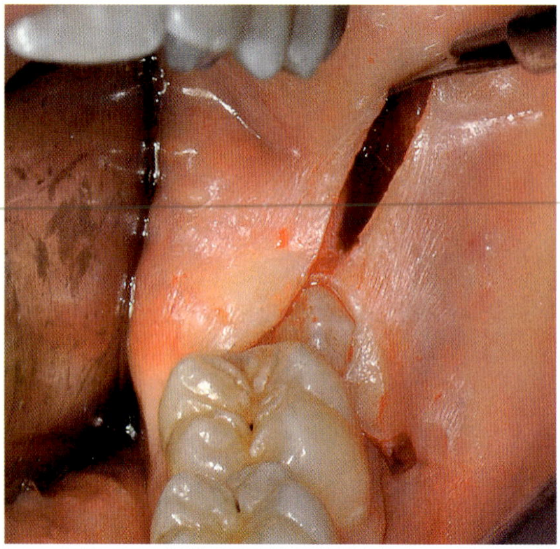

3.35 Correct incision technique: the scalpel blade is perpendicular to the soft tissues.

Surgical armamentarium for soft tissue incision

In the majority of cases, incisions are made with a No. 15 or 15C scalpel blade. For abscess drainage, the use of a No. 11 blade is indicated, while a No. 12 blade can be used for intrasulcular incisions on the lingual side of the mandible and the palatal side of the maxilla (3.34).

Whenever possible, it is preferable to incise the soft tissues over sound, well-vascularised bone: this precaution simplifies anatomic orientation and suture of the soft tissue at the end of the surgical procedure. The incision must be linear and continuous; conversely, an irregular or discontinuous incision can cause difficulties in the elevation and suture of the flap, as well as higher risks of flap necrosis and visible scar formation (3.35).

Flap elevation

Once incisions outlining the flap are made, the flap can be elevated. Elevation can be conducted along a subperiosteal or an epiperiosteal cleavage plane.

Subperiosteal flap elevation

Subperiosteal elevation corresponds to the elevation of a full-thickness (or mucoperiosteal) flap, which is typically used to expose the underlying bone. Periosteal elevators of different sizes and shapes can be used to separate the mucoperiosteal flap from the cortical bone (3.36a). The choice is mainly dictated by specific anatomic and surgical considerations, and also by personal preferences. Periosteal elevators can be either straight or curved, have a sharp or blunt edge, and numerous shapes and dimensions are available. During elevation, the free portion of the flap should be managed with the aid of anatomical or surgical pliers (3.36b), as it allows for better control of the soft tissues and over the tension that can be generated, thus reducing the risk of flap laceration. As blood vessels and nerves are found on an epiperiosteal plane (with the exception of the areas of the foramina), subperiosteal elevation generally protects from neurovascular lesions, facilitates creation of a well-vascularised flap with a high resistance to traction, and causes the reduction of intraoperative bleeding.

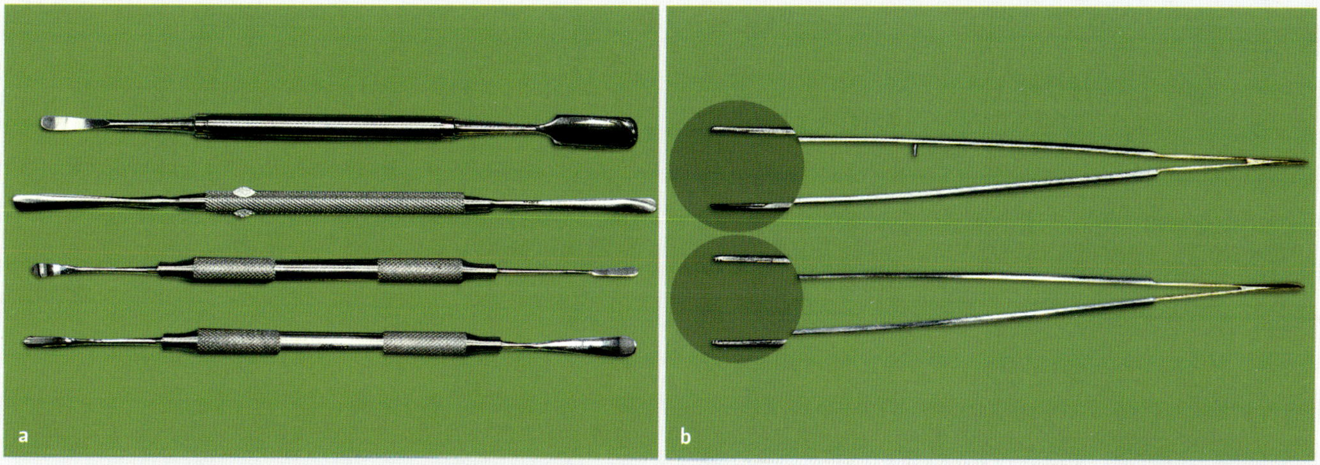

3.36 **a)** Periosteal elevators (different shapes and sizes). **b)** Surgical and anatomical pliers.

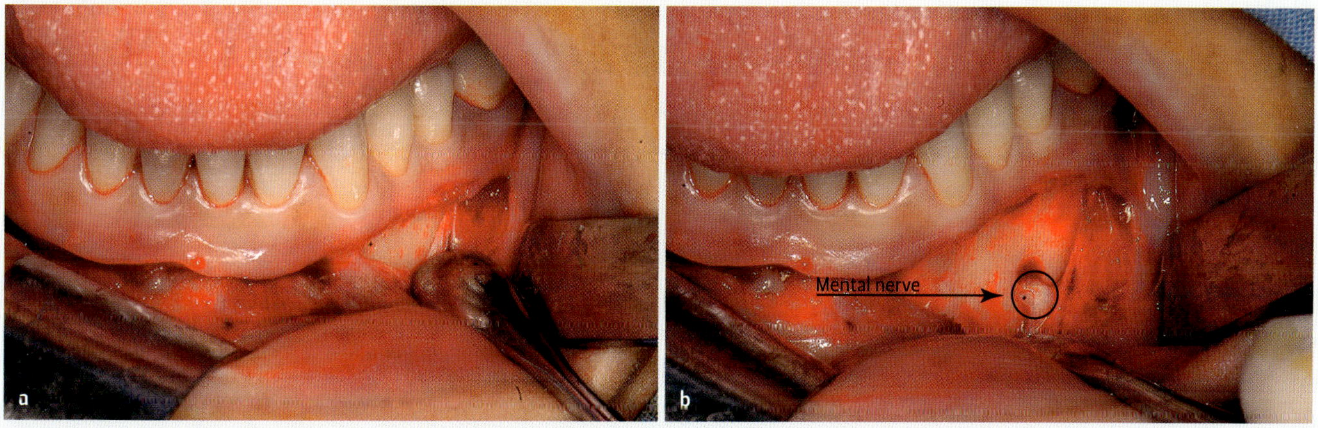

3.37 **a)** Elevation of a full-thickness submarginal flap in the anterior mandible. **b)** Identification of the mental foramen and the emergence of the mental nerve.

Superiosteal elevation should begin from the margins of the flap or from the interdental papillae, where soft tissues can be more easily reflected using the underlying bone as a supporting point (3.37a-b). If the cortical layer is eroded by an endosseous lesion (e.g. a cyst), the periosteum and the cystic wall can be adherent, thus risking penetration with the periosteal elevator inside the lesion. In these cases, elevation must begin far from the erosion where sound bone can be found, to facilitate progression towards the most critical area and allow an easier cleavage of the flap from the cystic wall.

Flap retraction

Once elevation of the soft tissues is completed, the flap must be retracted to allow adequate visibility and access to the surgical field. However, as the oral mucosa is relatively delicate, it should always be manipulated with care.

Excessive traction increases postoperative swelling and may cause flap laceration. A wide variety of retractors is available, and the choice is mainly dictated by specific anatomic and surgical considerations, including personal preferences.

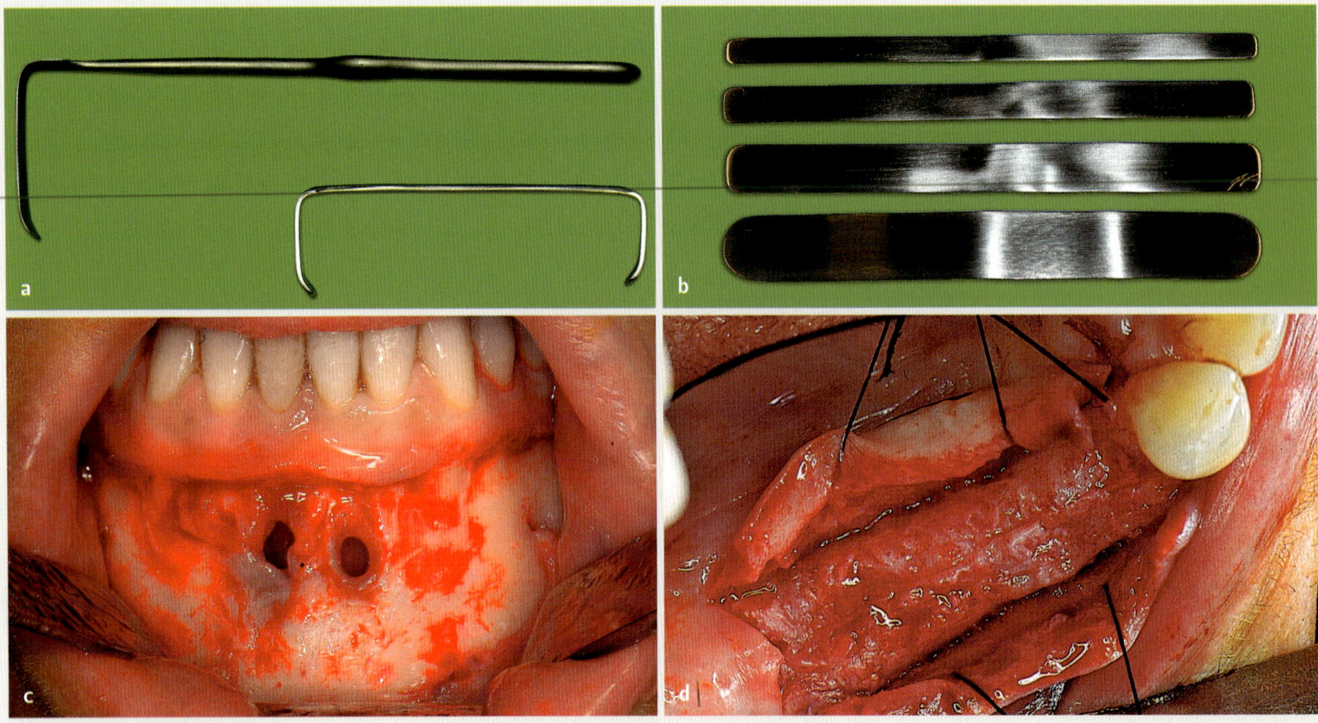

3.38 **a)** Langenbeck retractors for the posterior areas of the oral cavity, and Farabeuf retractors for the anterior areas. **b)** Malleable spatulas (different sizes and shapes). **c)** Example of adequate retraction and protection of the soft tissues on the buccal side of the anterior mandible. **d)** Flap retraction by means of sutures.

As a rule, longer retractors that can be used in the posterior areas of the maxilla and mandible are sufficient, with shorter retractors to manage flaps in the anterior areas (3.38a).

An alternative to commonly used retractors is represented by malleable spatulas. These instruments are made of thin, pliable surgical stainless steel, are available in different widths, and allow retraction and simultaneous protection of the soft tissues, particularly when important anatomic structures are at risk (3.38b). They can be used to retract and protect the soft tissues on the lingual side of the posterior mandible and avoid damages to the lingual nerve, or to retract and protect the soft tissues on the buccal side of the mandible and avoid damages to the facial artery and mental nerve (3.38c).

A simple and convenient method for flap retraction is represented by the use of sutures that can be tensioned using hemostatic forceps or interdental ligatures (3.38d).

Ostectomy

In the course of oral surgery procedures, the removal of a certain quantity of bone may be necessary to gain access to the area of intervention (e.g. for enucleation of an endosseous lesion, or extraction of an impacted tooth). This process, called ostectomy, should be conducted with extreme care, and with the aim to reduce trauma to the surrounding bone as much as possible. Three methods are generally used:

- ostectomy with manual instruments (chisels, bone rongeurs);
- ostectomy with rotary instruments;
- ostectomy with piezoelectric instruments.

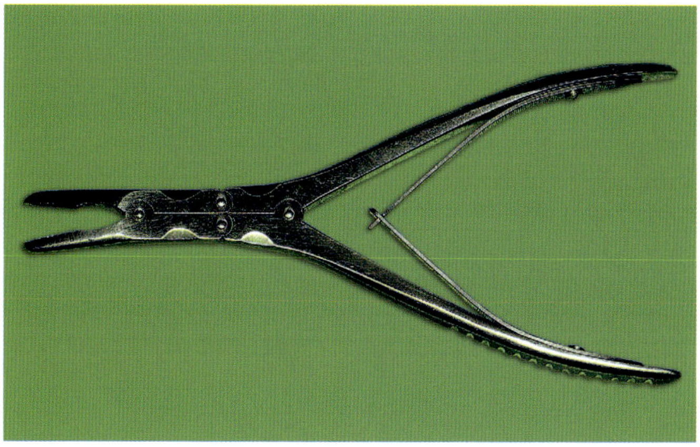

3.39 Bone rongeurs.

Ostectomy with manual instruments

This method is indicated when the cortical plate is thin (e.g. due to cyst expansion or erosion), or to even out the margins for ostectomy performed with rotary instruments (3.39).

Ostectomy with rotary instruments

This is the most frequently used method. Cooling is paramount, as bone cannot withstand thermal insults: if a temperature of 47°C is exceeded for more than one minute, bone necrosis may occur. To reduce friction and prevent uncontrolled temperature increases, slow-speed rotary instruments such as straight handpieces are used, mounted on surgical motors equipped with specific controls to set the adequate rotational speed; maximum speed must never exceed 40,000 rpm. Surgical burs must have good cutting capacity to allow delicate bone removal without excessive pressure being applied to the handpiece. During ostectomy, the bur and bone must receive adequate cooling by continuous irrigation with refrigerated (4-10°C) sterile saline. Specific peristaltic pumps, which are built into surgical motors, can provide irrigation when the bur is rotating, and offer the possibility of manually or automatically adjusting the coolant flow according to the rotational speed. However, disposable sterile syringes can also be used for irrigation whenever automatic systems are not available (3.40a-d). The use of high-speed rotary instruments, such as air turbines, is not recommended for oral surgery procedures, as they can cause the formation of submucosal or subcutaneous emphysema, and disperse bone fragments in the soft tissues.

Ostectomy with piezoelectric instruments

Piezoelectric surgery uses the ultrasonic (between 27 and 29 kHz) microvibration of dedicated metal inserts to perform ostectomy while leaving the soft tissues intact in case of accidental contact. This aspect has important implications in cases of neurovascular structures enclosed in the hard tissues, such as the inferior alveolar neurovascular bundle. Moreover, ostectomy inserts guarantee delicate and precise ostectomies due to their thinness, allowing better bone preservation. Furthermore, sterile saline used as a coolant exhibits a laminar flow along the insert, generating a physical phenomenon known as cavitation, which is characterised by the formation of bubbles at a very low pressure. When these bubbles implode, they cause an action of mechanical cleaning that reduces intraoperative bleeding (3.41).

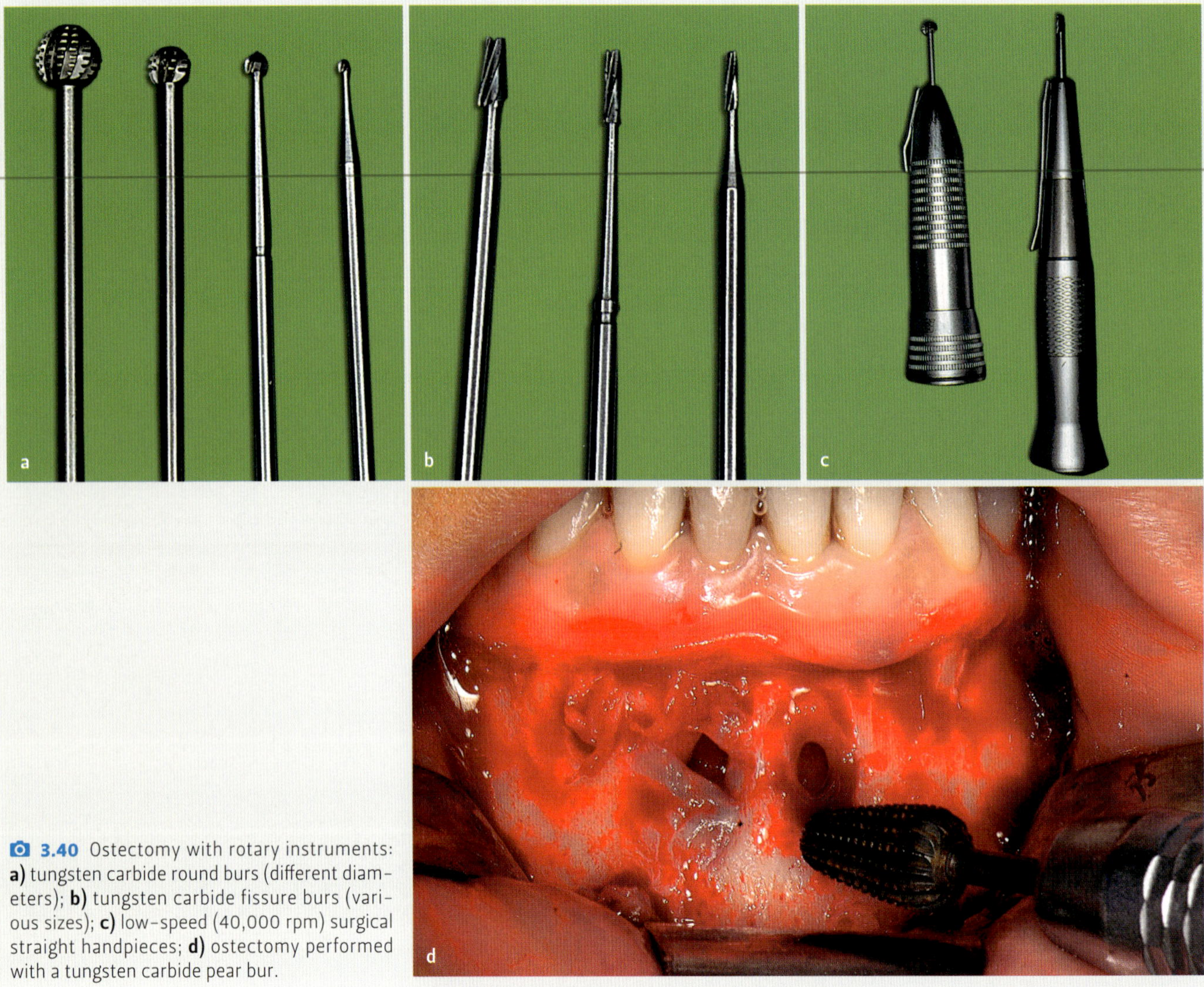

3.40 Ostectomy with rotary instruments: **a)** tungsten carbide round burs (different diameters); **b)** tungsten carbide fissure burs (various sizes); **c)** low-speed (40,000 rpm) surgical straight handpieces; **d)** ostectomy performed with a tungsten carbide pear bur.

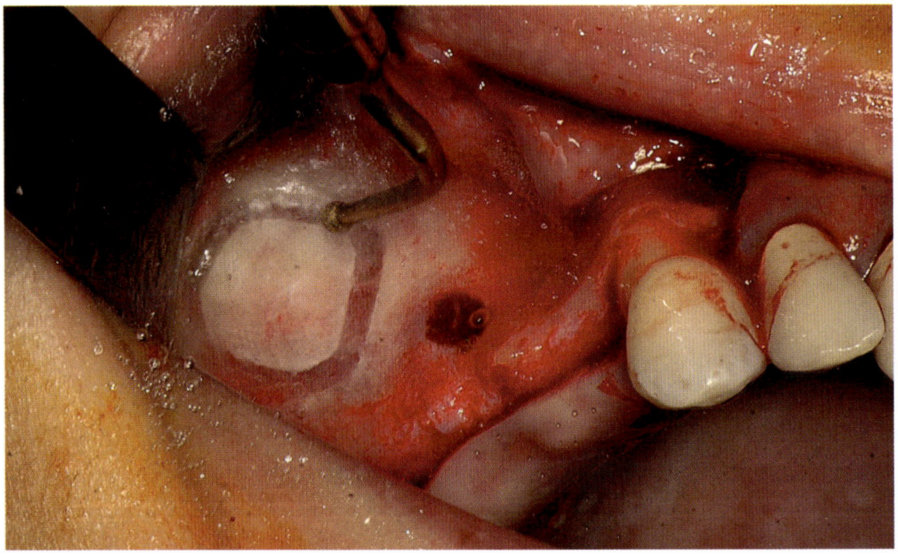

3.41 Ostectomy for the creation of a window on the lateral wall of the maxillary sinus is performed with piezoelectric instruments (diamond-coated round tip insert).

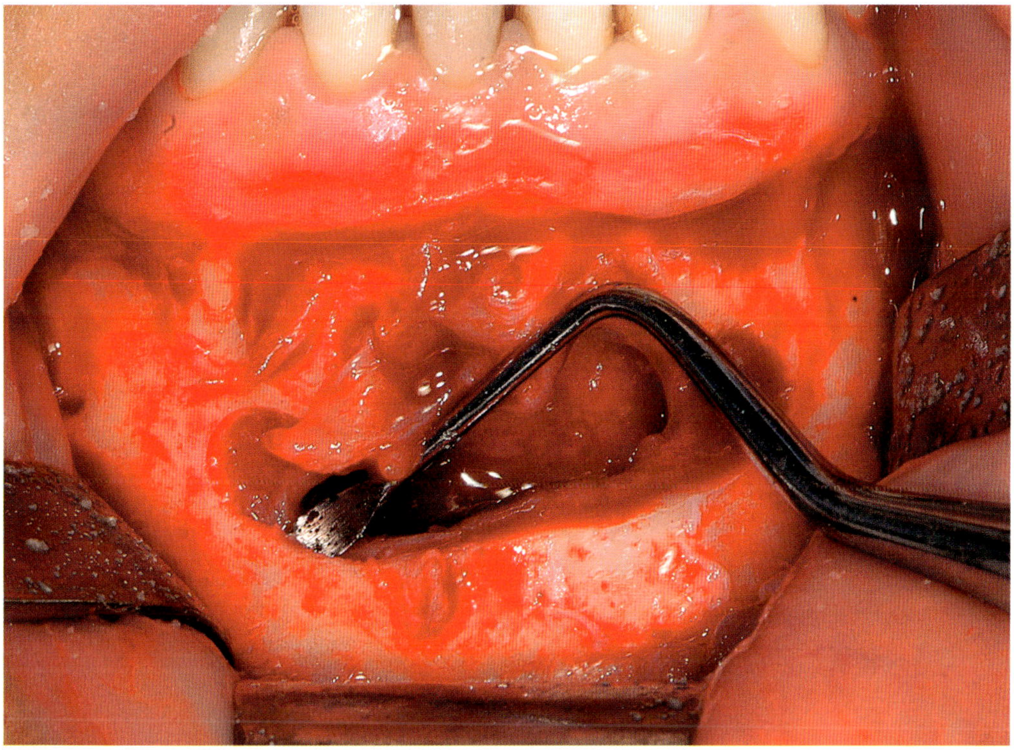

3.42 Revision of the cavity with a Lucas surgical curette after enucleation of an endosseous lesion.

Revision of the surgical field

A thorough revision of the surgical field is always recommended: surgical curettes or spoons may be used in association with sterile saline irrigation. This manoeuvre allows the area to be decontaminated, removes possible tissue remnants (e.g. tooth fragments), and reduces the bacterial load caused by contamination of the surgical field with oral fluids (3.42).

Haemostasis

Intraoperative bleeding always occurs during surgery. It represents a problem only if the haemorrhage is significant, as this may cause:

- reduced visibility;
- prolonged postoperative haemorrhage;
- formation of haematomas that represent an ideal culture media for the development of bacterial infections.

Conversely, the risk of severe complications such as hypovolemic shock due to profuse bleeding is rare in oral surgery, and it is always caused by evident technical errors involving arterial blood vessels such as the facial artery, the lingual artery, or the maxillary artery. The first and crucial precaution for preventing severe haemorrhage is represented by a detailed preoperative assessment aimed at excluding the presence of congenital or acquired coagulopathies, including those caused by drugs that interfere with platelet aggregation and blood coagulation (for details, see the specific section dedicated to the management of coagulopathic patients).

The second phase may be characterised by the use of vasoconstrictors in association with local anaesthetics, while the third phase includes intraoperative and postoperative manoeuvres to control bleeding.

The easiest method is compression of the bleeding area with a gauze swab soaked in sterile saline; the use of dry gauze is contraindicated as it absorbs blood, and once it is removed, the blood clot that has formed is removed with it. Compression should be exerted for at least 2 minutes, to allow coagulation. Typically, it is effective in cases of venous bleeding, or bleeding from small arterial vessels. Nonetheless, it also represents a fundamental operation during bipolar coagulation or ligature of arteries, allowing identification of the bleeding vessels (📷 3.43a-b).

When compression is insufficient to stop the haemorrhage, tamponade with resorbable haemostatic materials such as fibrin or collagen sponges and oxidised regenerated cellulose gauzes is indicated (📷 3.43c-d). Bone wax can also be used, except in close proximity to neurovascular bundles due to the risk of nerve compression.

These materials are particularly useful in cases of intraosseous bleeding (e.g. bleeding of the inferior alveolar artery), where bipolar coagulation is contraindicated due to the high risk of damaging adjacent nerves and when ligature of the bleeding vessels is impossible.

In cases of significant bleeding, diathermocoagulation can be used to manage the haemorrhage. Two methods are available:

- monopolar coagulation, whereby a single electrode transmits an electric current capable of creating a high temperature that causes local cautery of the involved tissues. The electrode should not be used directly, but positioned on hemostatic forceps blocking the bleeding vessel and acting as a conductor
- bipolar coagulation, whereby the tips of the dedicated forceps act as electric poles: an electric arc creates between the tips, and the clamped tissues are run through by the electric current and cauterised. The main advantage of bipolar coagulation is represented by the fact that the forceps act mechanically and electrically at the same time (📷 3.43e-g).

Diathermocoagulation must always be performed with great care in areas where nerve trunks are present to avoid damaging them irreversibly. As an example, attempts to control bleeding from the inferior alveolar artery with bipolar coagulation must never be made: compression and application of haemostatic materials should be performed instead.

In cases of severe bleeding, the most effective, albeit difficult, procedure is represented by the ligature of the bleeding vessel. Ligature is indicated for blood vessels with a relevant diameter, particularly arteries (e.g. the facial artery and its main branches) where compression and diathermocoagulation may prove ineffective. Ligature of the blood vessel can be performed before either sectioning it (when it interferes with the surgical manoeuvres) or when it is bleeding, upon prior clamping with hemostatic forceps (📷 3.43h-j). In the former case, the blood vessel must be identified, isolated and ligated with two non-absorbable or slowly absorbable sutures, while in the latter case the bleeding vessel must be located, clamped with hemostatic forceps 2-3 mm away from the interruption, and ligated just behind the hemostatic forceps.

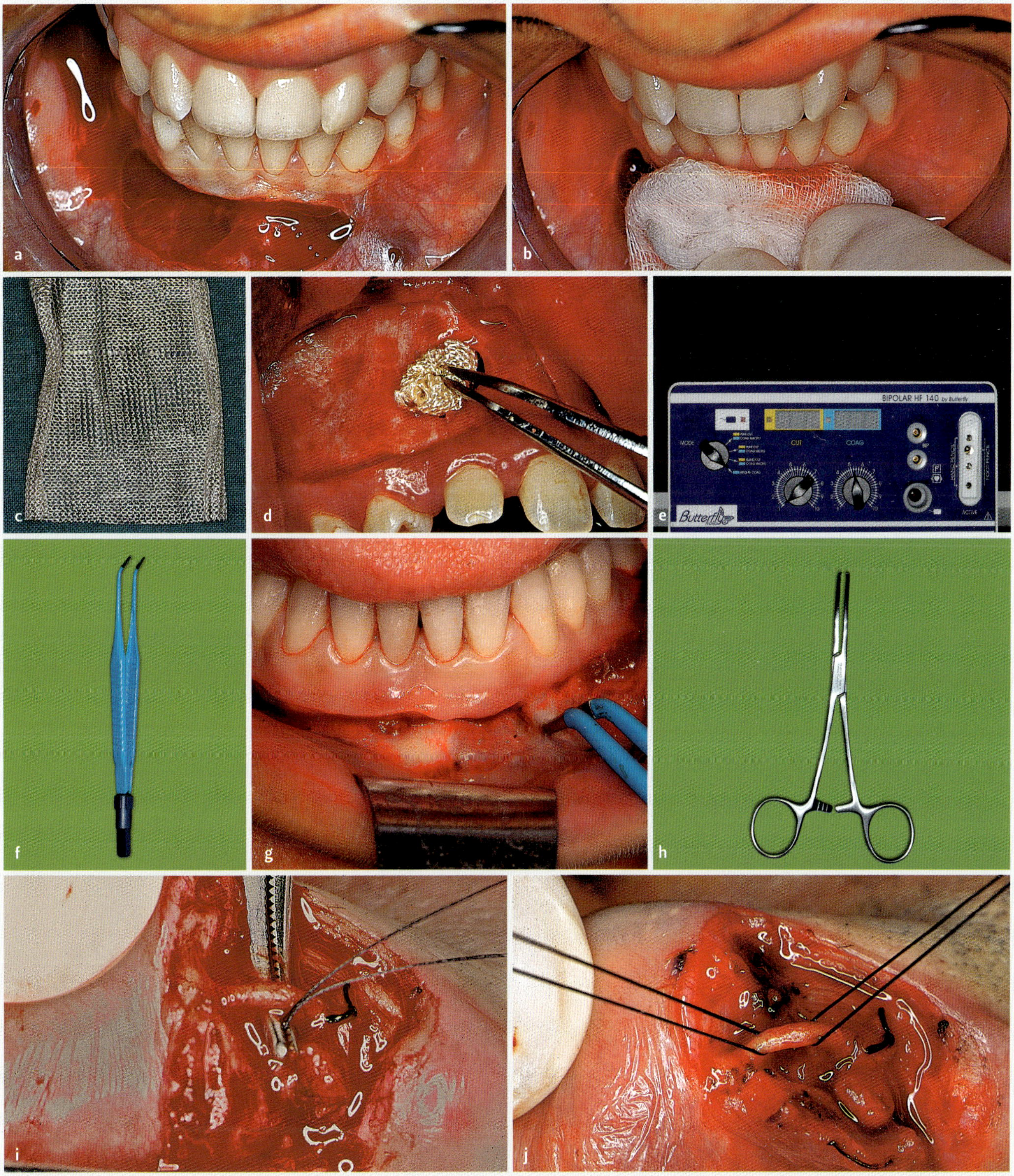

3.43 **a)** Intraoperative bleeding following incision of the soft tissues for the removal of an impacted mandibular canine. **b)** Compression with a sterile gauze swab soaked in sterile saline. **c)** Oxidised regenerated cellulose gauze. **d)** Haemostasis by means of compression with oxidised regenerated cellulose gauze. **e)** Electrosurgical unit for monopolar and bipolar coagulation. **f)** Bipolar coagulation forceps. **g)** Haemostasis by means of bipolar coagulation. **h)** Haemostatic forceps. **i)** Identification of the superior labial artery during the removal of an angioma of the lip. **j)** Suture loops for the ligature of the artery.

Suture

Suture of the access flap represents the final phase of surgery. Materials and techniques should be selected with the objective to optimising the healing process.

As far as materials are concerned, the following aspects of sutures should be evaluated:

- thread material and structure;
- thread diameter;
- needle shape and radius;
- needle body and tip.

SUTURE THREAD

Surgical sutures can be classified as absorbable or non-absorbable.

Absorbable sutures: they are generally for deep sutures (periosteum, muscle, submucosal tissues, and subcutaneous tissues). However, they can also be used to suture mucoperiosteal flaps in various situations, for instance when access to the sutured wound is difficult, or when odontophobic and non-cooperative patients are treated.

Resorbable sutures are made of either natural materials (e.g. small intestines of bovines, ovines, swines, and equines) like catgut, or synthetic materials (e.g. polylactic-polyglycolic acid or PLGA); each thread has peculiar characteristics as far as tensile strength and resorption time are concerned.

The choice between different sutures should be made not only according to personal preferences, but also primarily according to the importance of effectively keeping the tissues united until complete formation of a traction-resistant scar.

Absorbable sutures are more reactive than non-absorbable sutures: they can actually cause a local inflammatory reaction that may retard wound healing.

Non-absorbable sutures are made of either natural or synthetic materials. Among the first, the most widely used is silk which has good mechanical properties (tensile strength, knot strength), high elasticity, flexibility, and ease of use. The latter include nylon, polypropylene, polyester, and expanded polytetrafluoroethylene (e-PTFE), which reduce the risk of local inflammatory reaction, but exhibit lower knot strength. When avoiding local inflammatory reactions is paramount, the use of nylon and polypropylene monofilaments is recommended.

THREAD STRUCTURE

As far as the structure is concerned, sutures can be monofilament or braided (3.44a).

Braided sutures: braided sutures, such as silk and polyester, are more resistant than monofilaments, but they are also more abrasive on the soft tissues, and more prone to bacterial contamination.

To reduce the permeability, and thus the susceptibility to contamination, of braided sutures, the use of different coating materials (wax, polymers) has been introduced.

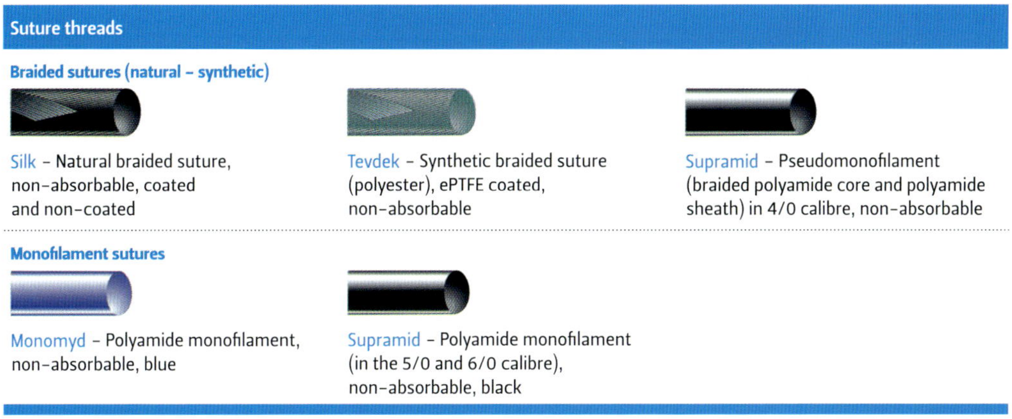

3.44a Different types of suture threads.

Monofilament sutures: monofilament threads, such as nylon and polypropylene, present opposite characteristics; in fact, they pass through the soft tissues without any friction, and they do not absorb the oral fluids or favour plaque deposition. However, they are more rigid and they can be a source of discomfort for the patients, particularly those exceeding 4/0 in diameter.

THREAD DIAMETER

Suture threads are available in different diameters, generally expressed in fractions of a millimetre. According to the international codification, this metric measurement is converted to a corresponding number of zeros that increases as the diameter of the thread decreases: for example, a 2/0 classification corresponds to a 0.3 mm diameter of the thread, and a 4/0 classification corresponds to a 0.15 mm diameter of the thread. In oral surgery, the use of small diameter sutures is indicated. Generally speaking, sutures ranging from 4/0 to 6/0 should be used.

The use of thinner threads exposes the patient to a lower risk of wound contamination and is generally associated with the formation of less visible scars, while on the other hand they have lower resistance to traction. However, as previously mentioned, the access flaps should always be closed with tension-free sutures. Therefore, thinner sutures should be sufficient to obtain adequate closure of the surgical wound. The use of thicker sutures is indicated only for the ligature of arterial vessels, for which a thread guaranteeing good knot strength should always be chosen.

NEEDLE SHAPE AND RADIUS

Needles are generally made of stainless steel. In the case of atraumatic sutures, the needle and thread are coupled according to their diameters. Small diameter needles are less traumatic, but more fragile.

Needles are available in different shapes and curvatures (1/4 circle, 3/8 circle, 1/2 circle, 5/8 circle): a pronounced curvature simplifies superficial soft tissue sutures, while a reduced curvature is more often indicated for interdental sutures (3.44b).

Atraumatic sutures: needles

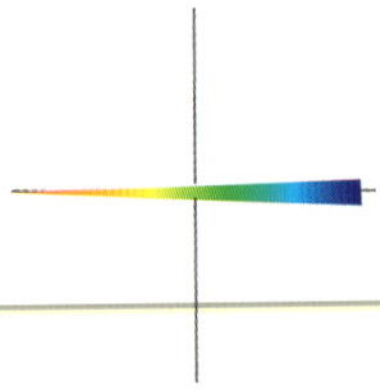	**Straight needle**	Use: cutaneous and intestinal sutures
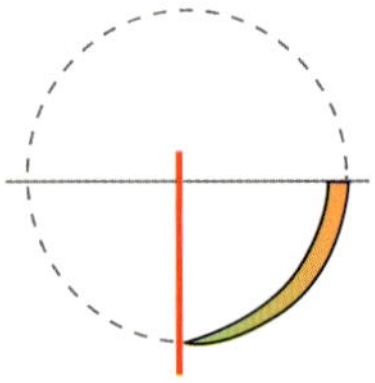	**1/4 circle needle**	Use: ophthalmic surgery, muscle repair
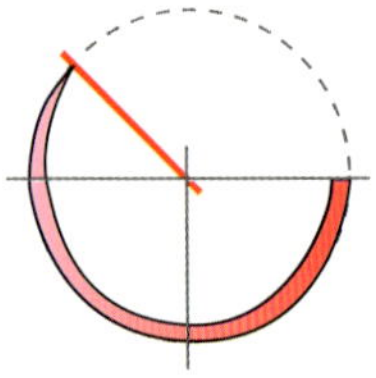	**5/8 circle needle**	Use: urology surgery
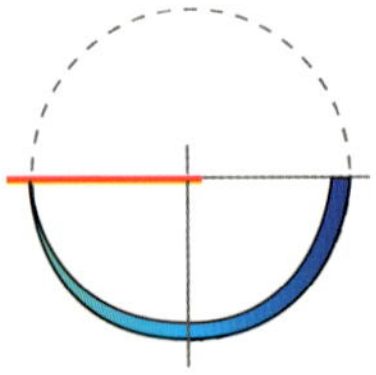	**1/2 circle needle**	Use: general surgery, oral surgery, maxillofacial surgery, gynaecological surgery, cardiovascular surgery
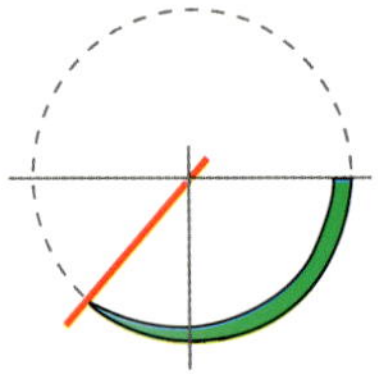	**3/8 circle needle**	Use: sutures of the skin and mucosa

3.44b Different needle curvatures.

NEEDLE TIP GEOMETRY

Needle tips have different tip geometry: in general, the first distinction is between needle tips with a round profile (atraumatic) and needle tips with a triangular profile (cutting). Needle tips with a round profile are less traumatic but penetration through the soft tissues is more difficult, particularly in the case of thick, keratinised mucosa; needle tips with a triangular profile have opposite characteristics.

The choice of needle tip geometry is mainly dictated by personal preferences. Nevertheless, round needle tips should generally be preferred when suturing thin or fragile tissues (3.44c).

Taper point (round)		
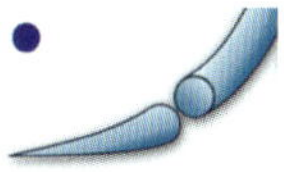	Used to suture thin soft tissues	Pros: does not cause lacerations in fragile soft tissues Cons: low penetration capacity in thicker tissues; as a result, the needle may bend or rotate
Reverse cutting		
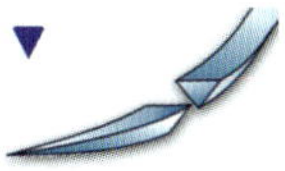	Used to suture soft tissues of different consistency	Pros: excellent penetration capacity Cons: can cause lacerations when suturing thin soft tissues
Taper cutting		
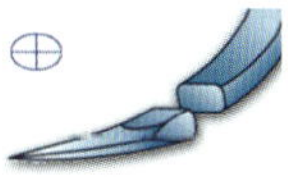	The tip has a square (or rectangular) pyramid profile with cutting edges	Pros: good penetration capacity, reduced trauma Cons: lower penetration capacity compared to reverse cutting needles, higher cost
Micro point reverse cutting		
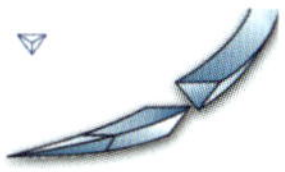	Sharp micro cutting tip, generally used in periodontal and muco-gingival plastic surgery	Pros: excellent penetration capacity and precision Cons: cost

3.44c Different needle tip profiles.

Suture removal

Intraoral sutures are generally kept in place for 6-8 days, but in specific cases they can be kept in place for 10-14 days (e.g. in the case of reconstructive/regenerative surgery). Conversely, extraoral sutures are kept in place for a shorter period (4-5 days). This precaution, along with the use of thin monofilaments, is aimed at reducing the risk of visible scar formation. Simple running (continuous) and interrupted sutures, as well as mattress sutures, are removed by tensioning the knot with anatomic pliers and cutting only one end of the thread loop under the knot itself with fine point scissors.

Subcuticular sutures are generally removed 2-3 weeks after surgery; a delicate, but firm and steady traction is exerted on one end of the suture.

Suturing techniques

The soft tissues and needle are manipulated using surgical pliers and a needle holder, respectively. For greater needle control and a correct penetration of the needle through the soft tissues, the needle should be firmly held at the distal portion of the body (ideally, three quarters of the distance from the tip), and perpendicularly to the needle-holder (3.45a-b).

The choice of the most appropriate suturing technique is essential to quick healing and a correct restoration of the soft tissues morphology. The knowledge and mastery of the different suturing techniques are fundamental to dealing with all clinical situations. Sutures are defined as everting when the margins of the flap, after the knot is tied, are everted, while they are defined as plane when the margins of the flap are juxtaposed in their original position (3.46a-d). It is worth remembering that everting sutures should be used when increasing the contact surface between the two sides of the access flap and obtaining a watertight closure of the surgical wound is necessary, as in the case of bone reconstruction/regeneration. Inverting sutures are never used in oral surgery (3.46d). Suture strength is caused by knot strength: when sutures providing good knot strength (e.g. silk) are used, three throws (two clockwise, the last counter-clockwise) are sufficient to tie a stable knot, while when sutures such as synthetic monofilaments (e.g. nylon) are used, four or five throws (alternating between clockwise and counter-clockwise) are recommended.

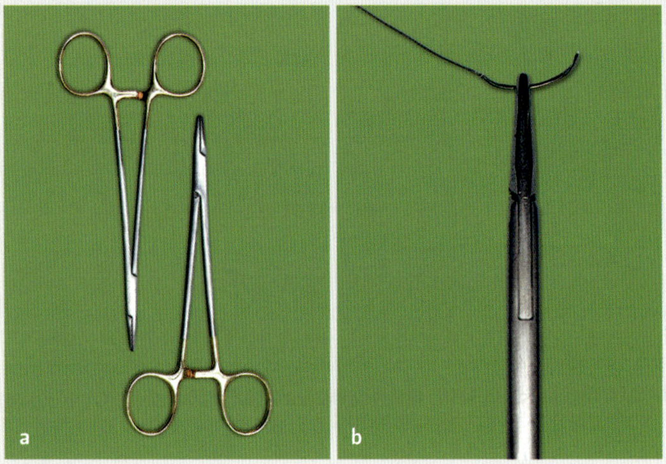

3.45 a) Different needle holders. **b)** Correct way to grasp the needle between the needle holder jaws.

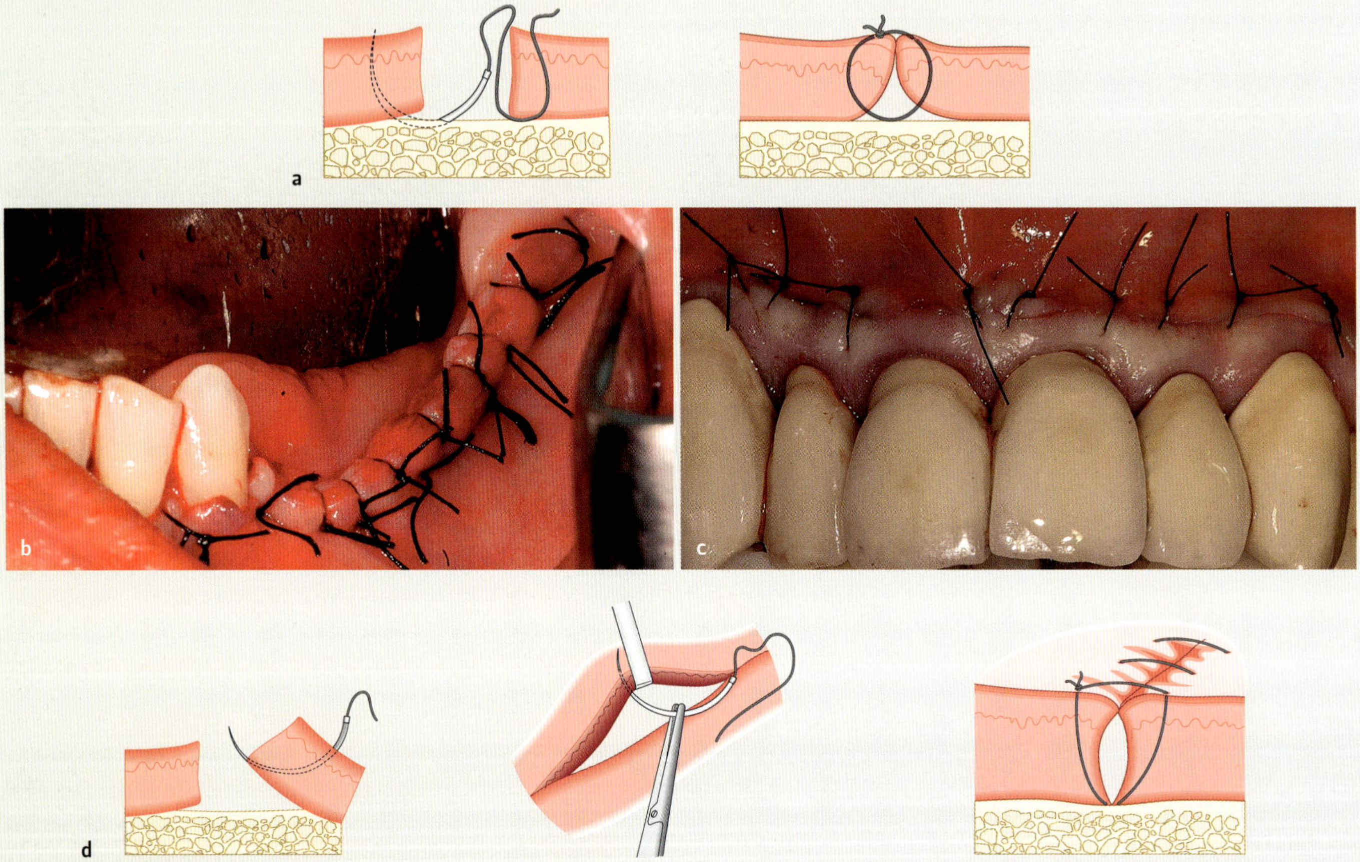

3.46 a–b) Example of everting suture. **c)** Example of plane suture. **d)** Example of inverting suture.

Simple interrupted suture

This is the most commonly used suture in oral surgery: it is indicated to close surgical wounds over sound, well-vascularised tissues, and when impermeability of the suture is important but not essential (e.g. after the extraction of erupted or impacted teeth or the enucleation of endosseous lesions) (3.47a–h).

Horizontal mattress suture ("U" suture)

This suture is particularly indicated when an airtight closure of the surgical wound is mandatory (e.g. bone reconstructive/regenerative surgery), or when the access flap cannot be sutured over sound, well-vascularised tissues (e.g. closure of oroantral fistulas). It is frequently used in periodontal surgery (3.48a–d).

Vertical mattress suture

The recourse to vertical mattress sutures is indicated when compression of the soft tissues is necessary. This type of suture is widely used in periodontal surgery, as it allows not only the interdental papillae to be adequately repositioned, but also firmly compressed against the underlying bone (3.49a–d).

Simple running (continuous) suture

This suture is typically indicated for single, linear incisions: it allows for quicker closure of the surgical wound, but in cases of knot failure, the entire suture is compromised (3.50a–e).

Subcuticular suture

In cases of surgical wounds or lacerations of the skin, to reduce the risk of visible scar formation, subcuticular sutures can be used. A subcuticular suture is a buried form of a running horizontal mattress suture; it is placed by taking horizontal bites through the papillary dermis on alternating sides of the wound. The simple tension applied at both ends of the thread is sufficient to keep the margins of the wound juxtaposed without the need for tying knots.

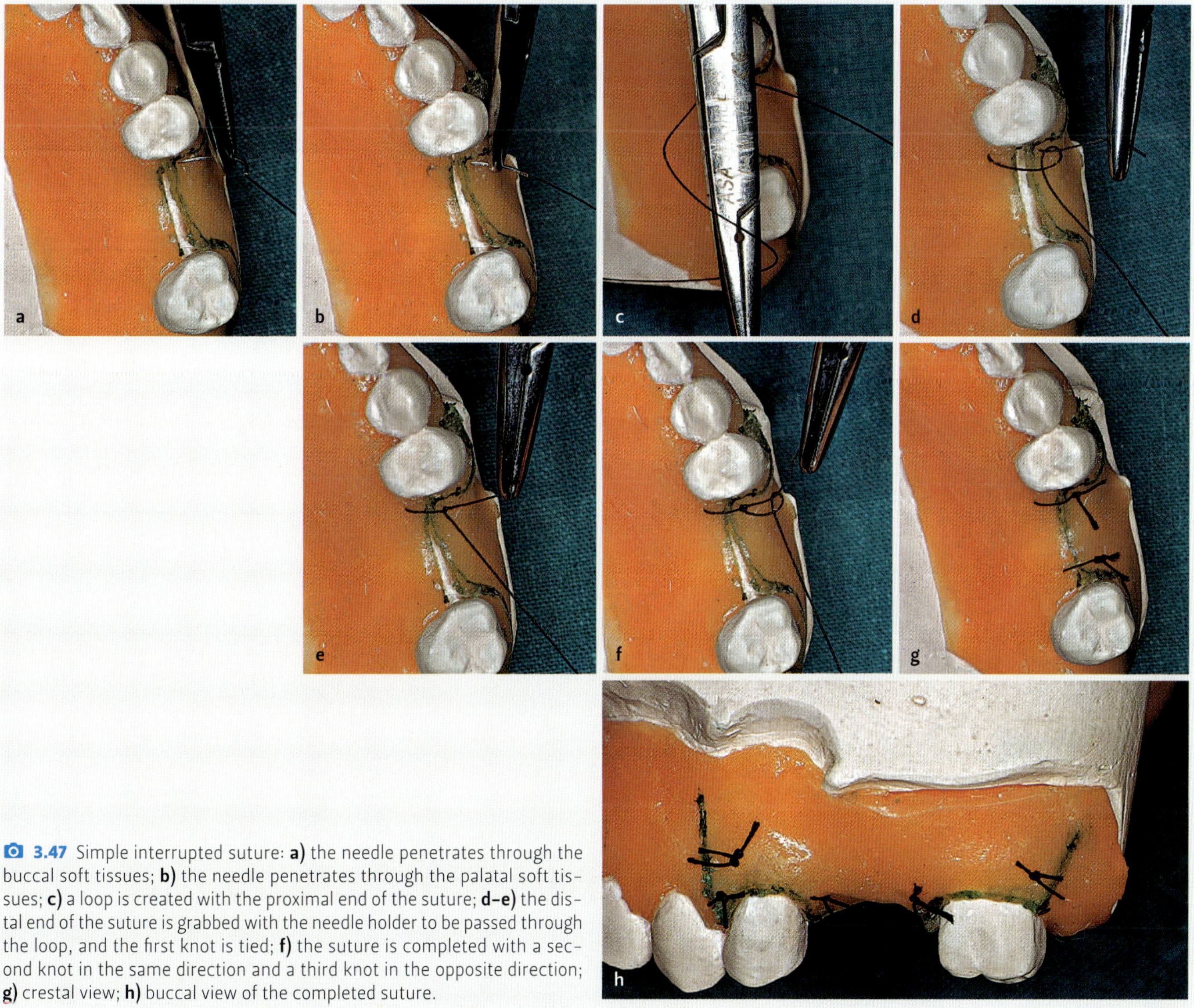

3.47 Simple interrupted suture: **a)** the needle penetrates through the buccal soft tissues; **b)** the needle penetrates through the palatal soft tissues; **c)** a loop is created with the proximal end of the suture; **d–e)** the distal end of the suture is grabbed with the needle holder to be passed through the loop, and the first knot is tied; **f)** the suture is completed with a second knot in the same direction and a third knot in the opposite direction; **g)** crestal view; **h)** buccal view of the completed suture.

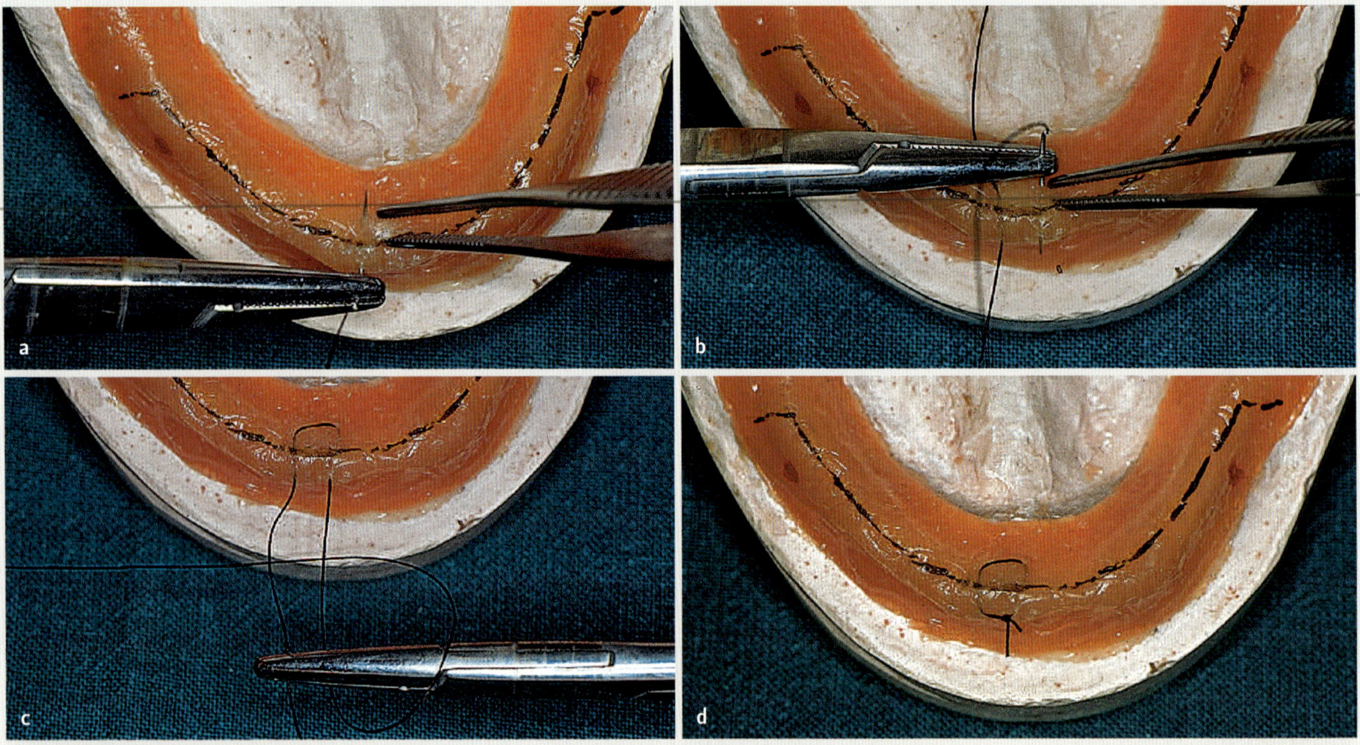

3.48 Horizontal mattress suture: **a)** the needle penetrates in the same way as for an interrupted suture; **b)** after passing through the lingual soft tissues, the needle penetrates again the lingual and then the buccal side of the flap a few millimetres laterally; **c)** first knot; **d)** the completed suture.

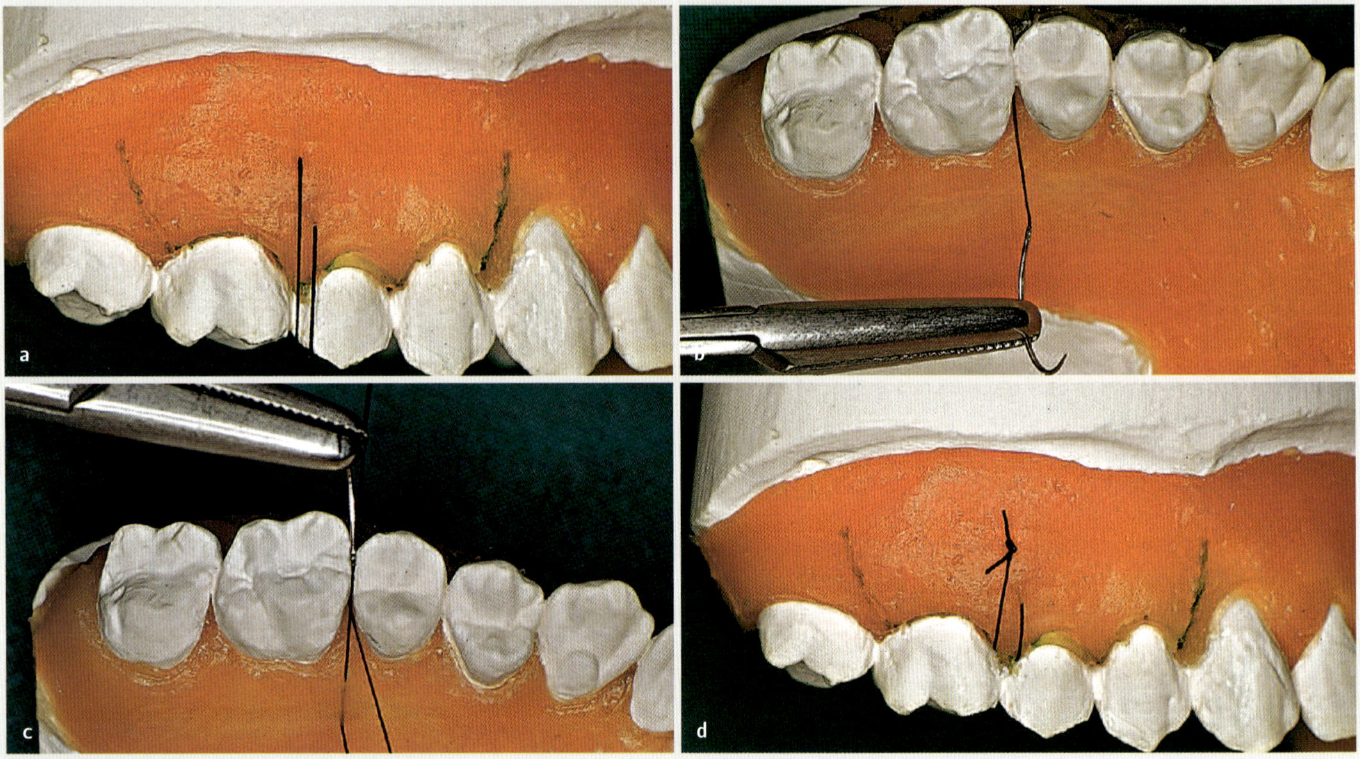

3.49 Vertical mattress suture: **a)** the needle penetrates and exits the buccal side of the flap (full-thickness); **b)** the suture is passed through the interdental space; **c)** the same manoeuvre is performed on the palatal side; **d)** the suture is brought back through the interdental space, three knots are tied and the suture is completed: the suture keeps the soft tissues (particularly the papilla) compressed over the underlying bone. The horizontal mattress suture is similar, the only difference being the direction of the needle as it penetrates the soft tissues.

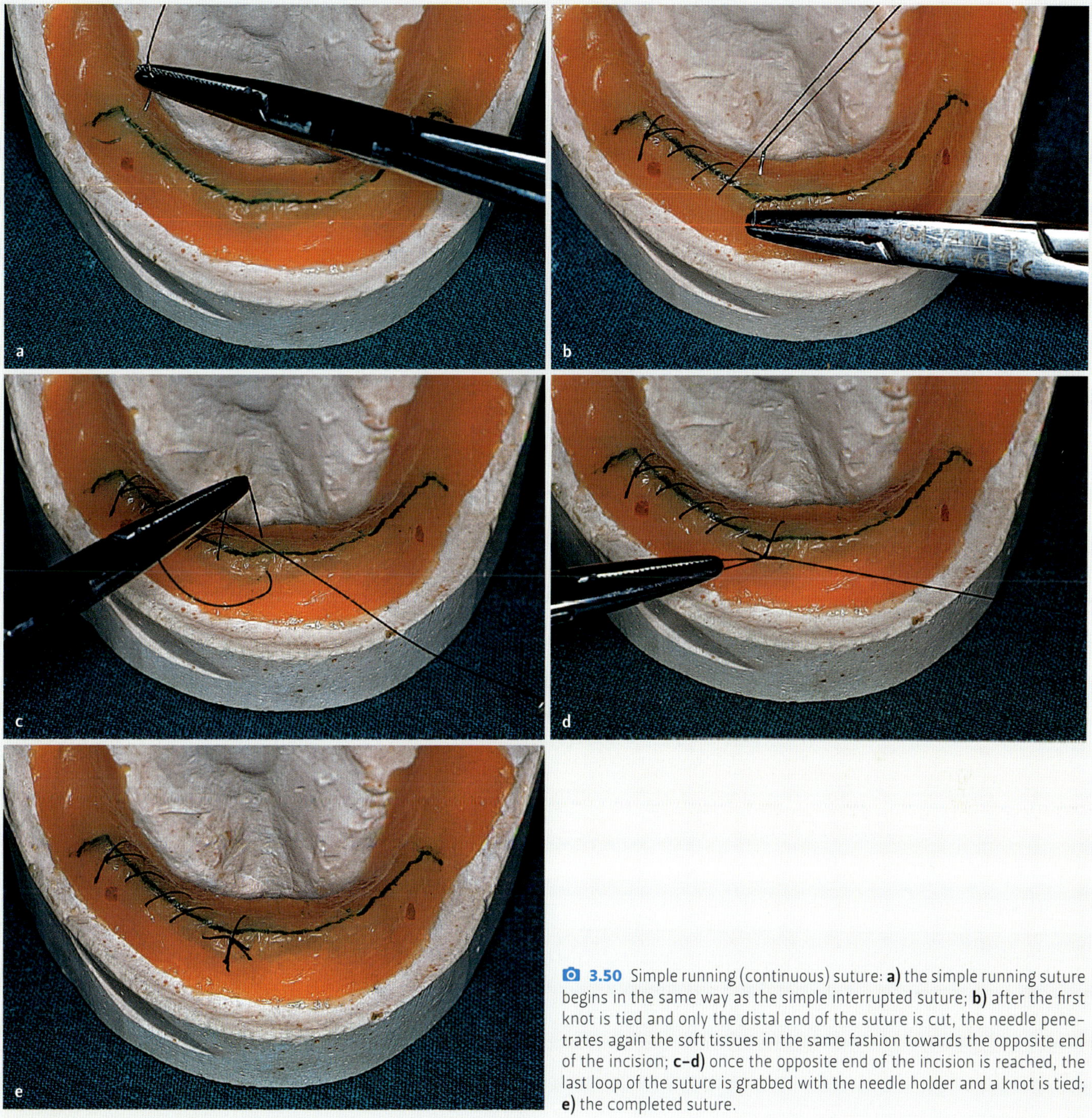

3.50 Simple running (continuous) suture: **a)** the simple running suture begins in the same way as the simple interrupted suture; **b)** after the first knot is tied and only the distal end of the suture is cut, the needle penetrates again the soft tissues in the same fashion towards the opposite end of the incision; **c–d)** once the opposite end of the incision is reached, the last loop of the suture is grabbed with the needle holder and a knot is tied; **e)** the completed suture.

Techniques for the incision and dissection of the soft tissues

As previously mentioned, the general rules described for prevention of ischaemia, soft tissue laceration, damages to important anatomic structures, and wound dehiscence apply also to surgical interventions involving only the soft tissues. However, some differences exist, particularly regarding incision, dissection, and elevation of the dissection planes.

Incision

Incisions should be made considering the absence of fixed reference planes such as bone. Therefore, a thorough knowledge of the thickness of the superficial tissues, the location of the lesion, and the local anatomy is essential. Manipulation must always be delicate, particularly when the lesion is located immediately below the mucosa (e.g. cysts of the minor salivary glands).

In cases of sessile or pedicled lesions (e.g. traumatic fibromas), a diamond-shaped excision is generally performed, as it allows for complete removal of the lesion with predetermined safety margins (📷 3.51a-b).

Conversely, in the case of submucosal lesions linear incisions are used: these should be made parallel with Borge's lines (relaxed skin tension lines) to reduce the risk of visible scar formation (📷 3.51c-d).

Elevation of the surgical flap

Due to the lack of a fixed reference plane, once the mucosal layer in incised with a scalpel the elevation of the superficial tissues should be performed by blunt dissection. With specifically designed scissors, the reverse of a cutting motion is used, starting with the scissor blades closed and gradually opening them, so that the working parts are the external (blunt) edges of the blades (📷 3.51 e-g).

Epiperiosteal elevation or dissection

Epiperiosteal elevation or dissection allows a mucosal flap to be raised, while leaving the periosteum untouched. This is needed to create an adequate recipient bed for free soft tissue grafts (e.g. keratinised mucosa graft) that can be used to correct soft tissue deficiencies affecting natural dentition, or to restore the anatomy of the soft tissues and buccal vestibule when used in association with vestibuloplasty after bone reconstruction procedures. Epiperiosteal dissection is also indicated in cases of surgical removal of lesions or anatomic structures of the superficial soft tissues such as epulides and frenula (📷 3.51h-j).

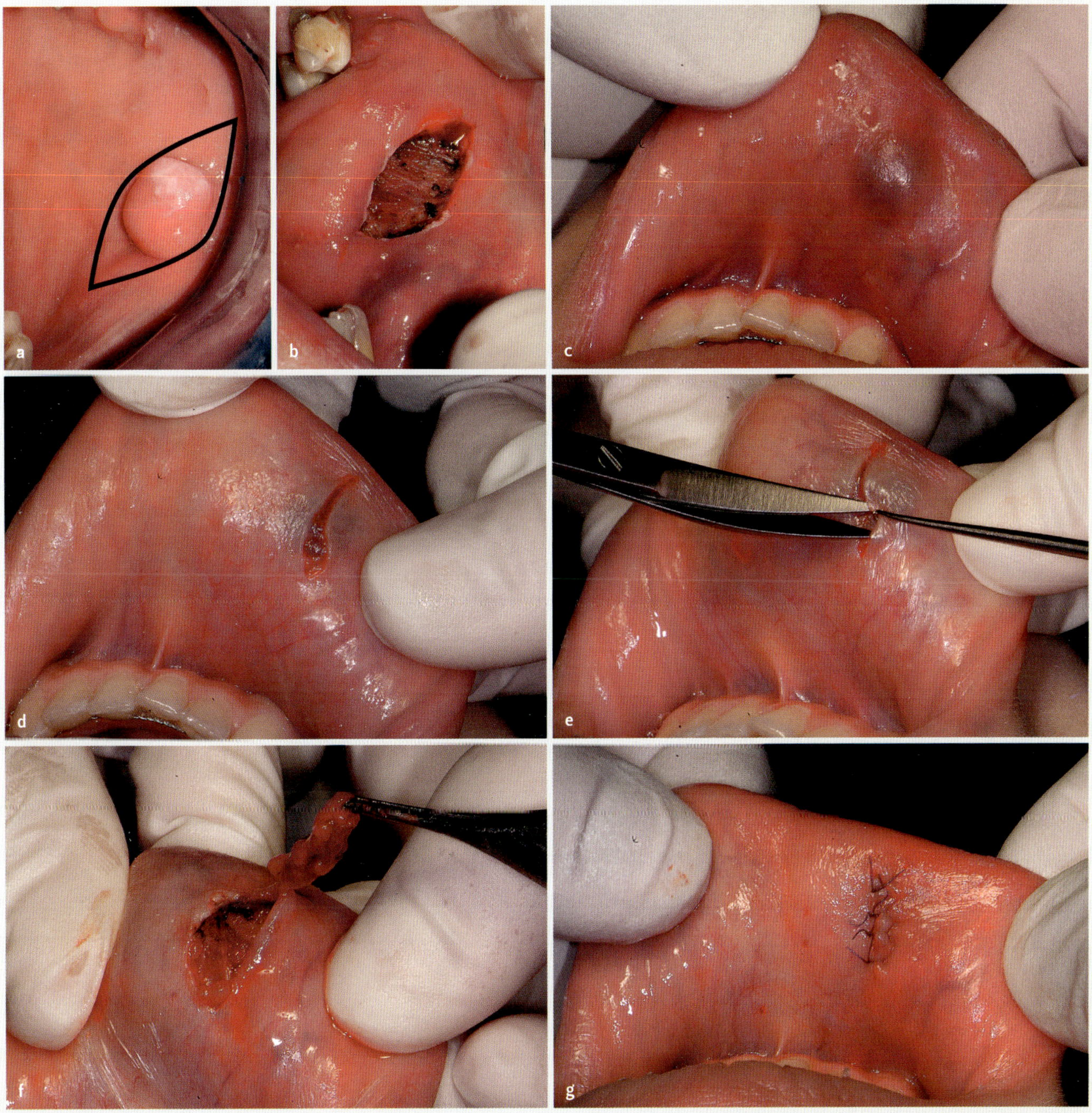

3.51 **a)** Fusiform incision for the removal (excisional biopsy) of a lesion on the malar mucosa. **b)** The operating field after the removal of the lesion. **c)** Mucocele involving the lower lip. **d)** Linear incision of the mucosa. **e)** Blunt dissection of the superficial mucosa is performed with dissecting scissors. **f)** The lesion is removed. **g)** Suture. (*continued*)

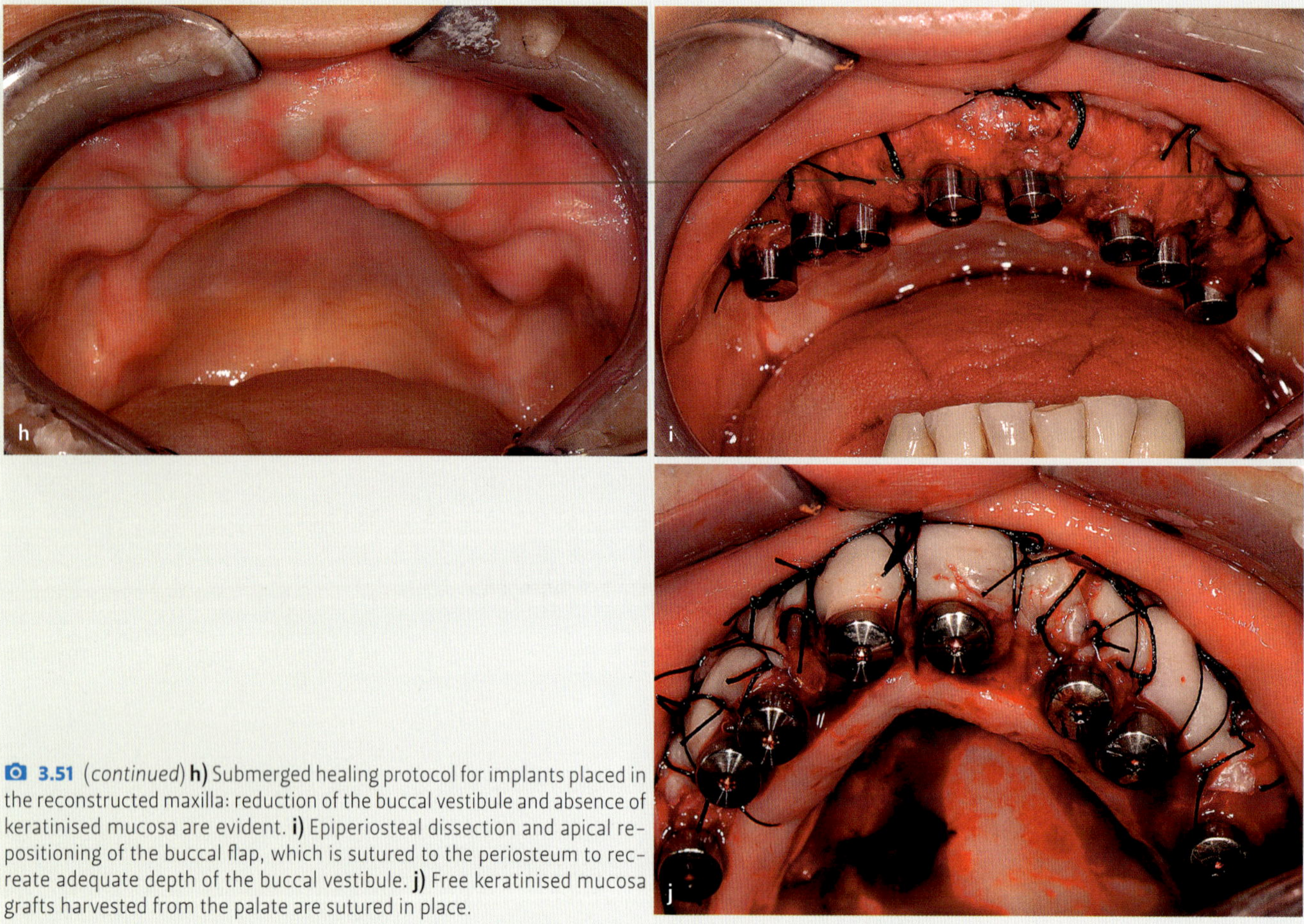

3.51 (*continued*) **h)** Submerged healing protocol for implants placed in the reconstructed maxilla: reduction of the buccal vestibule and absence of keratinised mucosa are evident. **i)** Epiperiosteal dissection and apical repositioning of the buccal flap, which is sutured to the periosteum to recreate adequate depth of the buccal vestibule. **j)** Free keratinised mucosa grafts harvested from the palate are sutured in place.

Principles of wound healing

The healing process of a surgical wound consists of three phases: the inflammatory phase, the proliferation phase, and the maturation (remodelling) phase.

Inflammatory phase: this phase develops in the first 5 days after surgery, and it is characterised by a vascular response that leads to haemostasis with blood clot formation and increased permeability of the blood vessels to permit infiltration of fluids, antibodies, growth factors, enzymes, and white cells (neutrophils, eosinophils, lymphocytes, and macrophages).

Proliferation phase: proliferation develops between 5 and 14 days after surgery, and consists of epithelial and connective repair:

- epithelial repair: migration and proliferation of epithelial cells cause superficial wound repair. However, in order for this process to occur, the support of a submucosal (or subcutaneous) plane is necessary;
- connective repair: collagen synthesis by fibroblast begins after 48-72 hours. The aggregation of collagen molecules leads to the formation of microfibrils organised in bundles, which go on to form mature collagen fibres.

Maturation (remodelling) phase: during the remodelling phase, which begins 14 days after surgery, fibroblasts are substituted by myofibroblasts responsible for tissue contraction. The presence of these cells causes remodelling and reorganisation of the collagen fibres, which take 6-7 weeks to complete.

Clinically, two healing modalities can be identified: healing by primary intention and healing by secondary intention.

HEALING BY PRIMARY INTENTION

Healing by primary intention occurs when the two margins of the surgical wound are kept in direct contact with a tension-free suture. It is the preferable healing modality, as it develops in a short time and reduces the risk of infection caused by penetration of bacteria in the submucosal or subcutaneous tissues.

Once the flap is sutured, the three phases of wound healing (described above) take place; after an initial inflammatory phase characterised by the formation of a fibrin scaffold, basal cells proliferate to close the wound. The migration and proliferation of the connective tissue lead to the formation of scar tissue that undergoes maturation and organisation.

HEALING BY SECONDARY INTENTION

Healing by secondary intention occurs when it is not possible to keep the margins of the wound in direct contact, as happens in the case of post-extractive sockets, laceration or traumatic soft tissue loss, or early wound dehiscence. In this event, the space that separates the margins of the wound is repaired by newly formed granulation tissue.

Initially, granulation tissue is rich in blood cells - it is well vascularised - and in 24-48 hours, fibroblasts migrating from the surrounding tissues colonise it to form scar tissue.

In the following days, granulation tissue evolves into dense fibrous tissue characterised by the presence of newly formed collagen fibres. The healing process ends with the complete transformation of the granulation tissue into scar tissue: myofibroblasts are responsible for the contraction of the wound.

However, it is worth remembering that healing of intraoral wounds is affected by bacterial colonisation and mechanical stresses to which the soft tissues are continuously subjected to during speech, chewing, and swallowing. Therefore, the healing process can be influenced by general and local factors. Among the former, factors that can impair tissue healing include debilitating diseases, systemic infections, the use of steroid medications, alterations of the immune response, radiotherapy, diabetes and other systemic conditions. Among the latter, factors that can impair tissue healing include the presence of foreign bodies and necrotic material inside the wound, excessive tension of the flap, ischaemia, infection, lack of flap support due to the absence of sound, well vascularised tissues.

Postoperative patient management

Adequate postoperative management of patients may significantly contribute to minimising postoperative morbidity and quicken healing. Factors that must be controlled are typically represented by swelling, pain, bleeding and infection. A satisfactory management of these factors can be obtained by inviting the patient to follow some simple rules, and with the correct medical therapy.

POSTOPERATIVE INSTRUCTIONS

Pain and swelling management: immediately after surgery, pain and swelling can be controlled with the application of ice packs. Ice packs should be applied above the treated area for 3-4 hours, alternating between 20 minutes of application and 10-15 minutes without the ice pack.

Management of postoperative bleeding: postoperative bleeding can be controlled with the application of gauze swabs soaked in sterile saline or water on the surgical wound; compression should be maintained for at least 10-15 minutes, to allow clotting. Rinsing should be avoided for 8-12 hours after surgery.

Infection control: infection control is obtained in the postoperative period by means of complete oral hygiene. Tooth brushing should be avoided for 8-12 hours after surgery, but it must be resumed immediately after. Care should be taken to avoid any insult to the surgical wound, which is kept clean by rinsing 2-3 times per day with chlorhexidine mouthwashes (0.2% chlorhexidine) until suture removal.

Diet: a fluid and cold diet should be followed for at least 24 hours after surgery. Until suture removal, a soft diet is indicated, and chewing should be limited to the untreated side of the mouth.

PHARMACOTHERAPY

Pain and swelling control: this is generally obtained with the administration of non-steroidal analgesics/anti-inflammatory drugs such as ketoprofen. It is worth noting that the dosage should be calculated according to the patient's weight, and that these drugs should always be taken on a full stomach and only if necessary.

In children under 12, the use of these drugs is not recommended; instead, paracetamol (or acetaminophen) can be used. However the correct dosage must be calculated with great care.

In case relevant swelling is expected, the administration of corticosteroids may be indicated: in this event, the first dose should be administered before surgery, or immediately after surgery at the latest.

Infection control: the basis for postoperative infection control is represented by the compliance with the postoperative instructions, particularly those regarding oral hygiene and antisepsis.

Notwithstanding the inevitable presence of bacteria in the oral cavity, and the interruption of the superficial tissues caused during surgery, the risk of postoperative infection is relatively low, particularly in the case of short and less invasive interventions, due to the tolerance of the body for these natural contaminants. Therefore, in these cases antibiotic therapy is not necessary.

Conversely, in cases where there is a significant risk of infection (long and invasive surgical procedures, bone reconstructive/regenerative procedures, immunocompromised patients, patients presenting conditions that cause a high risk of developing bacterial endocarditis) the recourse to a pre- and perioperative antibiotic regimen is indicated. The most effective scheme is represented by the administration of an antibiotic prophylaxis, according to the AHA (American Heart Association) protocols. Among antibiotics, the first choice is represented by penicillins and penicillin derivatives such as amoxicillin, alone or in association with clavulanate, while patients with a history of adverse reactions or allergy to penicillins should be treated with macrolides or tetracyclines.

The basic scheme entails administration of the maximum daily dosage of the antibiotic one hour before surgery in a single dose; administration can be repeated 6 hours after the first dose, and in cases of high risk of infection, the prophylaxis can be followed by a complete antibiotic therapy lasting 5-7 days. The rationale for antibiotic prophylaxis is to obtain peak levels of the drug in the patient's blood when the risk of microbial penetration through the access flap is higher. On the other hand, if antibiotic therapy is started after surgery, higher doses and a prolonged administration are necessary, increasing the toxicity and costs without improving the efficacy.

Basic scheme for antibiotic prophylaxis
Two grams (2 x 1 gram tablets) one hour before surgery, and 1 gram (1 tablet) 6 hours after the first dose.

REFERENCES

CHIAPASCO M. Manuale illustrato di Chirurgia Orale. 2ª ed. Elsevier Masson, Milano 2007.

LITTLE JW ET AL. Dental management of medically compromised patients. 5th ed. Mosby, S. Louis 1997.

PETERSON LJ, INDRESANO AT, MARCIANI RD, ROSER SM. Principles of oral and maxillofacial surgery. JB Lippincott Company, Philadelphia 1992.

SANTORO F, MAIORANA C. Chirurgia speciale odontostomatologica. Masson, Milano 2000.

TANNER J, SWARBROOK S, STURT J. Surgical hand antisepsis to reduce surgical site infection. *Cochrane Database Syst Rev* 2008 Jan; 23(1):CD004288.

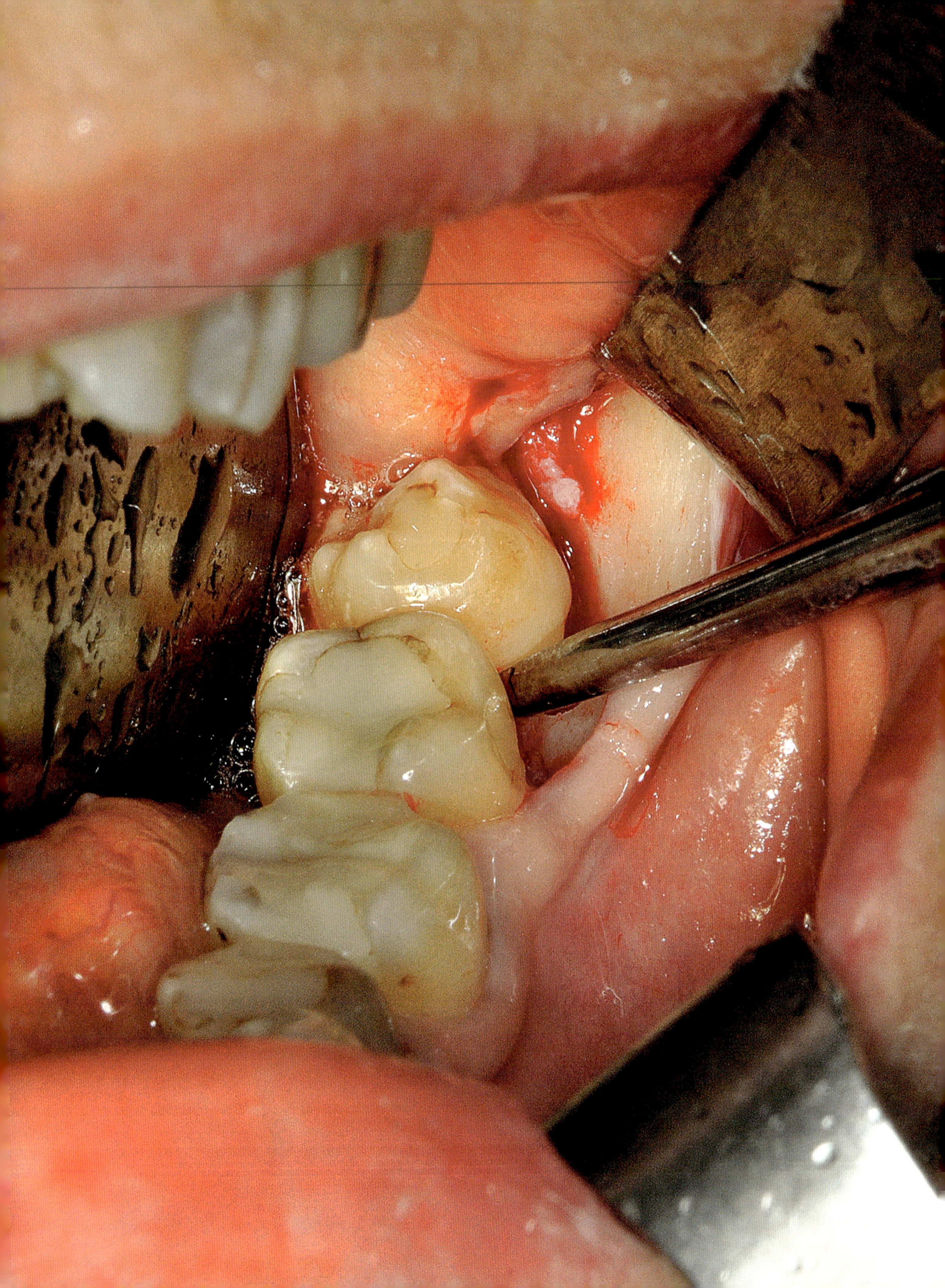

Dental extractions

M. Chiapasco ▪ M. Zaniboni ▪ A. Coggiola
P. Casentini

Introduction

The extraction of a tooth represents, for the majority of dentists, the first approach to oral surgery. As with any other surgical procedure, even the easiest extraction still requires careful analysis of the clinical case and the correct preoperative planning, followed by the application of a well-defined surgical protocol where nothing is left to chance. Moreover, it is worth noting that tooth extraction rarely represents a surgical act that is an end unto itself. Therefore, preservation of the alveolar bone, obtained by minimising surgical trauma as much as possible, is essential. Indeed, it makes it possible to preserve bone volume and morphology of the post-extractive site. These factors have relevant functional and aesthetic implications on the following prosthetic implications, either traditional or supported by endosseous implants.

Indications

The extraction of an erupted tooth is indicated when, due to lesions of various natures (traumatic, endodontic, periodontal, etc.), the tooth cannot be successfully restored or when its conservation does not appear appropriate in light of considerations on local conditions or the patient's general health status. To provide more detail, tooth extractions may be indicated in the following situations:

Ample carious lesions: particularly those extending to the roots, when restoring the tooth is difficult or impossible.

Periapical infection: when endodontic treatment fails to eliminate the periapical lesion, or when endodontic treatment (or re-treatment) is impossible due to the presence of non-removable obstacles in the root canals, or when surgical endodontic treatment is contraindicated due to the high risk of iatrogenic lesions to important anatomic structures.

Periodontal disease: in cases where periodontal disease has caused an excessive loss of periodontal support, particularly if the tooth exhibits significant mobility and the prerequisites for successful regenerative therapy are absent.

Combined periodontal-endodontic lesion: the prognosis is unfavourable due to the complexity of the treatment that renders the outcome less predictable (an apicoectomy would further reduce tooth support).

Horizontal and vertical root fractures: as they are untreatable, extraction of the tooth is unavoidable.

Orthodontic treatment: particularly in cases of teeth crowding, the orthodontist may refer the patient to an oral surgeon for strategic extractions. Typically, the first premolars are selected for extraction due to functional considerations, unless other teeth present incongruous restorations or root canal treatments that might impair their long-term prognosis. In this latter case, the teeth with the worst prognosis may be extracted. Other orthodontic indications for tooth extraction are described in Chapter 5 in detail (Extraction of impacted teeth).

Malpositioned teeth: when malposition causes trauma on the surrounding tissues. As an example, maxillary third molars exhibiting a buccal inclination may cause self-mastication of the cheek mucosa.
Extruded teeth should also be extracted when orthodontic intrusion is not feasible, when the presence of the extruded teeth prevents the rehabilitation of the opposing dentition, or when extruded teeth cause self-mastication lesions on the mucosa of the opposing arch.

Teeth involved in jaw fractures: whenever they represent an obstacle to the reduction of the fracture, or when untreatable lesions that may cause infection in the area, thus preventing adequate consolidation of the fracture, affect them.

Radiation therapy in the head and neck district for the treatment of malignant tumours: the extraction of teeth showing signs of endodontic and/or periodontal disease is indicated, as radiation therapy causes metabolic alterations in the involved tissues and a reduction of tissue perfusion that curtail the effect of medications (e.g. antibiotics, anti-inflammatory drugs) in the area. Moreover, tooth extraction in previously irradiated patients is associated with a higher risk of osteoradionecrosis.

Biphosphonate therapy (particularly for intravenous administration): as far as bone is concerned, it causes metabolic alterations and a reduction of tissue blood perfusion. These factors may predispose patients to a risk of osteonecrosis of the jaws after surgical manoeuvres, exposing the bone to contamination from bacteria that colonise the oral cavity. Therefore, all teeth affected by severe endoperiodontal lesions should be extracted before biphosphonate therapy is administered.

Caries or periapical infection of deciduous teeth: if exfoliation of the involved tooth is impending, extraction is indicated to prevent the extension of the pathologic process to the underlying permanent tooth.

Ankylosis of deciduous teeth: the ankylosis of a deciduous tooth can hinder the normal eruption of the permanent tooth and cause its ectopic eruption or impaction.

Possibility of replacing compromised teeth with endosseous implants: every effort should always be made to preserve natural teeth, but in selected cases, the replacement of a compromised tooth with an endosseous implant may represent the most reliable solution.

Financial issues: in some cases, the patient may refuse the conservative treatment of a tooth due to the cost of treatment.

Contraindications

Systemic contraindications

General contraindications are the same as described in Chapter 1, which apply to every oral surgery procedure.

Local contraindications

Acute inflammation of the periodontal tissues: particularly in the case of significant deposits of plaque and calculus, as this increases the incidence of infectious complications, lengthens the healing process, renders the manipulation of the soft tissues more difficult, and reduces the effectiveness of local anaesthetics. In these cases, an adequate etiologic treatment aimed at resolving the acute inflammation and reducing the bacterial load inside the oral cavity is indicated prior to tooth extraction. In particular, acute necrotising ulcerative gingivitis must be considered an absolute contraindication to tooth extraction. However, it is worth remembering that with acute abscesses, with the risk of diffusion of the infectious process, the extraction of the involved tooth may be indicated (if adequate antibiotic therapy is administered).

Acute pericoronitis of a partially impacted tooth and/or dentoalveolar abscess: antibiotic therapy and etiologic treatment should be performed before tooth extraction.

Stomatitis and acute inflammation of the oral mucosa: particularly in the case of viral origin (e.g. herpes virus), it represents a contraindication to tooth extraction due to the risk of diffusion of the viral infection and subsequent deterioration of the clinical presentation.

Continuity between a tooth and a malignant tumour: tooth extraction is absolutely contraindicated, due to the significant risk of dissemination of malignant cells.

Radiotherapy: special care must be taken for extraction of a tooth in an irradiated area of the jaws, due to the higher risk of infection and osteoradionecrosis (see Chapter 1 for details).

Surgical protocols for tooth extraction

Indications

- Caries
- Periapical periodontitis
- Periodontal disease
- Complex rehabilitations
- Malpositioned teeth, semi-impacted or impacted teeth, teeth involved in fractures of the jaws
- Orthodontic treatment
- Endoperiodontal lesions
- Root fractures
- Focuses of infection in immunodepressed patients, patients undergoing dialysis, and patients waiting for organ transplant
- Before radiotherapy
- Financial issues
- Deciduous teeth:
  - caries
  - periapical infection
  - ankylosis

Contraindications

- Systemic:
  - the same as described in Chapter 1 for all oral surgery procedures
- Local:
  - acute inflammation of the periodontal tissues
  - stomatitis
  - acute inflammation of the oral mucosa
  - acute pericoronitis
  - dentoalveolar abscess
  - continuity with malignant tumours
  - history of radiotherapy in the head and neck district

Preoperative evaluation

An adequate preoperative evaluation is necessary to assess the degree of difficulty of an extraction and, subsequently, to choose the most appropriate surgical technique. In fact, two different surgical approaches can be identified:

- *basic surgical technique*: elevation and extraction of the tooth are performed with the aid of root elevators and extraction forceps without the need of elevating an access flap. Therefore, the recourse to this approach is indicated for *simple extractions*;
- *open surgical technique*: it involves the elevation of an access flap, and ostectomy (the removal of a certain amount of alveolar bone) and odontotomy (the separation of a tooth in several fragments) may be indicated. This approach is indicated for *complicated extractions* (i.e. endodontically treated teeth, ankylosed teeth, erupted teeth with curved roots, fractured teeth, etc.).

Ideally, the choice between these surgical approaches should be made preoperatively based on an accurate evaluation of the clinical case to reduce the duration of the surgical session by choosing the most practical surgical technique and with an aim to minimising surgical trauma. Accurate preoperative planning is also important from an ergonomic point of view, to allow a precise evaluation of the duration of the surgical session and to select the most appropriate surgical armamentarium. In fact, a specific surgical armamentarium is necessary to perform complicated extractions with an open surgical technique. Moreover, it is worth noting that with unforeseen difficulties, the basic surgical approach should be converted into an open surgical approach.

The key factors to be considered in the preoperative clinical assessment to adequately plan tooth extraction are the following:

General preoperative evaluation: follows the principles detailed in Chapter 1.

Radiographic evaluation: it should always be performed, also for apparently simple extractions, as it allows visualising details that may not be clinically visible. For this reason, it represents a fundamental diagnostic tool and an important medico-legal document. In the majority of cases, when an erupted tooth is to be extracted, obtaining a preoperative periapical radiograph is sufficient. In peculiar situations, when it is indicated or necessary to gather detailed information regarding the relationships between the tooth and the adjacent anatomic structures, it is preferable to obtain a panoramic radiograph. The recourse to CT scans, on the other hand, is necessary only with the presence of anatomic or pathologic complicating factors, the latter of which should be evaluated tridimensionally, particularly in cases where potential risks or damaging relevant anatomic structures during surgery are significant.

Evaluation of the shape and number of the roots: the shape of the root (or roots) of a tooth is the preponderant factor to consider in evaluating both the grade of difficulty of the extraction and the most convenient surgical approach.

The number of roots is the first variable to consider; the presence of an abnormal number of roots, if diagnosed, allows modification of the surgical technique (e.g. performing odontotomy) to reduce the invasivity of the procedure and the risk of root fracture. The shape of the roots, and particularly their curvature, their length, and their divergence, are all factors that have a significant influence on the choice of the surgical protocol. The presence of a bulbous root with an enlarged apex, as well as the presence of long roots, diverging roots, or roots with sharp curvatures, are all complicating factors.

The presence of either internal or external root resorption renders the root more fragile and, thus, more prone to fracture, particularly if tooth extraction is performed with the sole use of extraction forceps. Endodontically treated teeth also present a higher risk of fracture during extraction, due to a loss of elasticity that renders these teeth more brittle and due to the higher frequency of ankylosis. In these cases, elevation of a mucoperiosteal flap, in association with ostectomy and odontotomy, provides a quicker and less traumatic extraction (4.1, 4.2).

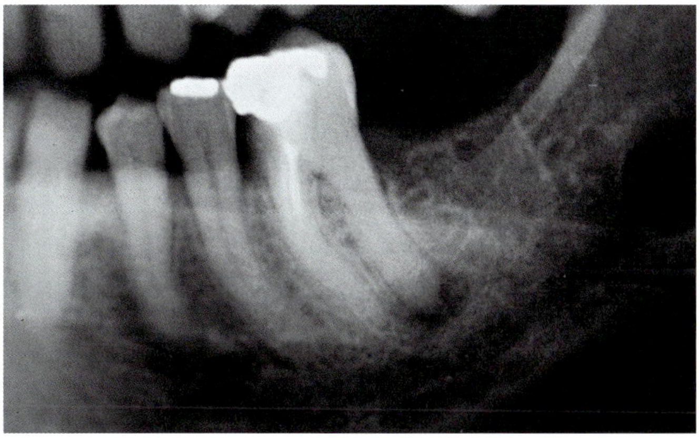

4.1 First mandibular molar with long and narrow roots: for extraction, odontotomy is indicated.

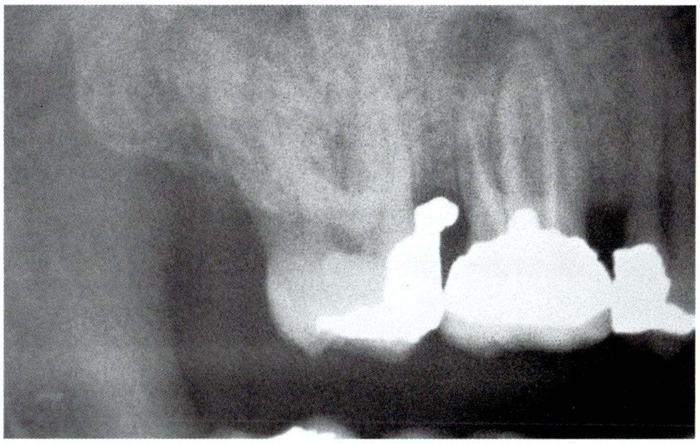

4.2 Second maxillary molar with divergent roots that may require odontotomy to avoid excessive trauma during extraction.

Evaluation of tooth mobility: the extraction of a tooth exhibiting significant mobility, a condition that is common in the case of severe periodontal disease, usually presents a low level of difficulty. Conversely, the complete absence of movement should raise the suspicion that the tooth is ankylosed, particularly when the absence of movement is associated with the absence of periodontal space around the roots of the tooth in preoperative radiographs (4.3).

Evaluation of the relationships with the neighbouring anatomic structures: before the extraction of a maxillary molar is performed, it is important to assess the relationships between the roots and the floor of the maxillary sinus. When only a thin layer of bone separates the root apexes from the sinus lumen (or when the apexes directly protrude inside the sinus lumen), surgical manoeuvres to extract the tooth may cause the formation of an oroantral communication. In these cases, the recourse to an open surgical approach with the elevation of a mucoperiosteal flap associated with the separation of the roots is indicated. This technique allows, in the majority of cases, preservation of the buccal cortical plate and interradicular septa, which may instead be fractured for luxation of the tooth performed with extraction forceps. Preservation of the integrity of the alveolar process is fundamental if an oroantral communication is produced, as it reduces its extent and facilitates its closure with local flaps (4.4). The relationships between roots of the mandibular molars (particularly, the third molar) and the mandibular canal should always be investigated (see below). For the same reasons, the position of the mental foramen should be considered when an access flap in the area of the mandibular premolars is to be elevated, and the relationships between roots of the maxillary incisors, the floor of the nasal cavities, and the nasopalatine canal.

Clinical evaluation of the crown: the presence of large carious lesions, particularly those extending below the gingival margin and involving the root, may render the use of extraction forceps difficult or impossible, thus representing an indication for the open surgical approach. Extraction forceps should always be used carefully for luxation of teeth bearing large restorations, to avoid fractures of the crown that may result in the loss of a valuable leverage point. In these cases, it is essential that the extraction forceps are positioned as far apically as possible, to allow the application of force on the most coronal portion of the root and thus avoid acting directly on the crown.

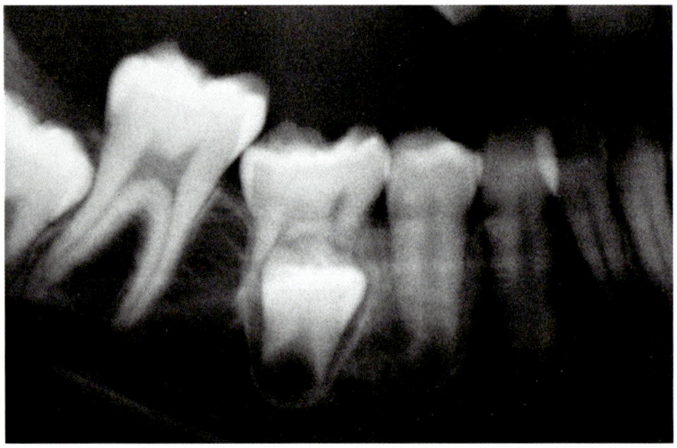

4.3 Ankylosis of a deciduous molar that may require ostectomy and odontotomy.

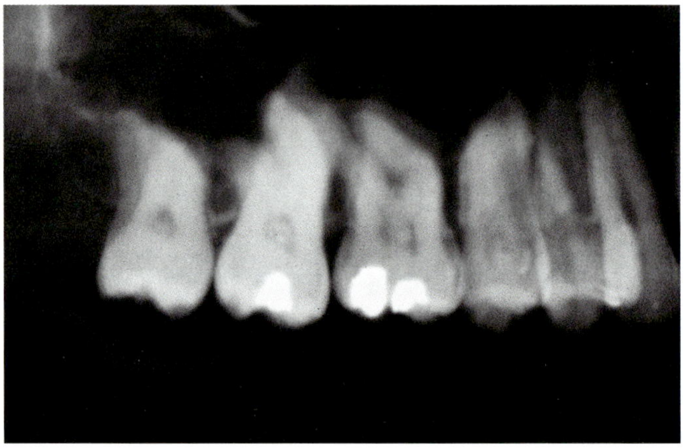

4.4 Maxillary molars presenting curved roots apparently protruding through the floor of the maxillary sinus.

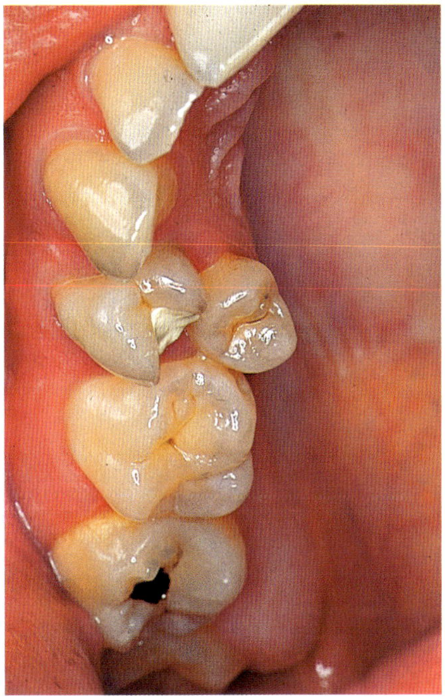

4.5 Malpositioned second maxillary premolar: extraction forceps cannot be used.

Preoperative clinical examination: factors to evaluate

- General preoperative assessment
- Radiographic evaluation
- Root anatomy
- Tooth mobility
- Neighbouring anatomic structures
- Condition of the tooth crown
- Position of the tooth
- Mineralisation of the surrounding bone
- Presence of periapical lesions

Evaluation of the tooth position in the dental arch: the extraction of a malpositioned tooth, particularly in cases of crowding, should not be performed with extraction forceps. In these cases, the recourse to an open surgical approach is indicated, as well as the use of alternative instruments (e.g. root elevators) to perform luxation and extraction of the malpositioned tooth (4.5).

Mineralisation of the surrounding bone: barely radiopaque bone (typically found in the posterior areas of the maxilla) is generally characterised by a lower density and a higher elasticity. These attributes render the extraction of the tooth easier, as the softer alveolar bone expands more easily under the pressure transferred with the luxation manoeuvres. Conversely, when the alveolar bone is very radiopaque (e.g. posterior areas of the mandible) the extraction is more complicated, due to the higher density and lower elasticity of the alveolar bone.

Presence of periapical lesions: the presence of a periapical lesion requires careful revision of the post-extractive socket and thorough bone curettage with specifically designed bone curettes, to prevent soft tissue remnants from proliferating and forming a residual cyst.

Preparation of the patient for the extraction

Generally, tooth extractions do not require a sterile environment to be performed: clean preparation of the patient and the room are described in detail in Chapter 3.

BASIC ARMAMENTARIUM (4.6)

- Materials for anaesthesia;
- Syndesmotome or periosteal elevator;
- Straight and angled root elevators;
- Extraction forceps;
- Bone curette;
- Periodontal curette;
- Scalpel handle and blade;
- Surgical tissue forceps;
- Surgical suction tip;
- Syringe for sterile saline irrigation and sterile gauze swabs;
- Needle holder, surgical scissors, and sutures.

Simple extractions

The basic surgical technique consists of the following phases:

- locoregional anaesthesia;
- syndesmotomy;
- papillae elevation;
- luxation of the tooth by means of straight root elevators;
- tooth luxation and socket expansion by means of extraction forceps;

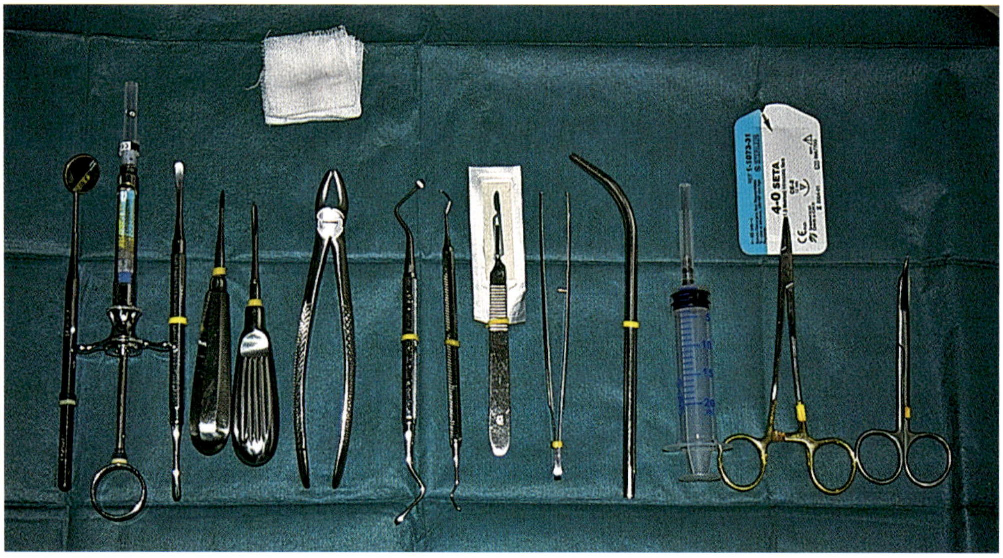

4.6 Example of a standard surgical kit for the extraction of erupted teeth.

- extraction of the tooth from the socket;
- verification of the integrity of the tooth;
- socket curettage and inspection of the cavity;
- elimination of excess soft tissues;
- irrigation of the socket with sterile saline;
- verification of possible oroantral communications;
- suture;
- check for blood clot formation;
- wound packing with a gauze swab soaked in sterile saline.

LOCAL ANAESTHESIA

For extraction of maxillary teeth, local anaesthesia in the buccal vestibule and on the palate is performed in the area of the tooth to be extracted. For extraction of mandibular incisors, canines, and first premolars, local anaesthesia is administered both on the buccal and the lingual side, while for extraction of mandibular second premolars and molars, the recourse to conduction anaesthesia of the inferior alveolar nerve is indicated, in association with conduction anaesthesia of the buccal and lingual nerve. In some cases, the use of intraligamentary anaesthesia may serve as a further support (see Chapter 3 for technical details).

SYNDESMOTOMY

It involves interrupting the most coronal portion of the periodontal ligament, to make the elevation of the papillae easier and atraumatic. Moreover, this manoeuvre allows a more apical positioning of the extraction forceps: this guarantees a better grip on the root and a more apical application of force, thus reducing the risk of crown or root fracture. Syndesmotomy is performed with a sharp periosteal elevator or with a dedicated instrument, the syndesmotome (4.7a-b); it can also be performed with a scalpel blade, although this action requires greater control of the instrument.

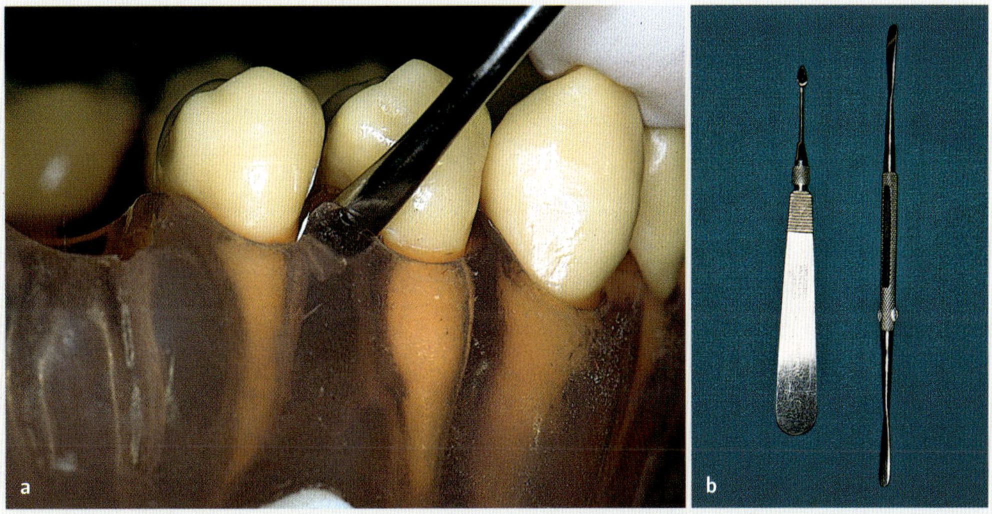

4.7 **a)** Syndesmotomy by means of a thin periosteal elevator. **b)** Syndesmotome and thin periosteal elevator.

PAPILLAE ELEVATION

Whenever the use of a straight root elevator is indicated to luxate the tooth, it is necessary to elevate the interdental papillae with a fine periosteal elevator. This manoeuvre frees the papillae and allows their displacement when the tip of the root elevator is placed in the interdental spaces for tooth luxation, avoiding any damage or trauma to the delicate soft tissues.

LUXATION OF THE TOOTH WITH A STRAIGHT ROOT ELEVATOR

The straight root elevator is used alternatively or in conjunction with the extraction forceps to luxate the tooth. The tip of the instrument is placed in the interdental spaces, perpendicular to the main axis of the tooth. Using gentle movements and applying controlled force, the instrument must be used carefully to avoid letting it slip towards the tongue or palate, as this can seriously damage to the soft tissues. The root elevator is held like a screwdriver, with the index finger, positioned near the tip, providing maximum control. It must never lie against the neighbouring tooth, but should act with a rotary movement between the alveolar crest and the tooth to be extracted to avoid accidental luxation or fracture of the adjacent tooth. To begin, an elevator with a narrow tip is indicated to engage the interdental spaces with ease; once the partial luxation of the tooth is obtained, the interdental spaces expand and root elevators with wider tips can be used. The use of root elevators should be considered with caution for extraction of a tooth with an intact crown if any neighbouring teeth also have an intact crown, due to the risk of accidental luxation of these latter. On the other hand, elevators are particularly useful for extracting roots, and their effectiveness is maximised when (mesially and/or distally) neighbouring teeth are absent (4.8a-b).

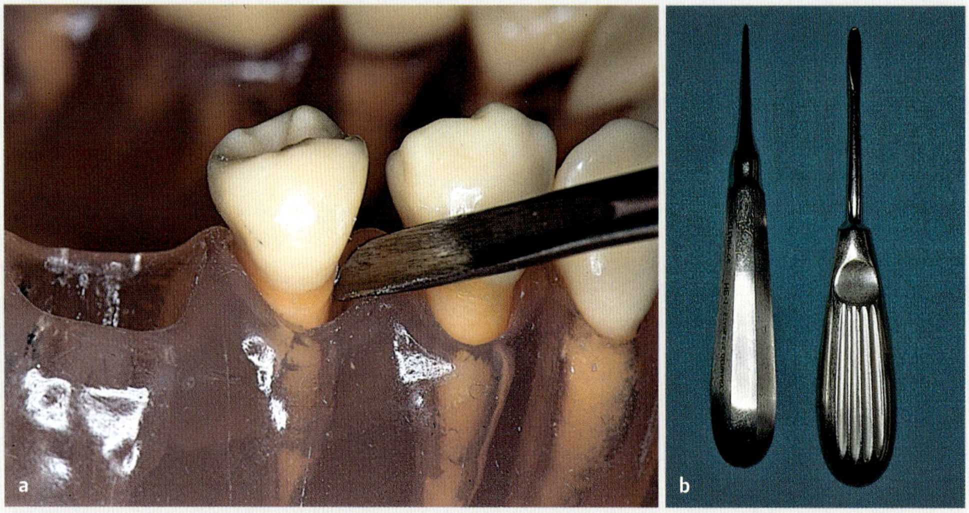

4.8 **a)** Use of the root elevator to luxate a tooth. **b)** Straight root elevators (smaller tip - larger tip).

LUXATION OF THE TOOTH AND EXPANSION OF THE SOCKET BY MEANS OF EXTRACTION FORCEPS

Extraction forceps are the most important instruments to perform simple extractions. The shape and dimension of each pair of forceps is specifically designed to match a peculiar tooth anatomy (incisors, canines, premolars and molars) and a specific area of the oral cavity (maxilla, mandible, anterior areas, and posterior areas). Therefore, the most appropriate extraction forceps to grab, luxate, and extract a tooth are those that enable the maximum contact surface between the forceps jaws with the tooth, guaranteeing in this way an adequate transmission of applied force. Moreover, the ideal angle between the jaws and handle provides the freedom to perform the ideal movements without interfering with the opposing arch dentition or the cheeks (4.9a-e).

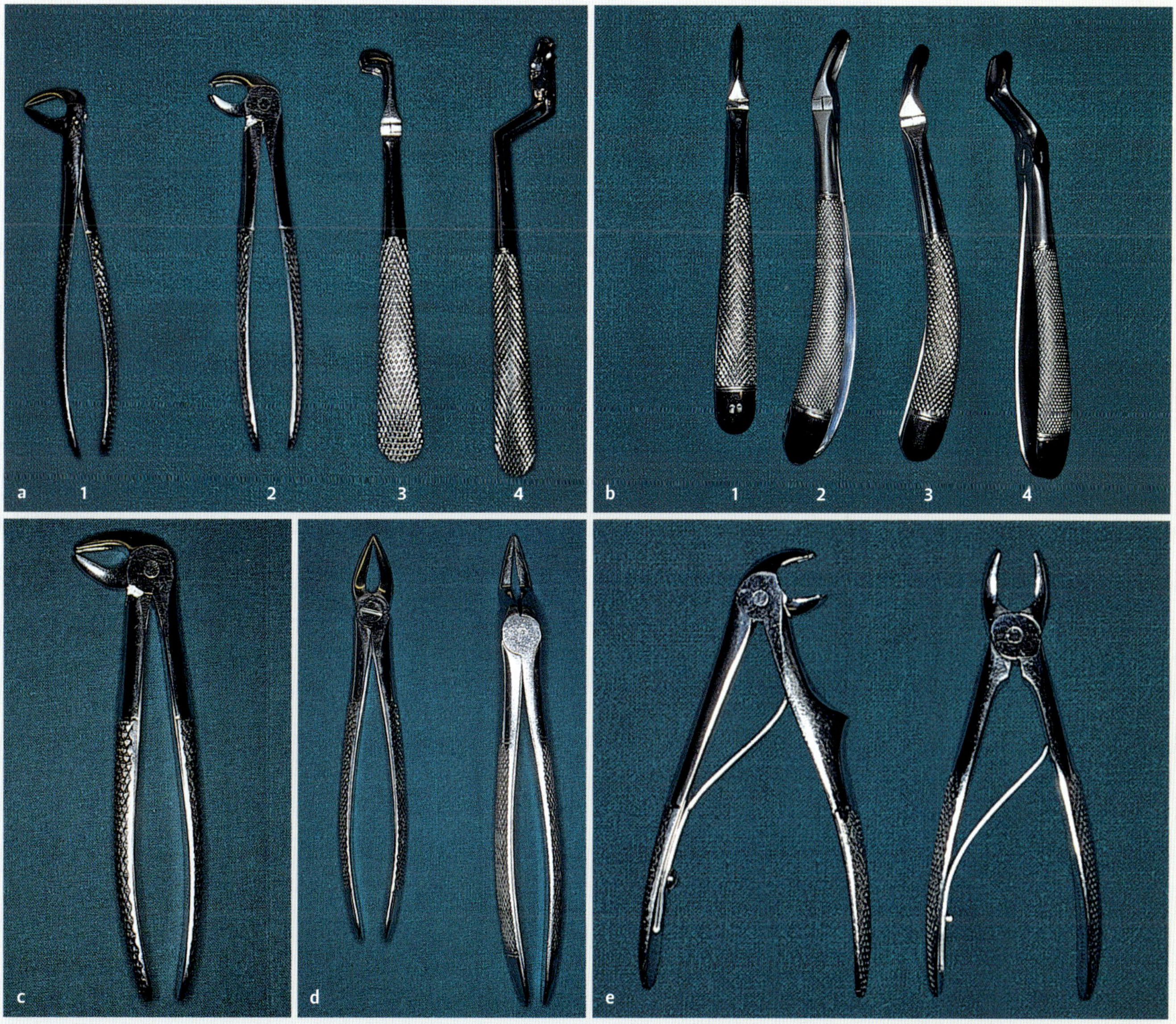

4.9 **a)** Examples of extraction forceps for mandibular teeth: **1)** incisors; **2)** premolars; **3)** molars (curved on the flat or anterior grip); **4)** bayonet. **b)** Examples of extraction forceps for maxillary teeth: **1)** incisors and canines; **2)** premolars; **3)** molars; **4)** bayonet. **c)** Extraction forceps for mandibular roots. **d)** Extraction forceps for maxillary roots. **e)** Extraction forceps for deciduous teeth.

Extraction forceps for mandibular teeth

Generally, these forceps have a 90° angle between the handle and the beaks. Those designed for incisor extraction have narrow beaks that adapt to the reduced diameter of the teeth, while those designed for canine and premolar extraction are similar in shape (although some models may have a 110° angle between handle and beaks), but are more robust and with wider beaks. Mandibular molar forceps have a pointed extension at the centre of the margin of the beaks to engage the furcation. The most widely used forceps for the extraction of mandibular molars are those curved on the back (lateral grip); the same forceps can be used on both the left and the right mandible. Different models are also produced which have a 45° angle between the handle and beaks to reduce tension on the lower lip during the luxation manoeuvres. Finally, extraction forceps curved on the flat (anterior grip) can be used to eliminate lip tension completely or to reach posterior areas in cases of limited access. However, the anterior grip does not provide the same range of movement and force as the lateral grip, thus rendering the use of these forceps more difficult (4.9a).

Extraction forceps for maxillary teeth

Extraction forceps for anterior maxillary teeth (incisors and canines) are straight, while those for premolars and molars have a 45° angle between the handle and beaks. Maxillary molar forceps have a pointed extension at the centre of the margin of the buccal beak to engage the buccal furcation; therefore, two symmetrical forceps are used in the right and left maxilla. Specifically designed forceps are also available for the extraction of maxillary third molars. These have a bayonet shape (two 90° angles between the handle and the beaks) to provide easier access and manoeuvrability in the posterior areas of the maxilla (4.9b).

Extraction forceps for roots and deciduous teeth

Forceps for the extraction of mandibular roots are similar to extraction forceps for mandibular incisors, but with narrower, touching beaks (4.9c). Bayonet forceps with long, narrow beaks are used for the extraction of upper roots, as by virtue of their shape they provide adequate access also in the posterior areas of the maxilla (4.9d). Extraction forceps for deciduous teeth are similar to their counterpart for permanent teeth, but are smaller in size (4.9e).

Basic techniques

The beaks of the extraction forceps should embrace the tooth while keeping parallel to its major axis, to provide effective transfer of applied force.
The extraction forceps should grab the tooth as far apically as possible, preferably below the cementoenamel junction. The lingual or palatal beak, which is less visible during the luxation manoeuvres, should be positioned first. For cervical caries, the forceps should be positioned on the involved side first, making sure that the beak rests on sound tissue. When, due to the extent of the carious lesion, this is not indicated for the high risk of crown fracture, it is better to perform the extraction with an open surgical approach.
Tooth luxation consists in the expansion of the socket and the complete interruption of the periodontal ligament fibres connecting the alveolar bone and the root cementum. Luxation is obtained with slow, ample movements performed with increasing pressure towards the buccal cortical plate first, due to its relative thinness, and then towards the palatal/lingual cortical plate. Pressure should be applied continuously for several seconds, to allow the socket to expand gradually. During tooth luxation, palpation of the alveolar ridge helps calibrate the pressure applied to the alveolar bone to prevent any excess that may lead to fractures of the cortical plates. When the socket begins to expand, the beaks of the extraction forceps can be positioned more apically, thus producing a more effective action. It is paramount that controlled force always be exerted during luxation to prevent crown fractures, particularly when the crown is damaged, or when it bears large restorations (4.10a-b).

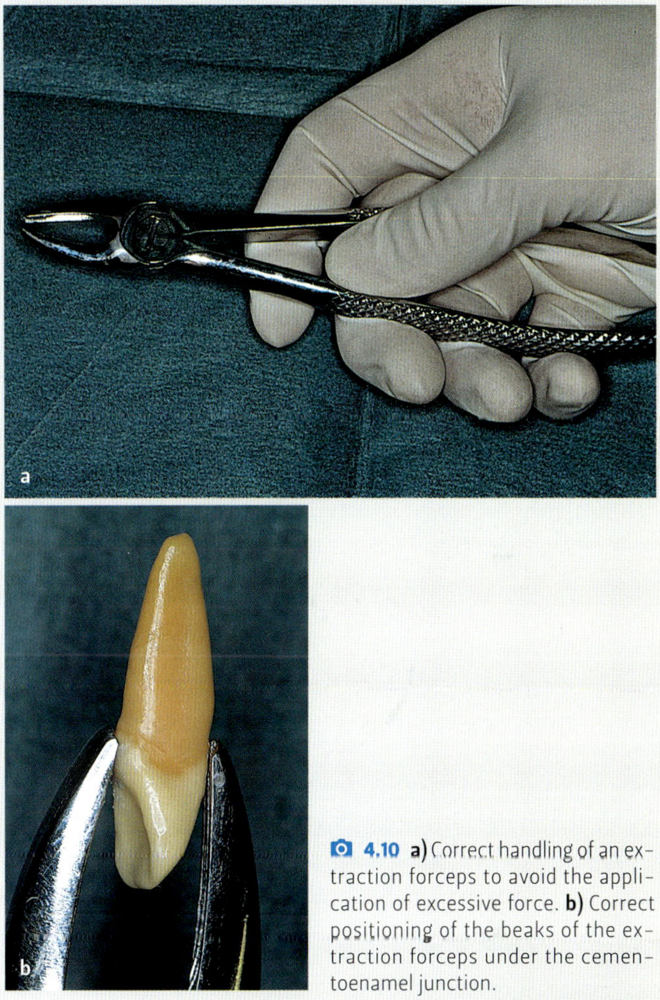

4.10 **a)** Correct handling of an extraction forceps to avoid the application of excessive force. **b)** Correct positioning of the beaks of the extraction forceps under the cementoenamel junction.

It is possible to identify five actions by means of which the extraction forceps expands the socket and luxates the tooth:

- *apical pressure*: the insertion of the beaks in an apical position allows the most coronal portion of the socket to expand (4.11a);
- *pressure towards the buccal cortical plate*: the buccal movement of the extraction forceps causes the expansion of the buccal cortical plate, particularly the most coronal part. In the maxilla, as well as in the anterior and lateral areas of the mandible, due to the thinness of the buccal cortical plate, this movement represents the main component of the luxation manoeuvre (4.11b);
- *pressure towards the palatal/lingual cortical plate*: the effects are similar to those of buccal pressure, and it is used mainly during extraction of mandibular molars due to the relative thinness of the lingual cortical plate in the posterior areas of the mandible (4.11c);
- *rotation*: this movement may be used only when extracting single-rooted teeth (e.g. incisors, canines, and lower premolars) if no signs of root anomalies are visible on the radiographic exams. Rotation should always be applied after all the other movements are performed, and allow the fibres of the periodontal ligament to be completely interrupted (4.11d-e).

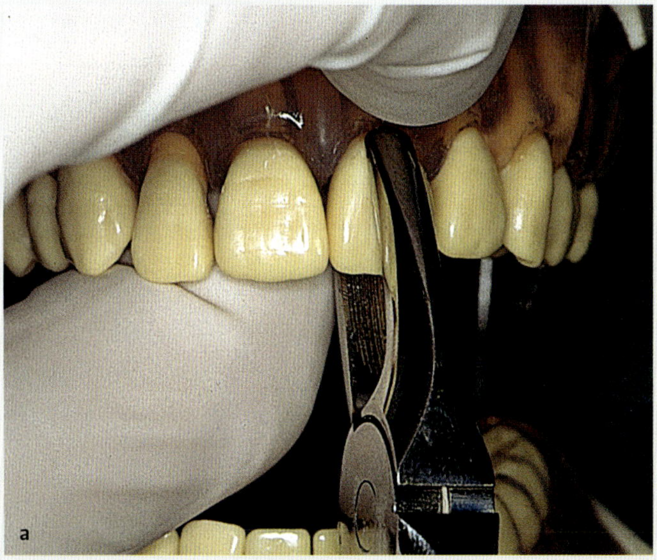

4.11 **a)** Positioning of the extraction forceps and palpation of the cortical plates to verify the controlled application of luxation force. (*continued*)

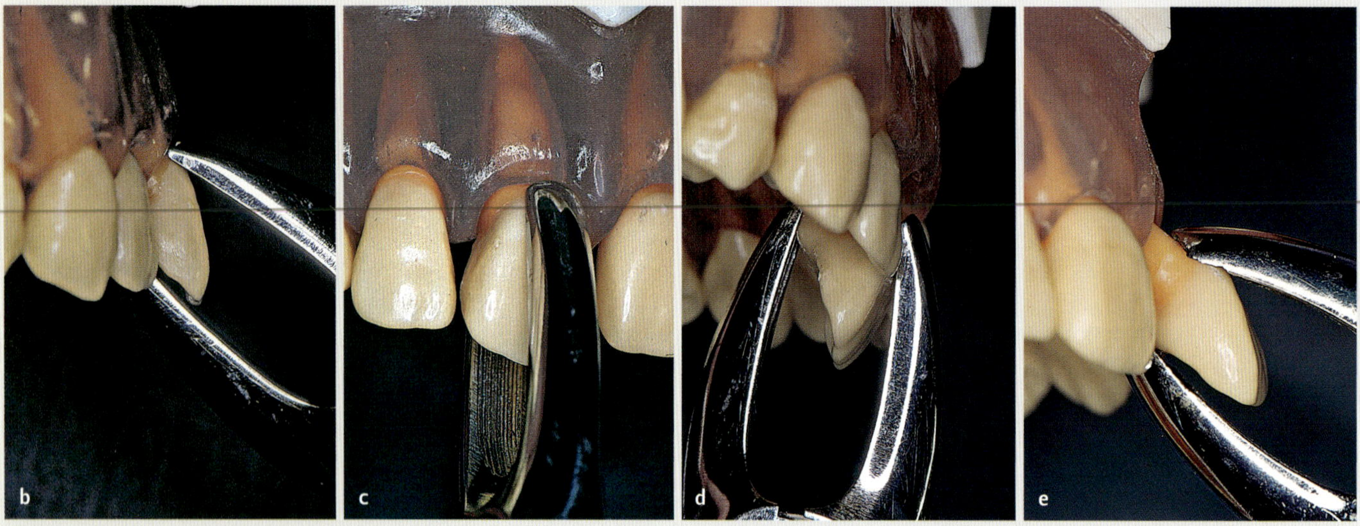

4.11 (*continued*) **b)** Luxation movement towards the buccal cortical plate. **c)** Luxation movement towards the palatal cortical plate. **d)** Rotational movement. **e)** Luxation and extraction.

Extraction of the tooth from the socket

After expansion of the socket and luxation of the tooth are completed, the tooth can be removed with a delicate coronal and buccal traction. The application of controlled force is fundamental for preventing sudden detachment of the tooth; uncontrolled movements of the extraction forceps may damage the opposing arch dentition.

Verification of tooth integrity

Once extraction is completed, the tooth should be cleaned and its integrity verified. If the fracture of one or more root fragments is suspected (e.g. a sharp noise during luxation may be indicative of root fracture), the fractured fragments must be located and removed (see specific section for details).

Socket curettage and inspection of the cavity

Soft tissue remnants (periodontal ligament, infectious tissue, etc.) that may be present on the bottom or walls of the post-extractive socket must be accurately removed to reduce the risk of infection, improve healing of the hard and soft tissues, and prevent the formation of residual cysts. The removal of these remnants can be performed with the aid of sharp bone curettes (e.g. Lucas surgical curette) or surgical spoons (e.g. Hemingway surgical curette) (4.12).

If the preoperative radiographic examinations show a close proximity between the bottom of the socket and the maxillary sinus or inferior alveolar canal, great care must be taken during bone curettage to avoid any complication.

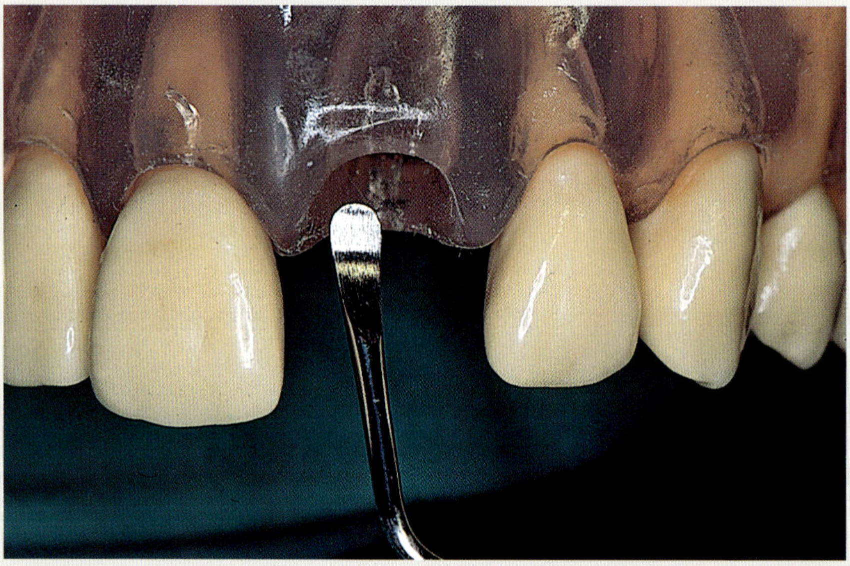

4.12 Socket inspection and curettage with a surgical curette.

Removal of excess soft tissues

When teeth with deep periodontal pockets are extracted, hyperplastic soft tissues may be found on the inner side of the gingiva. The removal of these excess soft tissues prevents the formation of flabby ridges; with the aid of surgical pliers and sharp instruments (e.g. scalpel, scissors) any excess is removed to obtain clean gingival margins. However, great care must be taken to avoid any loss of keratinised tissue, particularly when planning a substitution of the extracted tooth with an endosseous implant is planned (4.13a–b).

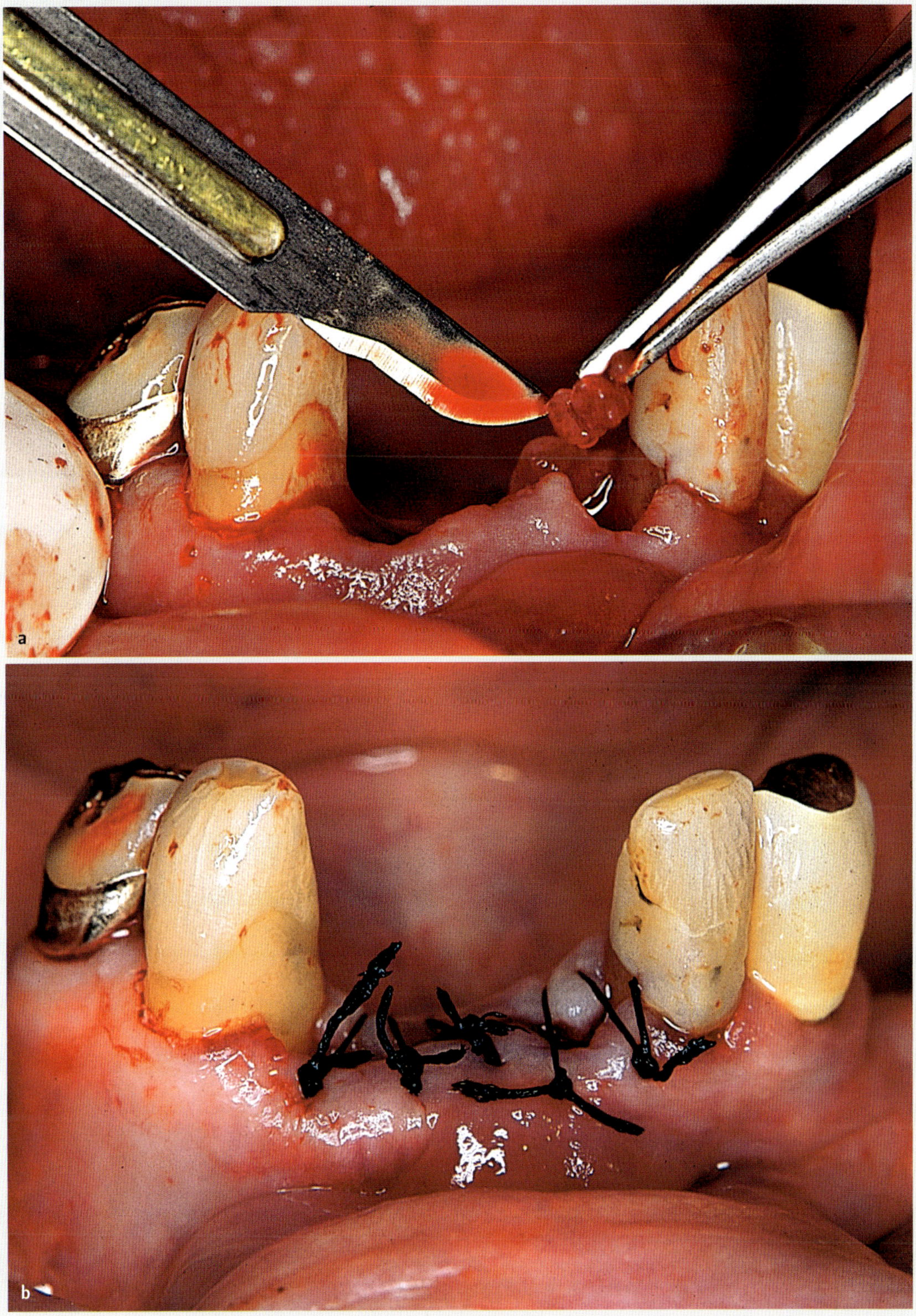

4.13 **a)** Removal of excess soft tissues. **b)** Suture.

Irrigation of the socket with sterile saline

After thorough bone curettage is completed, the socket is irrigated with sterile saline to remove possible contaminants. This simple manoeuvre has proven effective to reduce significantly the risk of post-extractive alveolitis.

Verification of possible oroantral communications

If preoperative radiographic examinations or intraoperative findings raise suspicions that an oroantral communication has been created following the extraction of maxillary molars and premolars, inspection of the socket can be performed using a buttoned probe. Direct irrigation of the bottom of the socket may also help to detect oroantral communications, as the patient will refer the feeling of water running down the nose or throat.
Communication can also be confirmed by the formation of bubbles in the blood that fills the socket.
The Valsalva manoeuvre, which involves the forced expulsion of air through the nose once the nostrils have been closed with the thumb and index fingers, is contraindicated: the increased air pressure inside the maxillary sinus may cause tears in the Schneiderian membrane and cause an oroantral communication, or increase a pre-existing membrane tear. The treatment of this complication is described in detail in Chapter 14.

Compression of the socket

The alveolar bone, previously expanded, may be taken back to its original volume by means of manual compression of the buccal and palatal/lingual cortical plate. The application of controlled pressure is required for avoiding excessive collapse of the socket or fracture of the cortical plates. However, this procedure is contraindicated when substitution of the extracted tooth with an endosseous implant is planned, as it reduces the width of the alveolar ridge.
Following the development and refinement of techniques for prosthetic rehabilitation supported by endosseous implants, the need for preserving adequate bone volume after tooth extraction has led to the introduction of new techniques for ridge preservation. The latter are described in detail in Chapter 13, but, in short, they involve the filling of the post-extractive socket with biomaterials such as particulate hydroxyapatites or xenografts associated with substrates such as collagen, with the aim of reducing the risk of volume reduction of the alveolar ridge during the healing period.

> If the substitution of the extracted tooth with an endosseous implant is planned, compression of the socket should be avoided to preserve the width of the alveolar ridge as much as possible.

Suture

For simple extraction, suture may be unnecessary. However, if the socket has been filled with resorbable haemostatic materials (collagen sponge, oxidised regenerated cellulose) to facilitate blood clotting, the use of crossed mattress sutures (X sutures) may be indicated to prevent materials from leaving the socket. For multiple extractions of adjacent teeth, the recourse to a continuous suture may be indicated.

Check for blood clot formation

Before discharging the patient, it is fundamental that a check for haemostasis be made. Ideally, the socket should be completely filled with a blood clot. In cases of insufficient bleeding, curettage of the bony walls of the socket with a surgical curette may stimulate adequate socket filling. The blood clot protects the exposed bone and stimulates healing and new bone formation and its absence may cause complications such as alveolitis, delayed healing, and incomplete bone formation inside the socket.

Wound packing with a gauze swab soaked in sterile saline

To promote haemostasis in the immediate postoperative period (15-30 minutes), the packing of the wound with a gauze swab soaked in sterile saline is indicated. The dimension of the gauze swab should not be excessive, as it should only exert a mild pressure on the involved area while being kept in place by the opposing arch dentition. The gauze swab must be soaked in sterile saline to prevent adhesion to the surface of the blood clot with the subsequent risk of clot dislocation once the gauze is removed.

> **What is the role of the non-dominant hand of the operator during tooth extraction?**
> The non-dominant hand can retract the soft tissues of the cheek, the lip, and the tongue. It can also be useful in the stabilisation of the patient's head during surgical manoeuvres. When luxation is performed, two fingers on the non-dominant hand should be used to palpate the buccal and palatal/lingual cortical plates to control the applied pressure and expansion of the alveolar ridge.

Extraction of maxillary teeth

Position of the operator and patient

The positions described are for right-handed operators who are used to sitting on the right-hand side of the patient. The seated position is preferable, as it provides better control of the applied force and reduces fatigue. For the extraction of maxillary teeth, the operating table (or dental chair) is kept flat so that the occlusal plane lies perpendicular to the floor. For the extraction of teeth in the lateral and posterior areas of the right maxilla, the patient's head should be rotated towards the left (4.14a), while for the extraction of teeth in the lateral and posterior areas of the left maxilla, the patient's head should be rotated towards the right. Finally, for the extraction of teeth in the anterior area of the maxilla, the patient's head is kept straight. For the right maxilla, the thumb of the left hand should retract the upper lip and the cheek and simultaneously palpate the alveolar ridge, while the left index finger should be positioned on the palatal side of the alveolar ridge. Therefore, the non-dominant hand is used to retract the soft tissues, stabilise the patient's head, and control the pressure applied during tooth luxation. For the left maxilla, the position of the thumb and index fingers is inverted: the thumb is positioned on the palatal mucosa, while the index finger is positioned on the buccal side (4.14b-c).

Luxation movements vary according to the tooth being extracted, as they are mainly dictated by root anatomy (4.15a-e).

For left-handed operators who always sit on the left-hand side of the patient, the positions described are reversed. However, it is worth remembering that the best view and easiest execution of surgical manoeuvres are obtained when operating on the side of the tooth being extracted. Therefore, it would be useful if the operator learned to operate on both sides of the patient and with both hands. The positions described above are applicable not only to tooth extractions, but to all oral surgery interventions.

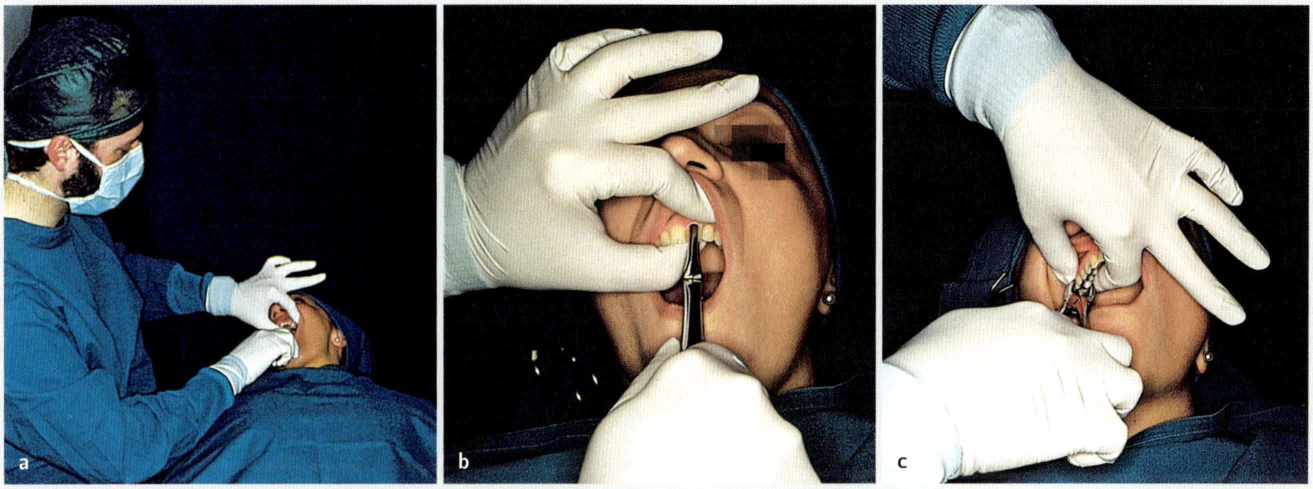

4.14 **a)** Position of the patient and operator for the extraction of a tooth in the left hemimaxilla. **b)** Control of the luxation movements, stabilisation of the head, and retraction of the soft tissues with the non-dominant hand. **c)** Correct positioning of the operator's hands to perform extractions in the right hemimaxilla.

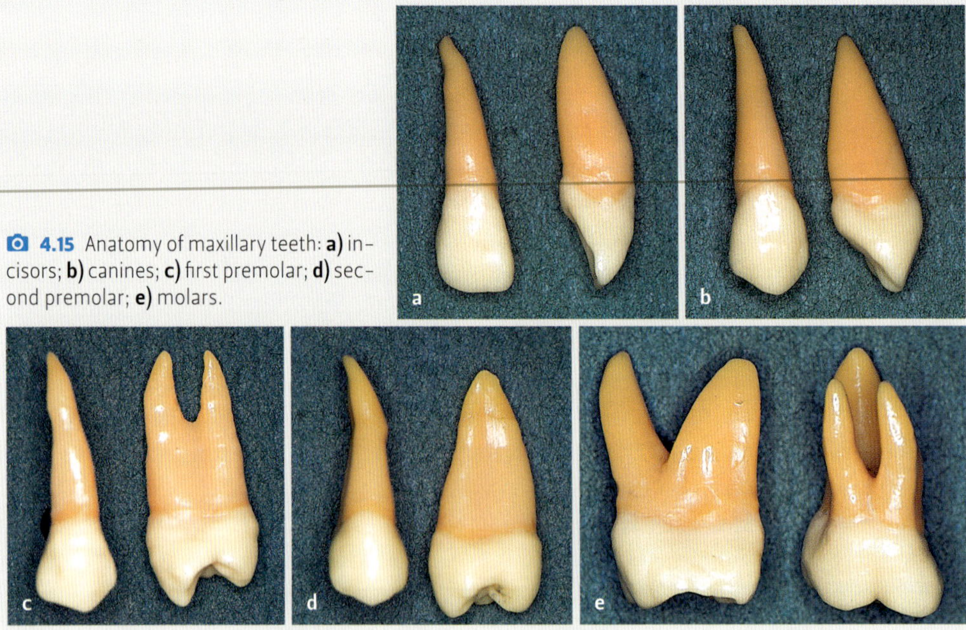

4.15 Anatomy of maxillary teeth: **a)** incisors; **b)** canines; **c)** first premolar; **d)** second premolar; **e)** molars.

UPPER CENTRAL INCISOR

Luxation movements: during tooth luxation, movements towards the buccal cortical plate and palatal cortical plate are performed in association with rotational movements that are possible due to the conical shape of the root. Rotational movements can be performed only if no signs of root anomalies are visible on the preoperative radiographic examinations.

Buccal-luxation movements are accentuated towards the buccal side, as the buccal cortical plate is thin and easily expandable; these movements should be performed slowly and gradually to prevent fractures of the alveolar ridge.

UPPER LATERAL INCISOR

Luxation movements: the main component of these movements is directed along the buccal-palatal axis, while the rotational movements should be limited to the final phase of luxation due to the oval section of the root and its smaller diameter. Preoperative radiographic examination can help identify the root anomalies that may sometimes occur.

Luxation movements should always be slow and controlled to prevent root fractures, which are possible given the relative fragility of the root.

UPPER CANINE

Luxation movements: they are similar to those described for the luxation of central and lateral incisors and they should always be performed with caution to avoid the fracture of the buccal cortical plate that, in the area of the canines, is particularly thin. Moreover, it is worth remembering that the root of the canine is longer and more robust than the roots of the other teeth, and as a further complicating factor, an accentuated curvature of the apical portion of the root may be present. The root has an oval section and a significant diameter, which cause the presence of canine eminence; in this area, the root is covered only by a thin layer of bone that, in some cases, may also be completely absent.

Luxation begins with a slow and controlled movement towards the buccal cortical plate to expand it, followed by a movement towards the palate. When the socket is expanded, mesial and distal rotational movements can be performed if no curvatures are present in the apical third of the root.

FIRST UPPER PREMOLAR

Luxation movements: in over 50% of cases the first upper premolar is characterised by the presence of two small roots (buccal and palatal) that are often fused in the coronal and middle thirds. Due to this peculiar root conformation, root fractures are more likely to occur; however, correct luxation manoeuvres can prevent this complication in the majority of cases. On the other hand, rotational movements are contraindicated as they can easily cause fracturing of the small apexes inside the socket. Luxation is performed with a slow movement towards the buccal cortical plate, followed by a movement of lesser amplitude towards the palate. In fact, accentuated palatal movements increase the risk of fracture of the palatal root, which is more difficult to reach and to remove. In some cases (e.g. short and fine roots), it may be indicated to perform the extraction of an upper first premolar with an open surgical approach; elevation of an access flap, odontotomy, and independent luxation of the two roots can prevent root fractures.

UPPER SECOND PREMOLAR

Luxation movements: only 15% of upper second premolars have two roots. Therefore, extraction of these teeth is generally easier than that of first upper premolars, since the presence of a single, bigger root reduces the risk of fractures. It is nonetheless indicated to begin luxation with a straight root elevator, and avoid rotational movements; the latter could be used in the last phase of tooth luxation, if the presence of a second root has been excluded by analysis of the preoperative radiographs. Luxation movements are mainly directed towards the buccal cortical plate, while gentle palatal pressure may contribute to socket expansion (4.16a-e).

FIRST AND SECOND UPPER MOLAR

Luxation movements: the complex root anatomy of the upper molars, characterised by three divergent roots, requires a careful preoperative evaluation, particularly as far as root length/curvature and their relationships to the floor of the maxillary sinus are concerned. Of the three roots, the palatal is the most robust, and often the longest: it typically diverges from the main axis of the tooth at a pronounced angle (circa 45°). In general, the mesio-buccal root has an oval section, while the disto-buccal root has a rounder section. The apexes of the buccal roots may exhibit symmetric curvatures that increase tooth retention. The roots of the second upper molar are usually less divergent and shorter compared to those of the first molar. In some cases, the buccal roots, or even all the roots, may be fused.

The extraction technique using forceps (similar to the one described for the extraction of premolars) mainly entails luxation movements directed towards the buccal cortical plate, which is typically thinner than the palatal cortical plate. The movements should be slow and ample, and it is necessary to maintain the pressure against the two cortical plates for several seconds to allow gradual compression of the alveolar bone and expansion of the socket to occur. However, in some cases, luxation manoeuvres performed with forceps may cause partial fractures of the buccal cortical plate and interradicular septa, particu-

Clinical case 1 – Extraction of the second maxillary premolar

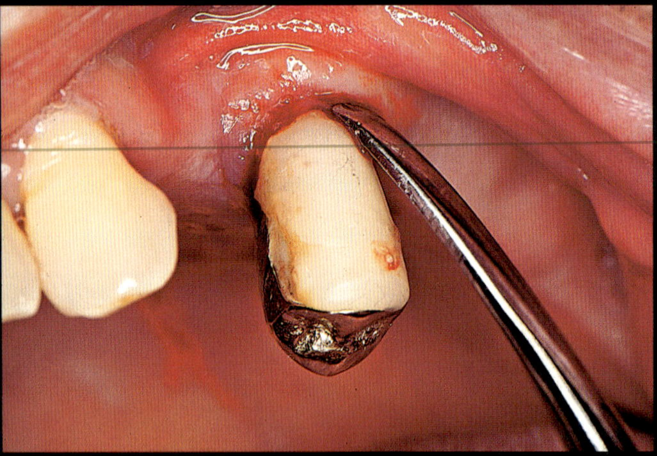

4.16a Extraction of 2.5: periotomy performed with a periosteal elevator.

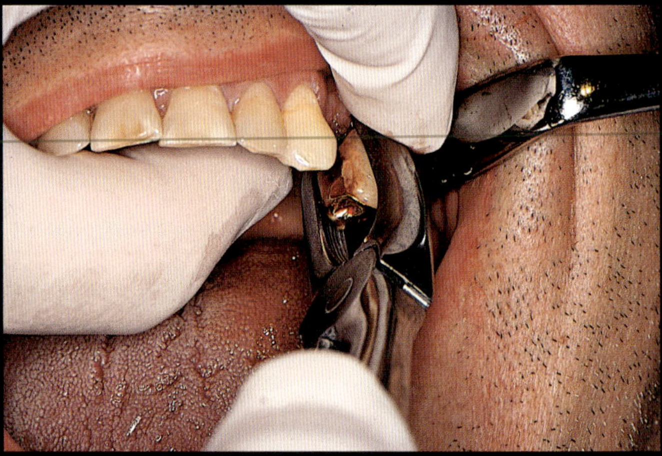

4.16b Luxation of the tooth with alternate movements towards the buccal and palatal cortical plates associated with stabilisation of the alveolar ridge with fingers on the non-dominant hand.

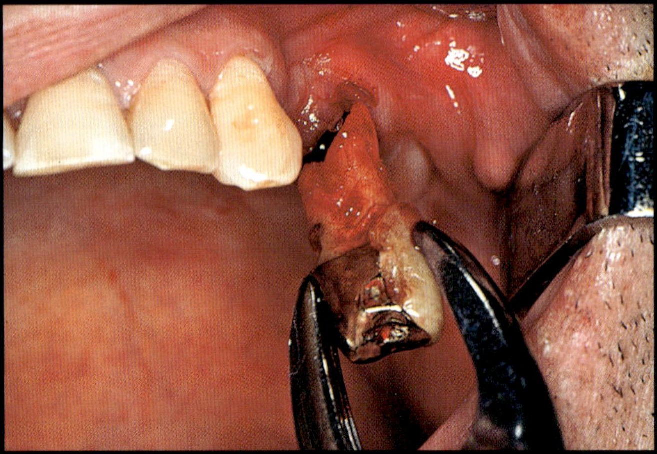

4.16c Extraction.

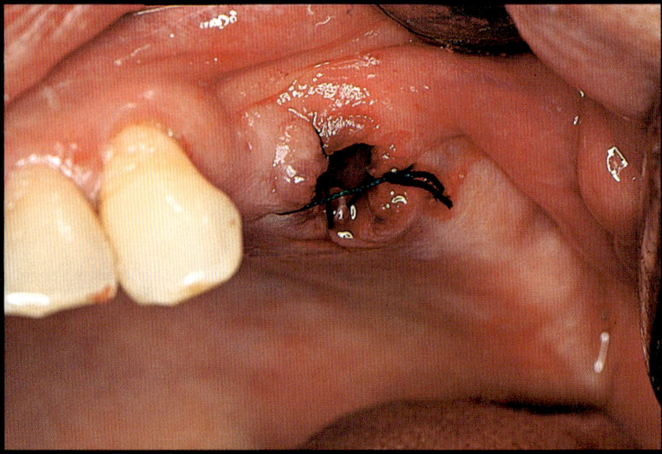

4.16d Suture after socket inspection and curettage.

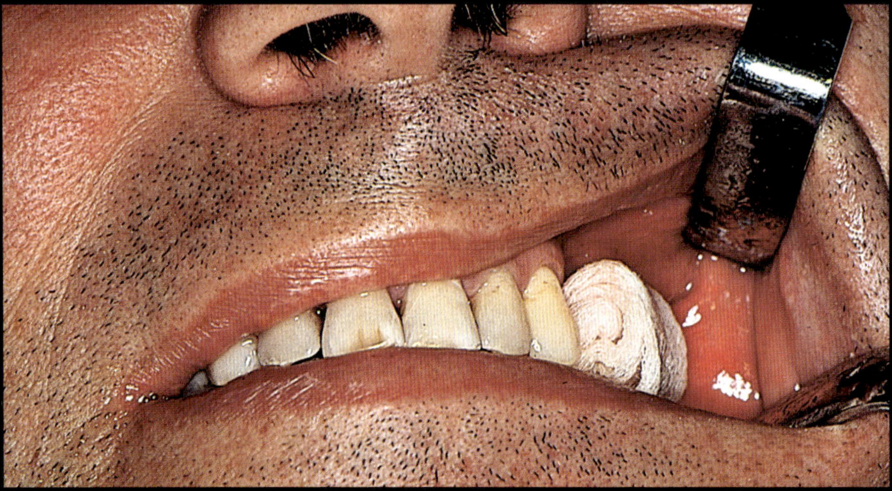

4.16e The wound is packed with a sterile gauze swab soaked in sterile saline to facilitate hae–

larly when these are thin. For this reason, especially when the roots diverge significantly or when the apexes are in close proximity to the floor of the maxillary sinus, the recourse to an open surgical approach involving the elevation of a mucoperiosteal flap and the separation of the roots is indicated. This approach makes it possible to reduce force, achieve tooth luxation and extraction and eliminate the risk of fracturing the buccal cortical plate, thus preserving the integrity of the interradicular septa. If an oroantral communication is created between the socket and the lumen of the sinus, the preservation of the interradicular septa improves the prognosis, as the buccal cortical plate acts as a support for the soft tissues, and the presence of the interradicular septa causes favourable anatomic conditions for blood clot stability and a quicker reossification of the socket.

UPPER THIRD MOLARS

Luxation movements: the upper third molar is often smaller than the first and second molars, but exhibits a great variety as far as root anatomy is concerned. In the majority of cases, the roots are fused into one single conical root, but it is not infrequent to see upper third molars with three or four roots in various lengths and curvatures. In many cases, the luxation can be completed with a root elevator, either straight or angled according to the accessibility of the area. In fact, after the papilla is detached, the tip of the root elevator should be wedged between the second and third molar and be kept against the interdental septum (not against the second molar) while luxation movements are applied in a distal and buccal direction. This technique is particularly indicated for upper third molars with a short conical root. In these cases, if the operator sits on the same side as the tooth to be extracted, the patient's head should be turned in the opposite direction and the mouth should be half-closed, to facilitate the correct location of the insertion point for the tip of the root elevator, and to reduce traction on the labial commissure. Luxation should always be cautious and gradual to prevent fracture of the maxillary tuberosity, which is a relatively frequent complication during the extraction of upper third molars. Luxation with the extraction forceps is achieved by alternating movements towards the buccal cortical plate and palate. Furthermore, pressure against the cortical plates should always be maintained for several seconds to allow gradual compression of the alveolar bone and expansion of the socket: this approach is particularly indicated in the presence of multiple divergent roots. The alveolar bone in the posterior maxilla is generally soft and elastic, due to its scarce mineralisation; therefore, it is frequently possible to complete the extraction of upper third molars with a complex root anatomy without separating the roots with rotary instruments.

Extraction of mandibular teeth

POSITION OF THE OPERATOR AND PATIENT

Ideally, for extraction of mandibular teeth, the mandibular occlusal plane should be parallel with the floor. A 45° angle between the seat and back of the operating table (or dental chair) is generally optimal for ensuring that the patient is correctly positioned. When performing extractions in the anterior area of the mandible and in the right mandible, the right-handed operator may sit on the patient's right-hand side, while to perform extractions in the left mandible the operator should sit on the patient's left-hand side, as this position provides a better view of the operating field, increases comfort for the patient, and facilitates execution of the surgical manoeuvres. Alternatively, the operator can sit at 12 o'clock, directly behind the patient. During extraction of mandibular teeth (particular-

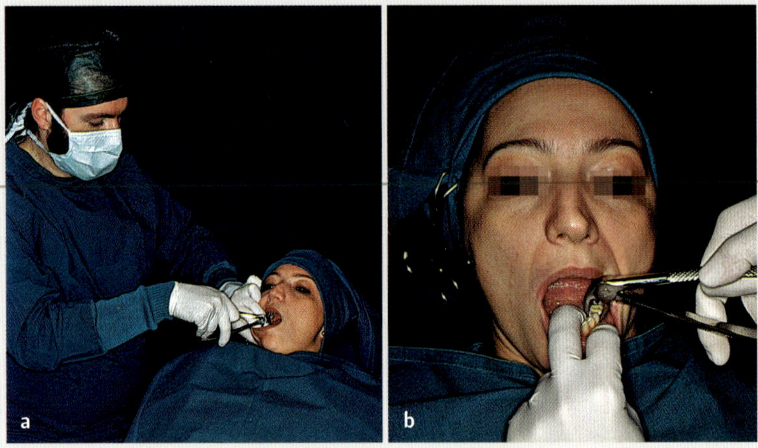

4.17 **a)** Position of the patient and operator for the extraction of teeth in the right hemimandible. **b)** Stabilisation of the mandible for the extraction of teeth in the left hemimandible.

ly molars), which requires the application of greater force, the operator's left hand is used to retract the soft tissues and to stabilise the mandible, to avoid transmission of excessive stress on the temporomandibular joints (4.17a).

For the right mandible, the thumb retracts the cheek and the other fingers on the left hand allow stabilisation of the mandible. For the left mandible, the index finger retracts the cheek, the middle finger can be positioned lingually to retract the tongue, and the thumb stabilises the mandible (4.17b). The luxation movements to extract mandibular teeth vary according to the thickness of the cortical plates in different areas and to the root anatomy of different teeth (4.18a-d).

As far as left-handed and ambidextrous operators are concerned, the same considerations reported in the section related to the extraction of maxillary teeth apply.

LOWER INCISORS

Luxation movements: luxation is performed with movements of equal amplitude towards the buccal and lingual cortical plates, followed by rotational movements: these latter should be performed with caution due to the reduced diameter of the root (4.19a-c).

LOWER CANINE

Luxation movements: the first luxation movement is performed towards the buccal cortical plate, which is very thin, and movements towards the lingual cortical plate follow to achieve expansion of the socket. Rotational movement should be used only in the last phase of the extraction, as the analysis of periapical or panoramic radiographs alone is not sufficient to exclude the presence of a doubling of the root.

LOWER PREMOLARS

Luxation movements: luxation is generally performed with alternating movements towards the buccal and lingual cortical plate of the same amplitude. Rotational movements can be used to loosen the fibres of the periodontal ligament, as the root of the mandibular premolars is usually single, straight, and almost conical in shape. If preoperative radiographic examinations show signs of possible forking of the root (typically in the apical third), rotational movements are contraindicated.

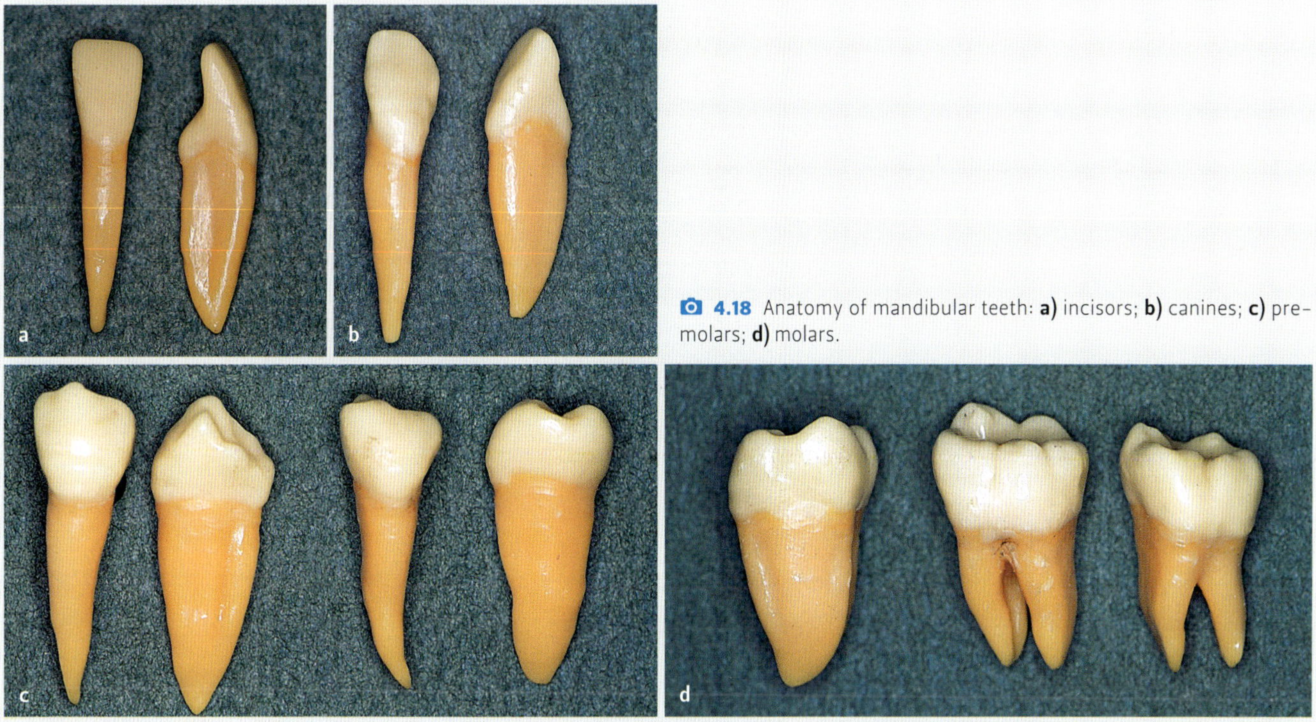

4.18 Anatomy of mandibular teeth: **a)** incisors; **b)** canines; **c)** premolars; **d)** molars.

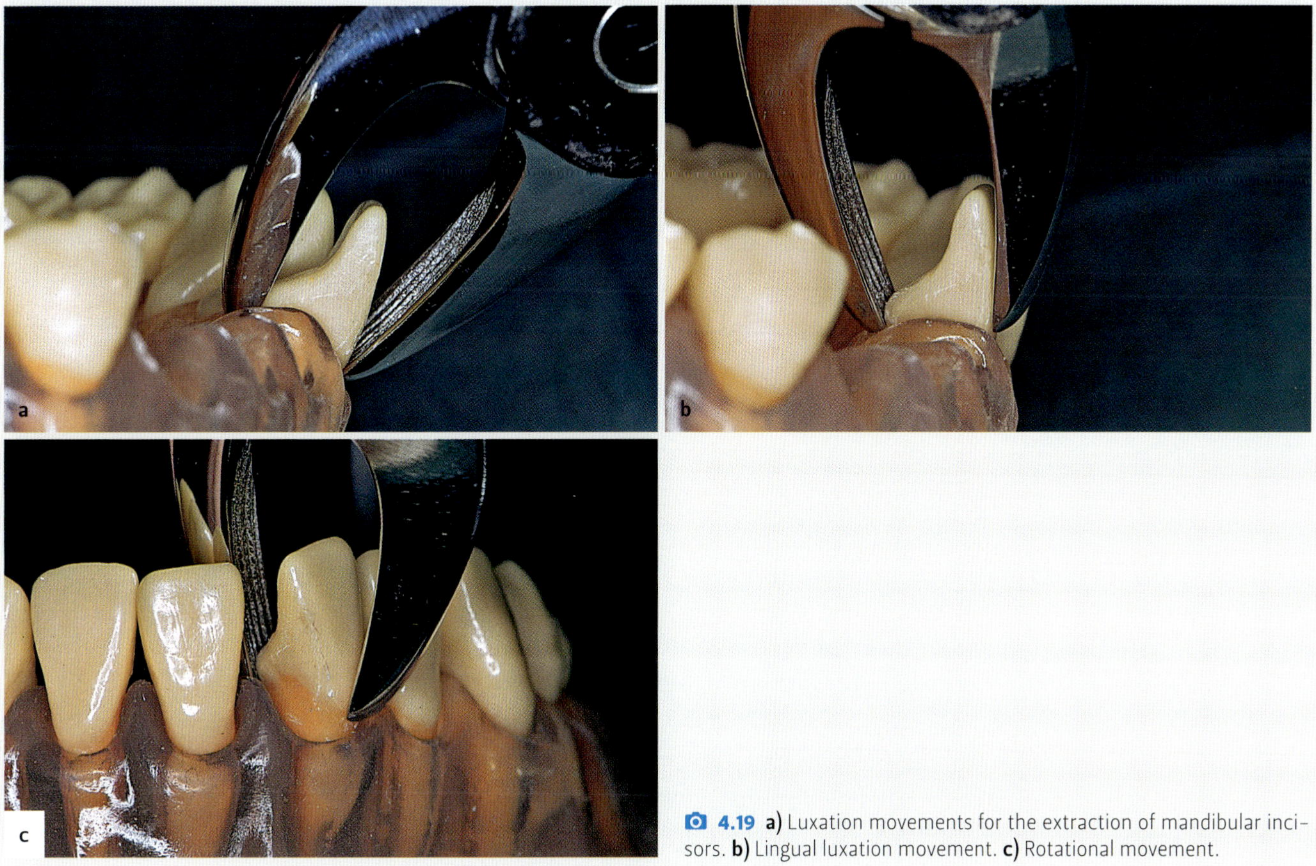

4.19 **a)** Luxation movements for the extraction of mandibular incisors. **b)** Lingual luxation movement. **c)** Rotational movement.

LOWER MOLARS

Luxation movements: mandibular molars typically have two robust roots, mesial and distal, which in some cases may be fused; both roots have an almost oval shape. Sometimes, instead of a single mesial root, a mesio-buccal and a mesio-lingual root are present.

The buccal cortical plate in the molar region is thick and dense, and corresponds to the mesial portion of the external oblique line of the mandible. The lingual cortical plate, although generally thinner, is nonetheless well represented. Root anatomy of the mandibular molars should always be analysed carefully. In the presence of fused or short roots, as well as in the case of tooth mobility, an open surgical approach may not be necessary. Conversely, in the case of multiple, long or curved roots, the elevation of a mucoperiosteal flap and the separation of the crown and roots with rotary instruments allows a significant reduction in the force needed to complete luxation and extraction of the tooth. This aspect is very important because it translates into greater comfort for the patient during the surgical manoeuvres and reduces the risk of lesions to the temporomandibular joint.

Luxation of mandibular molars requires ample movements towards the lingual and buccal cortical plate: increasing pressure should be exerted for several seconds against the cortical plates, particularly the lingual one that is thinner, to allow expansion of the socket. When no other teeth are present distally to the tooth to be extracted, initial luxation can be performed with a root elevator, which can be placed mesially to the tooth to apply a luxation force directed distally (4.20a-e).

Complex tooth extractions: open surgical technique

PREOPERATIVE EVALUATION

As previously mentioned, whenever complicating factors are identified in the course of the preoperative evaluation (endodontic treatment, ankylosis, crown and/or root fractures, etc.), it is indicated to opt for an open surgical approach in the first instance. When luxation with extraction forceps is unsuccessful, the elevation of a mucoperiosteal flap and separation of the crown and roots is recommended, to avoid unnecessary prolongation of fruitless surgical manoeuvres, and therefore of the operating time. The elevation of an access flap and ostectomy may be necessary in cases of accidental root fracture.

ADVANTAGES

Tooth extraction with the open surgical approach requires the application of lesser force to obtain luxation and extraction of the roots. Although apparently counterintuitive, the removal of a small quantity of bone and the separation of the roots facilitate the preservation of the alveolar bone, as these procedures significantly reduce the risk of fracturing the buccal cortical plate during luxation. Moreover, it is worth remembering that the preservation of the alveolar ridge is fundamental when substitution of the extracted tooth with an endosseous implant is planned.

The open surgical technique makes it possible to reduce the incidence of root fractures and the extent of possible oroantral communications, as well as the operating time if compared to repeated and fruitless attempts at extracting the tooth with extraction forceps.

Finally, in some cases the open surgical approach represents the only viable option for extracting a tooth, as in the case of decalcified or decayed roots.

Clinical case 2 – Extraction of an erupted mandibular third molar

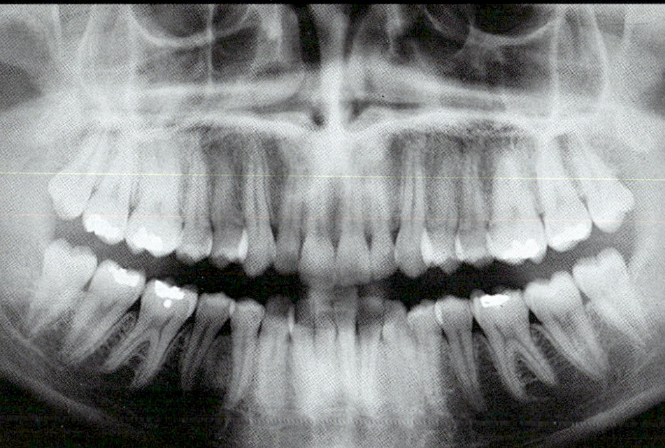

4.20a The panoramic radiographs shows a favourable anatomy of the root of 4.8.

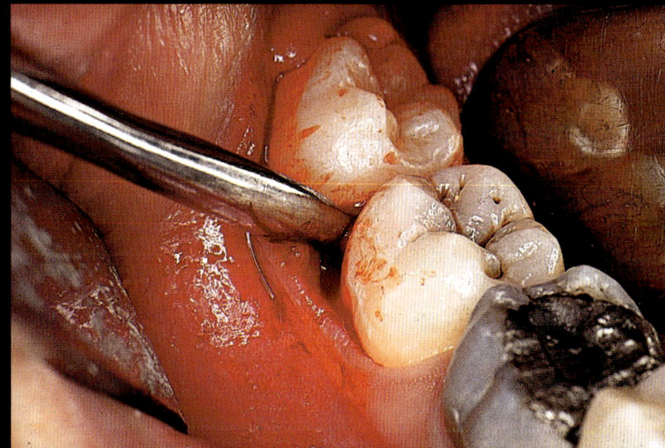

4.20b Initial luxation is performed with a root elevator.

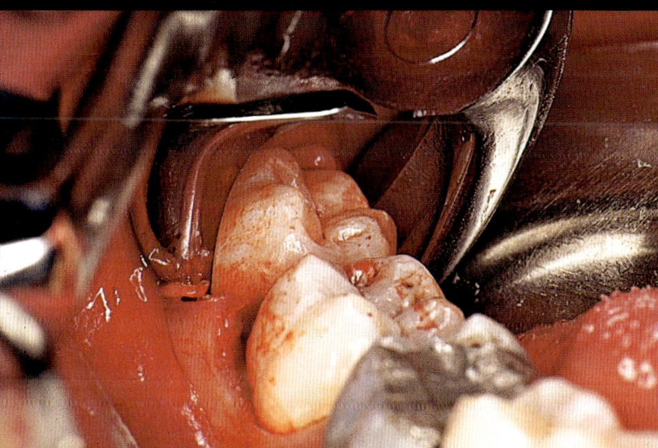

4.20c The beaks of the extraction forceps are placed below the cementoenamel junction.

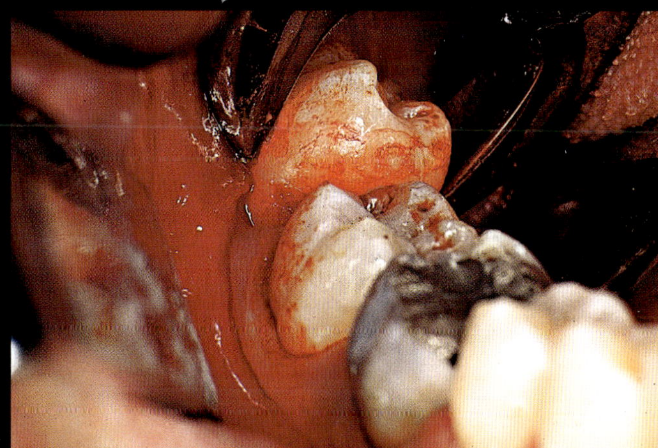

4.20d Luxation towards the lingual cortical plate.

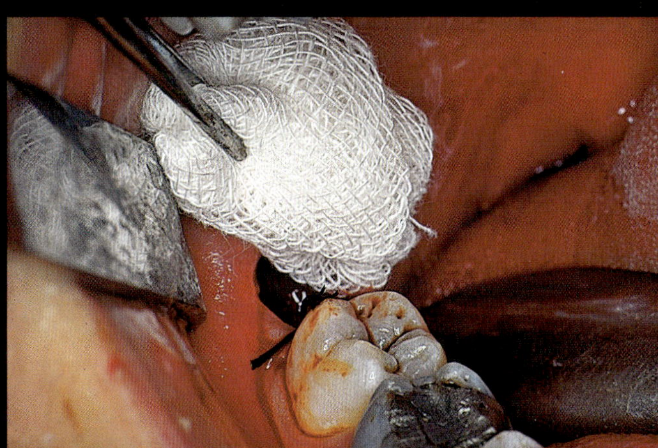

4.20e Haemostasis: compression with a sterile gauze swab soaked in sterile saline after the papilla between 4.7 and 4.8 is sutured.

Open surgical technique

Advantages
- Lesser force
- Preservation of the alveolar ridge
- Lower incidence of root fractures
- Reduced incidence of oroantral communications
- Time savings

Disadvantages
- Requires peculiar skills
- Requires specific armamentarium

DISADVANTAGES

Elevating an access flap and performing ostectomy and odontotomy, in addition to the use of specific surgical instruments, require a higher level of surgical skills.

Specific armamentarium (4.21a-b)

Besides the basic armamentarium (scalpel, periosteal elevators, retractors, etc.), performing tooth extraction with an open surgical approach requires specific surgical instruments:
- surgical straight handpiece and surgical burs to perform ostectomy and odontotomy;
- angled root elevators (Walter-Barry and or Pott elevators);
- apical pick elevators (Heidbrink elevators);
- root forceps;
- haemostatic forceps (Halsted-Mosquito or Kocher) that may be used to extract root fragments once they are luxated.

Technique

ANAESTHESIA

Anaesthesia follows the principles described in Chapter 3.

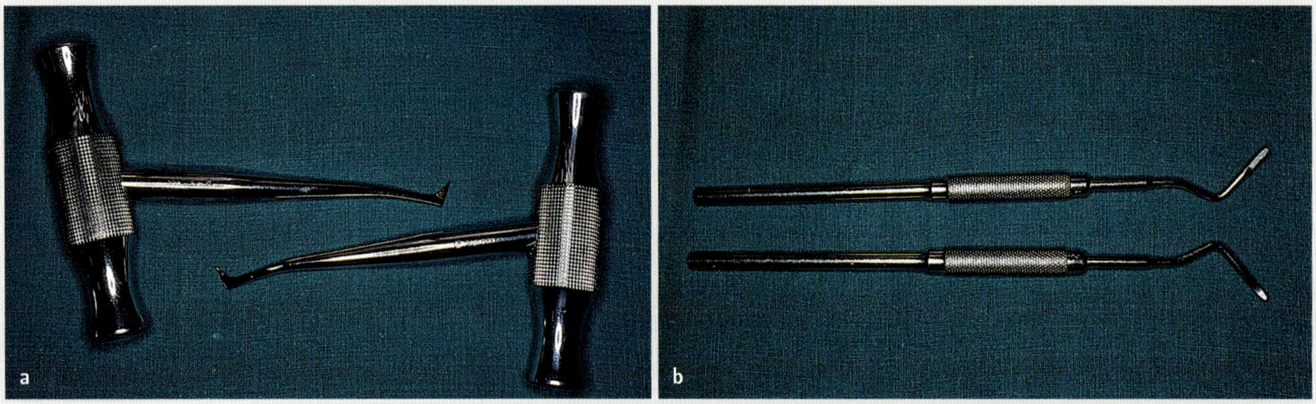

4.21 Specific armamentarium used for open surgical approach: **a)** Walter-Barry angled root elevators; **b)** Heidbrink angled apical pick elevators.

PREPARATION OF A MUCOPERIOSTEAL FLAP

Marginal (sulcular) incisions, in association with releasing incisions when required. Envelope flaps are used if limited access is sufficient for safely performing a marginal ostectomy. When greater exposure of the area is necessary, the envelope flap can be easily converted into a three- or four-corner flap, with the addition of one or two releasing incisions. It is worth noting that, once the releasing incisions are made, the shape and dimension of the access flap cannot be modified due to the risk of interrupting vascularisation of some soft tissue areas. Therefore, it is important to plan the extension and design of the flap with care before releasing incisions are made, to avoid technical difficulties caused by an inadequate operating field that cannot be modified.

OSTECTOMY

In some cases, the simple elevation of the access flap allows the positioning of the beaks of the extraction forceps more apically, on sound dental tissue, and to complete the tooth extraction. Root elevators can also be used more efficiently once the soft tissues are elevated from the crestal bone and retracted. When the exposed portion of the tooth is not sufficient to permit the completion of the extraction manoeuvres, it is necessary to remove a certain amount of bone.

Usually, ostectomy is performed on the buccal cortical plate, which is more easily accessible. A round or fissure bur mounted on a straight surgical handpiece (or, alternatively, piezoelectric instruments) can be used, and the quantity of bone removed should be the least possible, to guarantee adequate preservation of the alveolar ridge (4.22a-c). In some cases, in the presence of thick interdental septa, a more conservative option is represented by the removal of bone around roots in the interdental area. As a result, the space created between the root and interdental septum may be used to introduce the tip of a root elevator and alternately luxate the root mesially and distally until its complete mobilisation.

When molars are extracted, it may be useful to extend ostectomy to expose the furcation, to perform the following separation of the roots with greater precision (4.23a-c).

It is worth noting that the creation of an adequate space between the alveolar bone and the root can also be achieved by removing dental tissue instead of alveolar bone. This technique should be used particularly when immediate or delayed placement of endosseous implants is planned.

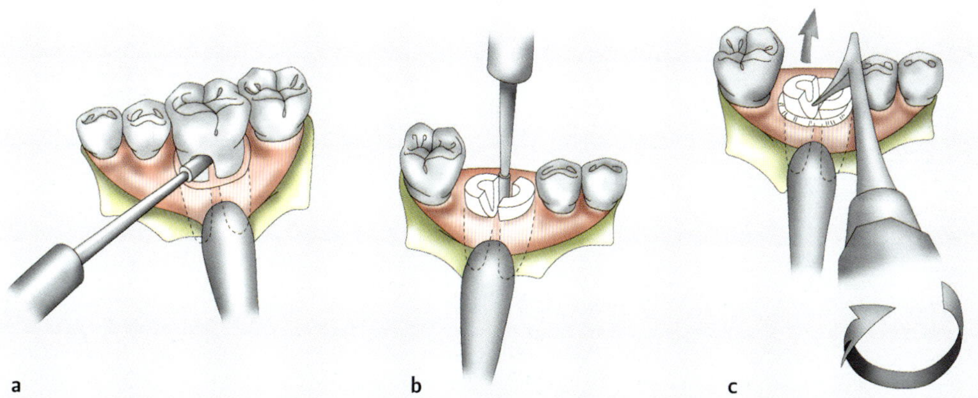

4.22 Extraction of a mandibular molar with an open surgical approach: **a)** buccal ostectomy and horizontal section of the crown with a fissure bur; **b)** separation of the mesial and distal roots; **c)** luxation of the roots with a root elevator.

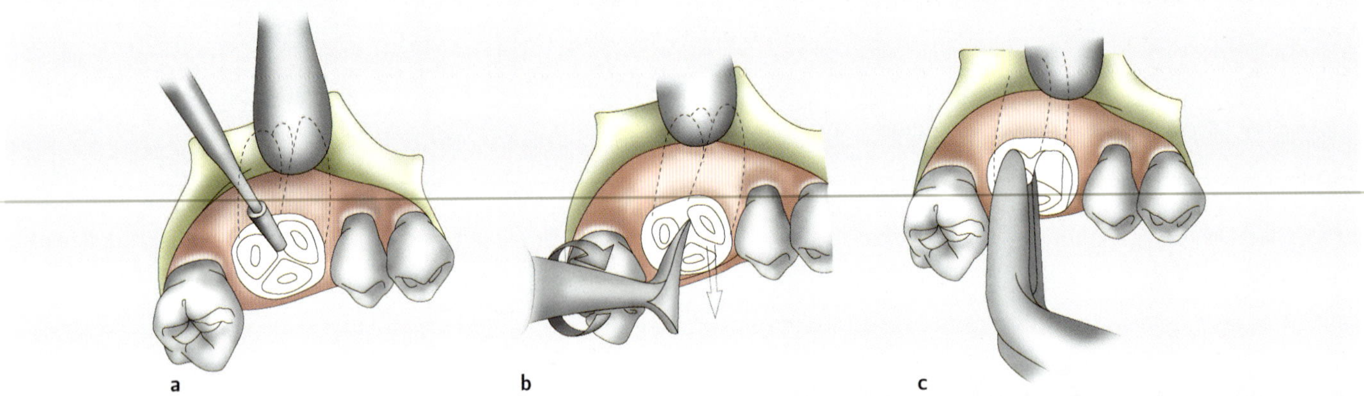

4.23 Extraction of a multi-rooted maxillary tooth with an open surgical approach: **a)** separation of the roots and removal of the most coronal portion of the interradicular septa; **b)** luxation with a root elevator; **c)** extraction of the roots with specifically designed root forceps.

ODONTOTOMY

The separation of the roots of multi-rooted teeth (odontotomy) enables the extraction procedure to be simplified.

In proximity to the mandibular canal or the floor of the maxillary sinus, separation of the roots should never be completed with surgical burs: the last septum of dental tissue should be interrupted by fracture separation, with the aid of a root elevator wedged between the roots to be divided.

This recommendation is particularly important when extracting maxillary molars, as the furcation may be in close proximity to the floor of the maxillary sinus. For decayed teeth, the corrupt portion of the tooth should be removed first, to expose sound dental tissue that can withstand the force applied with root elevators, and identify the pulp chamber, which represents an important reference point for the following root separation (4.23a-c). If the roots present an accentuated converging curvature, then separation and removal of the most coronal portion of the tooth provides space to perform luxation more effectively. It is preferable to begin root separation from the centre of the floor of the pulp chamber and proceed towards its periphery. Rotary (fissure burs) or piezoelectric instruments should always be used on dental tissue to avoid any damage to the alveolar bone. To prevent lesions of the surrounding soft tissues, the latter should always be retracted and protected with retractors or periosteal elevators, which act as barriers against possible contact with rotating burs.

When odontotomy is planned, amalgam restorations and cast or prefabricated metal posts should be removed before the access flap is elevated, to avoid dispersion of metal particles on the alveolar bone and soft tissues that may cause amalgam tattoos in the area.

LUXATION OF THE ROOTS

Generally, luxation of the roots is performed with straight or angled root elevators. These elevators may act between the alveolar ridge and the root, or between two roots to be extracted. This latter action should be performed with caution, to prevent the application of an apical pressure to one of the roots. Luxation should involve the root that presents a more favourable shape first: this can mean the shortest one, the one with the lesser curvature, or the one that presents a degree of mobility. Luxation may be completed with root forceps, which can also be used to complete extraction of the root (4.23a-c).

The open surgical approach can also be adopted for extraction of single-rooted teeth, when the anatomy of the root is unfavourable. Periradicular ostectomy provides easier mobilisation of the root and provides favourable insertion points for the tip of root elevators. In the presence of significant curvatures of the roots, or close proximity of the roots of the adjacent teeth, interproximal ostectomy may be contraindicated. In these cases, vertical separation of the root in two halves can be performed with a fissure bur, and completed with the aid of a small root elevator. The root elevator is then wedged between the wall of the socket and the two root fragments to luxate them towards the space created with the fissure bur (4.24).

POSSIBLE REMOVAL OF THE INTERRADICULAR SEPTA

In the presence of long roots exhibiting significant curvatures, their separation may not be sufficient to obtain adequate luxation and complete the extraction. In these cases, it is indicated to remove the most coronal portion of the interradicular septum with a round bur. Luxation attempts and ostectomy in an apical direction are alternated until adequate luxation is obtained with the application of controlled force.

BONE REMODELLING

Possible sharp edges resulted from ostectomy should be removed or rounded off with a bone rongeur or with rotary instruments (e.g. round bur). Moreover, it is important to verify the integrity of the interradicular septa: possible fractures should be identified and the fractured fragments removed.

SUTURE

Once the extraction is completed, the access flap must be correctly repositioned with sutures to restore the original anatomy of the soft tissues. Step-by-step clinical cases are presented in 4.25a-f, 4.26a-g.

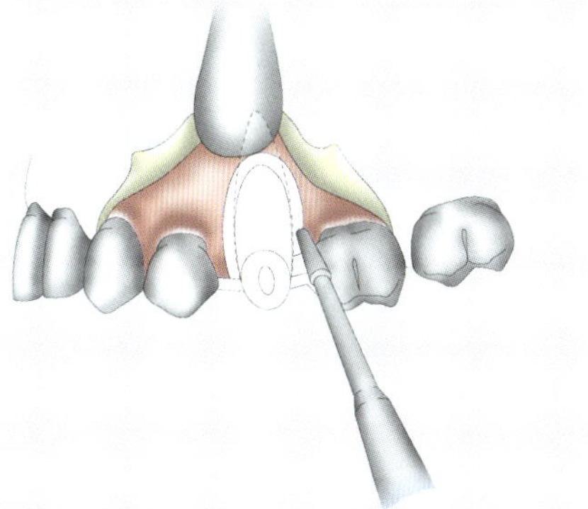

4.24 Extraction of a single-rooted tooth with an open surgical approach: periradicular ostectomy.

Clinical case 3 – Extraction of 3.6 presenting a large carious lesion

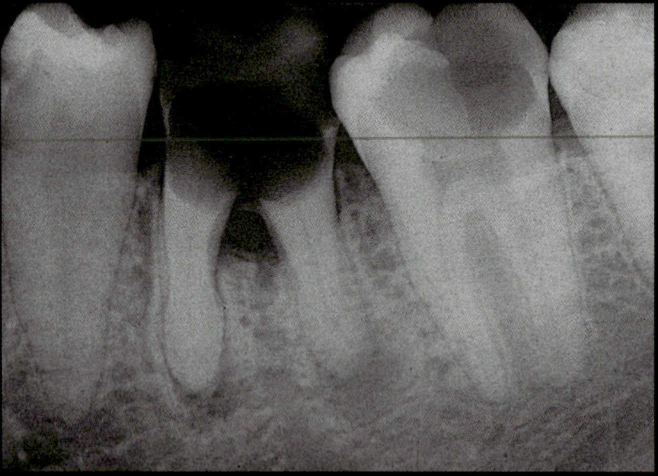

4.25a Large carious lesion on 3.6.

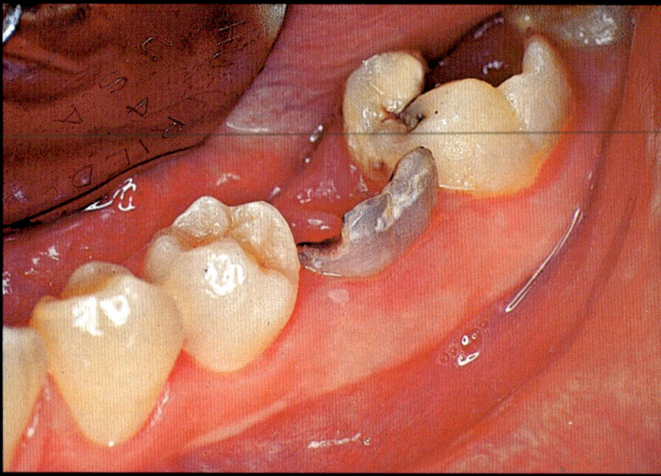

4.25b The crown is almost completely destroyed by the lesion: therefore, extraction forceps cannot be used.

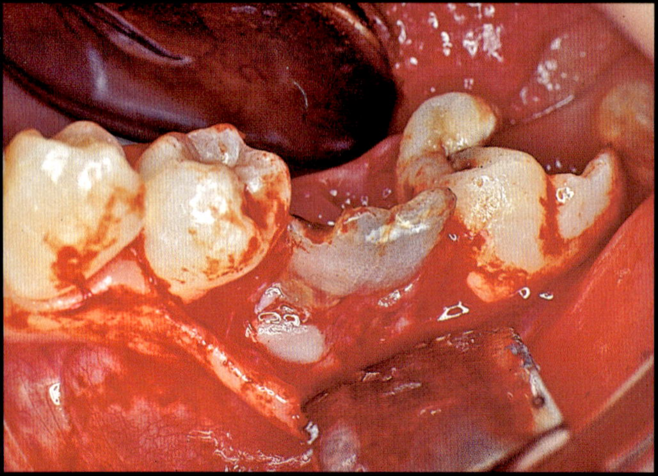

4.25c The buccal cortical plate is exposed.

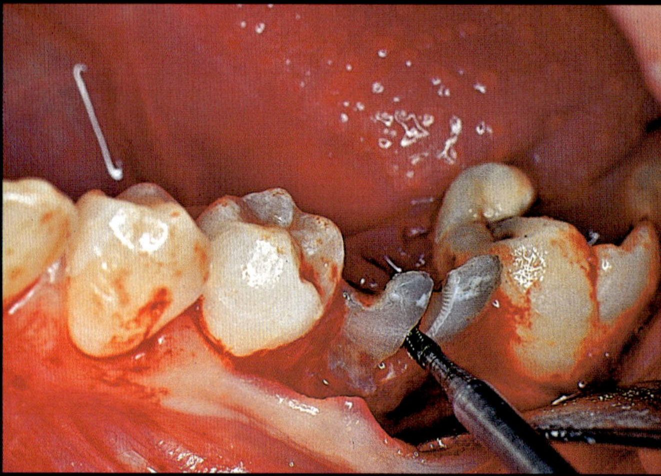

4.25d Vertical odontotomy.

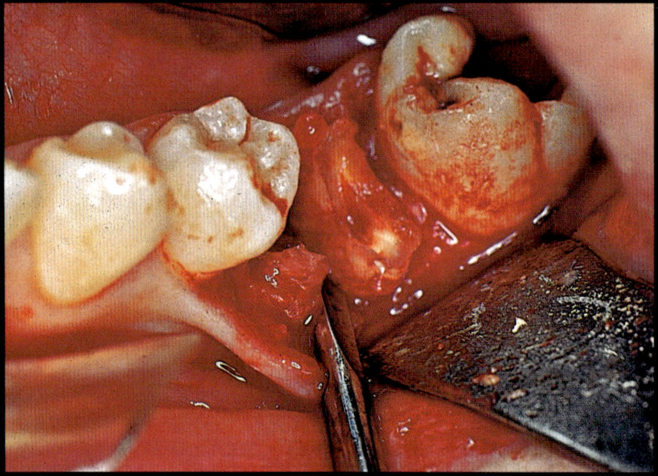

4.25e Luxation of the roots with a straight root elevator.

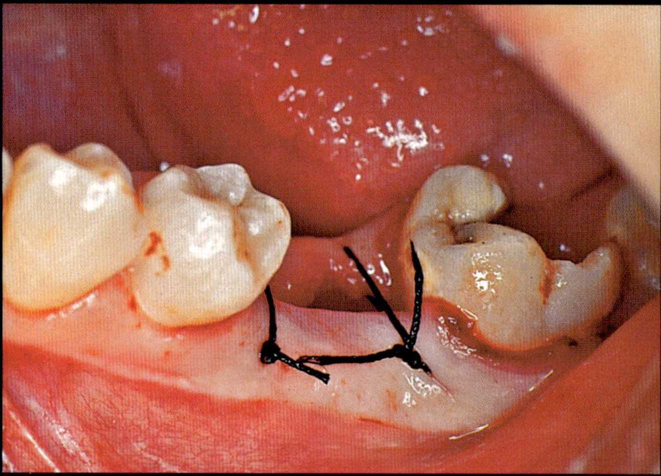

4.25f Suture.

Clinical case 4 – Extraction of erupted 3.8

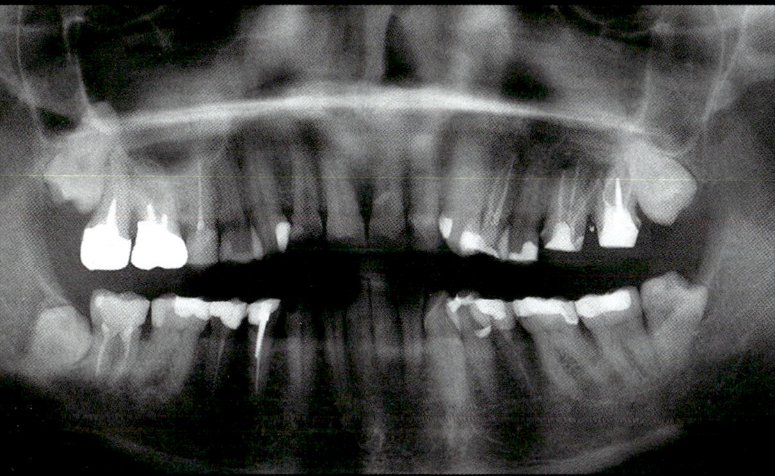

4.26a Panoramic radiograph showing a deep carious lesion on 3.8. Pulp vitality test response is negative.

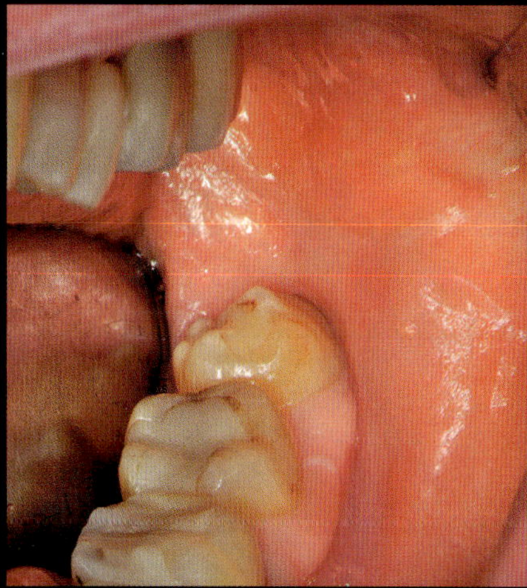

4.26b Initial clinical situation.

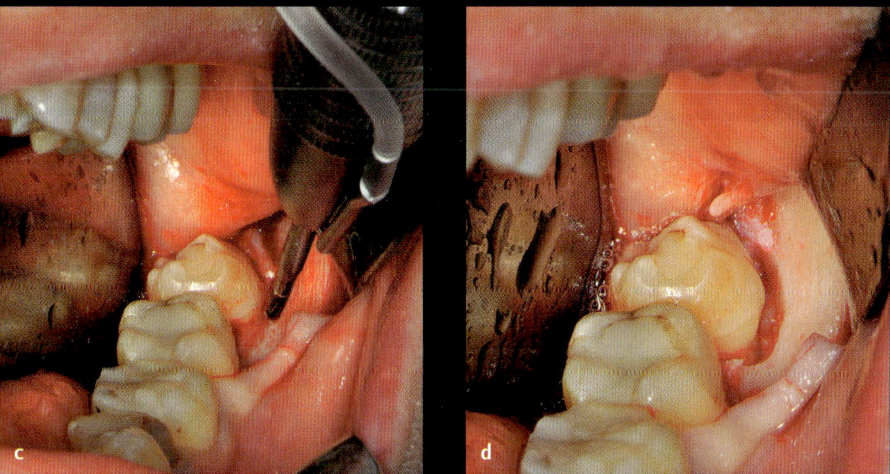

4.26c–d A mucoperiosteal flap is elevated and pericoronal ostectomy is performed with a fissure bur.

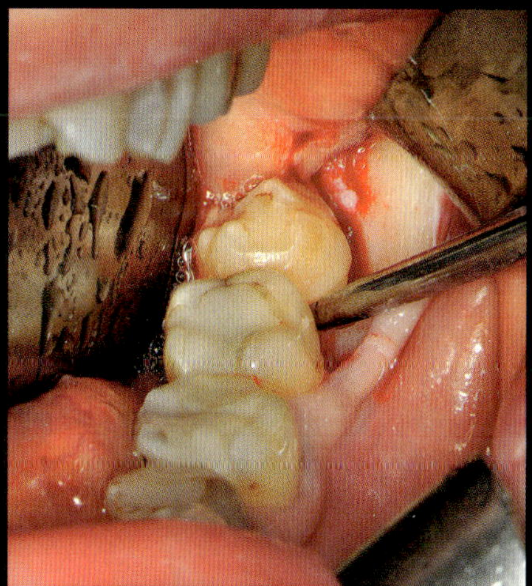

4.26e Luxation of the tooth with a straight root elevator.

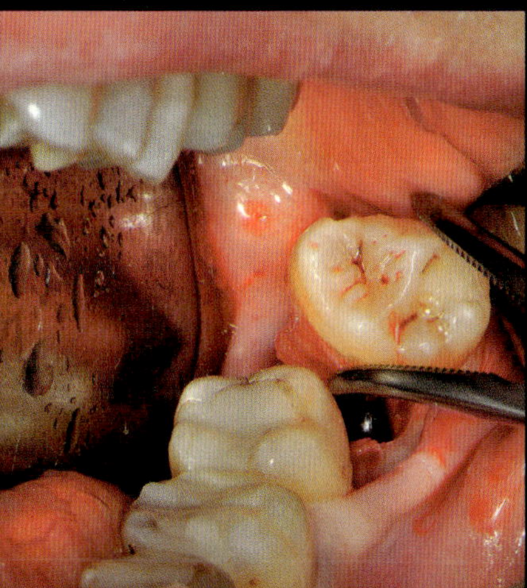

4.26f Extraction of the tooth.

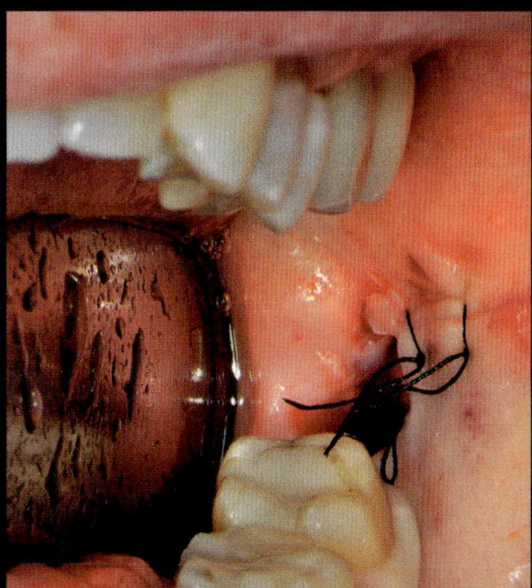

4.26g Suture.

Surgical technique for the removal of fractured root apexes

The fracture of the apical third of a root during tooth extraction is an uncommon complication. It is always recommended that extraction of fractured root apexes be completed, particularly in the presence of lesions caused by bacterial infection (e.g. periapical lesions, carious lesions with pulp necrosis, etc.), to prevent a local intraosseous infection that may lead to severe complications (e.g. osteomyelitis). Fragments of root apexes may be left inside the socket (although this is not an ideal solution) when their removal involves the associated risk of damaging important anatomic structures, such as the inferior alveolar nerve, and as long as no signs of infection of the tooth are present.

IDENTIFYING THE POSITION OF THE FRACTURED ROOT FRAGMENT

When a fracture of the root apex occurs, it is important to observe the extracted portion of the tooth: this inspection makes it possible to obtain valuable information about the dimension and shape of the fractured fragment. Furthermore, it is necessary to locate its precise position; ideal visibility of the socket should be obtained by means of profuse irrigation with sterile saline and suction with surgical suction tips. If there are any doubts on the precise location of the fragment or its relationship to adjacent anatomic structures, it is recommended that an intraoperative periapical radiograph be taken.

REMOVAL OF THE FRACTURED FRAGMENT

If the root fragment is sufficiently luxated when the fracture occurs, suction may be sufficient in some cases to remove it.

If the fragment shows no mobility, luxation with a thin apical pick elevator or periotome, wedged between it and the wall of the socket, should be performed. This manoeuvre must be performed circumferentially until complete mobilisation of the fragment is obtained. The fragment can then be removed with the aid of haemostatic forceps or with a surgical suction tip. Luxation with an apical pick elevator is easier if a space is created around a fragment in which the tip of the instrument can be wedged. Generally, a small fissure bur is used to complete this task, but special care must be taken to avoid any damage to anatomic structures such as the inferior alveolar nerve or the floor of the maxillary sinus, which may be in close proximity to the fractured apex.

If the root canal is visible, it is possible to attempt to engage it with the tip of an endodontic instrument (e.g. Hedstroem file) to exert traction; however, as root fractures frequently follow a diagonal path, this technique may not be applicable because the fractured surfaces are bevelled.

For ankylosed apexes, when all the manoeuvres described prove ineffective, the fractured fragment can be worn out with a round bur, taking care not to damage neighbouring anatomic structures. In such cases, it is indicated to take a postoperative periapical radiograph to verify successful elimination of the apex.

If none of the techniques described allow the complete removal of the fractured fragment, it is necessary to elevate a mucoperiosteal flap, and create an access ostectomy on the buccal cortical plate level with the apex. To identify the position of the apex with precision, the extracted tooth is measured with a periodontal probe, and the value obtained is reported on the surface of the buccal cortical plate. The fractured apex can then be luxated and extracted through the buccal ostectomy, or it can be lifted coronally with a root elevator and extracted through the socket (📷 4.27a–f).

If, in the absence of signs of infection, a root fragment is in close proximity to the mandibular canal, leaving it in situ may be an acceptable compromise to avoid the risk of damaging the inferior alveolar nerve.

A step-by-step clinical case is presented in 4.28a-g.

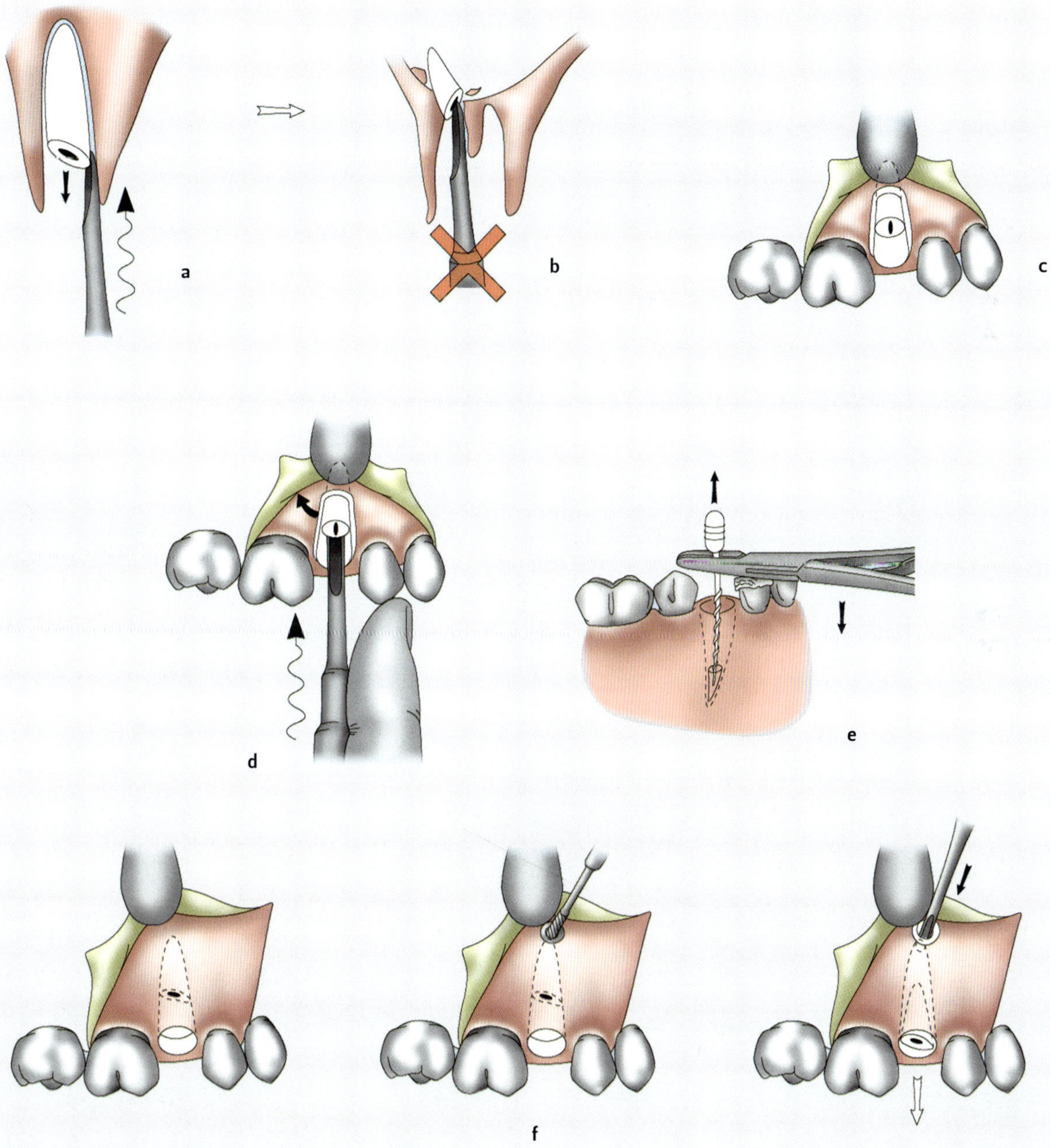

4.27 **a)** Extraction of a root fragment: luxation with an apical pick elevator. **b)** Incorrect movements may cause the dislocation of the root (e.g. inside the maxillary sinus). **c)** Conservative periradicular ostectomy. **d)** Luxation of the root fragment with a thin root elevator. **e)** Removal of the root fragment with an endodontic instrument (e.g. Hedstroem file). **f)** Removal of the root fragment after the elevation of a mucoperiosteal flap, periapical ostectomy with a round bur, and luxation through the access created.

Clinical case 5 – Extraction of 1.1 due to horizontal fracture

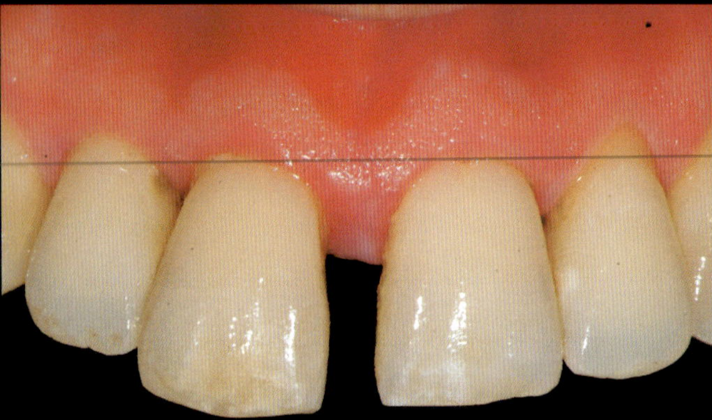

4.28a A horizontal fracture in the middle third of the root renders the extraction of 1.1 inevitable.

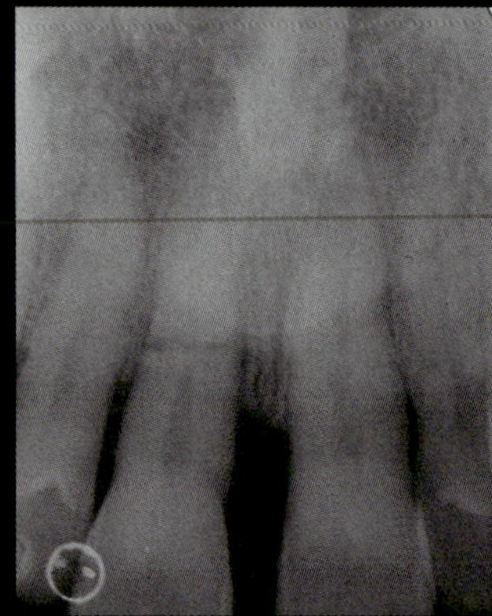

4.28b Periapical radiograph showing the line of fracture.

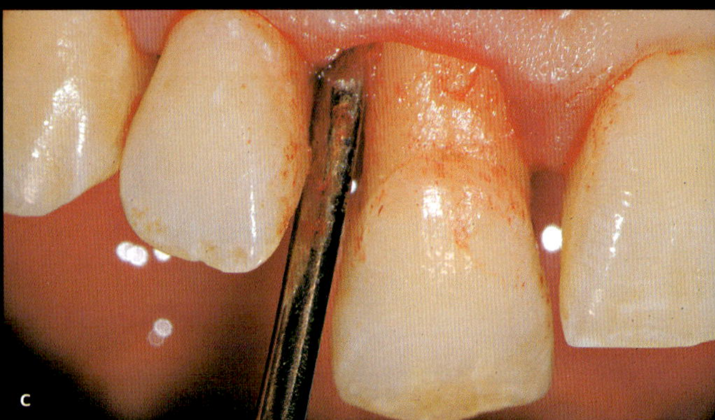

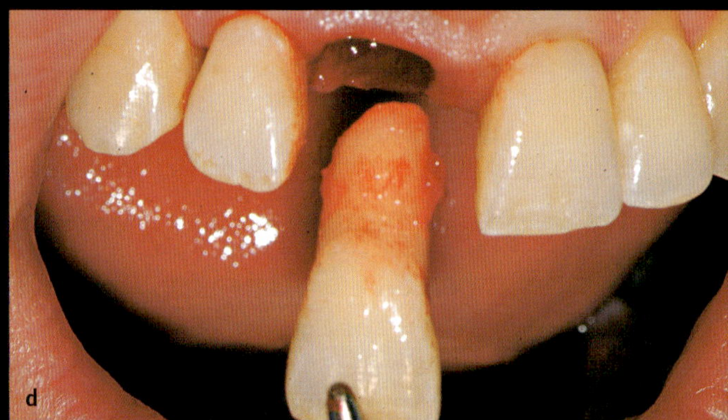

4.28c–d A periotome and a haemostatic forceps are used to extract the coronal fragment.

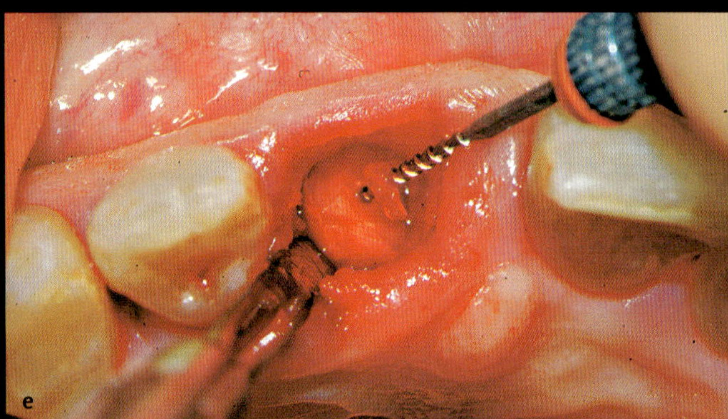

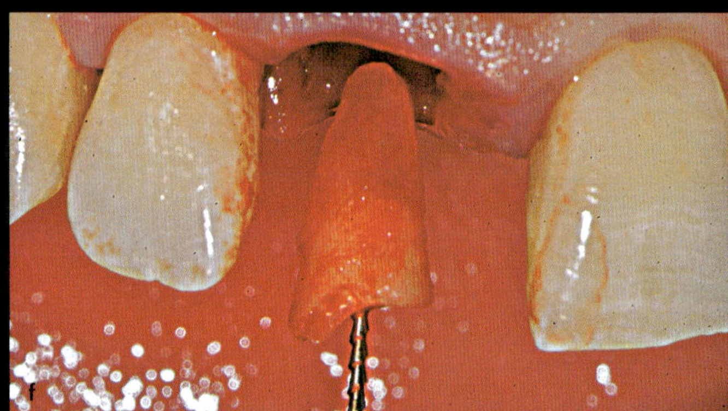

4.28e–f The combined use of an endodontic file and a periotome makes it possible to complete the extraction of the apical fragment.

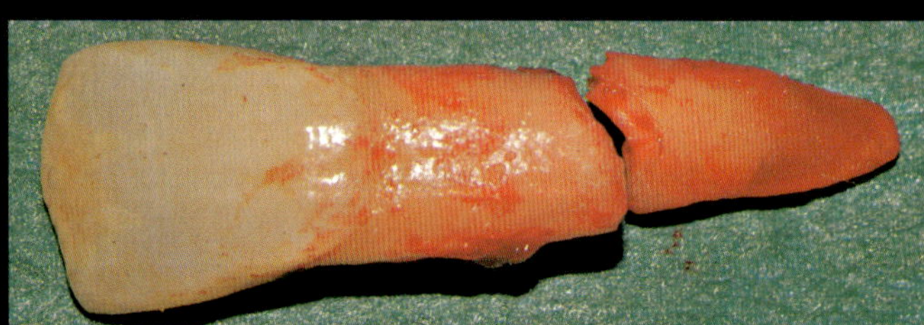

4.28g The extracted tooth.

REFERENCES

Byrd DL. Exodontia: modern concepts. Dent Clin North Am 1971; 15:273-98.

Jansma J, Schoen PJ, Raghoebar GM, Vissink A. Dentoalveolar surgery for the dentist: removal of teeth and root tips. *Ned Tijdschr Tandheelkd* 2004; 111(4):128-32.

Osunde OD, Saheeb BD, Adebola RA. Comparative study of effect of single and multiple suture techniques on inflammatory complications after third molar surgery. *J Oral Maxillofac* Surg 2011; 69(4):971-6.

Peterson LJ, Ellis III E, Hupp JR, Tucker MR. Contemporary oral and maxillofacial surgery. 2nd ed. Mosby, St. Louis, Missouri 1993.

Peterson LJ, Indresano AT, Marciani RD, Roser SM. Principles of oral and maxillofacial surgery. JB Lippincott Company, Philadelphia 1992.

Weiss A, Stern A, Dym H. Technological advances in extraction techniques and outpatient oral surgery. *Dent Clin North Am* 2011; 55(3):501-13.

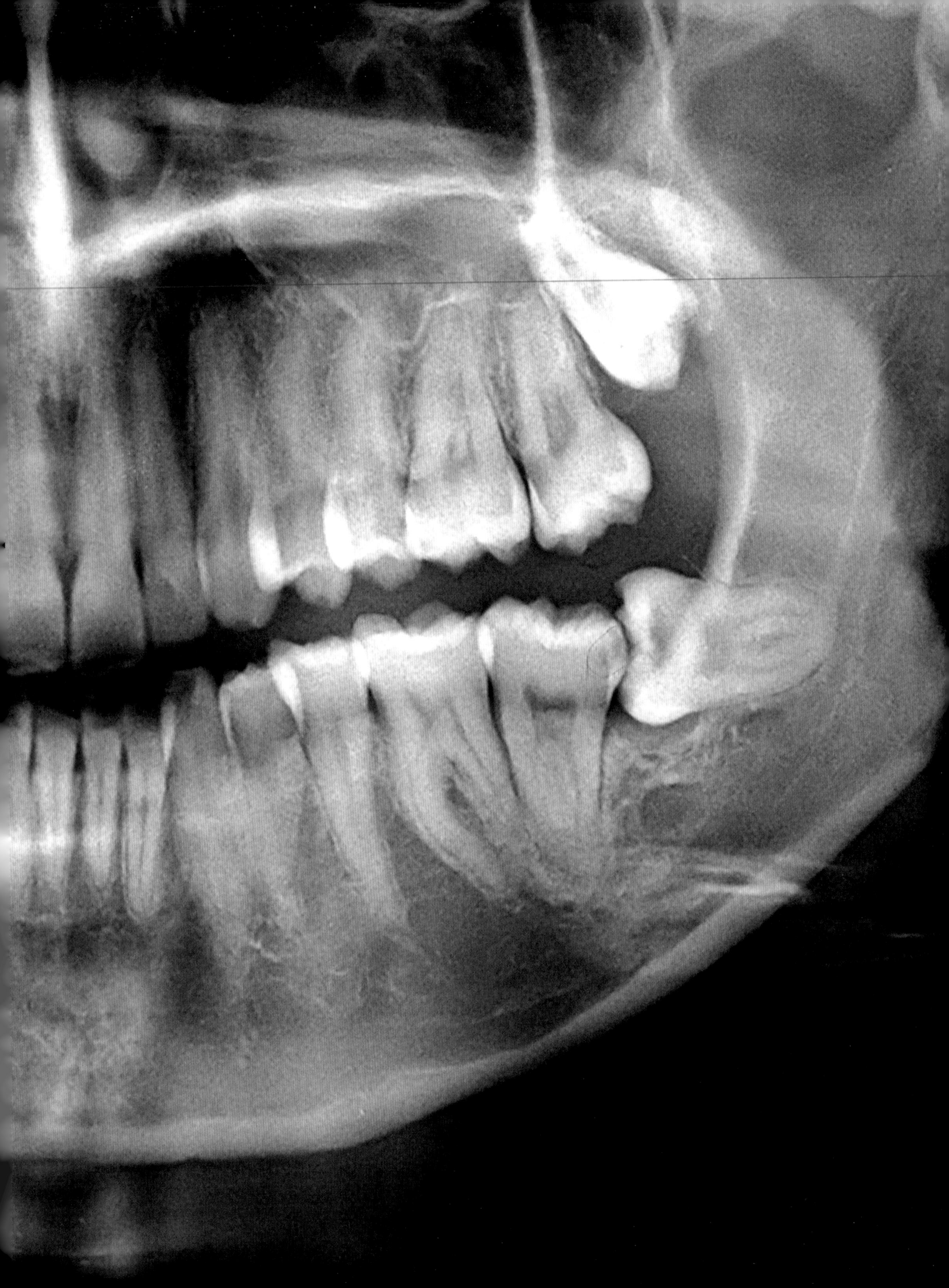

Impacted teeth

M. Chiapasco ▪ M. Zaniboni ▪ F. Gatti ▪ G. Garattini

Introduction

The eruption of permanent teeth is the final phase of a complex series of genetically controlled events, whereby a tooth germ develops inside the jawbones while migrating coronally and erupts in its functional position according to a predetermined timing and path. However, in the course of this evolutionary process, numerous events may interfere with the eruption of the tooth causing its impaction. Impaction represents a relatively common condition, particularly as far as vestigial elements such as third molars are concerned.

In fact, epidemiological studies demonstrate a 20% mean incidence of impaction in western countries, with a slight predilection for females. Mandibular third molars show the highest incidence of impaction, followed by maxillary third molars and canines; mandibular canines and the other teeth then follow in descending order of incidence.

Finally, multiple impaction (seldom associated with hypodontia) can be observed in some cases, as an independent finding or as one of the manifestations of a syndrome.

Etiopathogenesis

From an etiopathogenetic point of view, tooth impaction is ascribable to local and/or systemic factors.

LOCAL FACTORS

Early extraction of deciduous teeth: if a deciduous tooth is extracted more than two years prior to the physiological eruption of the corresponding permanent tooth, delays in the eruption of the latter and shortening of its roots may occur.

Caries in deciduous teeth: if caries are not associated with periapical inflammation, a delay in the exfoliation of the involved deciduous tooth may occur. If periapical inflammation is present, it may cause either a delay (75% of cases) or acceleration (25% of cases) of the exfoliation. In the maxilla, osteolysis caused by a periapical infection represents an area of reduced bone resistance that may cause the ectopic eruption of the permanent tooth (📷 5.1).

Malposition of the tooth germ: in some cases, despite a correct axis of eruption, the tooth germ is located in a deep position, and therefore must travel a longer distance to get to its final position in the dental arch. In these cases, it may exhaust its eruption force before reaching the arch. In other cases, the position and/or orientation of the tooth germ are incompatible with a correct eruption of the tooth (5.2).

Lack of sufficient space for a correct eruption: tooth impaction is frequently linked to the discrepancy between the available space (dimension of the jaws and alveolar ridges) and the space that is necessary to harbour all the permanent teeth. In the evolution of the human species, it is in fact possible to observe an evolution of the stomatognathic system characterised by the reduction of the permanent dentition and a concomitant dimensional contraction of the jawbones. This latter process seems to occur at a faster pace compared to the former, thus causing an increase in the incidence of crowding and impaction (5.3). Macrodontia also represents a predisposing factor for impaction, as it accentuates the dimensional discrepancy between teeth and alveolar ridges.

Presence of an obstacle along the eruption path: this obstacle can be represented by a supernumerary tooth or by a layer of dense bone that can form after the premature extraction of a deciduous tooth. Scars resulting from the surgical correction of orofacial cleft are also frequently associated with tooth impaction. Finally, due to their mass and localisation, several odontogenic tumours may cause impaction of teeth in the area where they develop (5.4).

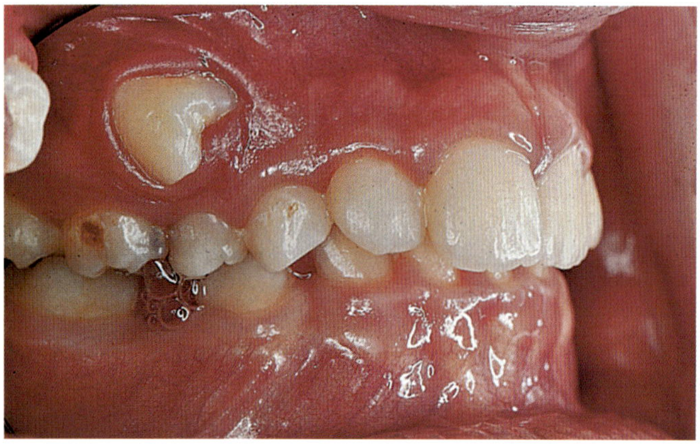

5.1 Ectopic eruption of the right maxillary first premolar secondary to endodontic infection.

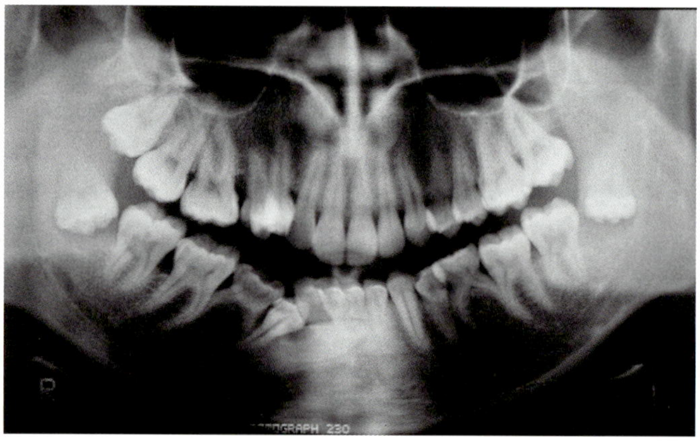

5.2 Ectopic impaction (mandibular ramus) of a left mandibular third molar.

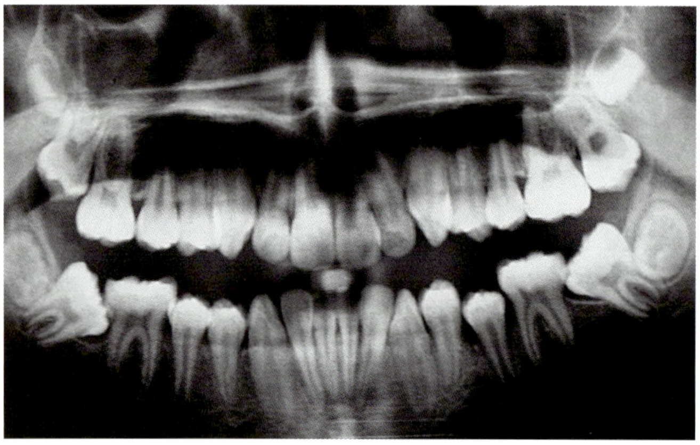

5.3 Evident crowding, particularly in the mandible, due to lack of space in the dental arch associated with multiple impactions.

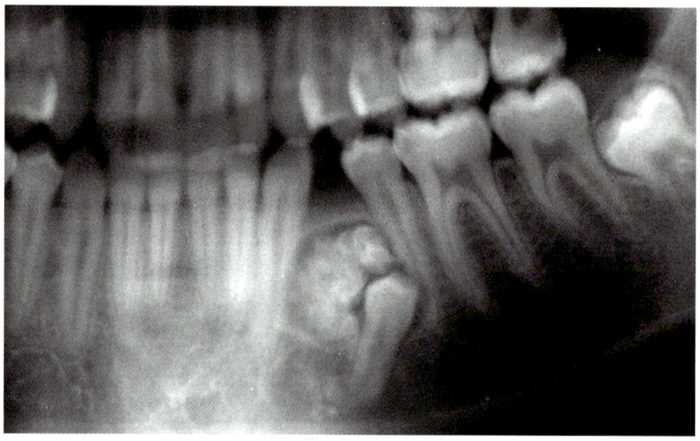

5.4 Odontoma preventing the eruption of 3.4.

Ankylosis of a deciduous tooth: this event may cause the impaction of the corresponding permanent tooth, but it is also frequently associated with the impaction of the deciduous tooth itself, particularly the mandibular molars.

Alterations of the dental follicle: a functional deficit of the dental follicle, a distinctive feature of amelogenesis imperfecta, is frequently associated with tooth impaction. The association between impacted teeth and dentigerous (follicular) cysts is also well documented (see Chapter 8 for details).

SYSTEMIC FACTORS

Genetic factors: monozygotic twins exhibit the same eruption characteristics in 90% of the cases, including those predisposing to tooth impaction. Genetic disorders involving bone catabolism, and particularly the osteoclastic functionality (e.g. osteopetrosis, cleidocranial dysplasia), are characterised by severe delay and defects in the eruption pattern.

Endocrine factors: hypopituitarism, hypothyroidism, and hypoparathyroidism cause a significant delay in tooth eruption.

Problems associated with tooth impaction

The presence of an impacted tooth may cause a series of problems and symptoms.

Pericoronitis: in 95% of cases, it is associated with a partially erupted mandibular third molar. This strict association seems to be caused by the peculiar anatomical characteristics of mandibular third molars. The absence of keratinised mucosa around the distal portion of the tooth is a common occurrence that facilitates bacterial colonisation of the gingival sulcus and may lead to the formation of a deep periodontal pocket. Pericoronitis represents the main cause of extraction for symptomatic third molars. Local predisposing factors such as poor oral hygiene, disto-version, and the presence of an ample distal follicular space have

Etiopathogenesis of tooth impaction

Local factors

- Extraction of deciduous teeth
- Caries in deciduous teeth
- Malposition of the tooth germ
- Lack of sufficient space in the alveolar ridge
- Presence of an obstacle along the eruption path
- Ankylosis
- Alterations of the dental follicle

Systemic factors

Genetic

- Monozygotic twins
- Autosomal dominant trait
- Osteopetrosis
- Cleidocranial dysplasia

Endocrine

- Hypopituitarism
- Hypothyroidism
- Hypoparathyroidism

been identified. The clinical presentation of acute pericoronitis includes localised pain, localised or extensive swelling, and trismus (caused by the diffusion of the inflammation to the muscles of mastication) (5.5). Pericoronitis shows a significant tendency to relapse, with increasing frequency and intensity, until the involved tooth is extracted.

Localised periodontal disease affecting the neighbouring teeth: the pericoronal space represents an ideal environment for the proliferation of bacterial flora; therefore, the presence of partially erupted teeth increases the risk of onset of periodontal disease involving the neighbouring teeth. In particular, an association between partially erupted mandibular third molars (particularly when mesially inclined or horizontal) and the presence of periodontal lesions affecting the distal aspect of the second molar has been observed (5.6). Damage to the periodontal tissues surrounding the second molar, together with pericoronitis, represents the most frequent indication for the extraction of mandibular third molars.

Caries affecting the partially or totally impacted tooth: studies published in the literature on caries in partially or totally impacted teeth report an incidence of this condition ranging from 3% to 15%. Caries can also affect teeth that appear completely covered by mucosa. In these cases, the presence of a communication between the follicular space of the impacted tooth and the periodontal space of the neighbouring teeth can be presumed (5.7).

Caries affecting neighbouring teeth: the presence of a partially erupted tooth often represents an obstacle to the daily oral hygiene manoeuvres, exposing the neighbouring teeth to a higher risk of developing carious lesions. Once caries is present, its removal and the restoration of the involved tooth can be performed only after the extraction of the impacted tooth (5.7).

Resorption of the roots of the neighbouring teeth: the pressure exerted by an impacted tooth on the roots of adjacent teeth may cause resorption of the root. The mechanism is still unclear, but a process similar to the one involved in root resorption of deciduous teeth is suspected. In these cases, extraction of the impacted tooth may favour a spontaneous reparative process, with apposition of newly formed cementum on the resorbed root and preservation of the tooth vitality.

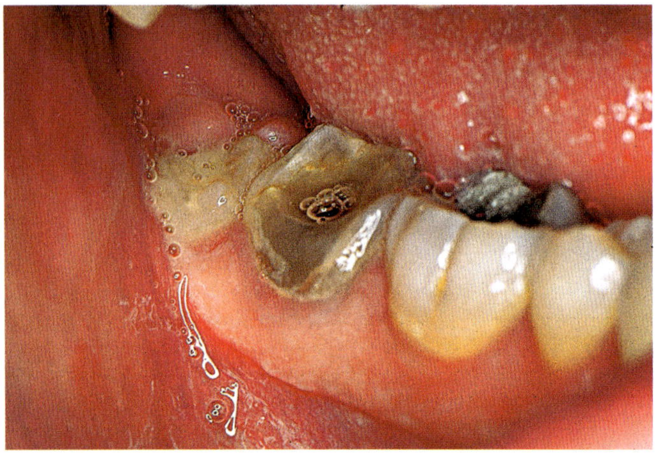

5.5 Pericoronitis associated with partial eruption of a mandibular third molar.

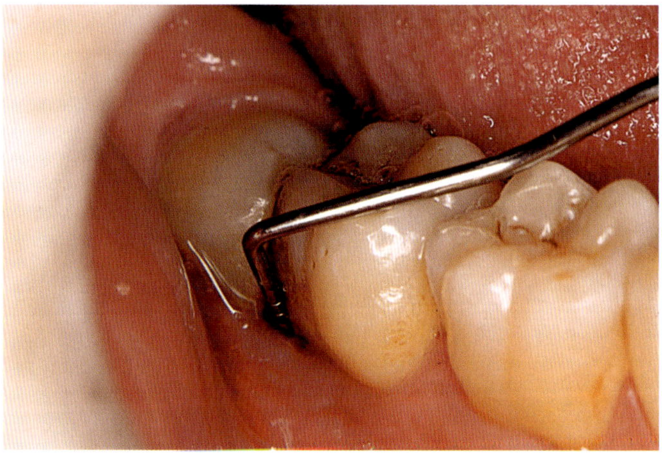

5.6 Periodontal lesion involving the distal surface of the second mandibular molar associated with a mesio-angular partially impacted third molar.

Odontogenic cysts: the dentigerous (follicular) cyst may cause tooth impaction, or be the consequence of it (5.8).

Odontogenic tumours: some odontogenic tumours, such as the keratocystic odontogenic tumour and ameloblastoma, may originate from the odontogenic epithelium that is present in the maxilla and mandible, and be associated with impacted teeth, particularly the mandibular third molar (5.9).

Orthodontic issues: in the past, crowding of teeth in the anterior area was often ascribed to the presence of third molars, particularly when mesially inclined. This interpretation is no longer deemed correct, as a number of clinical studies refute it. Crowding of the mandibular incisors seems to represent an adaptation that, under the restriction represented by the upper incisors, occurs when the growth of the mandible continues after that of the maxilla is completed. Therefore, the extraction of mandibular third molars to prevent or reduce crowding of the lower incisors seems to be unjustified. Conversely, extraction of the third molars may be indicated to allow distalisation of the other teeth, in case distalisation is necessary to complete orthodontic treatment successfully.

Prosthetic issues: when planning a fixed or removable prosthetic rehabilitation, impacted teeth that may be present in the edentulous area (except for those deeply impacted) should be extracted before the rehabilitation is completed. Bone resorption, in fact, may cause the emergence of the impacted tooth over time: this phenomenon is known as passive disinclusion. The presence of a partially erupted tooth may render the rehabilitation of the adjacent tooth with a prosthetic crown difficult, and jeopardise its long-term success due to the higher risk of periodontal disease caused by the partially erupted tooth (5.10).

Extraction of impacted teeth prior to orthognatic surgery: impacted third molars that may interfere with surgical manoeuvres are generally extracted prior to orthognatic surgery interventions such as sagittal osteotomy of the mandible, and Le Fort I maxillary osteotomy. It is recommended that the extractions be performed 6–12 months before orthognatic surgery, to facilitate complete bone healing.

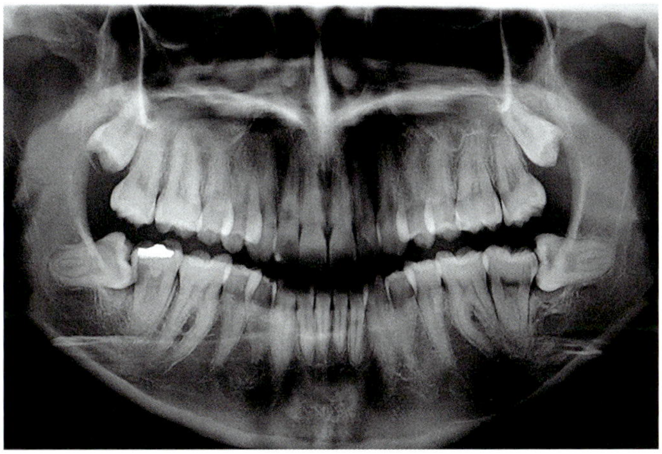

5.7 Panoramic radiograph showing the impaction of mandibular third molars in association with carious lesions involving the second molars.

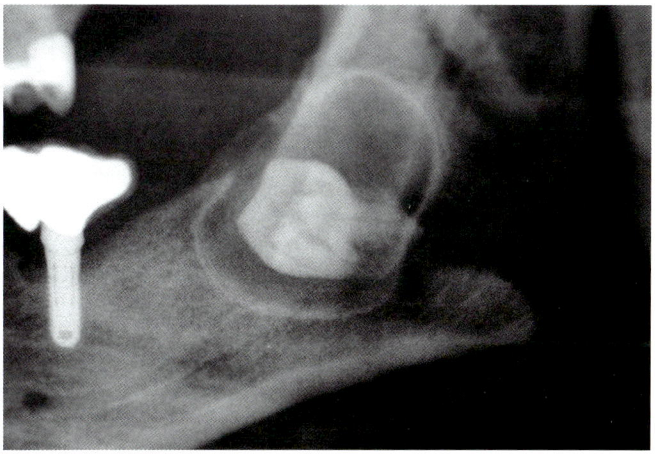

5.8 Radiograph showing a radiolucent endosseous lesion associated with an impacted tooth.

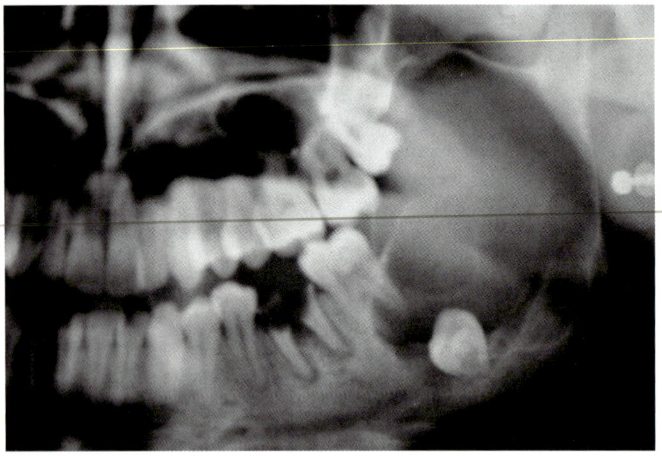

5.9 Large ameloblastoma developing inside the mandibular ramus associated with an impacted mandibular third molar.

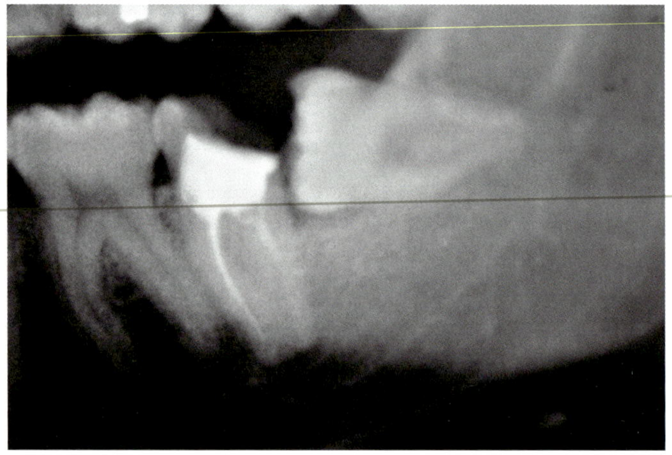

5.10 Impacted left mandibular third molar preventing a convenient prosthetic rehabilitation of the adjacent tooth.

Extraction

Indications

- Pericoronitis
- Periodontal disease affecting the neighbouring teeth
- Caries affecting the partially or totally impacted tooth
- Resorption of the roots of the neighbouring teeth
- Prosthetic rehabilitation of the neighbouring teeth
- Orthognatic surgery

Contraindications

- High risk of damaging important anatomic structures
- Compromised systemic conditions and age of the patient
- Possibility of surgical exposure and orthodontic treatment, or autotransplantation
- Poor patient compliance
- Orthodontic treatment

Treatment of eruption disorders

In general, the diverse approaches for the treatment of eruption disorders are included in the following categories.

Wait-and-see protocol: it is worth remembering that, when the decision to avoid surgical intervention is taken, the possible evolutions of the clinical picture may be diverse, and at times unpredictable. These, in fact, include all the aforementioned conditions, the lack of any evolution, or an unfavourable evolution in the absence of any symptom. Periodical radiographic and clinical examinations are important for monitoring the situation over time and, should it become necessary, to intervene appropriately.

Extraction of the deciduous tooth: the extraction of a deciduous tooth that does not spontaneously shed is indicated for a concomitant delay in the eruption of the corresponding permanent tooth. On the other hand, the premature extraction of a deciduous tooth may cause the formation of a layer of compact bone above the permanent tooth that can retard its normal eruption process. Therefore, the extraction of a deciduous tooth should not be performed, if possible, more than one year before the moment of natural eruption of the corresponding permanent tooth.

Surgical exposure and orthodontic alignment

Indications
- Ectopic eruption
- Dilaceration or post-traumatic root angulation
- Late orthodontic expansion

Contraindications
- Unfavourable inclination of the impacted tooth
- Scarce patient compliance

Orthodontic treatment: under this definition are considered all the preceding orthodontic treatments aimed at increasing the available space in the dental arch, thus facilitating the eruption of a tooth.

Surgical exposure alone or in association with orthodontic alignment: it is possible to obtain a successful outcome if the impacted tooth is moving along an eruption path that does not significantly (< 90°) deviate from the correct one, and if the tooth still maintains its eruptive potential.

Extraction: when impacted teeth cause problems, or are not functionally important (typically, maxillary and mandibular third molars), there is a clear indication for extraction.

Extraction and autotransplantation: see below for details.

As the clinical and prognostic picture, and consequent therapeutic approach, may significantly vary according to the tooth involved, different teeth are examined individually and the recommended treatment options for each situation are reported, considering the age of the patient as well. In the following sections of this chapter, all details regarding the surgical procedures for the extraction of impacted teeth are described.

Impacted incisors

PREVALENCE

The prevalence in the western population ranges between 0.1% and 0.5%. Impaction of the incisors is more frequent in the maxilla, and mainly involves the central incisors.

ETIOLOGY

The most frequent causes of impaction of the incisors are:
- physical obstacles to the eruption, such as the presence of supernumerary teeth (the presence of supernumerary teeth in the area of the incisors ranges between 1% and 4% in the western population), cysts, or odontomas;
- lack of space due to dentoalveolar discrepancy, or due to the insufficient growth of the premaxilla;
- premature loss of the deciduous incisors (with destruction of the follicle, or obliteration of the *gubernaculum dentis*);
- trauma to the deciduous incisors during the formation of the crown of the corresponding permanent teeth, with subsequent dilaceration or root angulation.

CLINICAL SIGNS

An asynchronous eruption of the incisors, with a delay of more than 4 months of one of them in the maxilla and 12 months in the mandible, requires a radiographic examination. The eruption of the lateral incisor before that of the central incisor should raise suspicions that an obstacle may be present along the eruption path of the central incisor. If the obstacle causes a deviation of the eruption path, the central incisor may be palpable below the mucosa: a buccal deviation is more frequent, while a palatal deviation is rare. However, the impacted tooth frequently maintains its position at the centre of the alveolar crest, and its exact position can be caused only with adequate radiographic examinations (5.11).

TREATMENT

Ectopic eruption: if the eruption of the permanent tooth does not take place within the 8th–9th year of age in a patient without associated pathologies, the extraction of the corresponding deciduous tooth is indicated.

If the position of the permanent tooth does not allow the eruption in a correct position, surgical exposure and orthodontic alignment are indicated.

If the ectopy is such that it is not possible to perform orthodontic alignment of the tooth successfully, or if the treatment would require an excessively long period of time, it is possible to plan an autotransplant.

If the diagnosis is made in adult patients, extraction of the tooth and prosthetic rehabilitation with a traditional bridge or with an endosseous implant supporting a crown can be considered as viable treatment options.

Presence of a supernumerary tooth: the extraction of the supernumerary tooth is always indicated, in association with the removal of the bone layer that may be present coronally to the impacted incisor. While performing this operation, extreme care must be taken to avoid any damage to its follicle. In 50% of cases, spontaneous eruption of the impacted incisor occurs within 6 to 24 months after the removal of the obstacle.

If surgery is unnecessarily delayed, the clinical picture can worsen and the orthodontic treatment may be more complex (5.12).

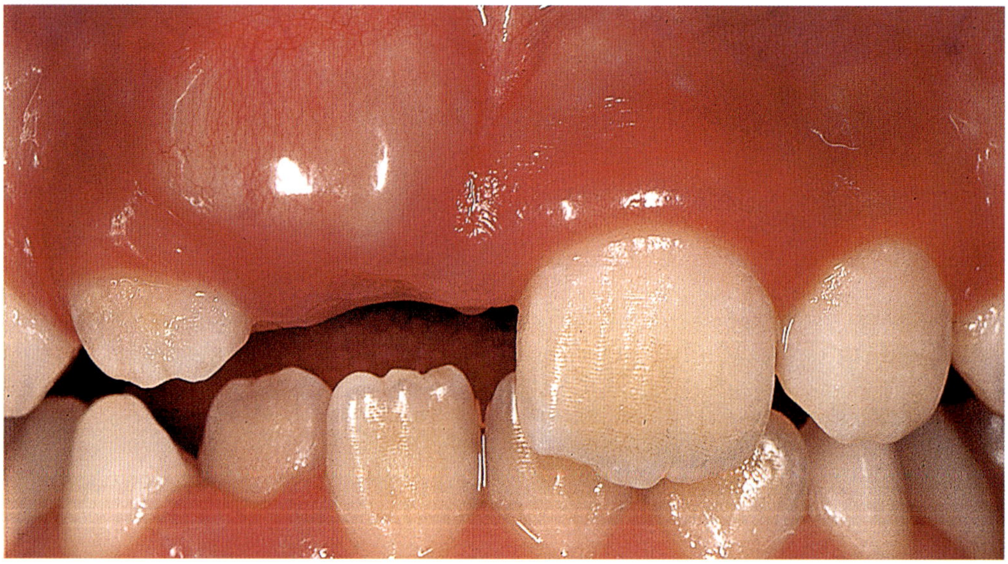

5.11 Buccal impaction of a maxillary central incisor.

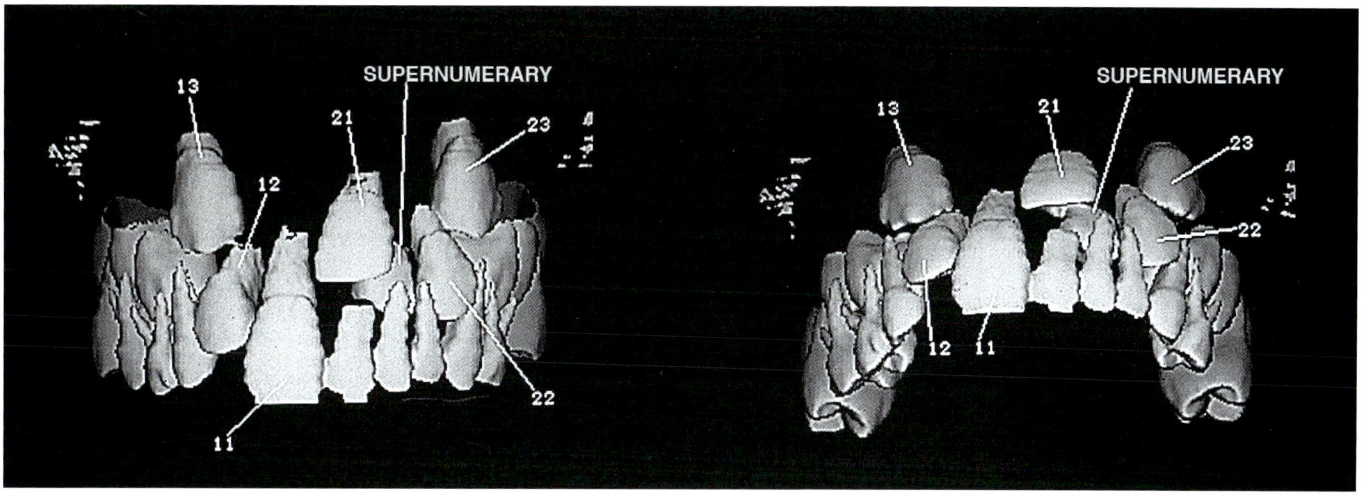

5.12 CT scan showing a supernumerary tooth hindering the eruption of 2.1 and 2.2.

Lack of available space: when impaction is caused by a lack of space in the maxillary alveolar ridge, an orthodontic palatal expansion may become necessary. Frequently, expansion is sufficient to obtain the spontaneous eruption of the impacted tooth, if it is performed before half of the root is formed. Conversely, if palatal expansion is performed at a later stage of root formation, subsequent surgical exposure and orthodontic alignment may become necessary.

Dilaceration or post-traumatic root angulation: in these cases, surgical exposure and orthodontic alignment are indicated. According to the gravity of the dilaceration or root angulation, orthodontic treatments may be more complex, and the results not always predictable.

Impacted maxillary canines

PREVALENCE

The impaction of maxillary canines is observed in 0.8%-2.9% of the population. It is more frequent in females, and in 85% of the cases, the impacted tooth is in a palatal position.

ETIOLOGY

The most frequent causes of impaction of the maxillary canines are:

- lack of resorption of the deciduous tooth or obliteration of the *gubernaculum dentis*, with loss of eruptive guidance;
- agenesia of the permanent lateral incisor, or presence of a conoid lateral incisor, with loss of eruptive guidance (40% of canine impactions seem to be caused by malformation, malposition, or agenesia of the permanent lateral incisor);
- ectopy of the tooth germ, or ectopic palatal migration;
- hereditary causes caused by a polygenic trait;
- presence of supernumerary teeth, cysts, odontomas that may represent an obstacle to the eruption of the canine;
- lack of space in the alveolar ridge, which can cause buccal impaction.

CLINICAL SIGNS

Specific clinical signs are:

- asynchronous eruption of the canines with a delay of more than 12 months;
- labial inclination of the lateral incisor;
- eruption of the premolar before eruption of the adjacent canine, and absence of canine eminence (in cases of normal eruption, eminence can be perceived upon palpation, on the buccal side of the alveolar ridge, in patients aged 8-10).

TREATMENT

No treatment: this can be considered a viable option in the absence of clinical problems related to impaction. In fact, with an unpredictable number of cases, spontaneous correction of the tooth axis inclination may occur, with the restoration of natural eruption.

Extraction of the deciduous tooth: this is necessary when eruption of the impacted permanent tooth is forthcoming.

Extraction of the deciduous tooth in association with exposure of the permanent tooth, and application of a space maintainer or orthodontic appliance to increase the available space in the alveolar ridge: in this case, spontaneous eruption of the impacted tooth is observed if deviation of the tooth axis from the normal inclination does not exceed 45°. Extraction of the deciduous canine should be performed between 10 and 12 years of age: if 12 months after extraction the permanent tooth is still impacted, the recourse to surgical exposure and orthodontic alignment is necessary.

Surgical exposure in association with orthodontic disimpaction (see further for details on the surgical techniques): this is indicated in cases of ectopic eruption when adjacent teeth are at risk, and when the delay in spontaneous eruption of the permanent canine exceeds 12 months.

The *risks* associated with this procedure are:

- loss of tooth vitality;
- root resorption;
- gingival recession and keratinised tissue defects;
- collateral effects and complications caused by the excessive duration of orthodontic treatment, which are difficult to predict.

The *prognosis* depends on several factors:

- age: notwithstanding the fact that treatment is also possible in adult patients, the presence of an open apex significantly improves prognosis;
- the extent of available space in the alveolar ridge and position of the root greatly influence the duration and difficulty of orthodontic treatment;
- the inclination of the main axis of the tooth (if it deviates more than 45° from the normal angle, the prognosis is less favourable);
- the proximity of the tooth crown to the palatine suture worsens the prognosis.

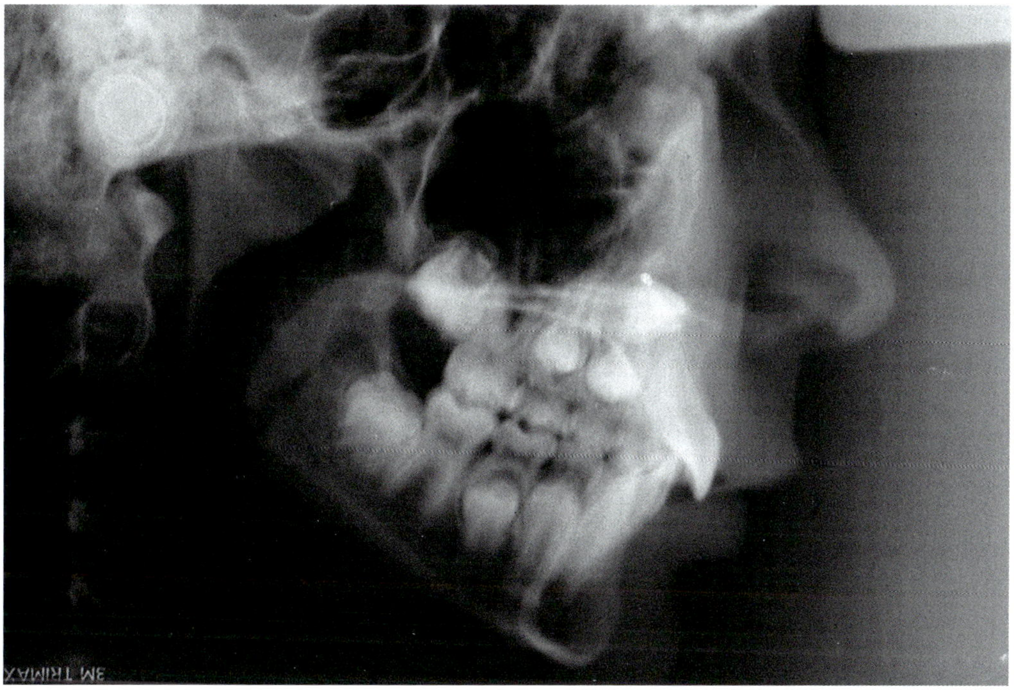

5.13 Horizontally impacted maxillary canine: surgical exposure and orthodontic alignment are contraindicated due to the unfavourable axis.

Autogenous tooth transplantation: can be evaluated when:

- the duration and complexity of orthodontic treatment might be excessive;
- the patient refuses orthodontic treatment;
- previous orthodontic treatments were not successful.

Extraction of the impacted tooth (see further for details on the surgical techniques): due to the fundamental strategic importance of canines, it is always recommended that the possibility of rescuing it with surgical and orthodontic techniques be evaluated. However, in some cases extraction can represent a viable option after all alternatives and the benefit-cost ratio have been thoroughly evaluated.

Extraction is indicated if:

- the tooth is horizontal and the apex is completely formed (5.13);
- a condition of severe lack of available space in the alveolar ridge, which would require extraction of another erupted permanent tooth, is present;
- resorption of roots of the neighbouring teeth is observed, and alternative treatment options are not accepted.

Mandibular canines

PREVALENCE

Impaction of mandibular canines is relatively rare, with a prevalence ranging from 0.05% and 0.4%.

ETIOLOGY

See above.

TREATMENT

No treatment: see above.

Surgical exposure in association with orthodontic disimpaction: apart from the considerations described for maxillary canines, the difficulties associated with this type of treatment are mainly correlated to the density and thickness of the mandibular bone. In fact, the cortical layer of the mandible is particularly thick, and the cancellous bone is dense. These factors render orthodontic movements more difficult to accomplish. Moreover, the frequently limited width of the alveolar crest in the area causes a higher risk of insufficient periodontal support at the end of treatment.

Autogenous tooth transplantation: see above.

Impacted premolars

PREVALENCE

The prevalence of impaction of mandibular premolars is 0.3%, while that of maxillary premolars is 0.2%.

ETIOLOGY AND TREATMENT

See above.

Impacted first and second molars

PREVALENCE

The prevalence of impaction of maxillary first molars is 0.02%, while that of maxillary second molars is 0.08%. As regards mandibular molars, the prevalence of impaction is 0.04% for the first molar, and 0.06% for the second molar.

ETIOLOGY

Besides common factors previously described for other teeth, in the case of molars a relationship between macrodontia and maxillary/mandibular hypoplasia is worth noting.

TREATMENT

No treatment: see above.

Impaction of the first molar cervically to the second deciduous molar: possible solutions are:

- subgingival placement of a metallic separator;
- active orthodontic distalisation of the permanent molar;
- extraction of the deciduous second molar followed by surgical exposure of the permanent first molar and application of a space maintainer or distaliser. This procedure is used when it is not possible to gain access to the permanent molar without first extracting the deciduous tooth.

Impaction with no apparent cause: here there are two viable approaches:

- surgical exposure and wait-and-see if the roots show good eruptive potential;
- surgical exposure and active orthodontic disimpaction of the permanent molar after adequate preparation of the orthodontic anchorage. The recourse to this approach is indicated when inclination of the permanent molar would not allow its spontaneous eruption. In both cases, the orthodontist should evaluate indications for the extraction of the third molar to facilitate mobilisation of the impacted tooth, without overlooking the possibility of its ankylosis, which may not be visible on the radiographs (as it is usually the case with molars presenting focal ankylosis).

Ankylosis of the permanent molar: choosing from the different solutions depends on the patient's age, as an ankylosis locally interrupts alveolar growth, and induces secondary movements of adjacent teeth.

With ankylosis of molar teeth at a prepubescent age, it is recommended that tooth extraction, and the subsequent spontaneous or guided alignment of the adjacent tooth, be performed. If the extracted tooth is a first molar, eruption of the second molar in its place is facilitated both by the promptness of the diagnosis and extraction, and by the presence of the third molar.

When ankylosis associated with partial eruption of molar teeth occurs at a postpubescent age, there are several therapeutic options:

- tooth extraction with subsequent spontaneous or guided alignment of the adjacent tooth: this is recommended when it represents part of a broader treatment plan (correct anchorage, necessity of extractions, etc.);
- heightening of the crown by means of a composite restoration: this represents a possible alternative to prevent uncontrolled movements of adjacent teeth while waiting for a definitive prosthetic solution once physical development is complete;
- extraction of the impacted tooth and autotransplantation of a third molar, or placement of a space maintainer in preparation for the later placement of an endosseous implant, are all recommended options when the exposed portion of the crown is insufficient to keep it in place and is unsafe from a periodontal point of view;
- tooth reimplantation: the partially or totally impacted tooth is extracted with great care to avoid any damage to the crown and roots, and it is reimplanted in the correct position.

Impacted third molars

PREVALENCE

The prevalence of impaction for third molars ranges from between 20% to 30%, with a gender predilection for females.

ETIOLOGY

See Etiopathogenesis, page 161.

TREATMENT

Impacted third molars have peculiar characteristics, as they rarely play a functionally significant role: for this reason, the treatment choice is essentially between *no treatment* and *extraction*.

The only exception is represented by the possibility of autotransplantation of the third molars (as germs or completely formed teeth) in cases where the first or second molars are absent or have been prematurely lost.

Given the problems related to tooth impaction (see page 163), an approach based on the concept of preventive extraction was once considered correct for the management of impacted third molars: as soon as a spontaneous eruption was considered impossible, the recourse to early extraction was chosen whenever no contraindications to tooth extraction were present.

In fact, early extraction makes it possible to prevent all the aforementioned pathologic conditions; they are generally less complex from a technical point of view, with a lower risk of damaging important anatomic structures, providing a better postoperative course, and thus a higher probability of achieving complete *restitutio ad integrum*.

However, with respect to the possible medico-legal implications of damage caused to the patient, a more cautious approach is currently favoured. In other words, this means not only the practical risks associated with the presence of the impacted tooth, but also a thorough analysis of the relationship between the biological costs related to the extraction of an impacted tooth – and the real benefits obtained, particularly in the absence of detectable pathologies.

Surgical exposure and orthodontic alignment

Advantages

- Complete aesthetic and functional recovery of the impacted tooth

Disadvantages

- Prolonged treatment period
- Complex treatment
- Good patient compliance is essential
- High benefit-cost ratio

Extraction

Advantages

- Short treatment
- Lower costs

Disadvantages

- Risk of damaging important anatomic structures
- More invasive treatment

Final considerations

Although the prevalence of impacted teeth in the general population is not particularly substantial, the presence of this condition often renders the diagnostic-therapeutic process quite complex. Choosing the most suitable treatment for each case depends on correct diagnosis, and on a thorough evaluation of the possibilities and limits of different treatment options.

A preventive approach, based on the clinical and radiographic evaluation of patients from the 6th year of age, permits the implementation of all the preventive measures, characterised by low biological and economic costs, which render the spontaneous eruption of the tooth possible according to physiologic criteria. A delayed diagnosis always leads to greater difficulties, and renders the prognosis unpredictable (if not negative), as far as recovery of the impacted tooth is concerned. Surgical exposure and orthodontic alignment may facilitate the recovery of an impacted tooth; however, some considerations must be made on this subject.

Surgical exposure and orthodontic alignment, when possible, frequently imply prolonged treatment periods and higher technical difficulties that occasionally require real "virtuosities of orthodontic biomechanics". Therefore, before undertaking these recovery procedures it is necessary to perform a precise analysis of the benefit-cost ratio for each case. In addition to the prolonged treatment period and the technical difficulties, the patient's compliance must be assessed: their motivation towards recovery of the impacted tooth might not be sufficient, but he/she must guarantee (or the family, in the case of paediatric patients) an optimal and consistent level of oral hygiene, and must respect scheduled appointments that, in these cases, can be frequent. Due to the level of refinement that materials and techniques in the field of oral implantology have reached today, the opportunity and benefit-cost ratio of saving an impacted tooth with a surgical-orthodontic approach should always be compared to those of an implantological approach involving extraction of the impacted tooth and its substitution with an endosseous implant.

The decision of saving an impacted tooth should always be taken in the light of a comprehensive orthodontic evaluation. In other words, it is not possible to consider the impacted tooth as a single problem involving only the tooth itself, but all orthodontic aspects of the case must be thoroughly evaluated to choose the most appropriate approach for individual cases. As such, close cooperation among orthodontist, dentist, and surgeon must be established from the first diagnostic phase, with the aim of jointly planning optimal treatment for every patient and considering both the possibilities and limitations of every clinical approach to tooth impaction. A detailed analysis of orthodontic treatments is beyond the scope of this manual. Therefore, only the following treatments are described:

- surgical exposure and orthodontic alignment;
- extraction;
- tooth transplantation.

Prevalence of inclusion

	%		%
Incisors	0.1-0.5	First maxillary molars	0.02
Maxillary canines	0.8-2.9	First mandibular molars	0.04
Mandibular canines	0.05-0.4	Second maxillary molars	0.08
Maxillary premolars	0.2	Second mandibular molars	0.06
Mandibular premolars	0.3	Third molars	20-30

Surgical exposure and orthodontic alignment

Surgical planning

Intervention involves surgically exposing the crown of the impacted tooth, applying an orthodontic attachment on the exposed crown with appropriate bonding techniques, and applying orthodontic force to obtain a correct positioning of the tooth in the dental arch. The indications of this approach are described in detail in the dedicated section of this chapter; the specific aspects needed for planning the surgical phase correctly are reported in the following paragraphs.

Preoperative evaluation: position of the impacted tooth and accessibility

Knowing the exact position of the impacted tooth is a key factor when planning the correct surgical approach and exposure of the crown. The easiest methods that can be used for superficial impaction are inspection and palpation. However, they do not provide information regarding the proximity of the impacted tooth to other anatomic structures. Therefore, the recourse to appropriate radiographic examinations is always necessary to plan surgical intervention in an adequate manner.

Radiographic examinations

Periapical radiograph: this is the simplest exam that provides information regarding the position of the impacted tooth. However, in the majority of cases, the information obtained is insufficient, particularly in the case of deep impaction, due to the small size of the film/sensor and the limitations associated with its intraoral positioning that frequently prevent a complete image of the tooth and the neighbouring anatomic structures. Moreover, periapical radiographs do not provide information on the position of the tooth on the buccal-palatal/lingual plane.

In the past, a simple method for evaluating the buccal-palatal/lingual position of the tooth consisted in taking two periapical radiographs with a different beam angle: first with an orthogonal beam angle, and secondly with a distal or mesial angle of the X-ray tube (Clark technique, or tube shift). If, in the second image, the impacted tooth appears to be shifted in the same direction as the X-ray tube, its position is nearer to the X-ray film/sensor (palatal/lingual position) (📷 5.14a-b). If the impacted tooth appears to be shifted in the opposite direction, its position is closer to the buccal cortical plate. This technique is rarely used today, as the evolution of digital CT scans gives more information and greater detail with a low radiation dose.

Panoramic radiograph: this exam offers a comprehensive display of both dental arches, but is generally unsuitable for obtaining adequate information on the exact position of the impacted tooth (📷 5.15).

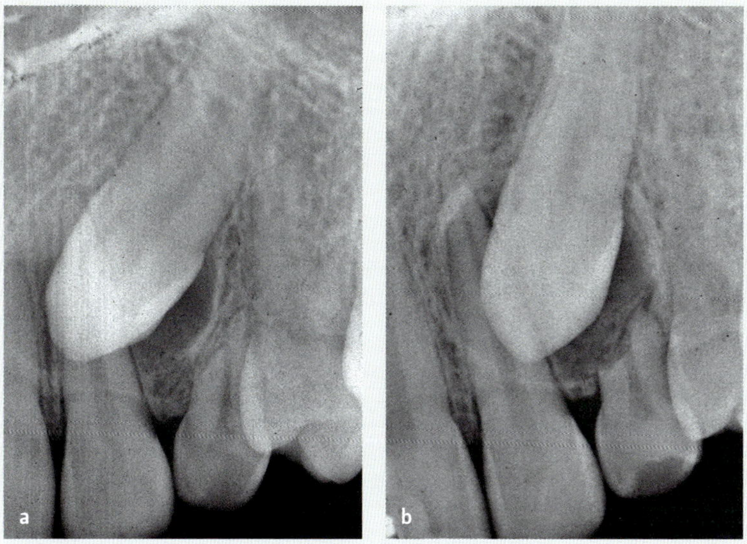

5.14 Clark technique: **a)** orthogonal projection: the crown of 2.3 completely overlaps the root of 2.2; **b)** the X-ray generator head is moved distally: the crown of 2.3 appears to be moving in the same direction, partially uncovering the root of 2.2. Therefore, the impacted tooth is in a palatal position.

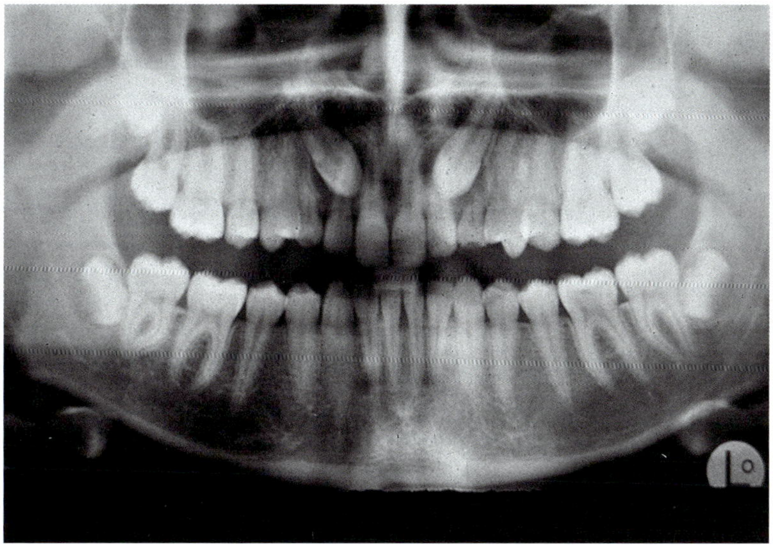

5.15 Panoramic radiograph of the same patient: impacted maxillary canines are clearly visible, but no precise tridimensional information on their position is available.

Lateral cephalometric radiograph: the lateral cephalometric radiograph can be useful for defining the buccal or lingual/palatal position of a tooth in cases of impaction in the anterior areas of the maxilla and mandible (5.16).

Occlusal radiograph: the occlusal radiograph of the palate or mandible can provide useful information on the buccal or lingual/palatal position of the impacted tooth (5.17).

Computed tomography: this is the radiographic exam of choice for obtaining precise tridimensional information on the position of the impacted tooth; the most recent digital cone-beam machines allow quick scanning and low radiation doses, thus contributing to the significant diffusion of this exam for the evaluation of clinical situations that, in the past, required the recourse to basic diagnostic exams (providing less information and detail) to limit the radiation dose.

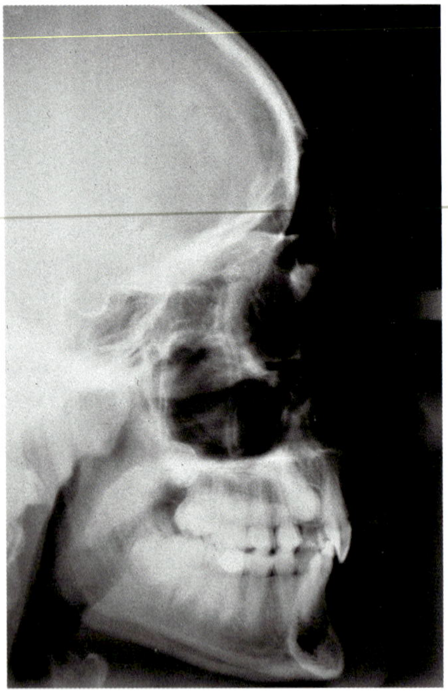

5.16 Lateral cephalometric radiograph of the same patient demonstrating the palatal position of the impacted canines.

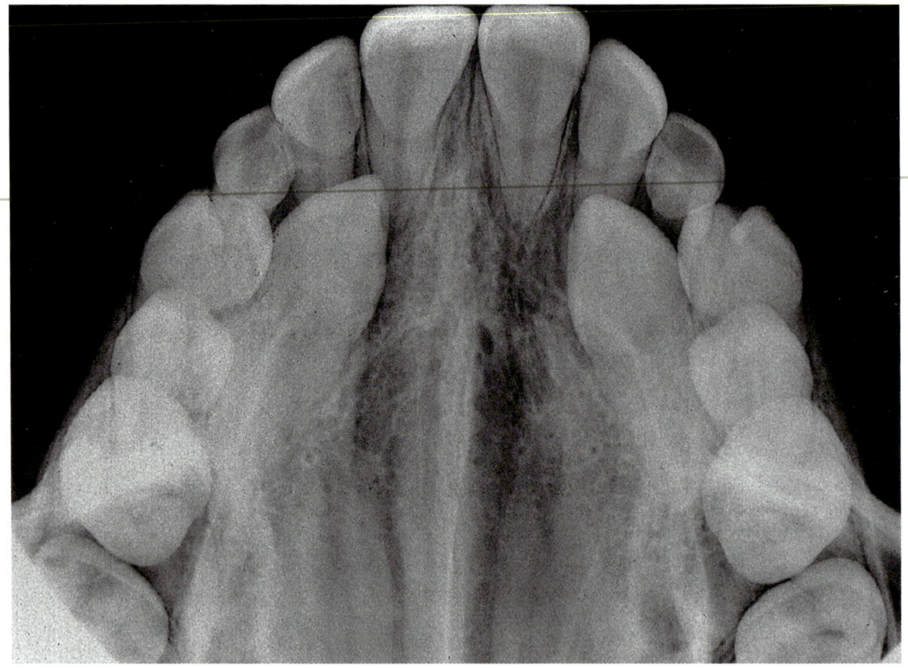

5.17 Occlusal radiograph of the same patient showing the palatal position of the impacted canines.

Radiographic examinations used to plan surgical exposure and orthodontic alignment of impacted teeth

	Advantages	Disadvantages
Periapical radiograph	Good individuation of the tooth position	Insufficient in cases of deep impaction
Panoramic radiograph	Good overall view	No indications on the buccal or palatal/ lingual position of the tooth
Double periapical radiograph with different projections	Simple to perform Good individuation of the tooth position	Insufficient precision in the individuation of the tooth position
Lateral cephalometric radiograph	Individuation of the buccal or lingual/ palatal position of the tooth	Difficult interpretation of the radiographic image
Occlusal radiograph	Individuation of the buccal or lingual/ palatal position of the tooth	Not useful in cases of impaction in the lateral-posterior areas of the jaws
CT scan	It guarantees optimal evaluation of the tooth position event in cases of deep impaction	Higher radiation dose

Surgical techniques

After the exact position of the impacted tooth is identified by means of radiographic images and its relationships with adjacent anatomic structures are defined, the most convenient surgical access is planned.

Specific armamentarium

- Phosphoric acid gel for crown etching.
- Self/light curing adhesives and composites for the fixation of the orthodontic attachment.
- Orthodontic attachments.
- Metallic wires.
- Wire cutter.
- If necessary, surgical kit for the placement of orthodontic implants used as anchor points to apply orthodontic tractions.

Locoregional anaesthesia

Anaesthesia follows the principles described in detail in the dedicated section.

Basic techniques

Access flaps

Access flaps should be designed with the aim of respecting periodontal tissues and guarantee the presence of a normal periodontium and adequate band of keratinised mucosa around the rescued tooth at completion of orthodontic alignment. For this reason, the closed orthodontic traction approach is currently preferred, because it ensures that guided eruption of the impacted tooth on the alveolar ridge is perfectly similar to natural eruption, thus optimising the morphology of periodontal tissues.

The term "closed orthodontic traction" is used when the access flap is sutured in its original position at the end of the surgical phase and the orthodontic wire connected to the tooth emerges from the most coronal margin of the flap. When this is not possible (buccal position or superficial palatal impaction), an open orthodontic traction approach is used; however, all necessary provisions must be implemented to create an adequate band of keratinised tissue around the saved tooth (see further for details).

Three types of access flaps can be used: crestal flap, removal of a circular portion of the soft tissues, and submarginal flap.

Marginal (crestal) flap

The use of this flap is particularly indicated with impaction in the middle of the alveolar ridge, when a covered orthodontic traction via a transalveolar approach is planned. Increasing flap mobility on the buccal side by means of periosteal releasing incisions is possible, while on the palatal side, these incisions should never be made to avoid damage to the branches of the major palatine neurovascular bundle (5.18a).

Removal of a circular portion of the soft tissues overlying the impacted tooth

This surgical access is indicated for the exposure of palatally impacted teeth, and consists in removing (with either a scalpel or acusector) the palatine mucosa overlying the impacted tooth. The recourse to this technique is especially indicated in cases of superficial impaction; however, it is worth remembering that the tooth should always be identified beforehand upon palpation, to avoid any sacrifice of soft tissues in an incorrect position (5.18b).

Submarginal (buccal) flap

The use of this four-cornered flap is indicated in cases of buccal impaction, and when an open orthodontic traction is planned. It is recommended that a band of keratinised tissue be included when designing the flap, which will be repositioned apically to the orthodontic attachment at the end of the surgical procedure. In this way, during the following phase of orthodontic alignment, the keratinised soft tissues will migrate together with the tooth to its correct position (5.18c).

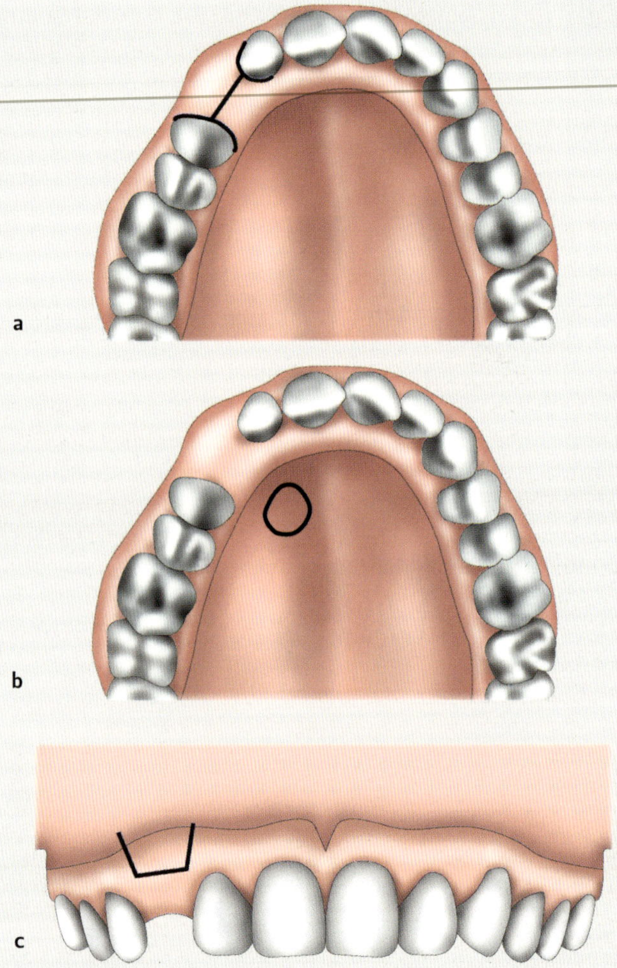

5.18 a) Crestal flap for the exposure of an impacted canine located in the middle of the alveolar ridge. **b)** Removal of a circular portion of palatine mucosa to expose a palatally impacted canine. **c)** Submarginal flap on the buccal side of the maxilla for the exposure of a buccally impacted canine.

Exposure of the impacted tooth

In cases of soft tissue impaction, the crown of the tooth is already visible after elevation of the access flap, while in cases of bony impaction ostectomy is necessary to expose the crown of the tooth once the access flap is elevated and retracted. When the crown of the impacted tooth is covered by a thick layer of bone, ostectomy is performed with a round bur mounted on a straight handpiece: in this case, care must be taken to avoid any damage to the tooth surface and to expose a portion of the crown that is sufficient for an adequate positioning of the orthodontic attachment. Furthermore, the position of adjacent teeth (particularly their roots/apexes) must be carefully assessed to avoid any manoeuvre that can compromise their vitality.

When the cortical layer is thin, the crown of the impacted tooth can be exposed using a surgical curette; if the follicle surrounds

the crown, its pericoronal portion can also be removed with the same instrument (5.19a–c).
When the corresponding deciduous tooth is still present, it is possible to create a tunnel in the alveolar bone between the apex of the deciduous tooth (which is extracted at the same time) and the crown of the impacted tooth, with a round bur mounted on a straight handpiece. Once the orthodontic attachment is bonded to the crown of the impacted tooth, the orthodontic wire is passed through the tunnel to guide the eruption of the permanent tooth in the middle of the alveolar ridge.

Positioning of the orthodontic attachment

Once the crown is exposed, the position of the orthodontic attachment is chosen. Ideally, it should be placed as far coronally as possible to facilitate traction and to guide eruption at the centre of the alveolar ridge. The orthodontic attachment should be selected according to the chosen position; round buttons or square brackets, with a concave or convex surface, can be used depending on the surface on which the attachment is to be bonded. A simple alternative consists in creating a loop with a piece of orthodontic wire and directly bonding it to the crown of the impacted tooth.
Among the proposed attachment systems, ligatures to the crown with orthodontic wires should be avoided due to the risk of root resorption and the use of parapulpar posts or crown perforations should be averted due to the risk of pulp injury. Maintaining a dry operating field is crucial for obtaining solid adhesion of the orthodontic attachment; the latter can be achieved by means of a combined use of intraoperative suction and specific techniques for adequate haemostasis (oxidised regenerated cellulose gauzes placed in the pericoronal space, bipolar coagulation/diathermy). Conversely, the use of an air spray to dry the crown should always be avoided, as it can easily cause contamination of the crown (blood, intraoral fluids). Etching is common with the application of phosphoric acid gel (34%–38%): the etchant is kept on the tooth surface for 30–60 seconds and is then suctioned away, and sterile saline is used to rinse the area. Suction is then used to dry the etched surface, which assumes the typical frosted appearance. A specific light cure composite adhesive is directly applied on the orthodontic attachment, while a thin layer of bonding agent is applied to the etched enamel surface (5.19d–f).
Once polymerisation is completed, the strength of the adhesion is verified with a pair of pliers, and the attachment is then connected to the orthodontic appliance (fixed to the neighbouring teeth) or to orthodontic implants with the chosen method (5.18g–h).
A few days after surgery, the orthodontist can initiate the traction phase that will last until the tooth is correctly positioned in the dental arch. Alignment of the tooth can take up to 12 months and is necessary for avoiding the application of excessive traction due to the risk of losing the tooth.

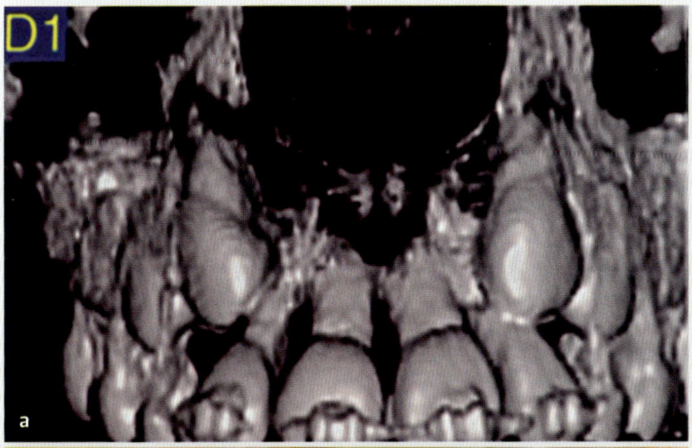

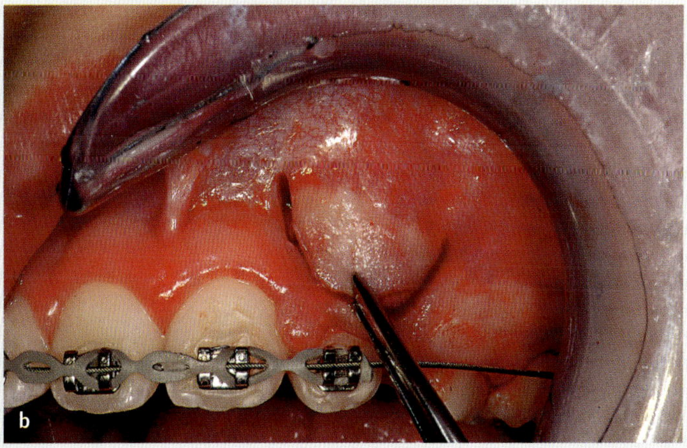

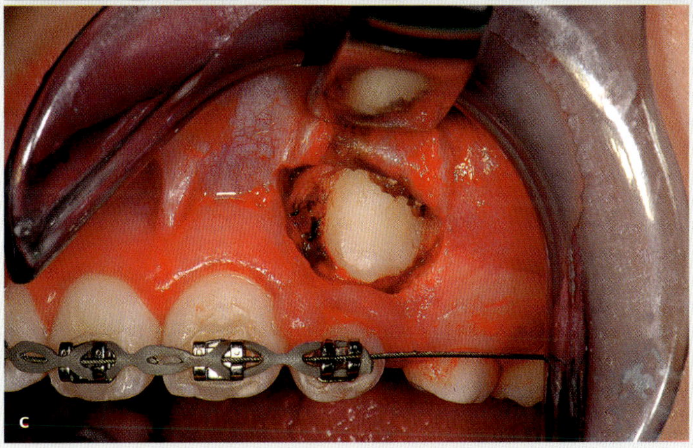

5.19 **a)** Surgical exposure and orthodontic alignment: tridimensional reconstruction of the maxilla showing fully impacted 1.3 and 2.3. **b)** Submarginal semilunar flap in the area of impaction. **c)** Exposure of the crown of the impacted canine. (*continued*)

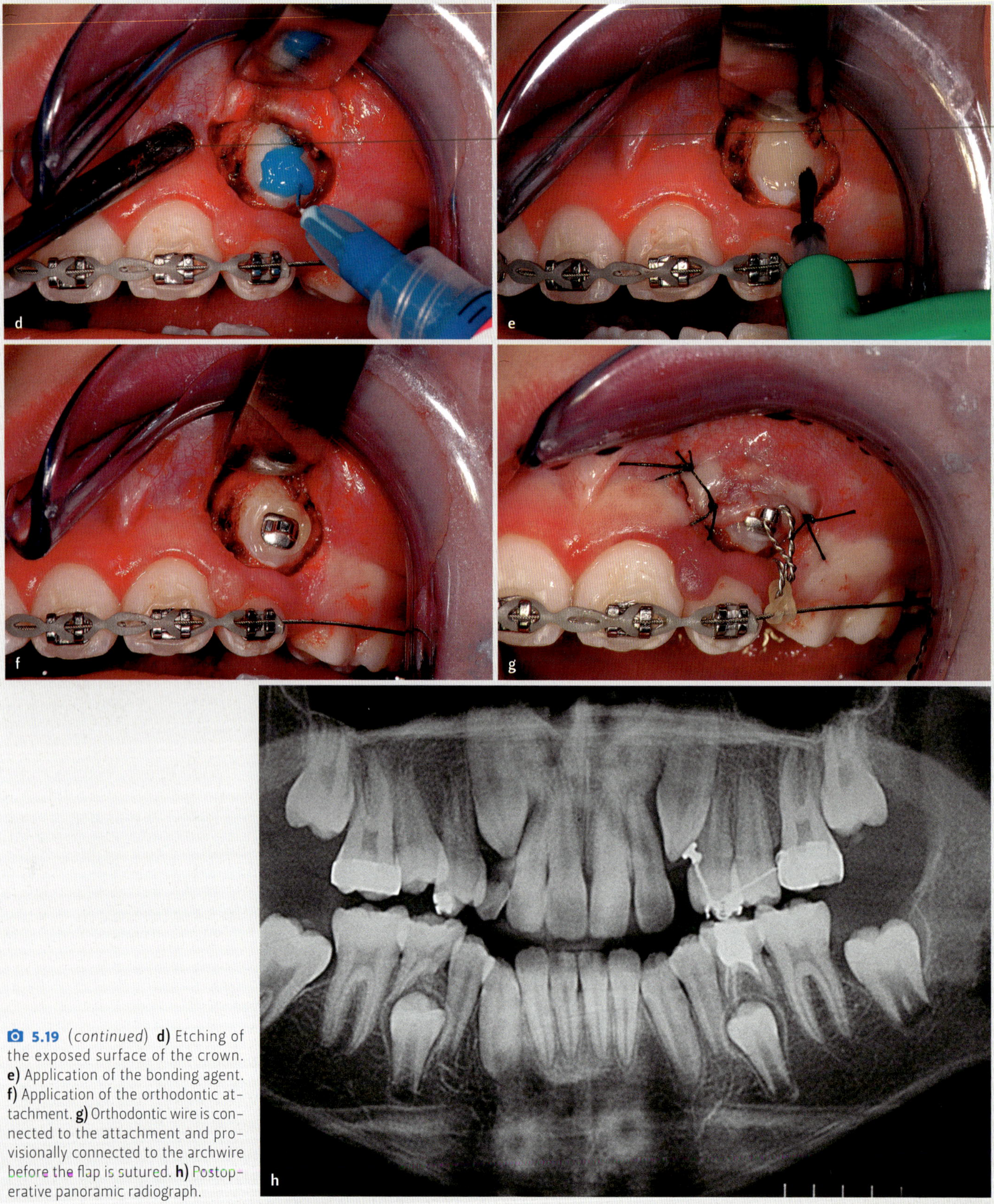

5.19 (*continued*) **d)** Etching of the exposed surface of the crown. **e)** Application of the bonding agent. **f)** Application of the orthodontic attachment. **g)** Orthodontic wire is connected to the attachment and provisionally connected to the archwire before the flap is sutured. **h)** Postoperative panoramic radiograph.

Clinical case 1 – Surgical exposure and orthodontic alignment of impacted 4.5

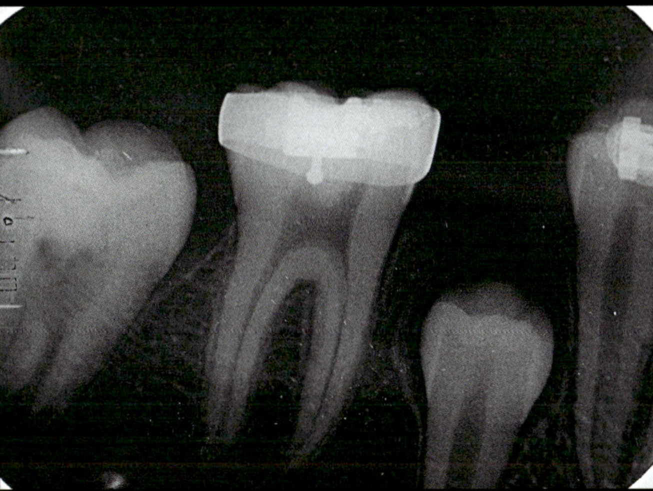

5.20a Periapical radiograph showing an impacted 4.5.

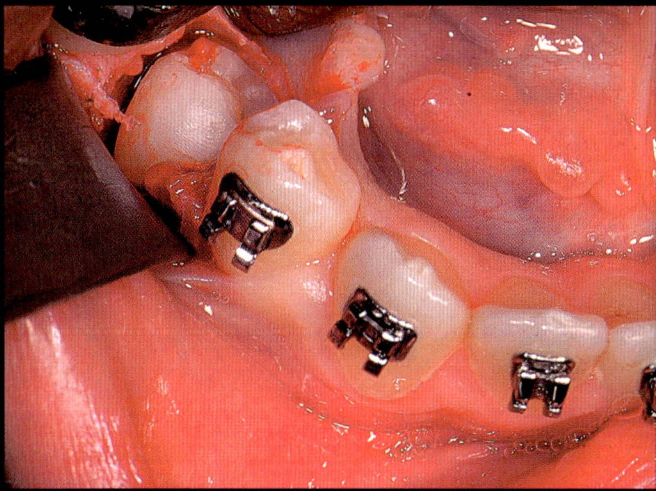

5.20b Access flap and exposure of the crown of 4.5.

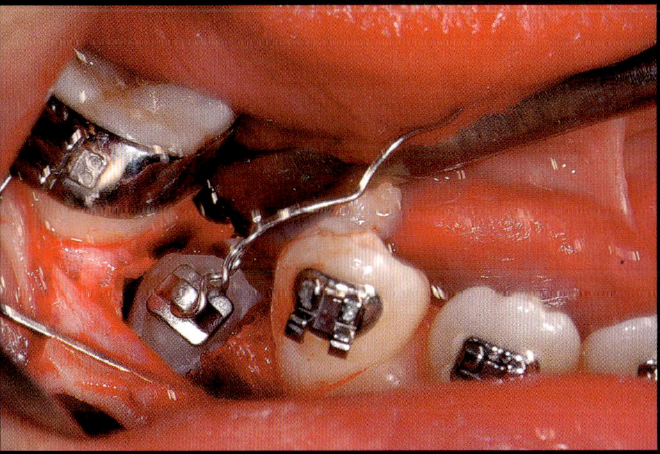

5.20c Application of the orthodontic attachment and wire loop.

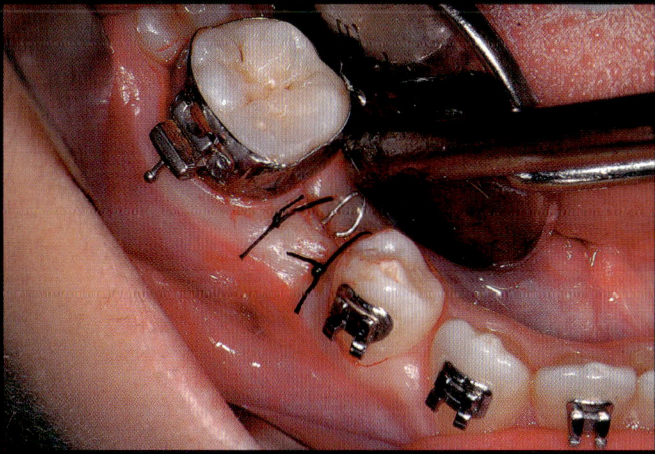

5.20d The access flap is sutured and the distal end of the wire loop protrudes through the sutured incision.

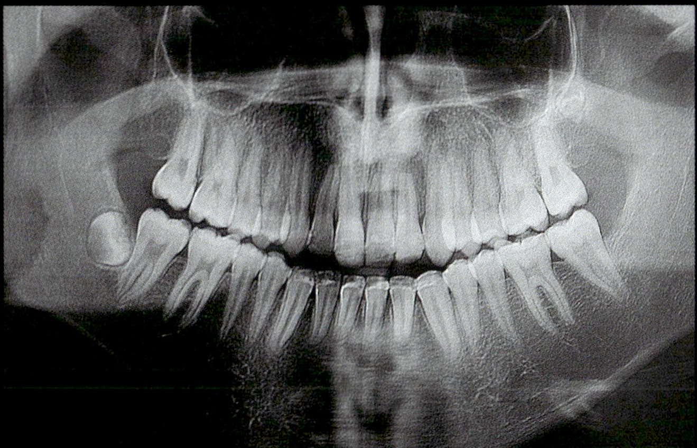

Extraction

Surgical planning

INDICATIONS

Indications are described in detail in the previous sections.

CONTRAINDICATIONS

In general, extraction of an impacted tooth is contraindicated when the potential risks of surgical intervention exceed the benefits that come from eliminating the tooth, or when the tooth can be saved and aligned with a surgical-orthodontic treatment.

More precisely, the contraindications to extraction of an impacted tooth can be schematised as follows.

High risk of damaging adjacent anatomic structures, in cases of asymptomatic impacted teeth with no signs of ongoing pathology (5.21): when a wait-and-see protocol is chosen, it is recommended that periodical follow-up radiographs are performed to verify the absence of pathological developments. Conversely, in the presence of any pathology, both symptomatic and asymptomatic (e.g. dentigerous cyst), planning the tooth extraction is necessary, even when the risk is high due to the proximity of important anatomic structures. In these cases, the radiographic exam of choice should allow the tridimensional reconstruction of the relationships between the impacted tooth and the involved anatomic structures. Consequently, the recourse to a CT scan is mandatory.

Systemic condition and advanced age of the patient: the general contraindications described for any oral surgery procedure are obviously valid in cases of extraction of impacted teeth as well. Moreover, in elderly patients this type of surgery can be more invasive due to the higher risk of tooth ankylosis. However, extraction of an impacted tooth can be necessary in patients with a partially compromised systemic condition. In these cases, close cooperation with the general practitioner or specialist in charge of the patient for the systemic problems is recommended. Furthermore, it is preferable to perform surgical intervention in a protected environment (e.g. hospital), with the possibility to monitor the patient's vital signs and with assistance from an anaesthetist/intensive care doctor.

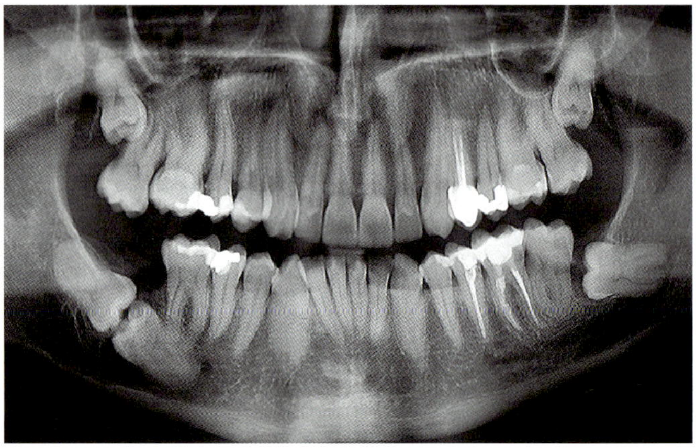

5.21 Panoramic radiograph showing deeply impacted 4.7 and 4.8 in close proximity to the mandibular canal. Due to the absence of symptoms, a surgical approach is contraindicated.

Impacted tooth that can be recovered and aligned by means of orthodontic therapy or replantation: see above and further for details.

Lack of patient's cooperation/compliance: this is a relative contraindication limited to surgical procedures performed under local anaesthesia, but it can be overcome by planning the recourse to general anaesthesia.

PREOPERATIVE EVALUATION

A thorough preoperative evaluation has a fundamental role in the planning of the surgical intervention: a precise assessment of the difficulty of the extraction makes it possible to predict the duration of the surgical session, evaluate possible difficulties or complications, and adequately inform the patient before performing the surgical procedure.

The preoperative evaluation is primarily based on the evaluation of accessibility, the patient's compliance/collaboration, and of the radiographic examinations.

Evaluation of accessibility and assessment of the patient's compliance/ collaboration

Adequate accessibility can be verified solely during the preoperative clinical examination, and represents an essential prerequisite. The assessment of the difficulty of a surgical treatment cannot be based exclusively on the evaluation of the radiographic exams: an extraction deemed "simple" can become extremely difficult with non-compliant patients or with patients who have limited accessibility (e.g. trismus).

Radiographic evaluation

Radiographic exams represent an important tool for evaluating the difficulty of an extraction and for planning the surgical procedure correctly. As regards choosing the most suitable exam for every clinical case, detailed indications are reported in the previous chapters/sections. Elements that cause difficulty during an extraction and that can be evaluated on radiographic exams are as follows:

Depth of impaction: deep impaction implies greater difficulty in exposing the tooth, and greater trauma on the surrounding tissues due to the necessity of a more extensive ostectomy (5.22).

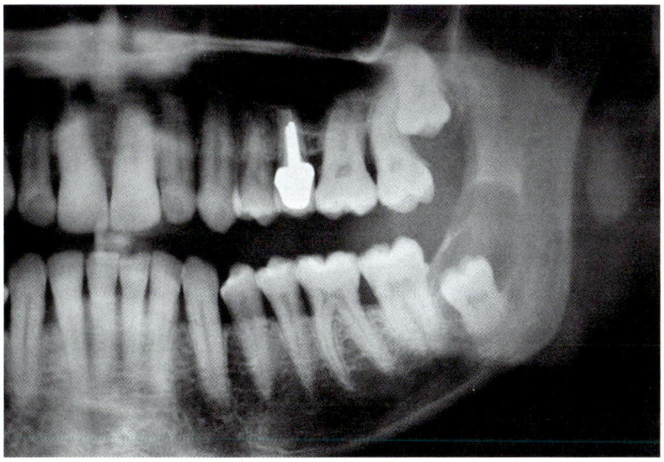

5.22 Radiolucent lesion associated with deeply impacted 3.8: careful planning and accurate surgical management are fundamental, due to the relationships of the impacted tooth with the mandibular canal.

Root anatomy: precise identification of the form, number, and length of the roots is essential, since all of these factors can influence the difficulty of the treatment, and the choice of surgical technique.

Length and degree of formation of the roots: these are the first factors to assess. The ideal moment to perform extraction of an impacted tooth corresponds to a stage of root formation ranging from a half to two-thirds (5.23). When the roots are only partially formed, or are not formed at all (as in germs), it is generally not necessary to separate them: in these cases, it is sufficient to separate the crown in two or more parts, thus reducing the risk of damaging adjacent anatomic structures.

Number of roots: the presence of a single root undoubtedly represents a favourable factor, while the presence of multiple roots, particularly when divergent, often requires their separation.

Moreover, it is important to evaluate the curvature of every root and the direction of the curvature in relation to the inclination of the tooth.

Size of the follicular sac: the presence of an ample follicular sac surrounding the crown of the impacted tooth is a favourable factor, as a larger available space around the tooth facilitates luxation manoeuvres.

Amplitude of the periodontal space/ligament: amplitude of the periodontal space is generally greater in young patients, and it progressively decreases with age. In adult patients, partial ankylosis of the impacted teeth is rather frequent, and may significantly complicate their extraction.

Degree of mineralisation of the bone surrounding the impacted tooth: in younger patients (< 20 years of age), the bone is less dense and less mineralised, thus presenting a greater elasticity. Therefore, during luxation it is subjected to partial deformations that facilitate the extraction of the impacted tooth. Irrespective of the age of the patient, the maxilla (with the exception of the palate) exhibits a lower bone density compared to the mandible. The luxation of maxillary impacted teeth is thus generally easier compared to the luxation of mandibular teeth.

Proximity of the impacted tooth to the adjacent teeth: the absence of a bony septum between the impacted tooth and the roots of the adjacent teeth represents a complicating factor, as it makes luxation more difficult and increases the risk of damaging the neighbouring teeth (5.24). In these cases, it may prove useful to use a bur to create a fissure on the impacted tooth, in which a root elevator can be inserted to facilitate luxation manoeuvres. The close proximity of the impacted tooth to the roots of adjacent teeth also complicates their periodontal prognosis, as after the 25th year of age the probability of a complete regeneration of the periodontal tissues around the neighbouring teeth decreases.

Proximity of the impacted tooth to important anatomic structures: the proximity or continuity of an impacted tooth with anatomic structures, such as the mandibular canal, the maxillary sinus, the floor of the nasal cavities, etc., represents a complicating factor that requires the implementation of all possible precautions to minimise the risk of intraoperative and postoperative complications (5.25a-b).

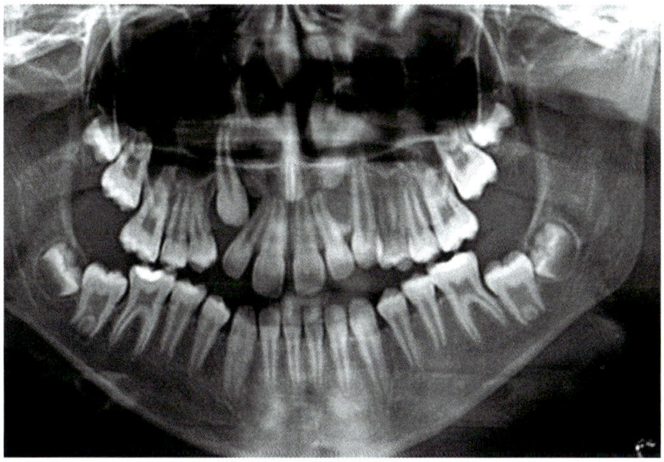

5.23 Panoramic radiograph showing an impacted 1.3: root anatomy is favourable, therefore surgical exposure and orthodontic alignment can be considered the treatment of choice.

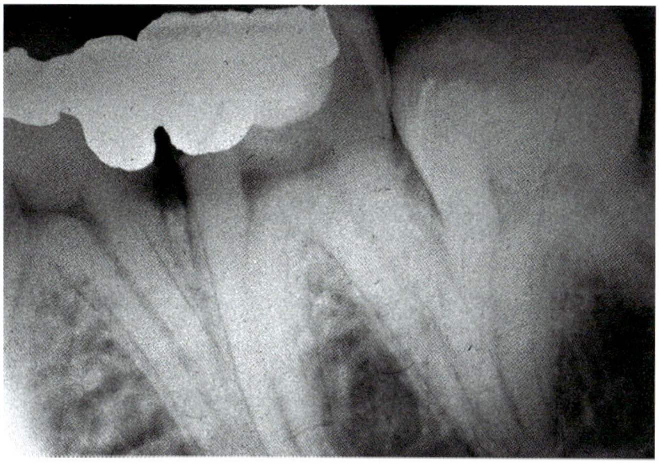

5.24 Impacted 3.8: divergent roots, absence of the periodontal space, and close proximity to the distal root of 3.7 render the extraction more complex.

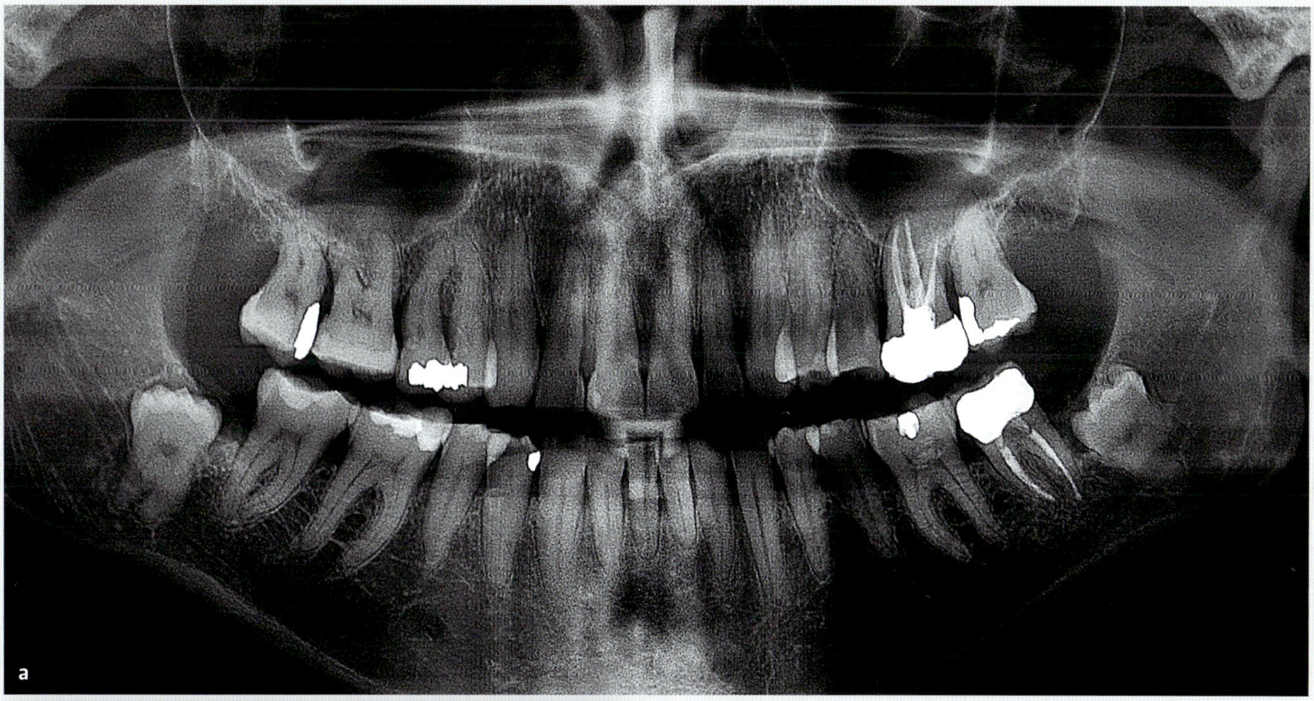

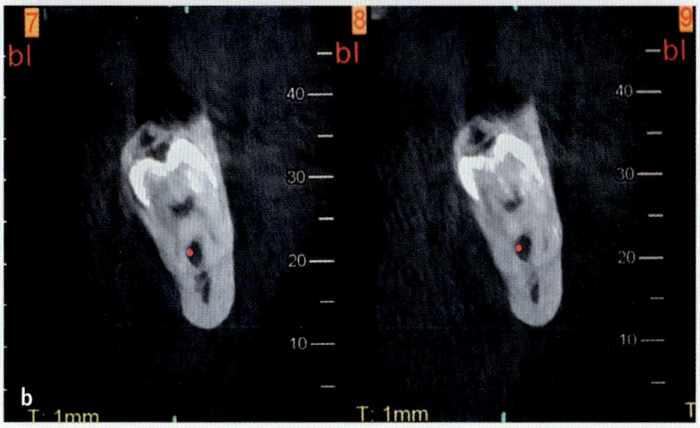

5.25 **a)** Panoramic radiograph showing a supposed direct relationship between 4.8 and the mandibular canal. **b)** CT scan demonstrating the exact relationship between 4.8 and the inferior alveolar nerve: the nerve runs between the roots of the impacted tooth.

Extraction of impacted teeth

Favourable factors	Complicating factors
Superficial impaction	Deep impaction
Incomplete root formation	Completely formed roots
Single, short, and conical root	Long, divergent roots with pronounced curvatures
Ample periodontal space	Narrow or absent (ankylosis) periodontal space
Ample dental follicle	Absence of the dental follicle
Elastic bone surrounding the impacted tooth	Dense, highly mineralised bone surrounding the impacted tooth
Sufficient distance from the adjacent teeth	Absence of space between the impacted tooth and the adjacent teeth
Safety distance from important anatomic structures	Close proximity or continuity between the impacted tooth and important anatomic structures

Surgical techniques

Several technical differences exist between the approaches used for extraction of impacted teeth and the approaches used for extraction of erupted teeth, even in the case of complex extractions performed with an open surgical technique. The first difference involves the access flaps, as impacted teeth require the elevation of larger mucoperiosteal flaps. A second difference is the necessity of removing greater quantities of bone, particularly in cases of deep impaction. Another peculiarity is the frequent necessity of separating the crown and roots (odontotomy), to make extraction less traumatic and to minimise bone removal.

Surgical armamentarium

This is similar to the armamentarium used to perform complex extractions of erupted teeth.

Technical details for impacted tooth extraction are described below, according to the type of tooth.

Mandibular third molars

PREOPERATIVE EVALUATION AND CLASSIFICATION

Mandibular third molars present peculiar characteristics that frequently render their extraction more difficult, compared to the extraction of other impacted teeth; therefore, a correct preoperative assessment is paramount. Various classifications based on radiographic observations have been proposed over the years to standardise this evaluation and to provide the preoperative definition, albeit approximate, of the complexity of the extraction.

Classification based on the inclination of the third molar relative to the axis of the second molar (Winter, 1926)

From a clinical point of view, it is a very important classification system, as it is the angulation of an impacted tooth that causes its "extraction path", which can be more or less anatomically/geometrically favourable. Based on this parameter, and in ascending order according to the complexity of their extraction, impacted mandibular third molars are classified as follows: a) mesio-angular teeth (the most frequent occurrence); b) horizontal teeth; c) vertical teeth; and d) disto-angular teeth. The difficulties in the surgical treatment of disto-angular impacted mandibular third molars are related to the fact that their "extraction path" is directed towards the mandibular ramus. Rarely, inverted impacted teeth can be observed in the mandible: these are rotated 180°, thus their crown is in an apical position and their roots in a coronal position. In addition to the different inclinations on the sagittal plane, mandibular third molars can also present a lingual inclination (the most frequent occurrence, due to the curvature of the mandible distally to the second molar), or a buccal inclination. The different positions/inclinations of impacted mandibular third molars allow ostectomy and odontotomy to be planned in a relatively predefined way (📷 5.26a) (see further for details).

Classification based on the position of the third molar relative to the anterior margin of the mandibular ramus, evaluated on a panoramic radiograph (Pell and Gregory, 1933)

Class I: the crown of the third molar is entirely mesial to the anterior margin of the mandibular ramus.
Class II: half of the crown of the third molar is covered by the mandibular ramus.
Class III: the crown of the third molar is entirely covered by the mandibular ramus.
The extraction of class III third molars is rendered more difficult by the scarce accessibility, thus requiring a more extensive ostectomy to gain adequate access to the impacted tooth (📷 5.26b).

Classification of the depth of impaction based on the relationship between the occlusal plane of the second and third molar (Pell and Gregory, 1933)

Class A: The occlusal planes of the second and third molar approximately coincide. In this case the impaction is superficial, often only a soft tissue impaction.
Class B: the occlusal plane of the third molar is comprised between that of the second molar and the enamel-dentin junction of this latter.
Class C: the occlusal plane of the third molar is entirely below the enamel-dentin junction of the second molar.
Class C third molars are the least accessible: therefore, extraction is more difficult and a more extensive ostectomy is necessary (📷 5.26c).

Different combinations of Pell and Gregory class I-II-III and A-B-C, together with different degrees of lingual or buccal inclination, cause different difficulty levels in the extraction of a mandibular third molar.

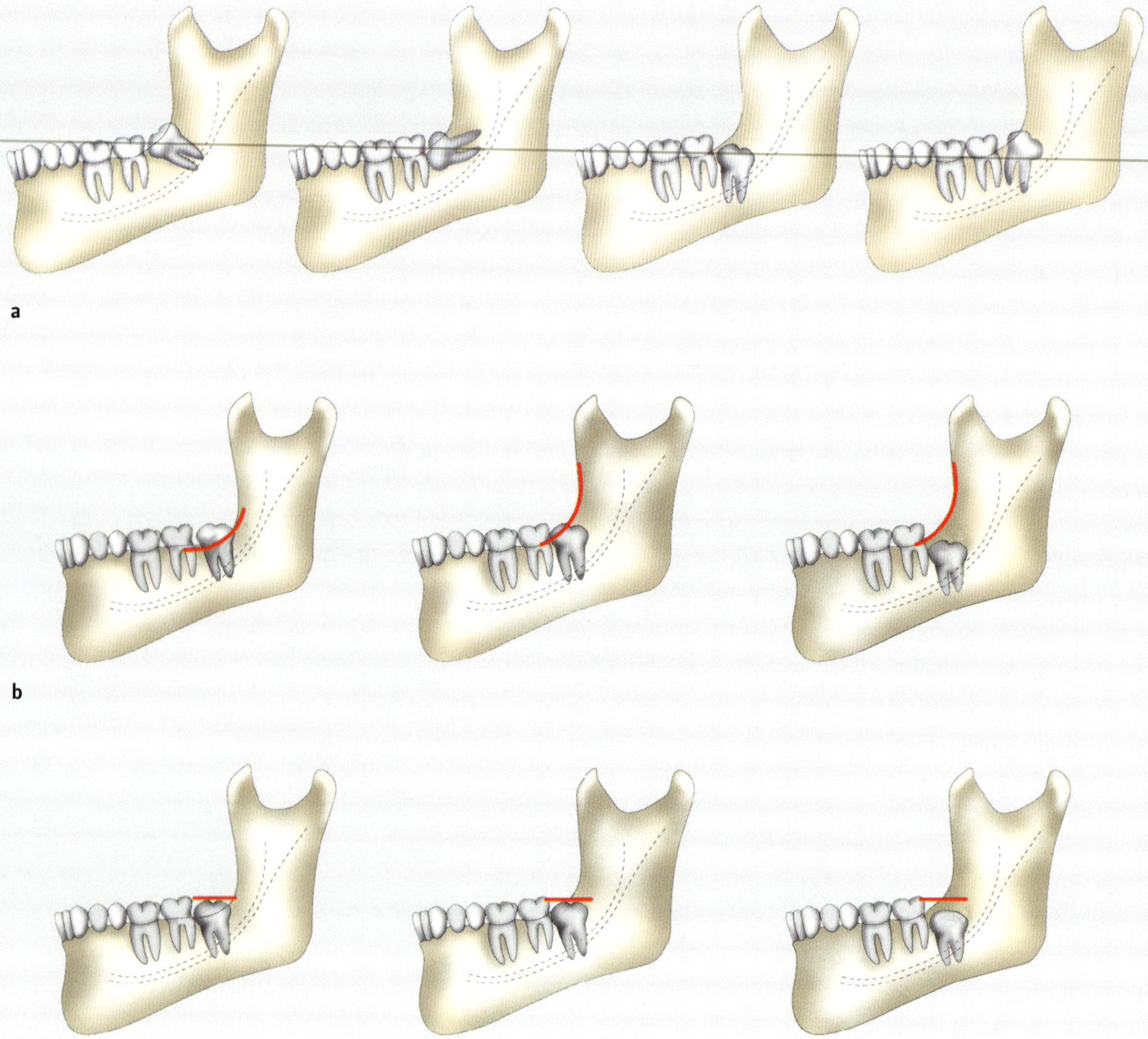

a

b

c

5.26 **a)** Classification based on the inclination of the third molar relative to the axis of the second molar (Winter, 1926). From left to right in ascending order of complexity: mesio-angular, horizontal, vertical, and disto-angular third molar. **b)** Classification based on the position of the third molar relative to the anterior margin of the mandibular ramus, evaluated on a panoramic radiograph (Pell and Gregory, 1933). From left to right in ascending order of complexity: class I, II, and III. **c)** Classification of the depth of impaction based on the relationship between the occlusal plane of the second and third molar (Pell and Gregory, 1933). From left to right in ascending order of complexity: class A, B, and C.

Relationships with the mandibular canal

Spatial relationships existing between an impacted third molar and the mandibular canal should always be clarified preoperatively through an accurate analysis of the radiographic images, as they represent a further factor influencing the complexity of the extraction. In general, the mandibular canal runs lingually to the third molar in 61% of cases, buccally to the third molar in 22% of cases, and in only 6% of cases is it in direct contact with the roots of the third molar.

Some radiographic images have been associated with a relationship of close proximity between third molars and the inferior alveolar neurovascular bundle:

Extraction of mandibular third molars

Favourable factors

- Mesio-angulation
- Pell and Gregory Class I
- Pell and Gregory Class A
- Safety distance from the mandibular canal
- All favourable factors in common with the extraction of other impacted teeth

Complicating factors

- Disto-angulation
- Pell and Gregory Class III
- Pell and Gregory Class C
- Close proximity of the tooth to the mandibular canal
- All complicating factors in common with the extraction of other impacted teeth

Interruption of the lamina dura of the mandibular canal and/or radiolucent band crossing the root where the root and mandibular canal are in close proximity: it is probable that the nerve runs in a groove on the root surface, or that it runs directly through the root (5.25a-b). Conversely, when the neurovascular bundle runs lingually or buccally to the roots, it is surrounded by a thin layer of radiopaque bone that can be clearly seen on the radiographic image.

Strictures or deviations of the mandibular canal in the area of the root apexes of the third molar: development of the roots and/or the apposition of cementum may cause the apical deviation of the mandibular canal or the presence of a stricture (5.25a).

Deviations of the roots of the impacted tooth in proximity to the mandibular canal: in this case, the presence of the neurovascular bundle represented a restriction to the development of the roots.

The presence of unfavourable radiographic findings represents a risk factor for possible neurologic complications in cases of extraction.

In some cases with a more unfavourable risk benefit ratio, it is appropriate to discuss the opportunity of performing the extraction with the patient, which may be performed only if symptoms or pathologies are associated with the impaction. If extraction is necessary, CT scans are surely an essential exam for clarifying the exact spatial relationships between the mandibular canal and the impacted tooth, thus helping to cause the best surgical approach to minimise the risk of intraoperative and postoperative complications. For example, knowing in advance that the neurovascular bundle runs in a groove on the lingual surface of the root will allow the ostectomy on the buccal side to be extended and the tooth to be luxated in a buccal direction. In this way, the tooth is moved away from the nerve, instead of being pushed towards it and causing its compression.

Surgical anatomy: notable anatomic structures

Mandibular canal

Evaluation of the existing relationships between the impacted mandibular third molars and the mandibular canal has already been discussed in detail.

Surgical implications. An involvement of the mandibular canal during the extraction of an impacted third molar may cause, in addition to neurologic complications, significant bleeding subsequent to the laceration of the inferior alveolar artery.

Lingual nerve

For anatomical details, see the dedicated paragraph (Chapter 2).

Surgical implications. The superficial course of the lingual nerve, in association with the thinness of the cortical plate, influences the design of the access flaps, which present distal releasing incisions directed buccally to avoid any damage to the nerve. Moreover, when odontotomy is necessary, the superficial course of the nerve must be considered and the lingual aspect of the access flap must be adequately elevated and protected (see further for details). Finally, when luxation manoeuvres in lingual directions cannot be avoided, adequate protection of the nerve must be guaranteed to avoid both direct and indirect damage.

Facial artery

For anatomical details, see the dedicated paragraph (Chapter 2).

Surgical implications. Vertical releasing incisions in the area of the first/second molar should not extend too apically towards the vestibular fornix, and they must never, in any case whatsoever, extend beyond its bottom.

Buccinator muscle

For anatomical details, see the dedicated paragraph (Chapter 2).

Surgical implications. The elevation of access flaps beyond the external oblique line is generally followed by greater postoperative swelling, pain, and trismus: therefore, it should be avoided whenever possible.

Buccal nerve

For anatomical details, see the dedicated paragraph (Chapter 2).

Surgical implications. The distal releasing incision can be performed full-thickness in the area of the retromolar trigone, but it should continue split-thickness distally to the trigone due to the risk of damaging the buccal nerve.

Surgical protocol for the extraction of impacted mandibular third molars

Specific armamentarium

Besides the basic armamentarium used to perform all complex extractions, some specific instruments are particularly useful:

- two straight root elevators, one with a fine and the other with a regular tip;
- angled elevators (e.g. Walter-Barry);
- apical pick elevators (straight and angled).

Locoregional anaesthesia

Inferior alveolar nerve block and buccal nerve block are used, while anaesthesia of the lingual nerve is frequently obtained together with the former, due to the proximity of the two nerves in the injection area.

Basic techniques

Access flaps

The choice of access flap is determined by the depth of impaction, and by the position of the impacted tooth. In general, complex extractions require a wider access flap, and it is therefore important to plan the design of the access flap preoperatively. However, it should be pointed out that the choice is also determined by personal preferences and by the surgeon's experience. In fact, it has been demonstrated that the type of incision does not significantly influence the long-term outcome as far as the periodontal condition of the adjacent teeth is concerned.

Envelope flap

A single incision is performed starting from inside the gingival sulcus of the second molar: once the blade has reached the middle of the distal face of the second molar, it is rotated distally and buccally to incise the soft tissues in the direction of the anterior margin of the mandibular ramus. This flap allows a limited retraction of the soft tissues, and its use should therefore be limited to less demanding extractions, where minimal ostectomy is required. The absence of mesial releasing incisions renders the elevation of this flap more difficult, particularly when periodontal soft tissues are thin. The main advantages offered by this type of flap are an easier and faster suture. To gain wider access to the surgical field, the sulcular incision can be extended to the first molar; in this case, to simplify suturing at the end of the intervention, it is recommended that interdental papilla between the first and second molar be preserved (📷 5.27).

Three-corner flap

This access flap associates a distal releasing incision similar to that of the envelope flap with a second (mesial) releasing incision that, starting from the disto-buccal corner of the second molar, is directed mesially towards the muco-gingival line at a 45° angle. The presence of a second releasing incision facilitates the elevation of the flap and improves retraction of the soft tissues, thus rendering this access suitable for the treatment of more complex cases. However, the correct repositioning of the flap may be more difficult compared to the repositioning of an envelope flap (📷 5.28).

Four-corner flap

This is a hybrid between the two flaps described above. The distal releasing incision is identical to that described for the previously described flaps, and it is associated with a sulcular incision involving the second molar (or both the second and first molar), and with a mesial releasing incision starting from the mesio-buccal corner of the second molar (or from the disto-buccal corner of the first molar) directed apically and mesially towards the muco-gingival line. Elevation of this flap is easier compared to elevation of an envelope flap, due to the second releasing incision that also grants wider access to the surgical field. Moreover, this flap is easier to reposition compared to a three-corner flap. Suturing is facilitated by starting the mesial releasing incision at the disto-buccal corner of the first molar (instead of starting it at the mesio-buccal corner of the second molar) and preserving the interdental papilla between the first and second molar (📷 5.29).

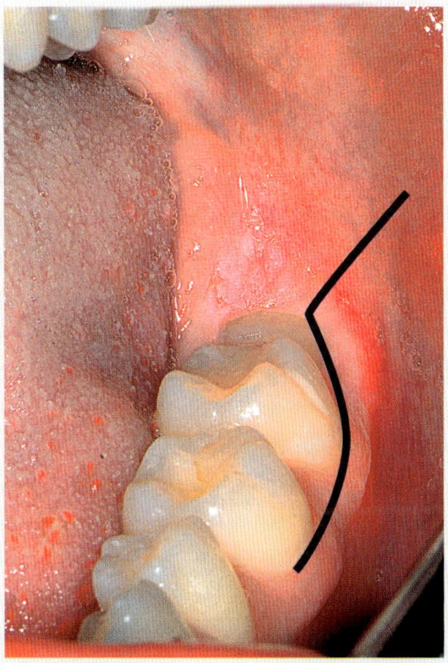

📷 **5.27** Marginal flap without a mesial releasing incision for the extraction of an impacted mandibular third molar.

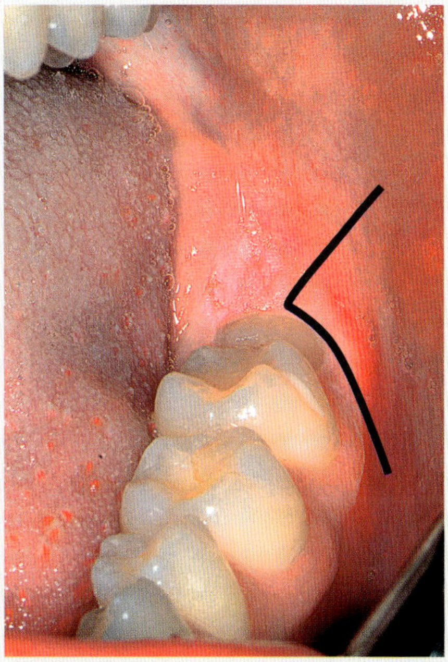

📷 **5.28** Three-corner flap.

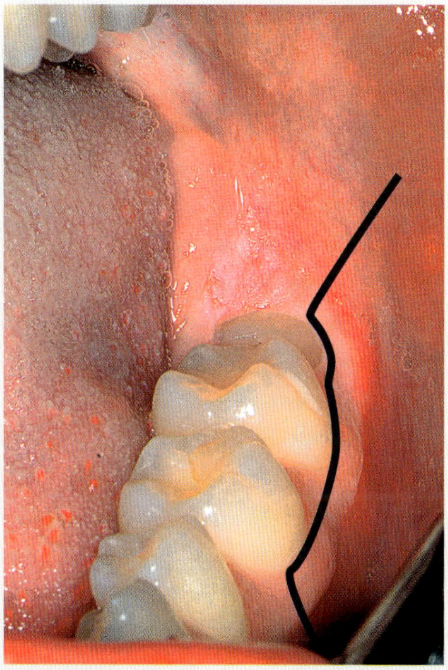

📷 **5.29** Four-corner flap.

Direction of the distal releasing incision

The distal releasing incision, which is identical for all three types of access flap, must be directed buccally as well as distally. In fact, the mandible does not develop along the line of the dental arch distally to the second molar, but it diverges laterally. If the distal releasing incision is directed distally, the scalpel blade loses contact with the mandibular bone and falls in the retromolar space, with the risk of sectioning the lingual nerve. Before carrying out the distal releasing incision, it can be useful to evaluate the anatomy of the retromolar area by palpation, to locate the lingual limit of the mandible precisely and carry out the incision in a safe zone. As a general rule, the distal releasing incision starts in the gingival sulcus of the second molar (at the middle of the distal face of the crown) and is directed distally and buccally at a 45° angle to the ideal continuation of the dental arch (5.30).

Modifications of the access flap for the extraction of partially erupted third molars

In cases of extraction of partially erupted mandibular third molars, the distal releasing incision is made in the same direction described above, but the starting point is at the disto-buccal corner of the erupted portion of the third molar (5.31).

Elevation and retraction of the access flap

The access flap must be elevated full-thickness. During the following phases of ostectomy and odontotomy, the lingual and buccal soft tissues must be protected from accidental contacts with rotary instruments to avoid possible damage to the lingual nerve and facial artery, respectively (5.32a-c).

Access ostectomy and exposure of the impacted tooth

The removal of bone around the impacted tooth should always be limited to the strict minimum necessary: it should help create favourable leverage points for the luxation of the tooth, and provide sufficient space to perform the following odontotomy manoeuvres. In cases of soft tissue impaction, once the flap is elevated, ostectomy may not be necessary; in cases of partial bony impaction, ostectomy is performed starting from the emerging portion of the tooth. Ostectomy can be extended, if necessary, to expose the entire buccal surface, the amelodentinal junction and, frequently, the distal surface of the crown of the impacted tooth. Conversely, ostectomy should never involve the thin lingual cortical plate, as the lingual nerve runs in close proximity to it.

In cases of complete bony impaction, ostectomy usually starts at the disto-buccal corner of the second molar: once the crown of the third molar is located, ostectomy is extended to expose it (5.32d-e). Only in cases of deep impaction, and particularly when the impacted tooth is in close proximity to the mandibular canal, can ostectomy be extended further. However, to avoid unnecessary loss of bone, the creation of a buccal bone lid (similar to the one used in bone harvesting from the mandibular ramus - see Chapter 13 for details) may allow easy access to the impacted tooth while keeping the inferior alveolar neurovascular bundle under direct control. Once the impacted tooth is extracted, the bone lid can be repositioned with the aid of titanium microscrews and plates.

Odontotomy

The factors determining the necessity of dividing the tooth in several parts are the position of the third molar and the anatomy of its roots. The oral surgeon must be able to balance the quantity of bone removed and the number of parts in which the tooth is divided in an adequate manner. In fact, extensive ostectomy may allow the tooth to be extracted without the need for odontotomy, but it may entail a relevant loss of bone causing an unnecessary weakening of the surrounding bony structures, potential periodontal damage to the adjacent tooth, and greater postoperative discomfort. Separation of the tooth is performed with a fissure bur and is not completed in the lingual, mesial, and apical directions. The bur penetrates at a depth of approximately two-thirds of the portion to be separated, and separation is then completed by fracture, with the aid of a root elevator. In this way, the risk of damaging the lingual nerve, inferior alveolar nerve, and root of the second molar is significantly reduced (5.32f-g).

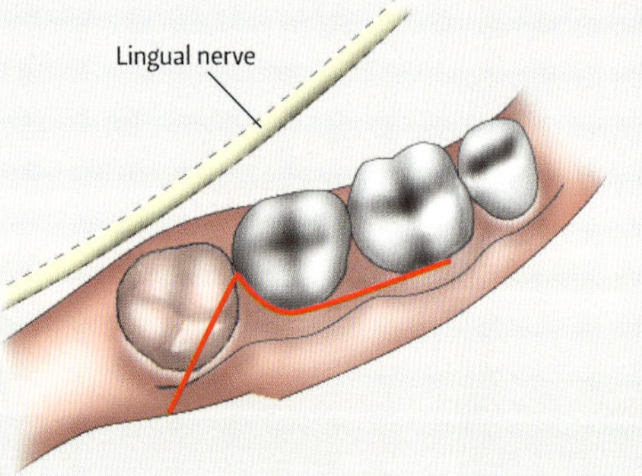

5.30 The distal releasing incision must always be directed buccally to prevent the lesion of the lingual nerve.

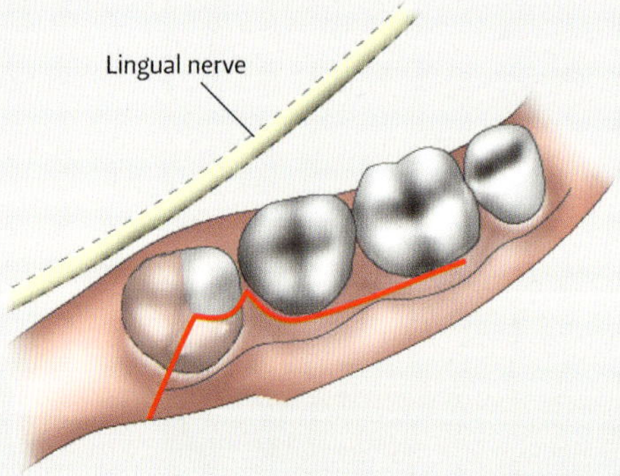

5.31 Access flap for the extraction of partially erupted mandibular third molars: the distal releasing incision starts at the disto-buccal corner of the erupted portion of the tooth.

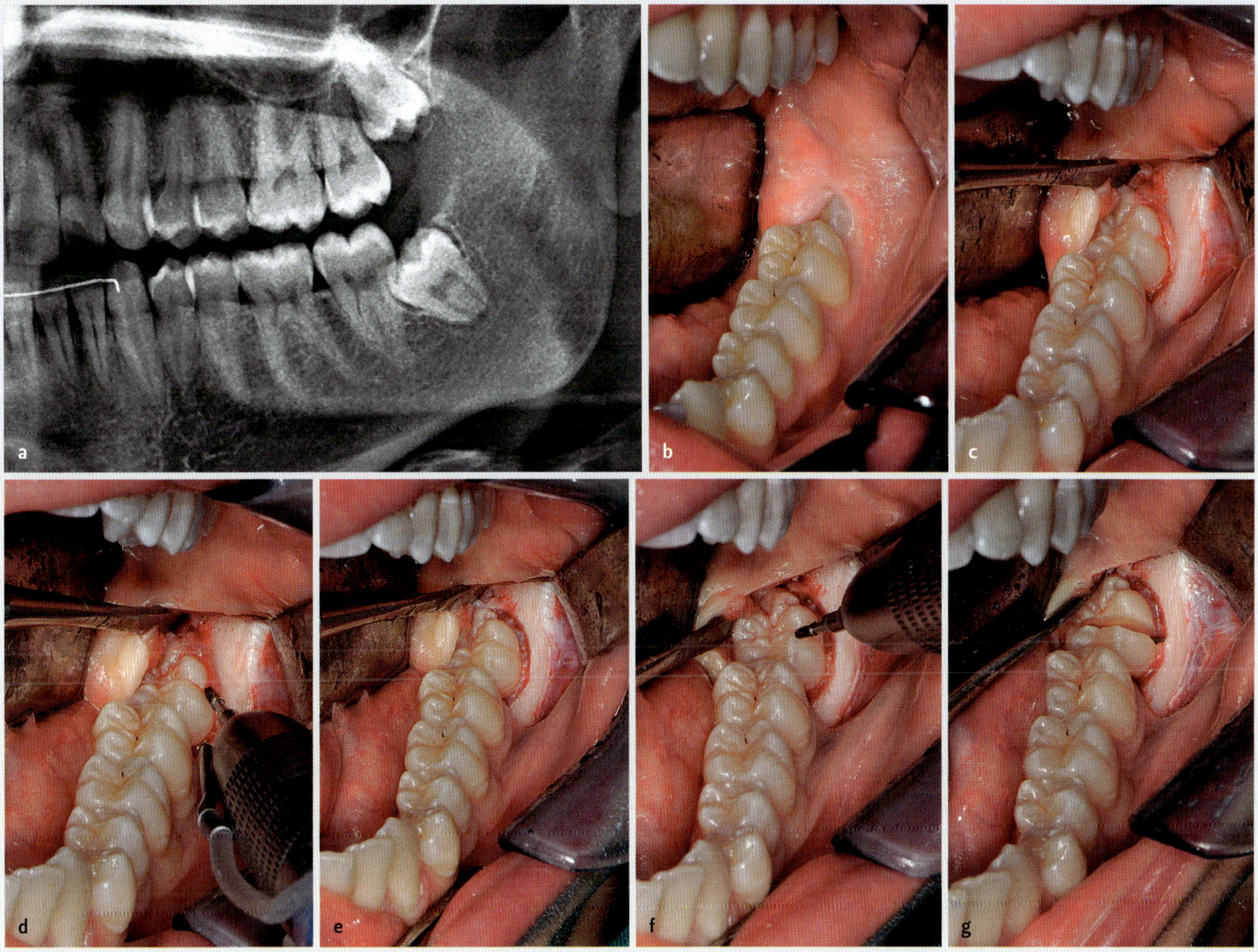

5.32 **a–b)** Partially impacted 3.8. **c)** Protection of the lingual and buccal soft tissues after flap elevation. **d)** Bone removal with a fissure bur mounted on a straight handpiece to expose an adequate portion of the crown. **e)** The exposed crown. **f–g)** Separation of the crown with a fissure bur mounted on a straight handpiece. (*continued*)

Odontotomy of vertical impacted third molars

If the tooth has a single root and its extraction is impeded by a distal obstacle, it is sufficient to remove the distal part of the crown. If the tooth has two retentive roots, the removal of the crown in its entirety by means of a horizontal odontotomy precedes the separation of the roots. The greater complexity in the extraction of these teeth is caused by the necessity of a wider buccal ostectomy to compensate for the reduced accessibility caused by the proximity to the second molar.

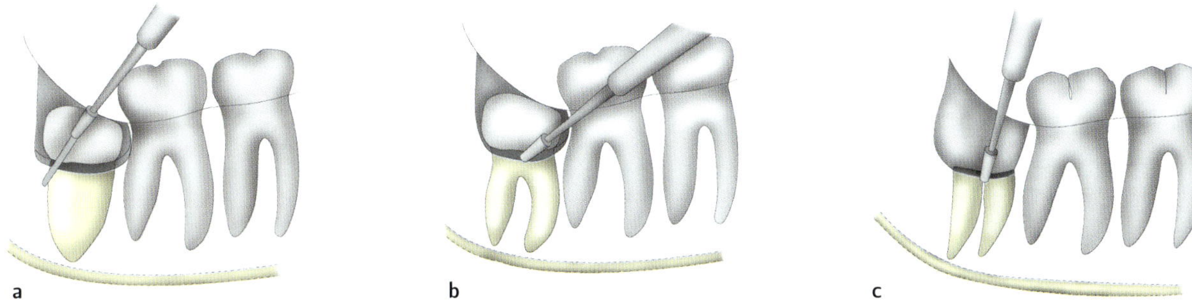

Odontotomy of the vertical impacted mandibular third molars: **a)** distal separation; **b)** crown separation; **c)** root separation.

Odontotomy of the mesio-angular impacted third molars

To perform extraction of these teeth, it is generally necessary to separate the distal part of their crown, the removal of which frees the space that allows the distal luxation of the tooth. If the tooth has divergent roots, removal of the crown in its entirety precedes separation of the roots.

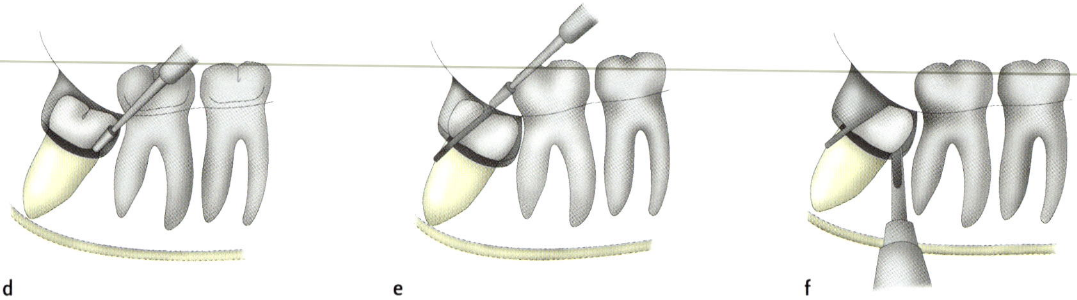

d e f

Odontotomy of mesio-angular impacted mandibular third molars

Odontotomy of horizontal impacted third molars

In this case, it is necessary to separate the crown from the roots at the amelodentinal junction. Separation of the crown should be conducted with a slightly oblique (mesial) inclination, to facilitate the subsequent removal of the separated crown. In some cases, particularly when the impacted tooth has pronounced cusps that are stuck in the undercut on the distal surface of the second molar, removal of the crown is possible only after its further separation in a mesio-distal direction. Removal of the crown allows the luxation of the roots in a mesial direction. Finally, in cases of divergent or retentive roots, it is necessary to proceed to their separation.

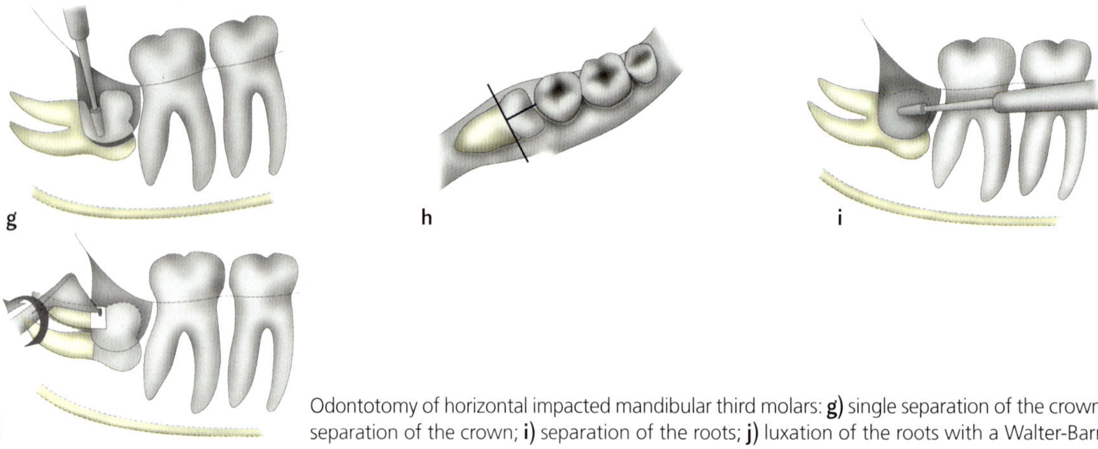

g h i j

Odontotomy of horizontal impacted mandibular third molars: **g)** single separation of the crown; **h)** multiple separation of the crown; **i)** separation of the roots; **j)** luxation of the roots with a Walter-Barry elevator.

Odontotomy of the disto-angular impacted third molars

Extraction of disto-angular impacted mandibular third molars is frequently more complex, as the crown of the second molar hides the roots of the impacted third molars, thus rendering their separation very challenging. A second reason is represented by the fact that the "extraction path" of disto-angular third molars causes these teeth to get stuck against the mandibular ramus: in these cases, removal of a greater quantity of bone is required. The crown, or at least the distal part of it, must be separated from the roots and removed, to allow luxation of the roots in a distal direction. Multiple, divergent roots must be separated to complete their extraction atraumatically.

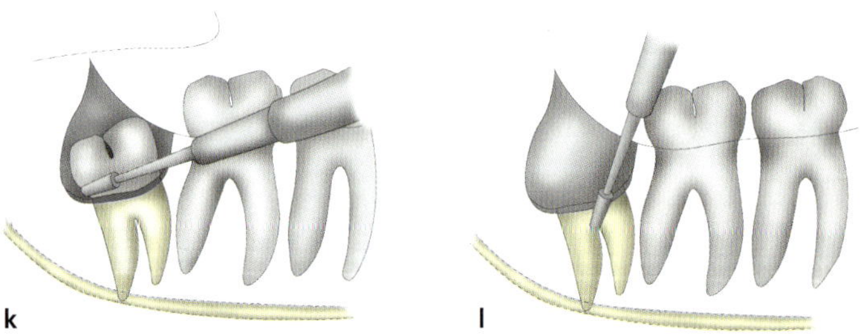

k l

Odontotomy of disto-angular mandibular third molars: **k)** separation of the crown; **l)** separation of the roots.

Extraction

After ostectomy and odontotomy (if necessary) are completed, the tooth or its parts are delicately luxated. Luxation requires the application of controlled force, to reduce the patient's discomfort and to avoid root fractures or, in extreme cases, the fracture of the mandible. Luxation is typically performed with a straight root elevator or with Walter-Barry elevators; it can also be facilitated by creating a notch on the tooth surface with a fissure bur into which the tip of the elevator can be inserted. Extraction is completed by removing the tooth or its parts with the aid of curved haemostatic forceps (5.32h-i).

Socket curettage and inspection of the post-extractive cavity

Socket curettage is performed to remove possible leftovers of the dental follicle, which are grasped with haemostatic forceps and detached with a surgical curette. The post-extractive socket is then profusely irrigated with sterile saline and the distal portion of the second molar is checked (5.32j-k).

Suture

Interrupted sutures performed with 4/0 or 5/0 filaments are generally used to reposition the access flap so that the anatomy of the soft tissues is restored. Healing will occur by primary or secondary intention according to the initial situation (complete or partial impaction). Complete closure of the access flap is contraindicated in cases of partial eruption or relevant infection (5.32l).

It is recommended that a gauze swab soaked in sterile saline be kept on the surgical wound for 10-15 minutes after the end of the intervention, to exert a moderate compression that reduces postoperative bleeding and promotes blood clotting.

Cold packs applied on the cheek can be very useful immediately after surgery, to relieve pain and swelling: the patient should be instructed to alternate 15 minutes of application and 15 minutes of rest in the first 4-5 hours after surgery.

Postoperative administrations of non-steroidal anti-inflammatory drugs and, in selected cases, the recourse to corticosteroids such as desamethasone, complete the protocol for the management of postoperative pain and swelling.

On the other hand, the role of antibiotic prophylaxis is still controversial: some studies have demonstrated that the incidence of postoperative infection does not present statistically significant differences between groups of patients who received an antibiotic prophylaxis and groups of patients who did not receive it.

The authors of this manual follow the guidelines periodically published by the AHA (American Heart Association) on this subject: the latest recommendations can be found on the association website.

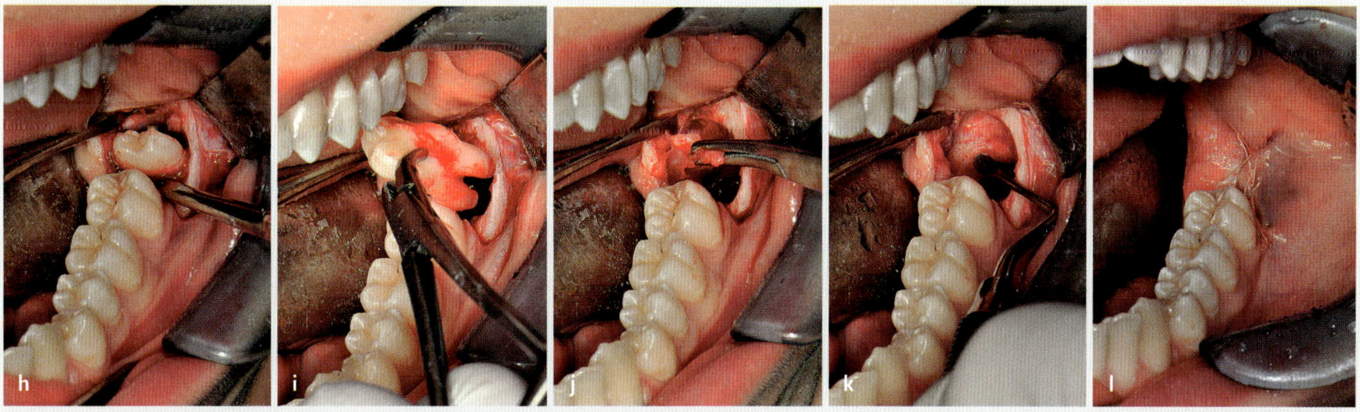

5.32 (*continued*) **h)** Luxation of the tooth with a straight root elevator. **i)** Extraction of the tooth with curved haemostatic forceps. **j)** Socket inspection and removal of possible leftovers of the dental follicle. **k)** Bone curettage of the post-extractive socket. **l)** Suture.

Clinical case 2 – Extraction of mesio-angular impacted 4.8

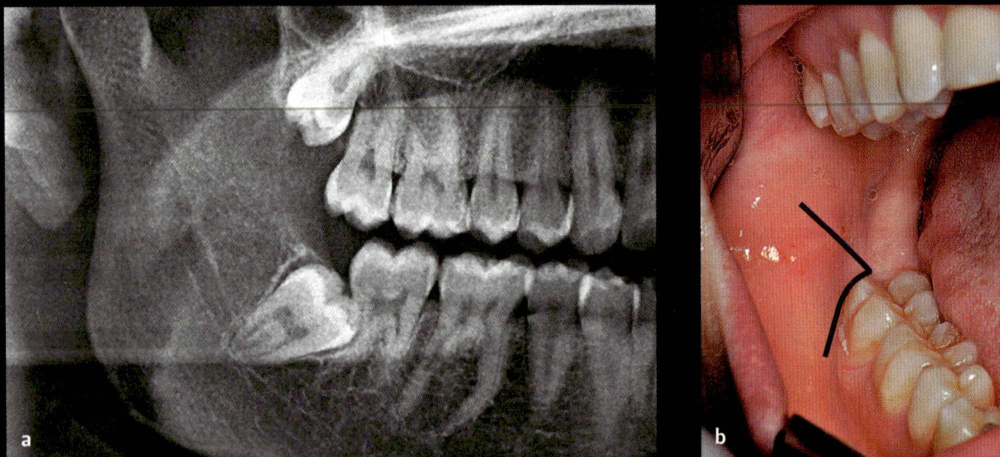

5.33a–b Fully impacted mesio-angular 4.8, and design of the access flap.

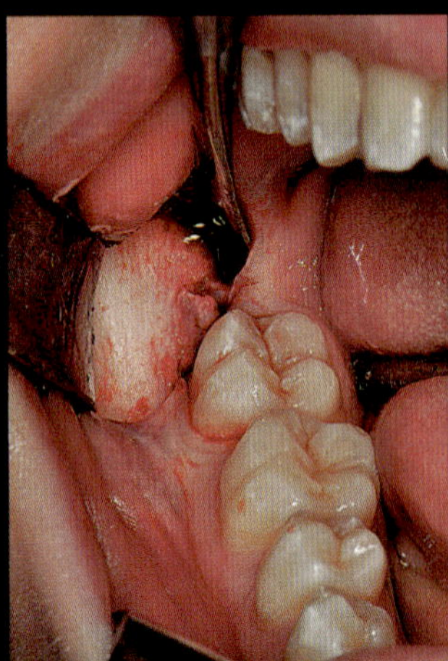

5.33c Elevation of a full-thickness flap and protection of the lingual and buccal soft tissues.

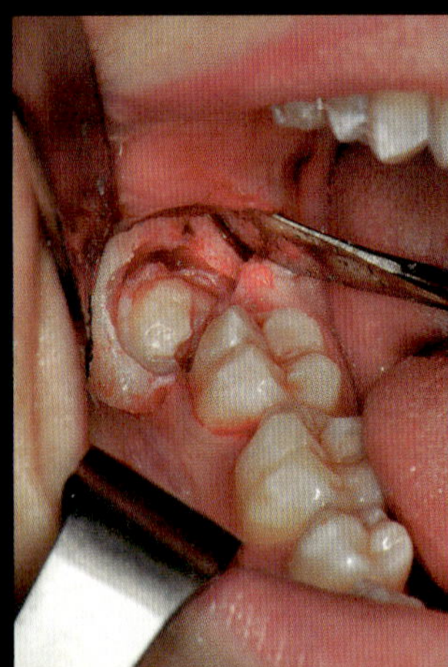

5.33d Exposure of the crown of the tooth.

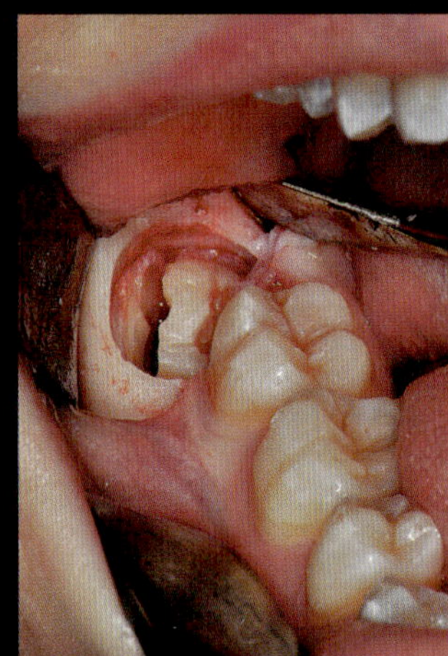

5.33e Separation of the crown from the roots.

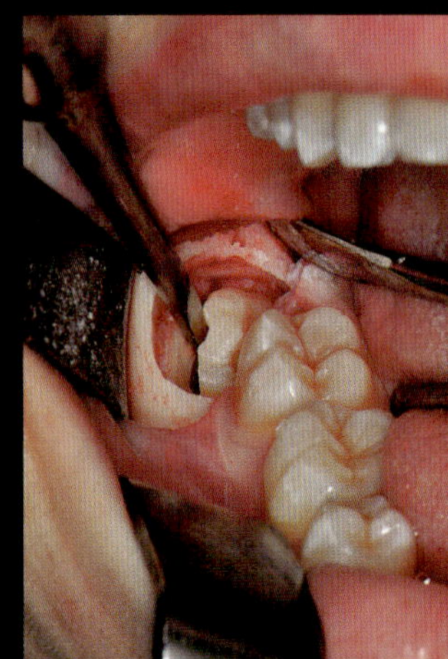

5.33f Luxation of the crown.

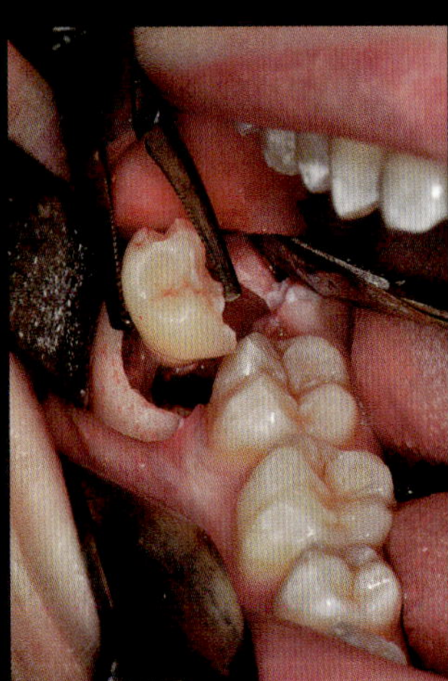

5.33g Removal of the crown with haemostatic forceps.

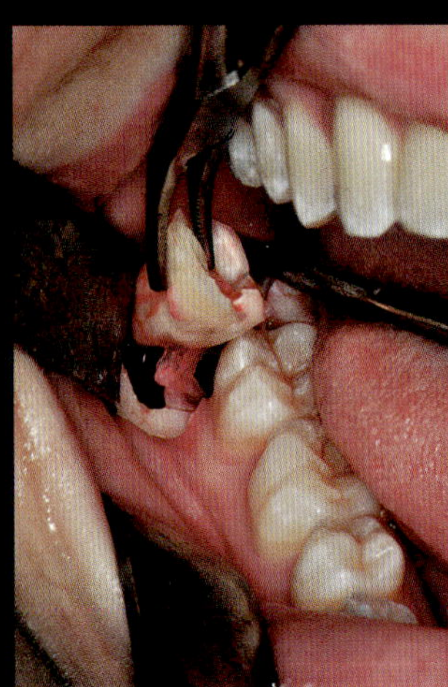

5.33h Removal of the roots with haemostatic forceps.

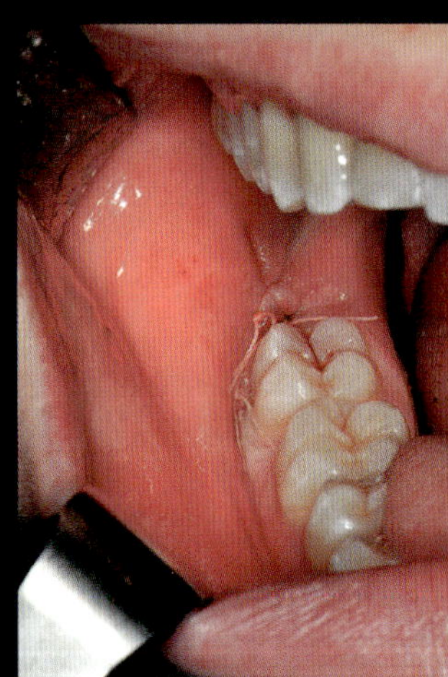

5.33i Suture.

Clinical case 3 – Extraction of impacted 4.8

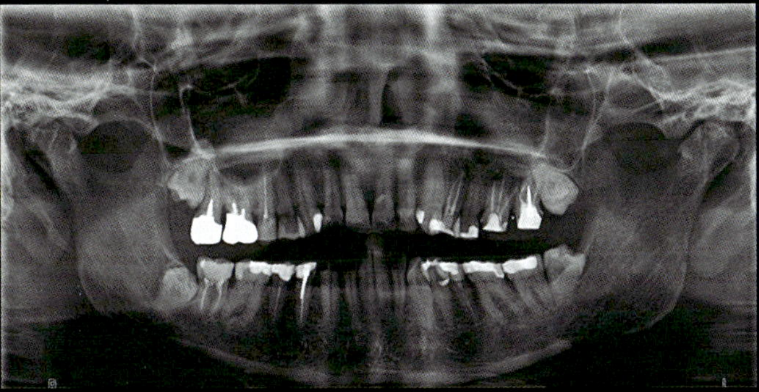

5.34a Preoperative panoramic radiograph showing a deeply impacted 4.8.

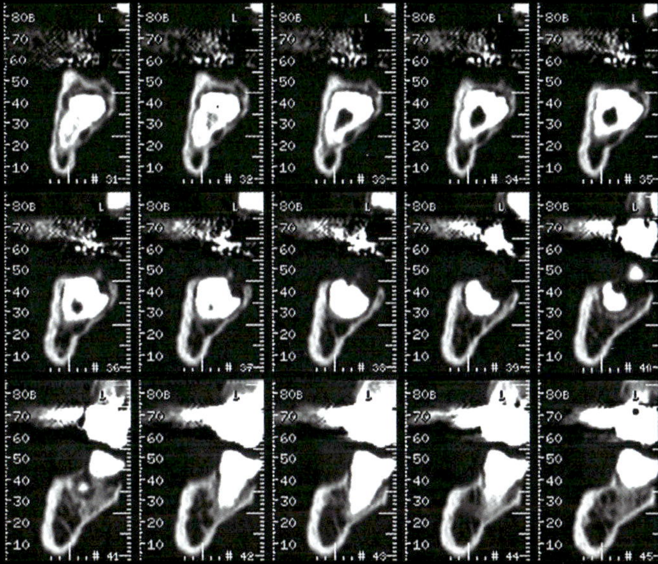

5.34b CT scans clarifying the relationships of the impacted tooth with the inferior alveolar nerve. Due to the depth of impaction, a surgical approach involving the creation of a bone lid on the buccal cortical plate of the mandible is chosen, to provide a greater control of the surgical field.

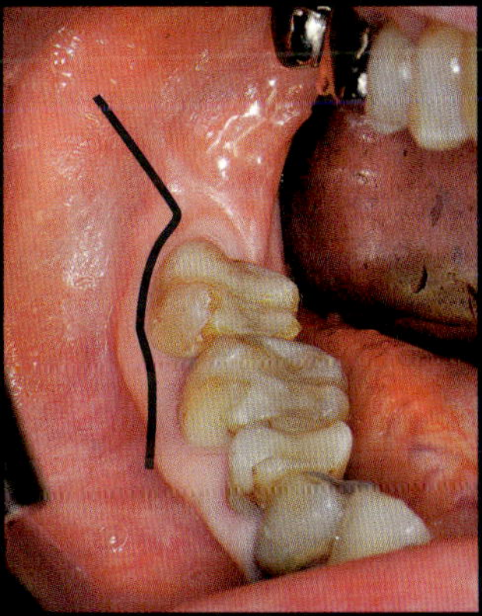

5.34c Preoperative clinical situation and design of the access flap.

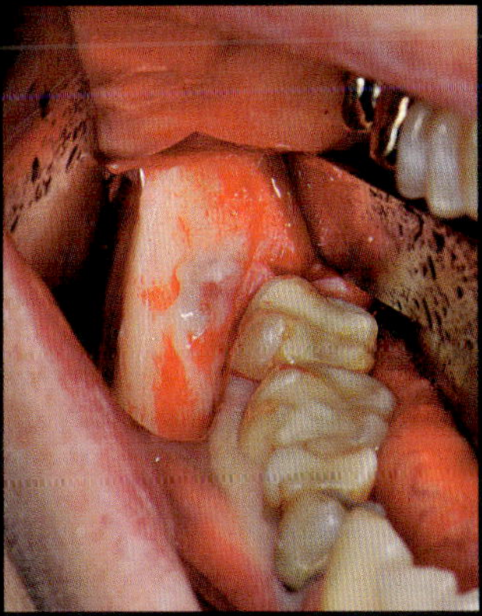

5.34d Elevation of a mucoperiosteal flap and protection of the lingual and buccal soft tissues.

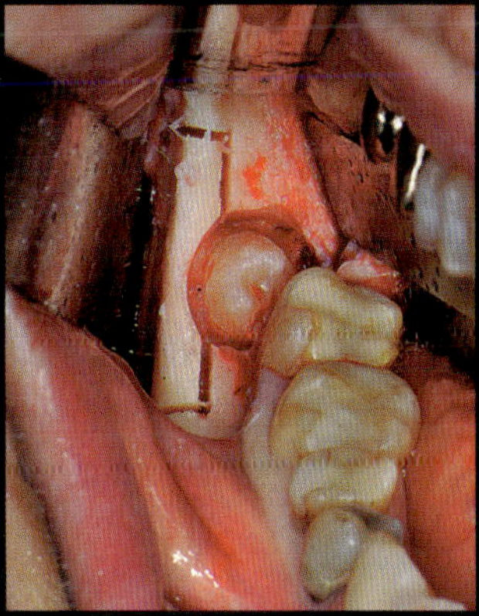

5.34e Ostectomies are performed to isolate a bone lid that, once removed, provides better access to the impacted tooth.

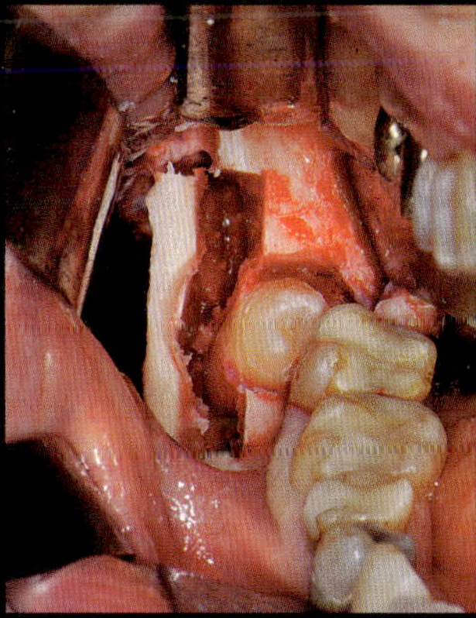

5.34f Separation of the bone lid with a surgical chisel.

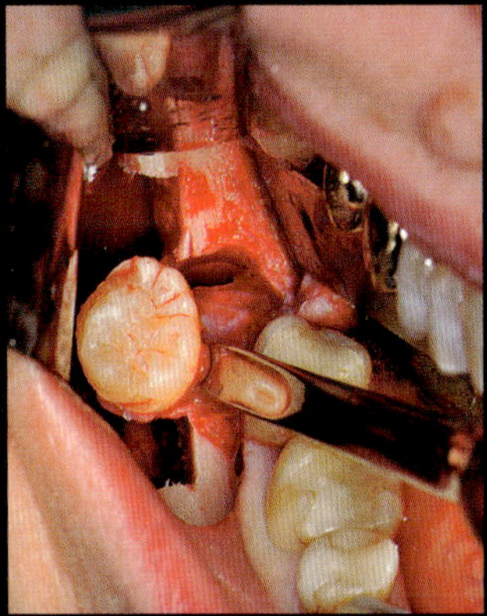

5.34g Luxation of the impacted tooth.

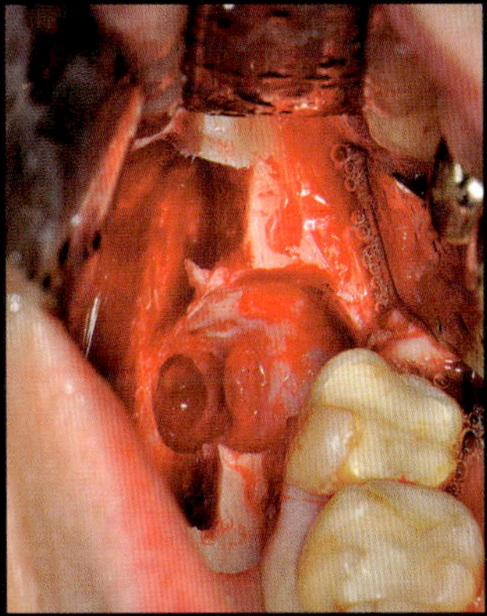

5.34h The post-extractive socket. The inferior alveolar nerve is visible on the lingual surface.

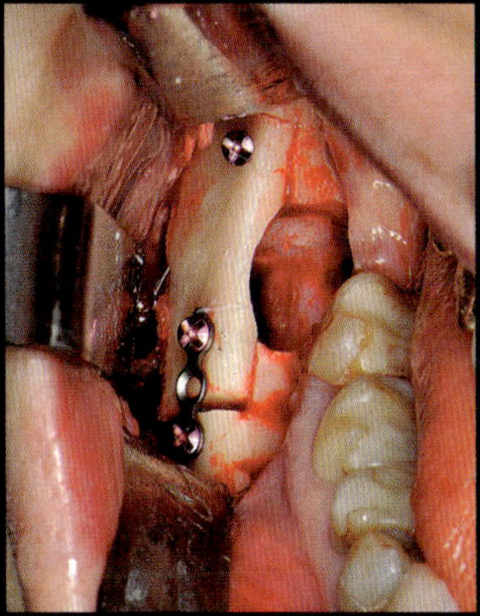

5.34i The bone lid is fixed back in place by means of titanium microscrews and plates.

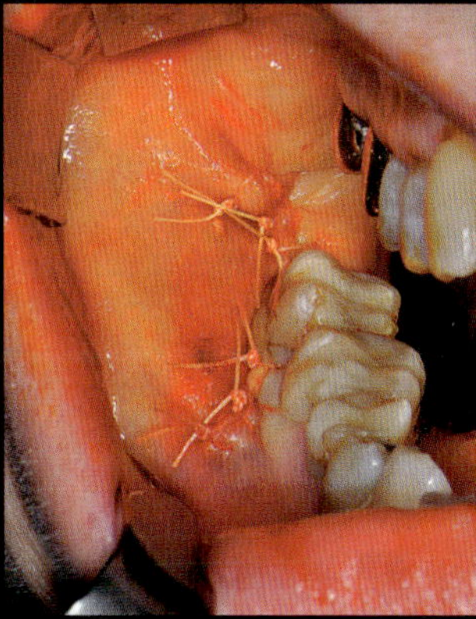

5.34j Suture.

Risk factors influencing the health of the periodontal tissues surrounding the second molar after third molar surgery (from Kugelberg, 1990)

- More than 25 years of age
- Visible presence of plaque distally to the second molar
- Probing depth > 6 mm distally to the second molar
- Presence of an intraosseous defect > 3 mm distally to the second molar
- Mesio-angulation of the third molar > 50°
- Presence of an ample contact area between the second and third molar
- Resorption of the roots of the second molar
- Pathologic enlargement (> 2.5 mm) of the dental follicle of the third molar
- Smoking habit

Extraction of the third molar and periodontal health of the second molar

As regards third molar extraction on the periodontal health of the second molar, a number of factors have been identified that can influence the healing process of the periodontal tissues.

The evaluation of risk factors may provide a criterion to manage situations in which third molars should be extracted as a preventive measure.

The analysis performed by Kugelberg (1990) suggests that the extraction of third molars before the 25th year of age in patients considered at risk is ideal, as extraction at an older age implies a lower probability of a complete *restitutio ad integrum*.

Germectomy of the mandibular third molar

The term germectomy defines the extraction of an impacted tooth at an early stage of its development, when only the crown, or coronal third of the roots at most, are formed.

INDICATIONS

Orthodontic treatment: germectomy of the mandibular third molars is indicated to make space in the dental arch when an orthodontic treatment involving the distalisation of the first and second molar is planned. In other cases, germectomy is indicated to treat anomalies in the position of the second molar (e.g. rotation, buccal migration).

Prevention of third molar impaction: when crowding is already observable, it is unlikely that third molars may find sufficient space to erupt correctly. In these cases, germectomy helps prevent the onset of all pathologic conditions associated with the eruptive process of third molars.

Alterations in the anatomy and position of the germ: in these cases, extraction of the germ helps prevent impaction.

Interference of the third molar with the eruption of the second molar: when the presence of the third molar represents an obstacle to the normal eruption of the second molar, the latter can take place only after the germ of the third molar is extracted.

Odontogenic lesions associate with the germ: early extraction is indicated when a dentigerous cyst or neoplasm (e.g. ameloblastoma) is associated to the germ.

CONTRAINDICATIONS

General contraindications to surgery: see dedicated section.

Absence or loss of other teeth: tooth agenesia or previous extractions of other permanent molars represent a contraindication to germectomy, as third molars are potential substitutes for missing teeth. With early deterioration of the second molar (e.g. destructive caries), its extraction may allow the spontaneous eruption of the third molar (if the germ is in an early developmental stage) in the place originally occupied by the second molar. The germ of the third molar can also be extracted and transplanted in the position of the second molar (see further for details).

SUITABLE AGE FOR GERMECTOMY

Choosing the best age to perform a germectomy should be mostly influenced by the degree of cooperation that the patient can guarantee during surgery, as these types of surgical interventions are generally performed under local anaesthesia. Some authors advocate the recourse to early germectomy, when the patient is between 9 and 12 years of age, since removal of the germ at the initial stages of its development would simplify surgical intervention and improve postoperative recovery. However, at this young age a correct evaluation of real indications (besides cases of severe dentobasal discrepancy, dysplasia, ectopy, or obvious pathology) may be difficult, as with obtaining adequate cooperation from the patient. Therefore, as a general rule, it is recommended that a germectomy be performed in patients between 13 and 16 years of age.

PECULIAR TECHNICAL ASPECTS OF GERMECTOMY

Germectomy of mandibular third molars does not substantially differ from the extraction of the completely formed corresponding teeth, thus involving the same phases (incision, flap elevation, access ostectomy, odontotomy, and extraction). The only difference concerns the access flaps. In fact, the most distal position of the germ avoids involvement of the periodontal soft tissues around the second molar in the flap.

Basic techniques

Access flaps

Submarginal flap

This flap is similar to the three-corner flap previously described. The only difference is that, in this case, the incision is made 2-3 millimetres distally to the gingival sulcus of the second molar, therefore avoiding its involvement in the elevation of the flap. This approach can be used when the germ of the third molar is at a relatively early stage of its development and is located at a distance from the second molar (5.35a-c).

Traditional access flaps

When the germ of the third molar is in close proximity to the second molar, the recourse to one of the previously described marginal flaps (envelope flap, three-corner flap, four-corner flap) is recommended.

Access osteotomy

In cases of germectomy, the creation of an access osteotomy as small as possible is essential to obtaining a complete *restitutio ad integrum* and an uneventful postoperative recovery. Access can be made either above the germ or laterally to it (5.35d).

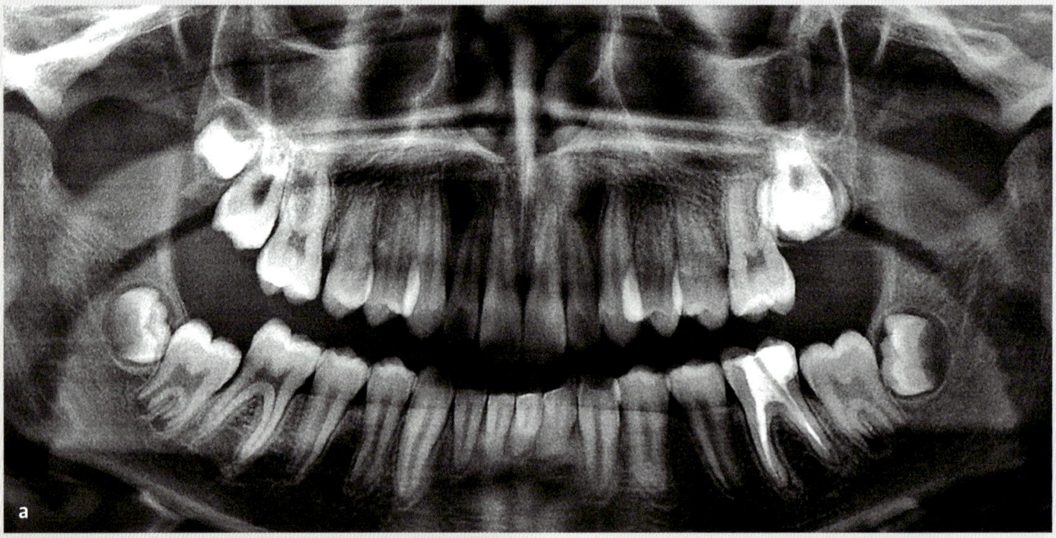

5.35 **a)** Panoramic radiograph demonstrating the presence of the germs of all four third molars. The correct alignment of the second molars is possible only after the extraction of the germs of the third molars. **b)** Three-corner submarginal access flap. **c)** Elevation of the access flap. **d)** Identification of the germ after access ostectomy. *(continued)*

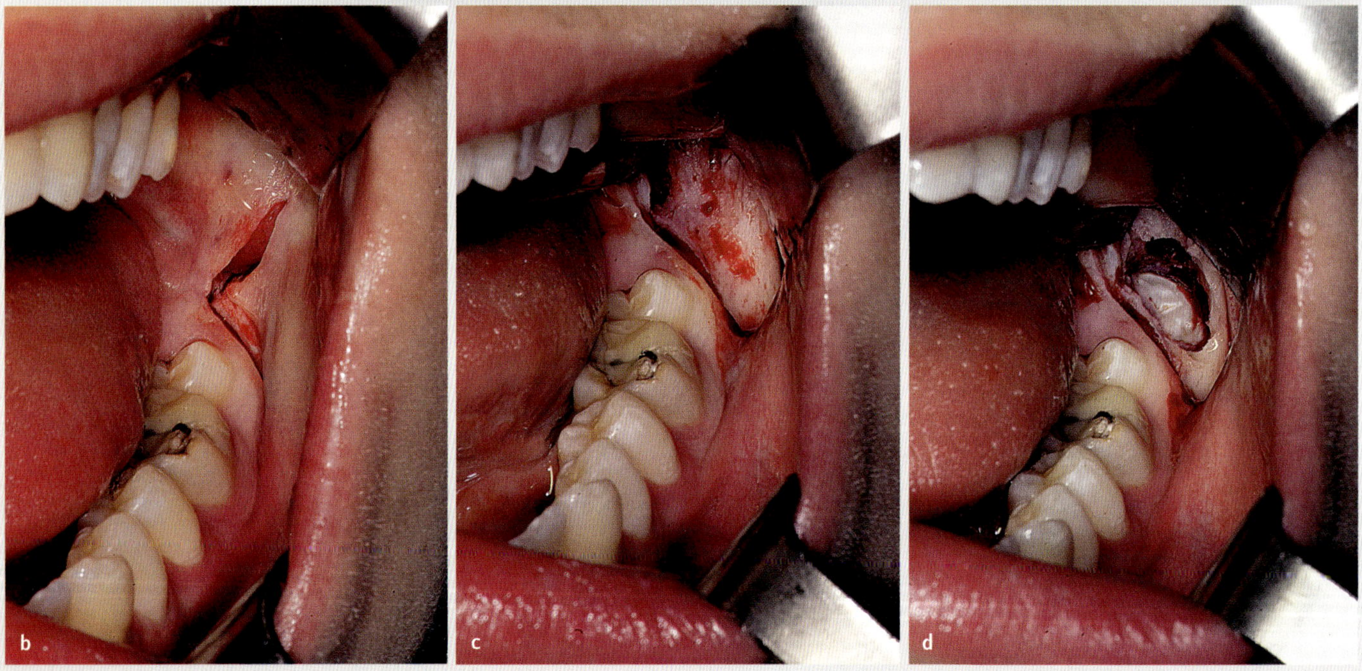

Odontotomy

To minimise the quantity of removed bone, the germ is extracted after being separated into two or more pieces. This operation may present some difficulties, as the germ is surrounded by its follicle and tends to rotate upon itself inside the surrounding bone cavity. To facilitate odontotomy, the germ can be immobilised with the tip of a root elevator or with a curette (5.35e).

Extraction

Extraction follows the principles previously described for other impacted teeth (5.35f).

Cavity inspection and suture

It follows the same principles described above. However, special care must be taken to remove the follicular sac in its entirety and to avoid the risk of formation of a residual cyst (5.35g–h). Suture of the access flap follows the principles previously described (5.35i).

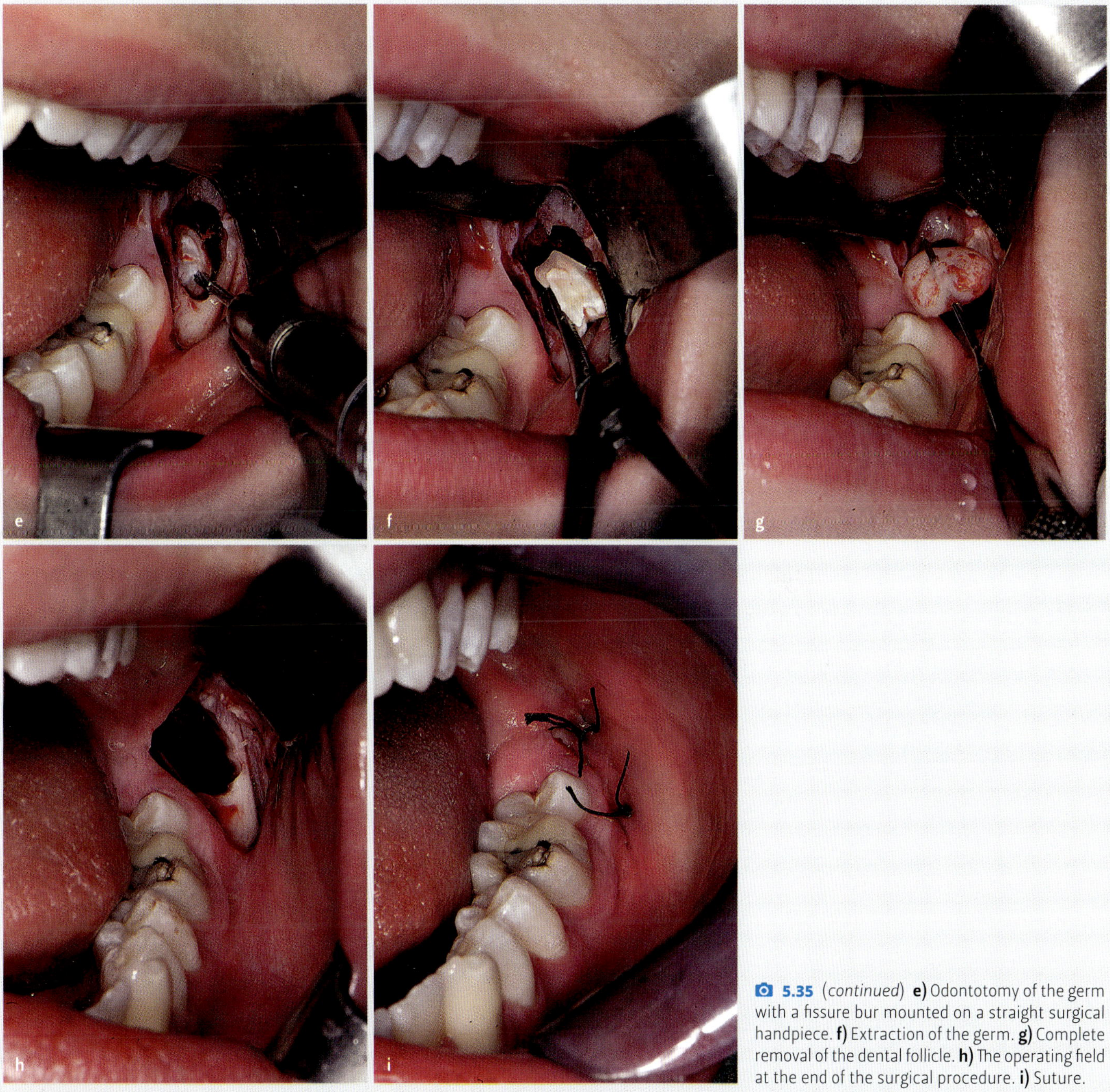

5.35 (*continued*) **e)** Odontotomy of the germ with a fissure bur mounted on a straight surgical handpiece. **f)** Extraction of the germ. **g)** Complete removal of the dental follicle. **h)** The operating field at the end of the surgical procedure. **i)** Suture.

Maxillary third molars

PREOPERATIVE EVALUATION AND CLASSIFICATION

Specific factors to assess the level of difficulty of an extraction also exist for impacted maxillary third molars.

Classification of impacted maxillary third molars

Classification according to angulation is also valid for maxillary molars, but some differences do exist. Vertical and disto-angular impacted maxillary third molars are observed more frequently. Unlike mandibular third molars, the extraction of mesio-angular impacted maxillary third molars, as well as horizontal and inverted ones, is frequently more difficult. As far as the inclination on the buccal/palatal direction is concerned, the majority of maxillary third molars present a buccal inclination and their extraction is generally easier. Palatal inclination (quite rare) reduces accessibility and may render extraction more difficult, as it frequently entails the creation of a palatal access. Class A-B-C, which defines the depth of the inclusion and therefore the accessibility (5.36), are also applicable to maxillary third molars.

Radiographic evaluation

A panoramic radiograph, associated with palpation of the maxillary tuberosity, may be sufficient for identifying the inclination of a superficially impacted third molar in the buccal/palatal direction. In cases of deep impaction, the recourse to a CT scan may be indicated. Radiographic images help evaluate not only the parameters required to plan the extraction of every impacted tooth (anatomy and length of the roots, width of the periodontal space, etc.), but also the relationships of the impacted tooth with the maxillary sinus and the maxillary tuberosity (for details on the surgical implications, see further) (5.37).

a

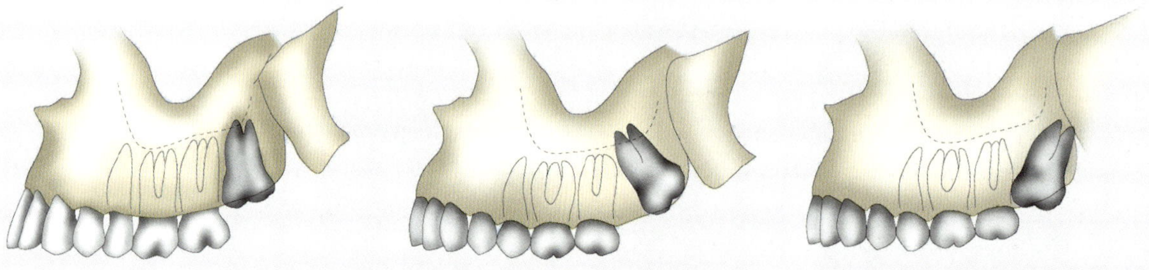

b

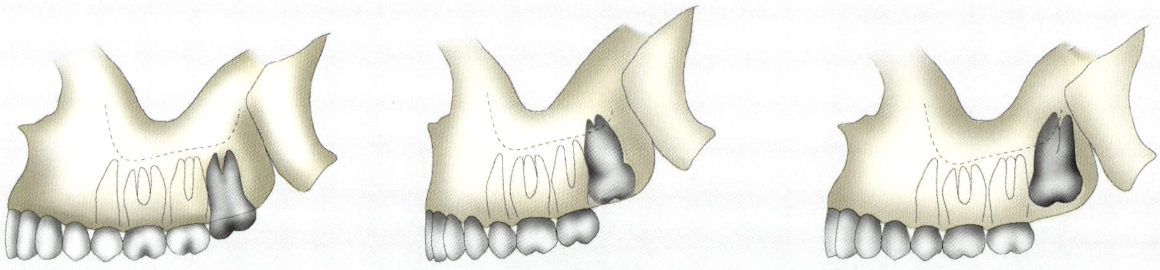

5.36 a) Classification of the impacted maxillary third molars based on their inclination relative to the axis of the second molar: from left to right in ascending order of complexity: vertical, disto-angular, and mesio-angular third molar. **b)** classification of the depth of impaction based on the relationship between the occlusal plane of the second and third molar: from left to right in ascending order of complexity: class A, B, and C.

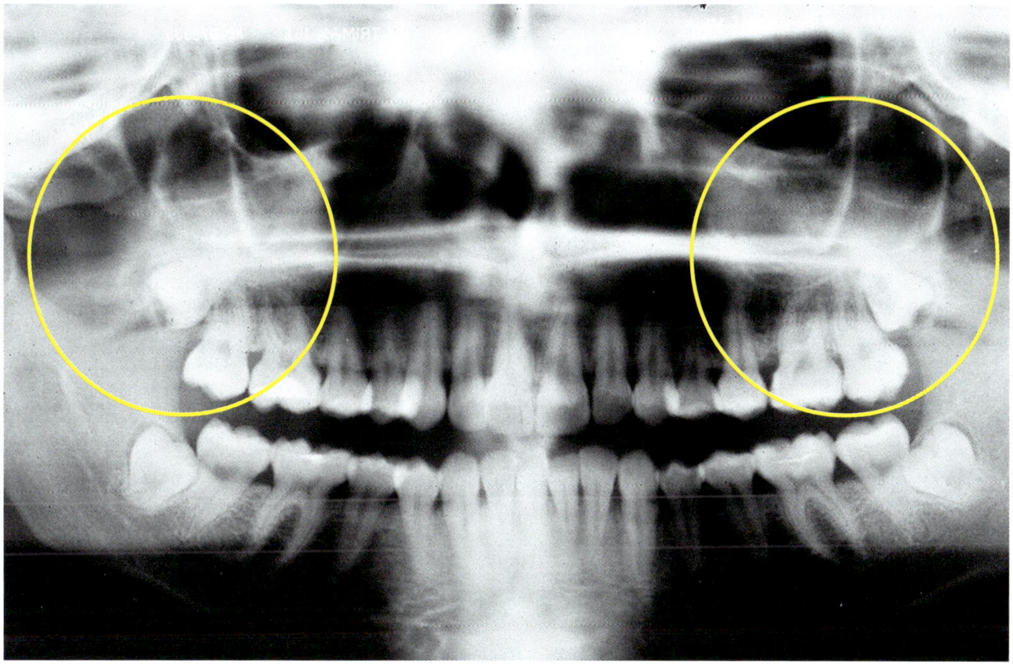

5.37 Disto-angular impacted 1.8 and 2.8: the roots of the impacted teeth visibly protrude inside the lumen of the maxillary sinus.

Extraction of impacted maxillary third molars is generally less demanding than that of their mandibular counterpart: maxillary third molars, in fact, frequently present a single root (or a buccal and a palatal root mimicking a single root on periapical and panoramic radiographs), while the presence of multiple roots is a rare occurrence. Buccal inclination, which is common for maxillary third molars, causes the presence of a thin buccal cortical plate that requires only minimal ostectomy to expose the crown of the impacted tooth. Finally, impacted maxillary third molars are surrounded by a more elastic, less dense bone, which is more easily deformed during luxation. However, in some cases the extraction of impacted maxillary third molars may prove more complex than the extraction of their mandibular counterpart, due to the limited accessibility and visibility of the operating field. In fact, it is essential that the patient keep the mouth half-closed during surgery, as a wider mouth aperture causes an advancement of the coronoid process of the mandible, thus limiting the access to the operating field. When necessary, odontotomy may be difficult to perform, due to the limited dimensions of the operating field and the reduced angles for the introduction and management of the necessary surgical instruments. Favourable and complicating factors are similar to those described for the extraction of impacted mandibular third molars (see dedicated section for details).

Surgical anatomy: notable anatomic structures

Maxillary sinus

Maxillary third molars may be in close proximity to the maxillary sinuses, particularly in adult patients, due to the progressive expansion of these paranasal cavities towards the alveolar ridge (5.37).

Surgical implications. When a thin bony septum separating the socket of the impacted third molar from the maxillary sinus is present, luxation must be performed with controlled movements, avoiding the exertion of apically directed force to minimise the risk of dislocating the tooth inside the maxillary sinus. The possible formation of an oroantral communication should be anticipated, to allow modification in the design of the access flap for its closure (see Chapter 14 for details).

Maxillary tuberosity

Surgical implications. The fracture of maxillary tuberosity is a relatively frequent complication, particularly when the impacted third molar has multiple divergent roots, when the bone is dense and stiff, or the tooth is ankylosed (see Chapter 14).

Pterygopalatine fossa

Surgical implications. The distal releasing incision should never extend beyond the confines of the maxillary tuberosity to avoid causing damage to the pterygoid plexus, which may otherwise cause significant bleeding. During luxation manoeuvres, the exertion of excessive distally directed force must be avoided as this may cause dislocation of the impacted third molar inside the pterygopalatine fossa.

Buccal fat pad (Bichat's fat pad)

Surgical implications. Periosteal releasing incisions or accidental perforation of the periosteum may cause herniation of the buccal fat pad. This event is not a serious complication per se, nor is it followed by relevant sequelae. However, it may cause further reduction in already limited visibility of the small operating field. In other cases, deliberate exposure of the buccal fat pad may be useful for the closure of an oroantral communication caused during extraction of the impacted tooth (see Chapter 14 for details).

Surgical protocol for the extraction of maxillary third molars

The different phases of extraction are very similar to those described above for mandibular third molars; therefore, only particular aspects exclusive to maxillary third molars are described.

Specific armamentarium

Besides the basic armamentarium used to perform all complex extractions, some specific instruments are particularly useful:

- straight root elevator with a fine tip;
- angled root elevators (Pott);
- angled apical pick elevators.

Locoregional anaesthesia

Anaesthesia of the superior-posterior alveolar nerves is obtained by submucosal infiltration of the anaesthetic in the vestibular fornix, while major palatine nerve block is obtained by injecting the anaesthetic directly into the major palatine foramen.

Basic techniques

Access flaps

The flaps are very similar to those described for the extraction of impacted mandibular third molars, implying a buccal approach (5.38a,e,f). Only in cases of markedly palatal position of the impacted tooth can a palatal approach be indicated.

Envelope flap

This flap entails a single sulcular incision involving the second molar (and the first molar, if necessary) and a distal releasing incision starting from the distal surface of the second molar and directed distally and buccally across the maxillary tuberosity (5.38a-b).

Four-corner flap

The addition of a mesial releasing incision starting from the mesio-buccal corner of the second molar (or first molar, if necessary) and directed apically towards the vestibular fornix helps create a wider access, and is therefore indicated in cases of deep impaction (5.38c).

Three-corner flap

This is formed by a distal releasing incision similar to that described above in association with a mesial releasing incision starting distally to the second molar. It prevents interference with the periodontal tissues of the adjacent teeth, but offers more limited access to the operating field (5.38d).

Palatal access flap

If the impacted third molar is in a palatal position, a buccal approach may prove insufficient, thus necessitating the recourse to a palatal approach. The incision is performed inside the palatal gingival sulcus of the first and second molars, while the distal releasing incision runs across the maxillary tuberosity starting from the middle of the distal aspect of the second molar. Elevation of this flap requires great caution, and it is imperative that it be performed full-thickness to avoid any damage to the major palatine artery and nerve.

Access ostectomy and exposure of the impacted tooth

Generally, the superficial position of the impacted maxillary third molars and the reduced thickness require that a modest quantity of bone be removed to expose the crown of the tooth. Frequently, removal of the thin buccal cortical layer can be performed with a surgical curette, thus avoiding the use of rotary instruments. Ostectomy should involve the buccal surface of the impacted tooth, to allow insertion of the tip of the root elevator between the second and third molars. When a more extensive ostectomy is necessary, a round bur mounted on a straight handpiece is recommended, but extreme care must be taken to avoid flap laceration and herniation of the buccal fat pad.

Odontotomy

Separation of impacted maxillary third molars is quite difficult to perform, but it is very rarely needed to complete their extraction. Only in cases of mesio-angular or disto-angular teeth, or in cases of extremely divergent roots, may separation of the crown from the roots be indicated, particularly if the crown of the third molar is stuck in the distal concavity of the second molar.

Luxation of the impacted tooth (or its parts)

Luxation is performed with the same modalities described for mandibular third molars, typically exerting force directed apically and buccally, while being careful not to fracture the maxillary tuberosity or dislocate the impacted tooth in the maxillary sinus or pterygopalatine fossa. Luxation is typically performed with straight or angled root elevators. Once the tooth is completely luxated towards the buccal vestibule, it can be easily grabbed with haemostatic forceps or extraction forceps. During the latter phase, the patient is asked to occlude to avoid accidental swallowing of the extracted tooth (5.38g-h).

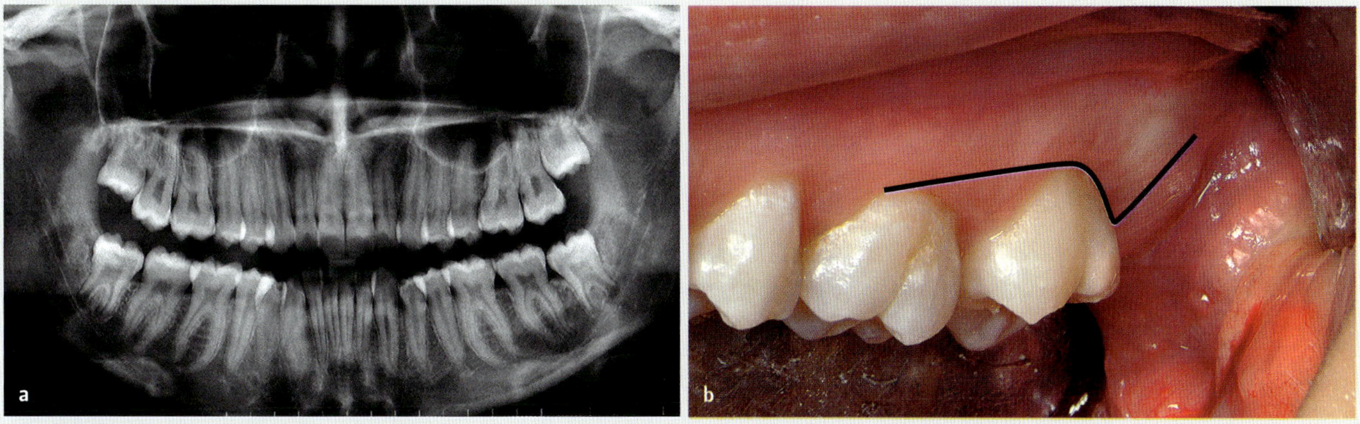

5.38 **a)** Panoramic radiograph showing impaction of the maxillary third molars. **b)** Design of an envelope flap for the extraction of maxillary third molars. (*continued*)

Cavity inspection and suture

Besides the common inspection manoeuvres, it is important to verify the possible presence of oroantral communications by gently probing the bottom of the extraction socket. Small oroantral communications have a high probability of healing spontaneously. Conversely, in cases of ample oroantral communications, proceeding immediately to their surgical closure with local flaps is indicated (see Chapter 14 for details).

The suture of the access flaps does not present relevant peculiarities (5.38i).

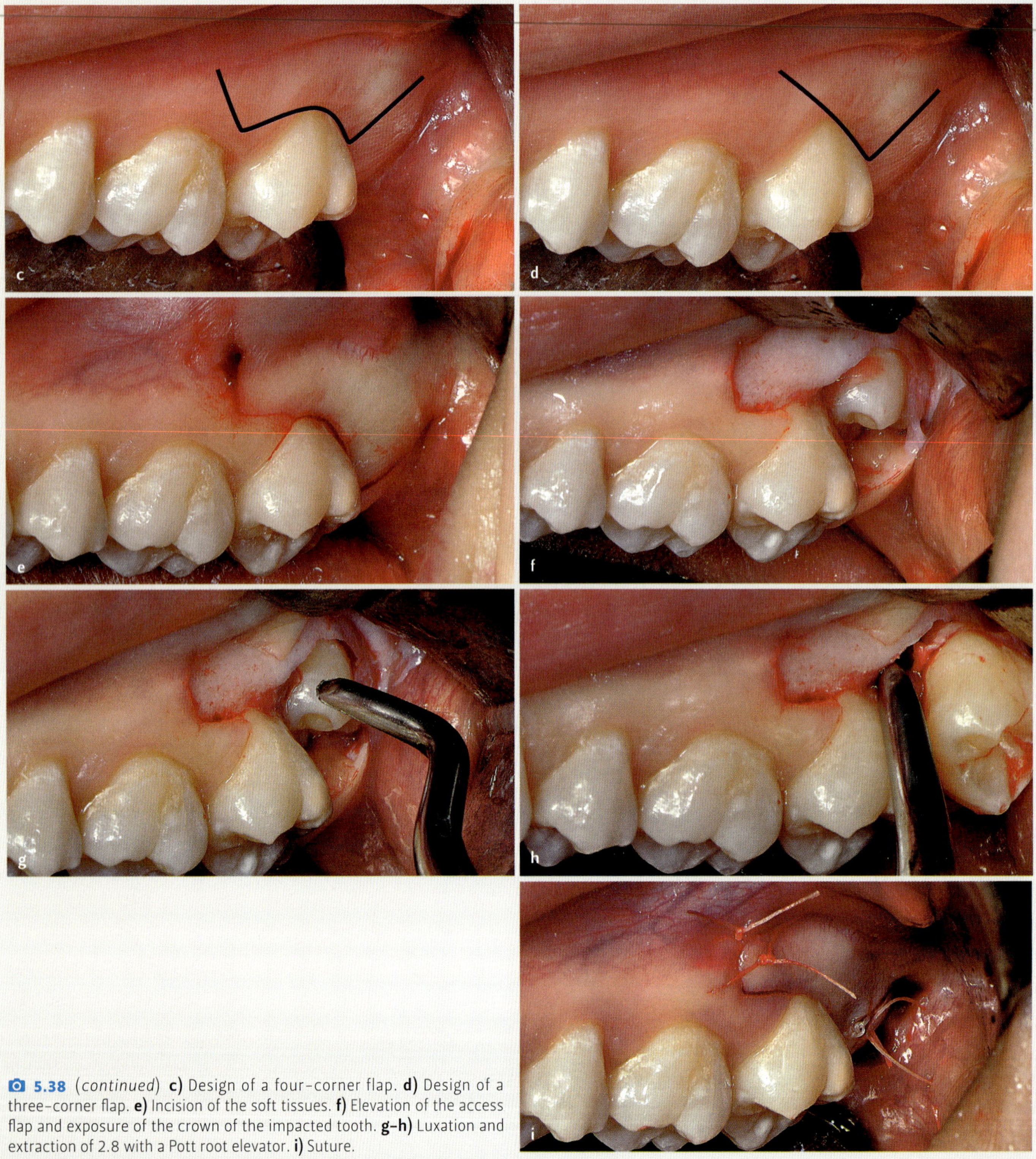

5.38 (*continued*) **c)** Design of a four-corner flap. **d)** Design of a three-corner flap. **e)** Incision of the soft tissues. **f)** Elevation of the access flap and exposure of the crown of the impacted tooth. **g–h)** Luxation and extraction of 2.8 with a Pott root elevator. **i)** Suture.

Germectomy of the maxillary third molars

The indications for the germectomy of maxillary third molars are the same as those described for the germectomy of mandibular third molars. Likewise, access to the germ field can be obtained either with a marginal three- or four-corner flap, or with a submarginal flap. A palatal approach is indicated only in cases of palatally impacted germs. Exposure of the germ and its extraction do not present relevant peculiarities. In fact, the germs of maxillary third molars are generally extracted intact, due to the greater elasticity of bone surrounding the follicle (5.39a–e).

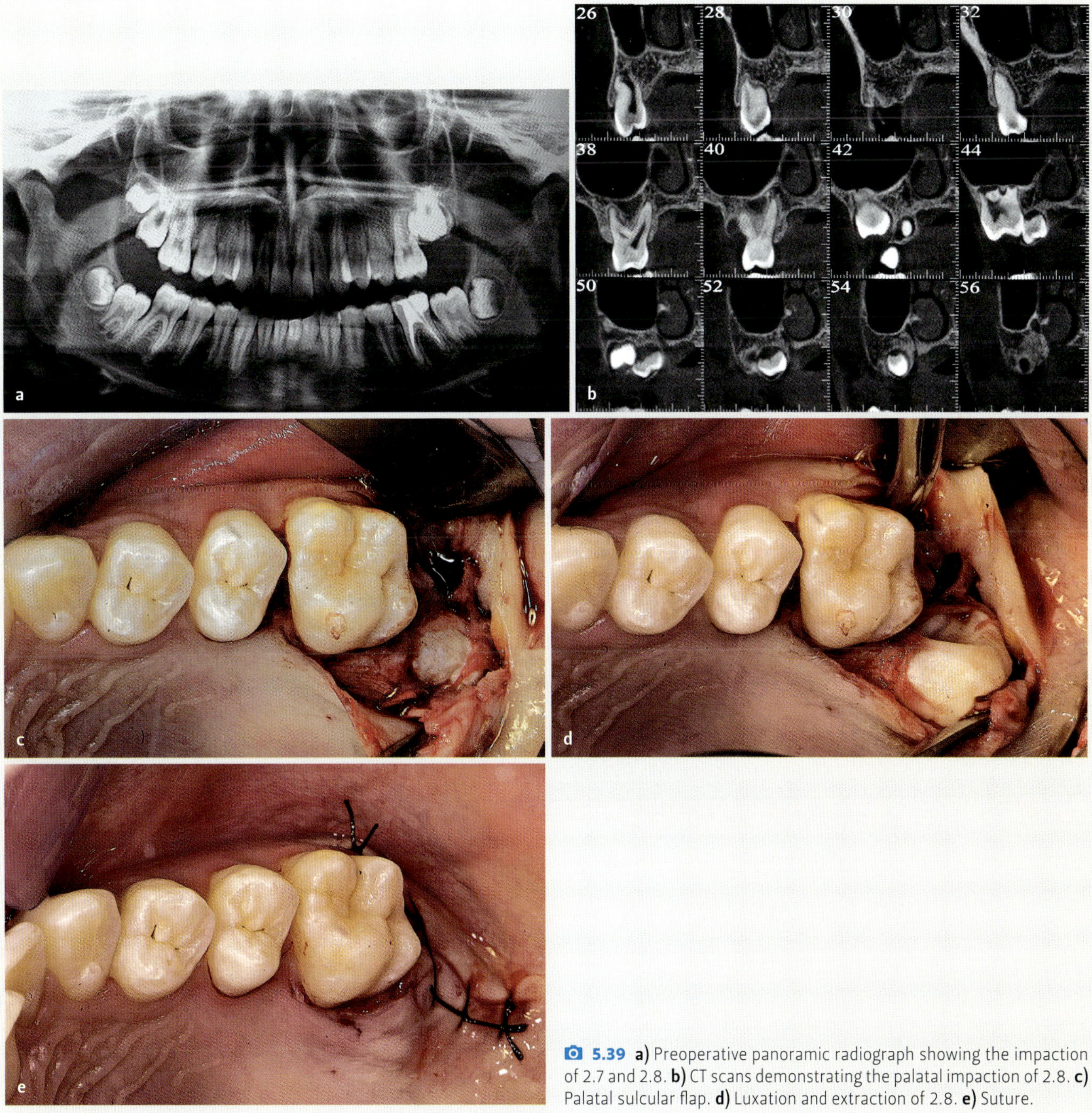

5.39 **a)** Preoperative panoramic radiograph showing the impaction of 2.7 and 2.8. **b)** CT scans demonstrating the palatal impaction of 2.8. **c)** Palatal sulcular flap. **d)** Luxation and extraction of 2.8. **e)** Suture.

Impacted maxillary canines

PREOPERATIVE EVALUATION

There are two main objectives:

- to exclude the possibility of surgical exposure and orthodontic alignment, which always represents the first therapeutic option due to the functional importance of the canines;
- to identify with precision, by means of clinical examination and radiographic exams, the position of the impacted canine and its relationships to adjacent teeth. In this way, it is possible to plan the most suitable surgical access and minimise the risk of damaging neighbouring anatomic structures.

Surgical anatomy: notable anatomic structures

Palatine artery

Surgical implications. When a palatal approach is chosen, full-thickness elevation of the access flap is mandatory to avoid damage to the major palatine neurovascular bundle; for the same reason no releasing incisions can be performed.

Nasopalatine neurovascular bundle

Surgical implications. Interruption of the nasopalatine neurovascular bundle does not generally cause relevant sequelae, as the anterior portion of the palate is also innervated by the terminal branches of the major palatine nerve. Bleeding caused by the accidental rupture of the artery can be controlled by means of bipolar coagulation or with ligature of the artery itself.

Nasal fossae

Surgical implications. In some cases, an impacted maxillary canine can be in an apical position, in direct contact with the lateral wall of the ipsilateral nasal fossa. In these cases, it is recommended that the nasal mucosa be gently detached and protected with malleable spatulas or retractors, particularly when rotary instruments are in use.

Infraorbital nerve

Surgical implications. If a buccal approach is chosen, and the impacted canine is in an apical position, it is imperative that the elevation and retraction of the access flap be performed with great care to avoid any damage to the infraorbital nerve.

Surgical protocol for the extraction of impacted maxillary canines

Locoregional anaesthesia

The area of the canines, particularly in cases of deep impaction, receives its innervation from different nerve branches arising from the infraorbital nerve, the major palatine nerve, and the nasopalatine nerve. Moreover, when the canine is located in close proximity to the median line it can receive additional innervation from nerve branches coming from the opposite side.

Generally, where a buccal approach is chosen, it is sufficient to perform a submucosal injection in the buccal vestibule, but where a palatal approach is chosen, block anaesthesia of the nasopalatine nerve is necessary. In cases of deep impaction, the recourse to infraorbital nerve block via an intraoral or percutaneous approach is indicated.

ACCESS FLAPS

Marginal palatal flap (5.40a): a single palatal incision extends from the area of the contralateral incisors/canines to the area of the ipsilateral premolars/molars, according to the position of the impacted canine. In cases of bilateral impaction, the incision extends to the area of the premolars/molars on both sides of the maxilla. The palatal soft tissues are strongly adherent to the underlying bone; therefore, the elevation of this flap requires the application of a certain force. However, as previously emphasised, the elevation must be strictly subperiosteal to minimise the risk of damage to the branches of the palatine artery. The neurovascular bundle can be cut, if necessary, after it is cauterised by means of bipolar coagulation or ligated with a resorbable suture. Atraumatic retraction of the palatal flap can be obtained with the aid of a suture anchor around the crown of the premolars.

Submarginal palatal flap (5.40b): the incision is similar to that described above for the marginal palatal flap, but it runs 2-3 millimetres below the free gingival margin. Some authors advocate the use of this flap based on the assumption that preserving the integrity of the papillae and periodontal soft tissues surrounding the erupted teeth improves wound healing and facilitates a complete *restitutio ad integrum*. Actually, the elevation and suture of this flap are more difficult, and may cause even greater trauma to the soft tissues. Moreover, the recourse to this flap is contraindicated in the case of close proximity of the impacted canine to the palatal surfaces of the adjacent teeth.

Buccal access flaps (5.40c): the size of the flap depends on the tooth position. The choice between marginal and submarginal flap is also determined by the corono-apical position of the tooth. The presence of prosthetic restorations represents another critical factor in the choice between marginal and submarginal flaps: as a rule, when proper restorations are present, the submarginal flap involves a lower risk of exposure of the prosthetic margin. One or two releasing incisions are generally associated to the marginal or submarginal incision.

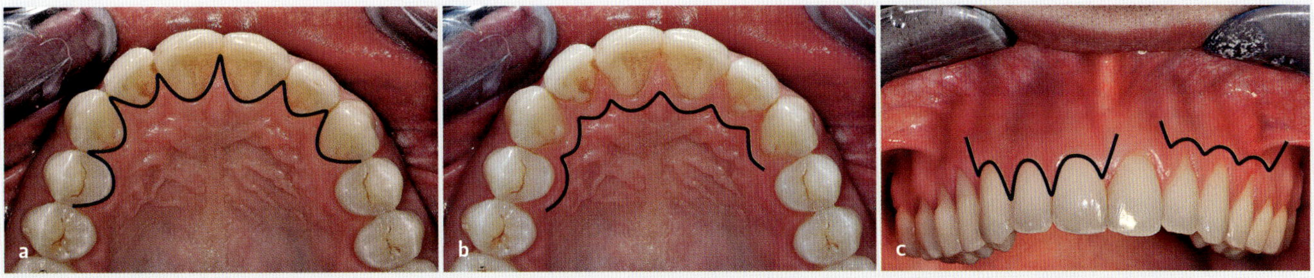

5.40 a) Design of a marginal palatal flap. **b)** Design of a submarginal palatal flap. **c)** Design of marginal (first quadrant) and submarginal (second quadrant) buccal flaps.

Clinical case 4 – Extraction of buccally impacted 1.3

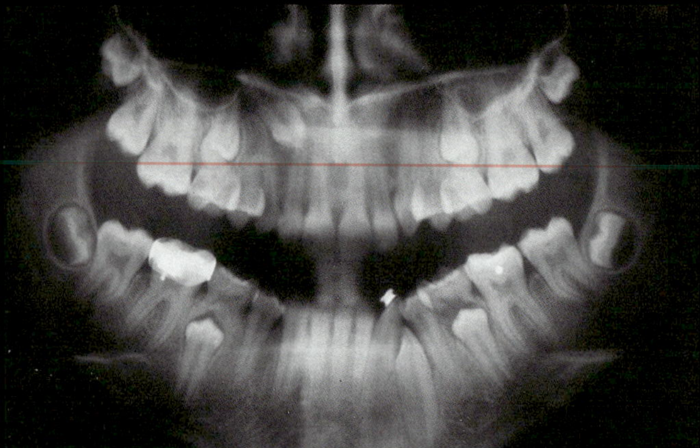

5.41a Extraction of buccally impacted 1.3: the panoramic radiograph is not sufficient to define accurately the exact position of the impacted tooth and its relationships with neighbouring anatomic structures.

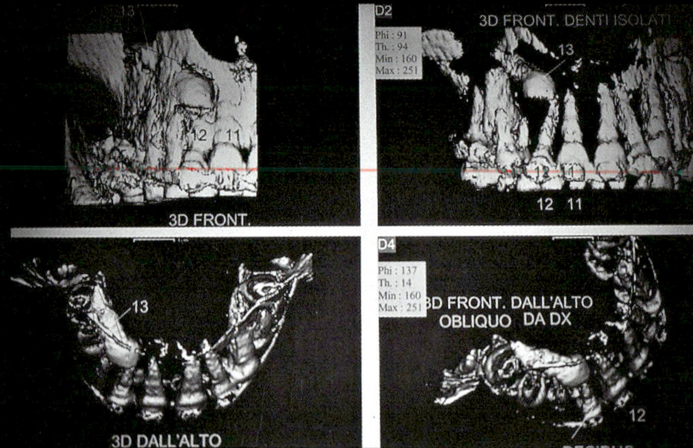

5.41b Tridimensional reconstruction obtained from the axial images of the CT scan showing the exact position of the impacted tooth.

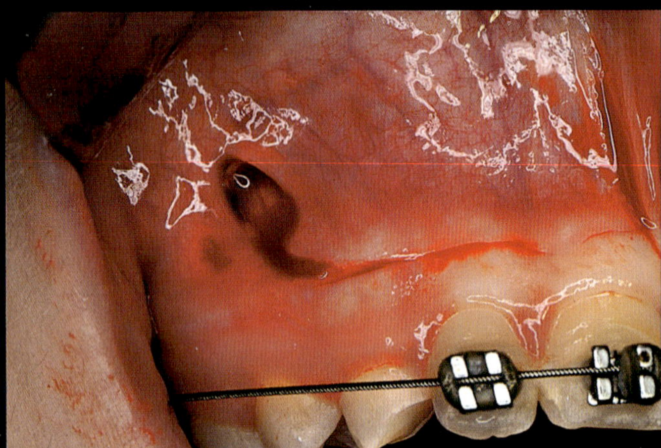

5.41c Submarginal four-corner access flap.

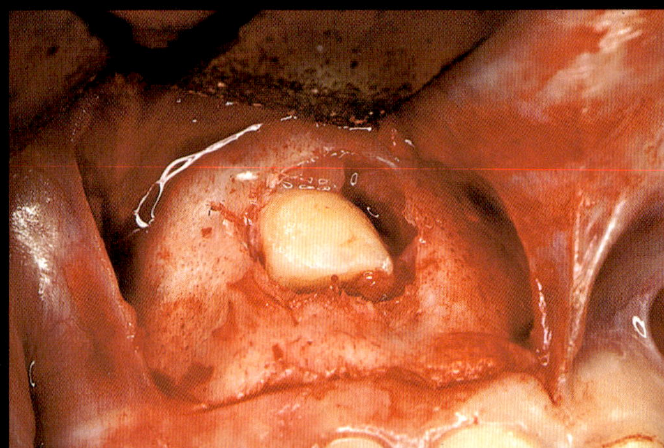

5.41d Exposure of the crown by means of ostectomy.

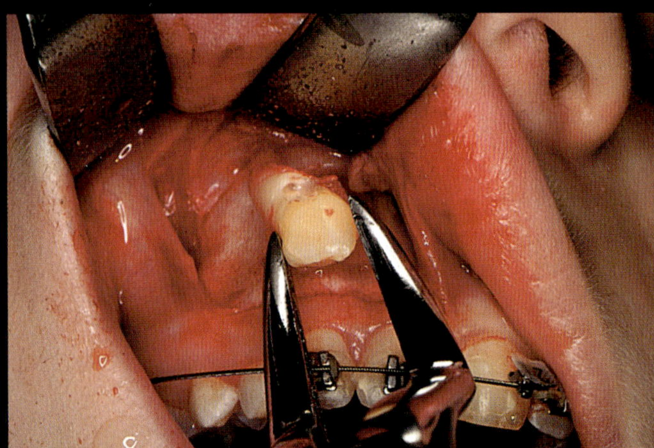

5.41e Extraction of the impacted tooth.

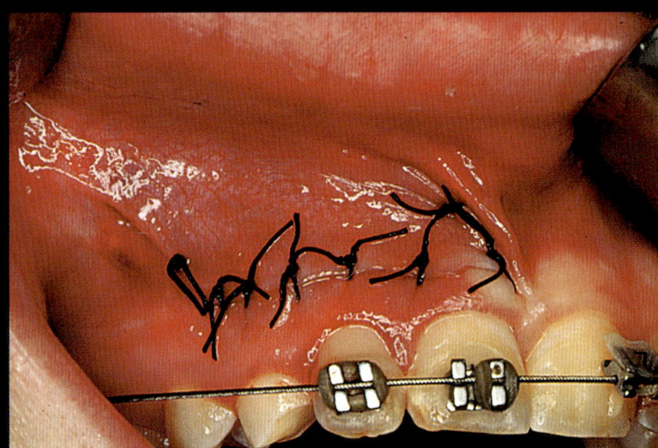

5.41f Suture.

OSTECTOMY, ODONTOTOMY, LUXATION, AND EXTRACTION

Once the flap is elevated, the position of the impacted canine is frequently revealed by the presence of a visible convexity on the cortical bone. However, a precise radiographic assessment is necessary both with superficial and deep impaction. Ostectomy is performed according to the principles described in previous sections.

After adequate exposure of the crown is obtained, it is recommended that a preliminary luxation of the tooth be performed, which, in some cases, may be sufficient to complete the extraction, particularly when the canine is relatively small. If preliminary luxation does not allow adequate mobilisation of the tooth, instead of extending ostectomy it is preferable to separate the crown from the root with a fissure bur. If the crown of the impacted canine is very large, its separation into two parts along the main axis may be necessary. Removal of the crown creates space for the luxation and extraction of the root, thus eliminating the need for excessive bone removal.

CAVITY INSPECTION AND SUTURE

These follow the principles described in previous sections.

Impacted mandibular canines

Surgical anatomy: notable anatomic structures

Mental foramen

Surgical implications. When the crown of the impacted canine is in close proximity to the mental foramen, elevation of a buccal flap should be performed with caution due to the presence of the emergence of the mental nerve. In these cases, it is preferable to identify and protect the nerve.

Lingual soft tissues

Surgical implications. When a lingual approach is necessary (a rare circumstance), elevation of the access flap should be performed with gentle manoeuvres due to the thinness of the lingual mucosa, and the presence of muscle insertions, neurovascular structures and salivary glands in the floor of the mouth (lingual nerve, sublingual veins and arteries, and submandibular duct).

Incisive nerve

Surgical implications. Extraction of an impacted mandibular canine may cause the interruption of the incisive nerve and the subsequent paraesthesia/anaesthesia of the ipsilateral mandibular incisors. While this may not be considered a severe sequela, it can be nevertheless annoying for the patient. Therefore, the possible occurrence of this complication must always be discussed preoperatively with every patient.

Surgical protocol for the extraction of impacted mandibular canines

LOCOREGIONAL ANAESTHESIA

In cases of superficial impaction, field block may be sufficient to allow adequate anaesthesia of the tissue involved in the surgical intervention; conversely, in cases of deep impaction the recourse to inferior alveolar nerve block is necessary. Lingual nerve block is indicated in cases of lingual approach to the impacted tooth.

ACCESS FLAPS

Buccal marginal flap: typically extending from the first molar to the incisors, and with a mesial releasing incision. If the deciduous canine is missing, the incision of soft tissues in the edentulous space is performed on top of the alveolar ridge.

Buccal submarginal flap: the use of this access flap is indicated in cases of deep impaction.

Lingual flap: in the rare circumstance of lingual impaction, a marginal or submarginal incision running from the molars to the incisors is made to create an envelope flap. Releasing incisions are contraindicated, due to the concave surface of the lingual side of the mandible and the presence of important anatomic structures in the floor of the mouth.

OSTECTOMY, ODONTOTOMY, LUXATION, AND EXTRACTION

These follow the principles described in previous sections.

Other impacted teeth

The incidence of impaction of the first and second molars, premolars, and incisors is significantly lower than that of third molars and even canines and the techniques used to extract them are very similar to those previously described for the latter.

However, as mentioned earlier, it is worth remembering that surgical exposure and orthodontic alignment must always be considered the treatment of choice in cases of impaction of functionally important teeth, and that extraction should only be considered when recovery of the impacted tooth is impossible or presents an unfavourable cost-benefit ratio.

Impacted incisors

Extraction of impacted maxillary and mandibular incisors requires a surgical approach identical to that described for the extraction of impacted canines. The considerations regarding local anatomy, which influences possible intraoperative and postoperative complications, are also identical.

Impacted premolars

SURGICAL ANATOMY: IMPORTANT ANATOMIC STRUCTURES

The anatomic structures that can usually be involved in extraction of impacted premolars are the same as those described for impacted canines. Nonetheless, it is worth pointing out the close relationship that usually exists between impacted mandibular premolars and the mental nerve. The recommendations reported in the paragraph dedicated to elevation of buccal flaps in the area and relative to the importance of identifying the mental nerve and protecting it are even more important in this case. The same considerations apply to the extraction of lingually impacted mandibular premolars: full-thickness elevation of the access flap significantly contributes to prevent accidental damage to the neurovascular anatomic structures in the floor of the mouth.

Impacted maxillary premolars, and particularly the second premolar, generally exhibit a close relationship with the maxillary sinus and must always be assessed preoperatively. Atraumatic surgical manoeuvres are thus essential for avoiding dislocation of the impacted tooth inside the sinus lumen and the creation of an oroantral communication. When a buccal flap is chosen to gain access to the impacted tooth, releasing incisions should never extend beyond the bottom of the vestibular fornix, and elevation of the soft tissues should always be conducted subperiosteally to avoid the risk of herniation of the mesial pole of the buccal fat pad.

SURGICAL PROTOCOL FOR THE EXTRACTION OF IMPACTED PREMOLARS

Access flaps, ostectomy, odontotomy, luxation, and extraction: these follow the principles described in previous sections concerning the extraction of other impacted teeth (limited ostectomy, multiple odontotomy to simplify luxation and extraction, controlled luxation, etc.). The only additional precautions that are important to take when extracting impacted mandibular premolars are:

- avoiding buccal releasing incisions in the area to prevent any damage to the mental nerve at the mental foramen;
- as previously mentioned, identifying and protecting the mental nerve during surgery.

A step-by-step clinical case is presented in 🔍 5.42a-e.

Impacted first and second mandibular molars

From a surgical point of view, extraction of these teeth has many aspects in common with the extraction of impacted third molars; however, it may sometimes prove more difficult due to some characteristics that are peculiar to the impaction of first and second molars.

Depth of impaction: impacted mandibular first and second molars are frequently located in a very deep position (particularly in cases of late diagnosis), which may require a more invasive approach, implying a higher incidence of complications such as damage to the inferior alveolar nerve.

Clinical case 5 – Extraction of lingually impacted 4.5

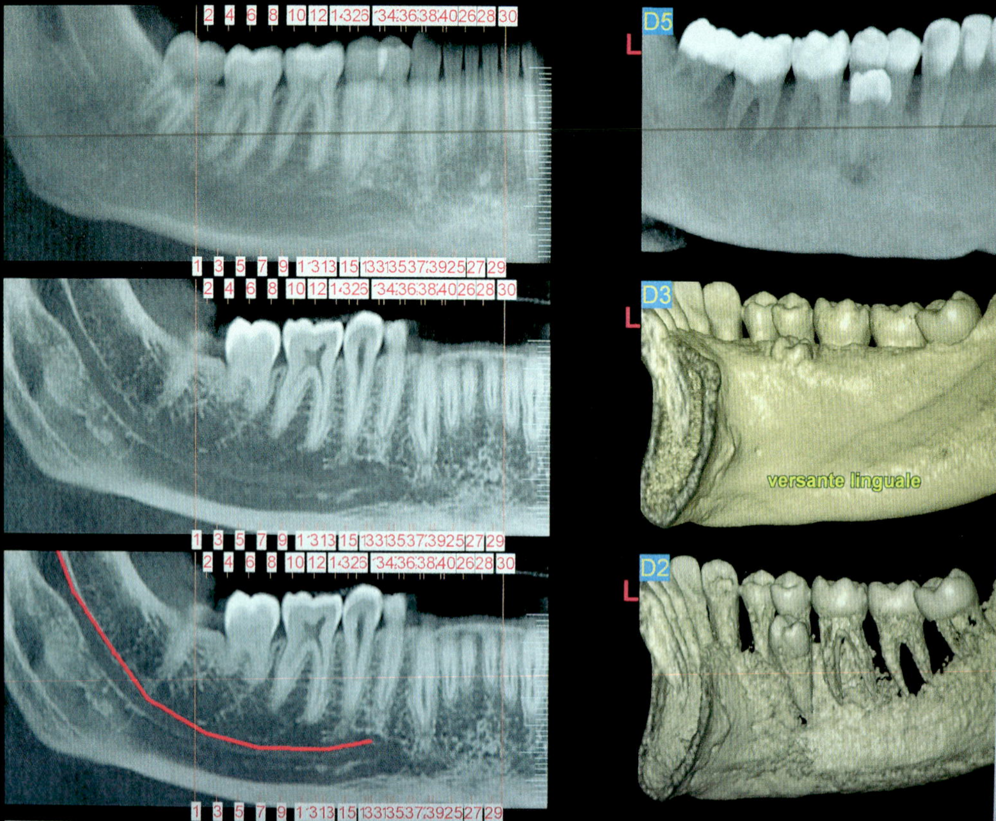

5.42a CT scans (panorex and tridimensional reconstruction) of the mandible showing a lingually impacted supernumerary tooth.

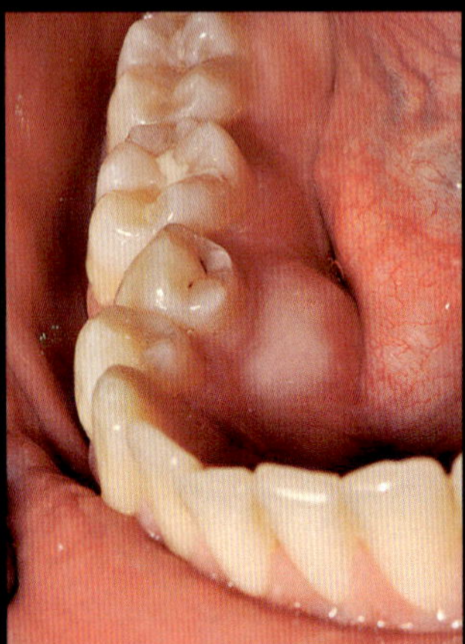

5.42b Preoperative clinical situation.

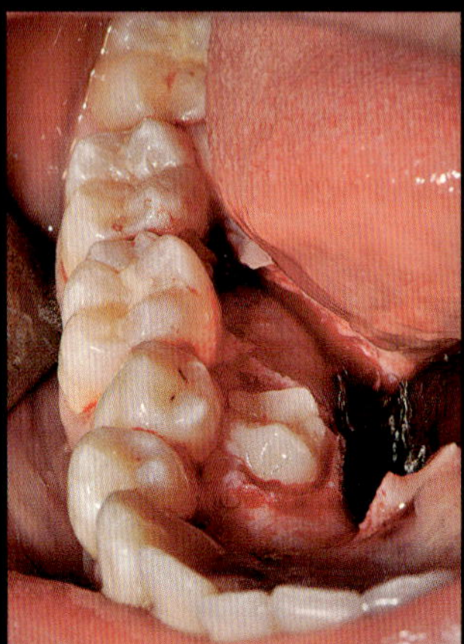

5.42c Elevation of a mucoperiosteal flap, protection of the lingual soft tissues, and identification of

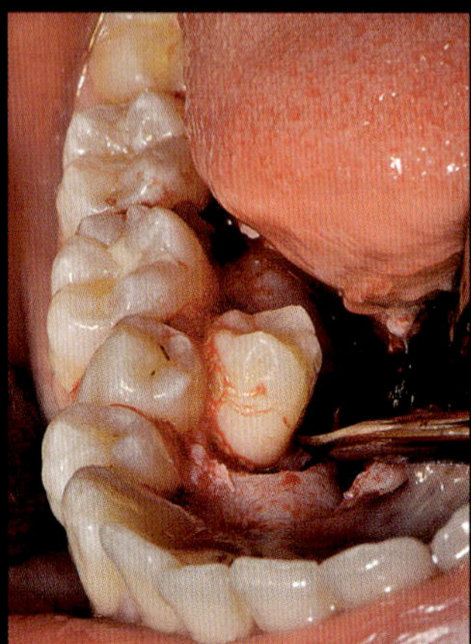

5.42d Luxation and extraction of the impacted supernumerary tooth.

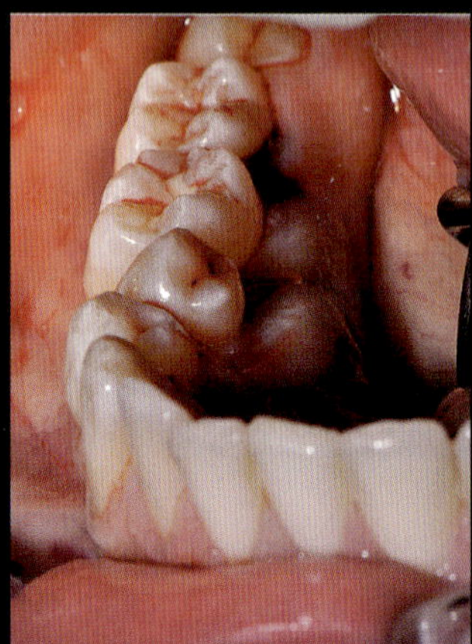

5.42e Suture.

Tooth ankylosis: ankylosis complicates the extraction, as the tooth has no mobility and its removal is possible only after the point of ankylosis is fractured. Ankylosis can be both the cause and the consequence of impaction, but it does not influence the development of the roots, which continues in an apical direction. Occasionally, when the roots are completely formed, the apexes may be in close proximity to the mandibular canal or the inferior border of the mandible.

Migration of other teeth above the impacted tooth: in the absence of an early diagnosis, the space destined to accommodate the impacted tooth is partially occupied by adjacent teeth. In these cases, the space available for performing the necessary surgical manoeuvres is very small; therefore, multiple odontotomy is generally required to complete removal of the impacted tooth.

Relationships with the mandibular canal: impacted mandibular first and second molars generally exhibit a close relationship with the mandibular canal. Therefore, extraction can be performed only if a thorough preoperative investigation allows clarification of the spatial relationships between the mandibular canal and the roots of the impacted tooth: these can be typically evaluated in great detail on CT scans. However, in these cases, the risk of direct or indirect damage to the inferior alveolar nerve cannot be completely ruled out. Hence, the patient must be adequately informed and every precaution must be taken to avoid this contingency.

SURGICAL PROTOCOL FOR THE EXTRACTION OF IMPACTED MANDIBULAR FIRST AND SECOND MOLARS

With the exception of the aforementioned peculiarities, the surgical anatomy, anaesthetic techniques, and phases of the surgical intervention are similar to those used for the extraction of third molars (see the dedicated section for details). The possible complications and their management are also similar. A last peculiar aspect of the extraction of impacted mandibular first and second molars, however, is the necessity of wide surgical access to compensate for the significant depth of impaction that is typical of these teeth. Four-corner access flaps are generally used and care must be taken to avoid any releasing incision to fall in the area of the premolars to prevent damage to the mental nerve (📷 5.43a-g).

Impacted first and second maxillary molars

The peculiarity of these impacted teeth is their relationship of contiguity or continuity with the maxillary sinus. Therefore, the closure of a possible oroantral communication caused by the removal of the impacted tooth must be planned preoperatively. Details on the surgical techniques for the closure of oroantral communications are reported in Chapter 14.

Multiple impactions

Multiple impactions may render the treatment significantly more complex due to the relevant functional and aesthetic implications, particularly when they involve the majority of teeth. In these cases, a thorough preoperative assessment should be conducted with the

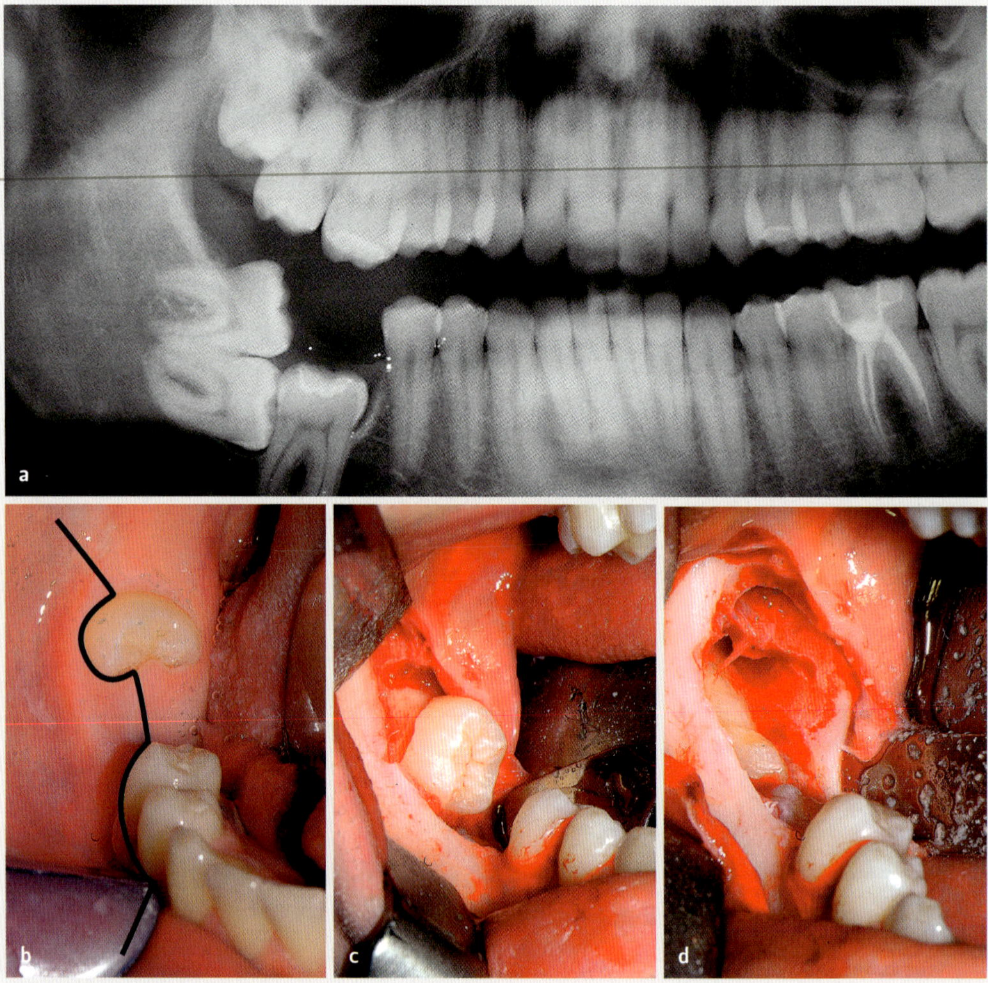

5.43 **a)** Preoperative panoramic radiograph showing malposition and impaction of 4.6, 4.7, and 4.8. **b)** Preoperative clinical situation and design of the access flap. **c)** After elevation of the access flap and identification of the impacted teeth are performed, separation of the crown of 4.8 is performed. **d)** Once the extraction of 4.8 is completed, deeply impacted 4.7 is more clearly visible and is subsequently extracted. (*continued*)

aim of evaluating the possibility of recovering the functionally important impacted teeth by means of surgical exposure and orthodontic alignment. If this is not possible, extraction of the impacted teeth may be inevitable: missing teeth can subsequently be replaced with oral implants and implant-supported rehabilitations.

A detailed description of the etiology and syndromes associated with multiple impactions (such as cleidocranial dysplasia, anhydrotic ectodermal dysplasia, etc.) is beyond the scope of this manual.

Supernumerary teeth

ETIOLOGY

The exact etiology of supernumerary teeth is still unknown, even if several studies suggest an association with the hyperactivity of the embryonic epithelial cells of the dental lamina, or with an accidental separation of the dental follicle.

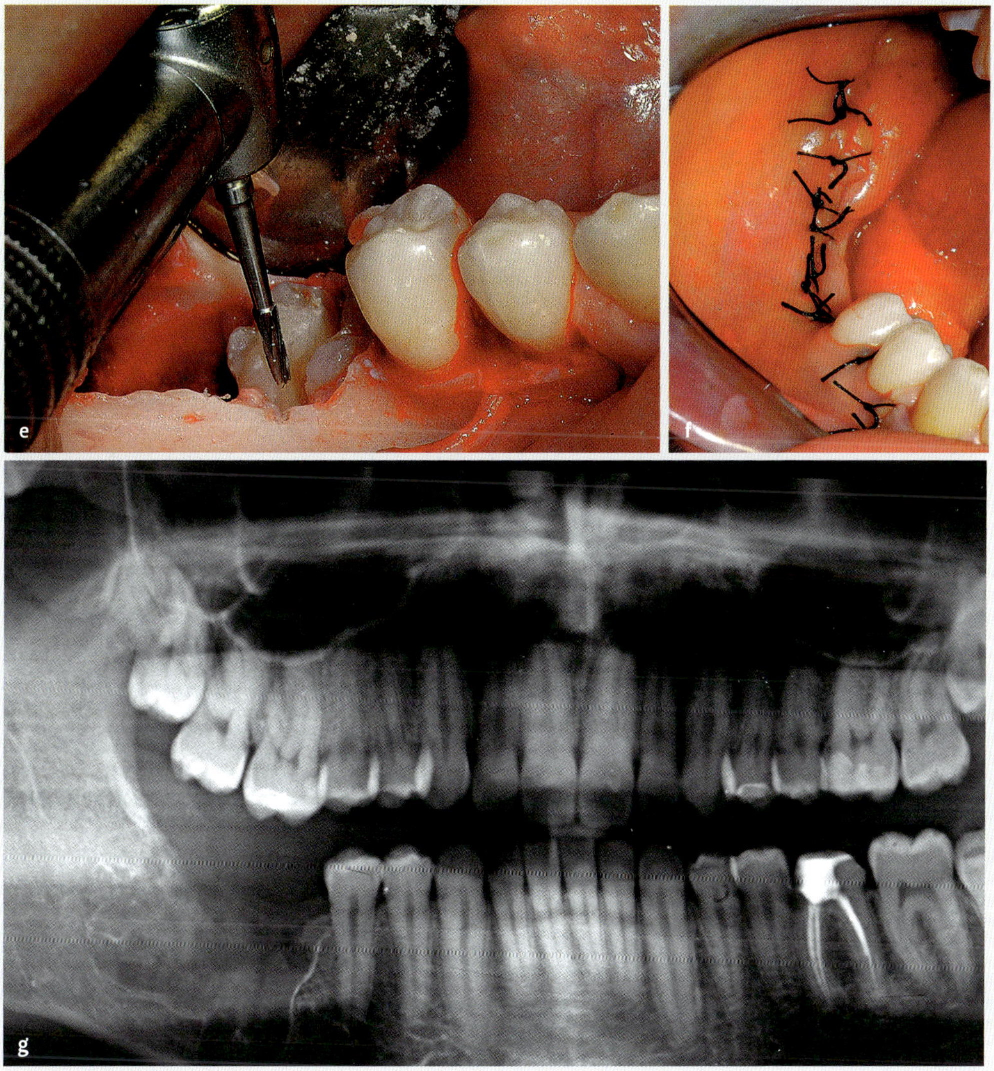

5.43 (*continued*) **e)** Odontotomy of 4.6. **f)** Suture. **g)** Postoperative radiographic follow-up.

PREVALENCE

Supernumerary teeth are a relatively frequent finding, with an overall incidence ranging from 1% to 4% and a significant gender predilection for men. They are more frequently found in the maxilla, particularly in the area of the incisors, but the presence of supernumerary teeth in the area of the premolars and distally to the third molars is not rare. Conversely, supernumerary deciduous teeth are a very rare finding (5.44).

MORPHOLOGY

Supernumerary teeth can be similar to the permanent teeth that are present in the same area, or present an atypical anatomy; they are often smaller than other teeth. In the area of the maxillary incisors, conoid supernumerary teeth (also known as mesiodens) can be observed, while in the molar and premolar area supernumerary teeth generally imitate the shape of the corresponding permanent teeth, even though they are usually smaller.

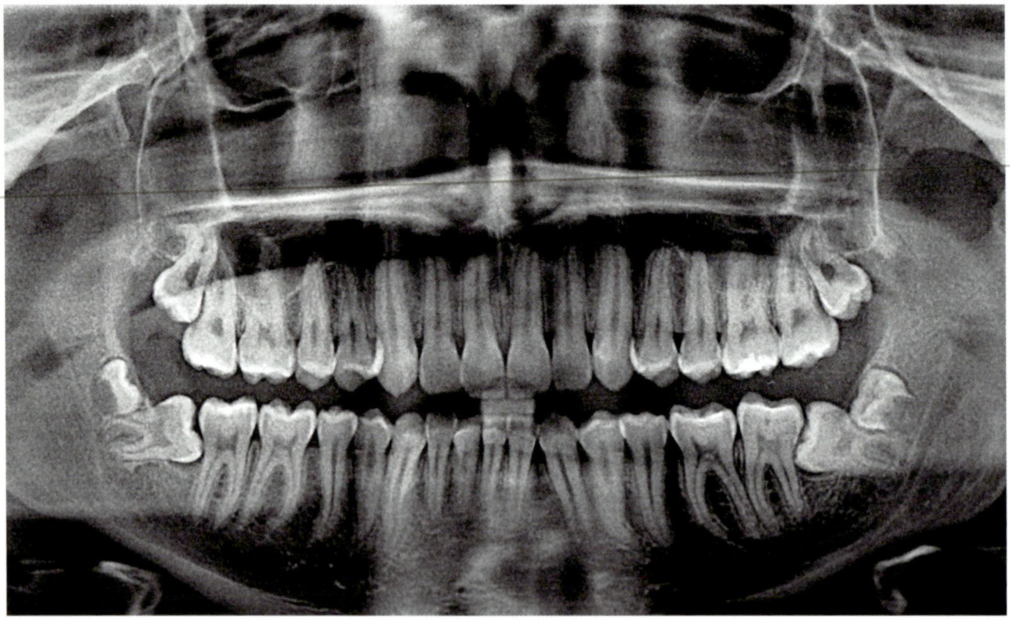

5.44 Panoramic radiograph showing the presence of supernumerary teeth distal to the third molars.

PROBLEMS

Only a quarter of all supernumerary teeth manage to erupt, while impaction of the remaining three quarters may cause problems such as interference with the eruption of permanent teeth (thus leading to impaction, malposition, or ectopy), the presence of diastemata or the cystic or neoplastic degeneration of its follicle.

SURGICAL PROTOCOL FOR THE EXTRACTION OF SUPERNUMERARY TEETH

The surgical techniques for the extraction of supernumerary teeth are similar to those described for other impacted teeth.

Usually, extraction is facilitated by the small size of these teeth and by the frequent presence of a single root and an ample follicular space (5.45a-f).

Autogenous tooth transplantation and tooth reimplantation

Surgical planning

Several studies published in the last decades have demonstrated, thanks to a better understanding of several phenomena (e.g. etiopathogenesis of root resorption, repair and regeneration of the periodontal tissues and their relationships with infectious processes), the reliability of tooth transplantation and tooth reimplantation techniques.

Tooth reimplantation (see Chapter 12 for details on the reimplantation of a tooth following traumatic avulsion): a semi-impacted or fully impacted tooth is extracted, and is then placed in a correct position immediately after extraction.

Clinical case 6 – Extraction of an inverted mesiodens

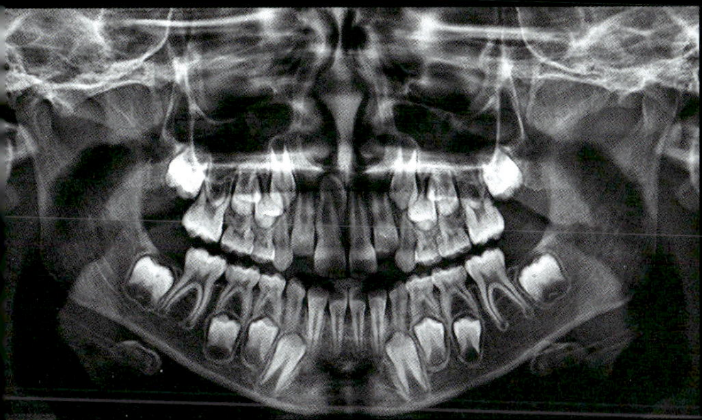

5.45a Panoramic radiograph showing an inverted mesiodens located between 1.1 and 2.1.

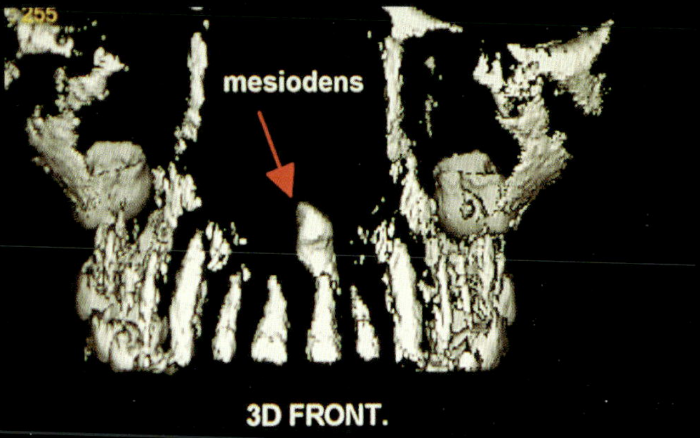

5.45b CT scan showing the exact anatomy and position of the impacted supernumerary tooth.

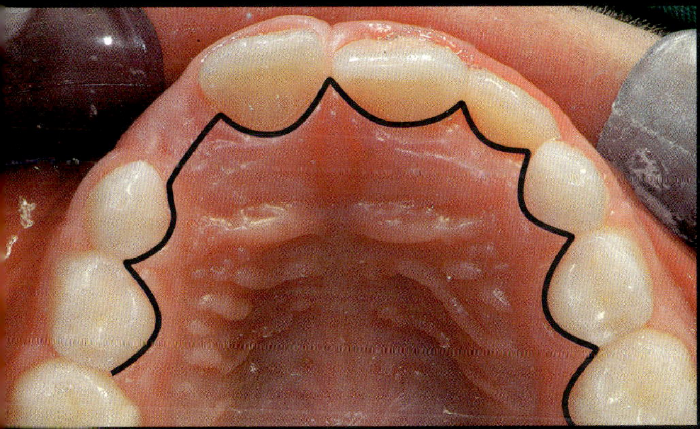

5.45c Preoperative clinical situation and design of the access flap.

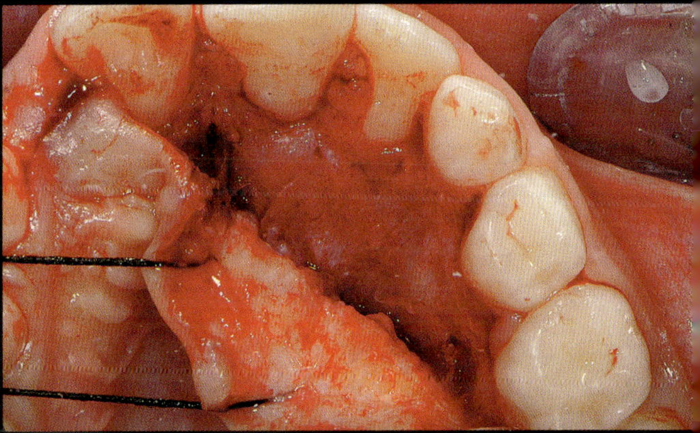

5.45d The access flap is elevated full-thickness and retracted with the aid of sutures anchored to the crowns of the contralateral teeth.

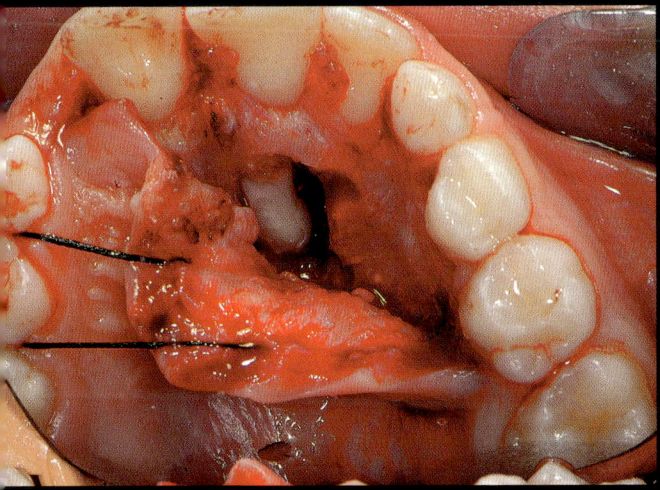

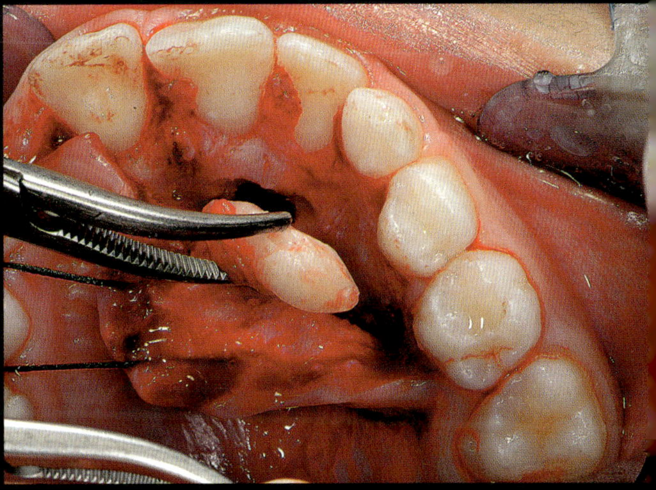

Autogenous tooth transplantation: an impacted, functionally irrelevant tooth (generally, a third molar) is extracted with an atraumatic approach and is then transplanted in an edentulous area as a substitute for a missing permanent tooth.

Tooth reimplantation and transplantation are treatment options to consider whenever they are technically feasible, but it is essential to evaluate all the benefits that can genuinely be obtained in every single case, as well as the possible complications, in the context of an accurate analysis of the benefit-cost ratio.

Identification of the tooth position and orientation of the impacted tooth, and morphology of the recipient site

See previous section.

SURGICAL TECHNIQUES FOR AUTOGENOUS TOOTH TRANSPLANTATION AND REIMPLANTATION

Surgical armamentarium

The surgical armamentarium is the same as that used for the extraction of other impacted teeth.

Locoregional anaesthesia

Follows the principles previously described for the extraction of impacted teeth.

HARVESTING OF THE IMPACTED TOOTH TO BE TRANSPLANTED/REIMPLANTED

The techniques used for the extraction of impacted teeth are described in detail in the previous sections of this chapter. For the correct application of these surgical techniques, it is essential that the integrity of the impacted tooth be safeguarded during extraction. Preserving the vitality of the cells of the periodontal ligament is essential for avoiding postoperative complications, such as root resorption and ankylosis.

REIMPLANTATION/TRANSPLANTATION

These procedures are easier to perform when the tooth that needs to be replaced is still present, whether it is a permanent or deciduous tooth. In this case, in fact, it is important that the morphology of the recipient site be similar to that of the post-extractive socket. For this reason, modifying the shape of the recipient site is often required, with the aid of surgical burs mounted on a straight handpiece. If the tooth to be replaced is already missing, it is essential to evaluate accurately the residual bone volume and the possible surgical morbidity associated with extensive bone removal, which is a prerequisite for the positioning of the harvested tooth.

STABILISATION OF THE TRANSPLANTED TOOTH

If the primary stability of the transplanted tooth is already satisfactory, it is possible to stabilise it only with compression sutures; mattress sutures crossing over the occlusal surface of the tooth are used to keep it in close contact with the socket.

Conversely, if it is not possible to achieve adequate primary stability, the tooth must be stabilised by splinting it to the neighbouring teeth (two on each side, if applicable).

Four weeks are generally sufficient to obtain stabilisation of the transplanted tooth.

RESTORATION OF THE TRANSPLANTED TEETH

As far as pulp vitality of the transplanted tooth is concerned, dedicated tests can provide results 3-4 months after surgery. However, a waiting period of 6-8 months is recommended to improve the reliability of responses to the tests. On the other hand, due to the unlikelihood that the pulp of a completely formed tooth remains vital after extraction and transplantation, it is recommended that an appropriate endodontic treatment be performed during surgery or in the following weeks. The anatomy and position of the transplanted tooth are frequently less than ideal to achieve acceptable occlusion and aesthetics; the recourse to restorative treatments such as inlays, veneers, or direct composite restorations allows all inconsistencies to be corrected. In some cases, after a 3-month waiting period, orthodontic treatment can be implemented to obtain small movements that may allow optimal results from a functional and aesthetic point of view.

REFERENCES

ANDREASEN JO, KOLSEN PETERSEN J, LASKIN DM. Textbook and color atlas of tooth impactions. Munksgaards, Copenhagen 1997.

ARAKERI G, ARALI V. Tooth section technique and pain upon elevation in third molar removal. *Int J Oral Maxillofac Surg* 2010 Jan; 39(1):98-9.

BEDOYA MM, PARK JH. A review of the diagnosis and management of impacted maxillary canines. *J Am Dent Assoc* 2009 Dec; 140(12):1485-93.

CHIAPASCO M, CRESCENTINI M, ROMANONI G. Germectomy or delayed removal of mandibular impacted third molar teeth? The relationship between age and incidence of complications. *J Oral Maxillofac Surg* 1995; 53:418-22.

CHIAPASCO M, DE CICCO L, MARRONE G. Side effects and complications associated with third molar surgery. *Oral Surg Oral Med Oral Pathol* 1993; 76:412-20.

ESPOSITO M. Impacted wisdom teeth. Review. *Clin Evid* 2006 Jun; (15):1868-70.

GROVER PS, LORTON L. The incidence of unerupted permanent teeth and related clinical cases. *Oral Surg Oral Med Oral Pathol* 1985; 59:420-5.

KUGELBERG CF. Impacted lower third molars and periodontal health. An epidemiological, methodological, retrospective and prospective clinical study. *Swed Dent J* 1990; 68(Suppl):1-52.

LUBBERS HT, MATTHEWS F, DEMERAU G, KRUSE AL, OBWEGESER JA, GRATZ KW, EYRICH GK. Anatomy of impacted lower third molars evaluated by computerized tomography: is there an indication for 3-dimensional imaging? *Oral Surg Oral Med Oral Pathol Oral Radiol Endod* 2011 May; 111(5):547-50.

LYSELL L, ROHLIN M. A study of indications used for removal of the mandibular third molar. *Int J Oral Maxillofac Surg* 1988; 17:161-164.

MIZRAHI E, MIZRAHI B. Mini-screw implants (temporary anchorage devices): orthodontic and pre-prosthetic applications. *J Orthod* 2007 Jun; 34(2):80-94.

PELL GJ, GREGORY BT. Impacted mandibular third molars: classifications and modified tecniques for removal. *Dent Digest* 1933; 39:330.

PETERSON LJ, INDRESANO AT, MARCIANI RD, ROSER SM. Principles of oral and maxillofacial surgery. JB Lippincott Company, Philadelphia 1992.

RAGHOEBAR GM, JANSEN HWB, JONGEBLOED WL, BOERING G, VISSINK A. Secondary retention of permanent molars: an assesment of ankylosis by scanning electron and light microscopy. *Br J Oral Maxillofac Surg* 1992; 20:50-5.

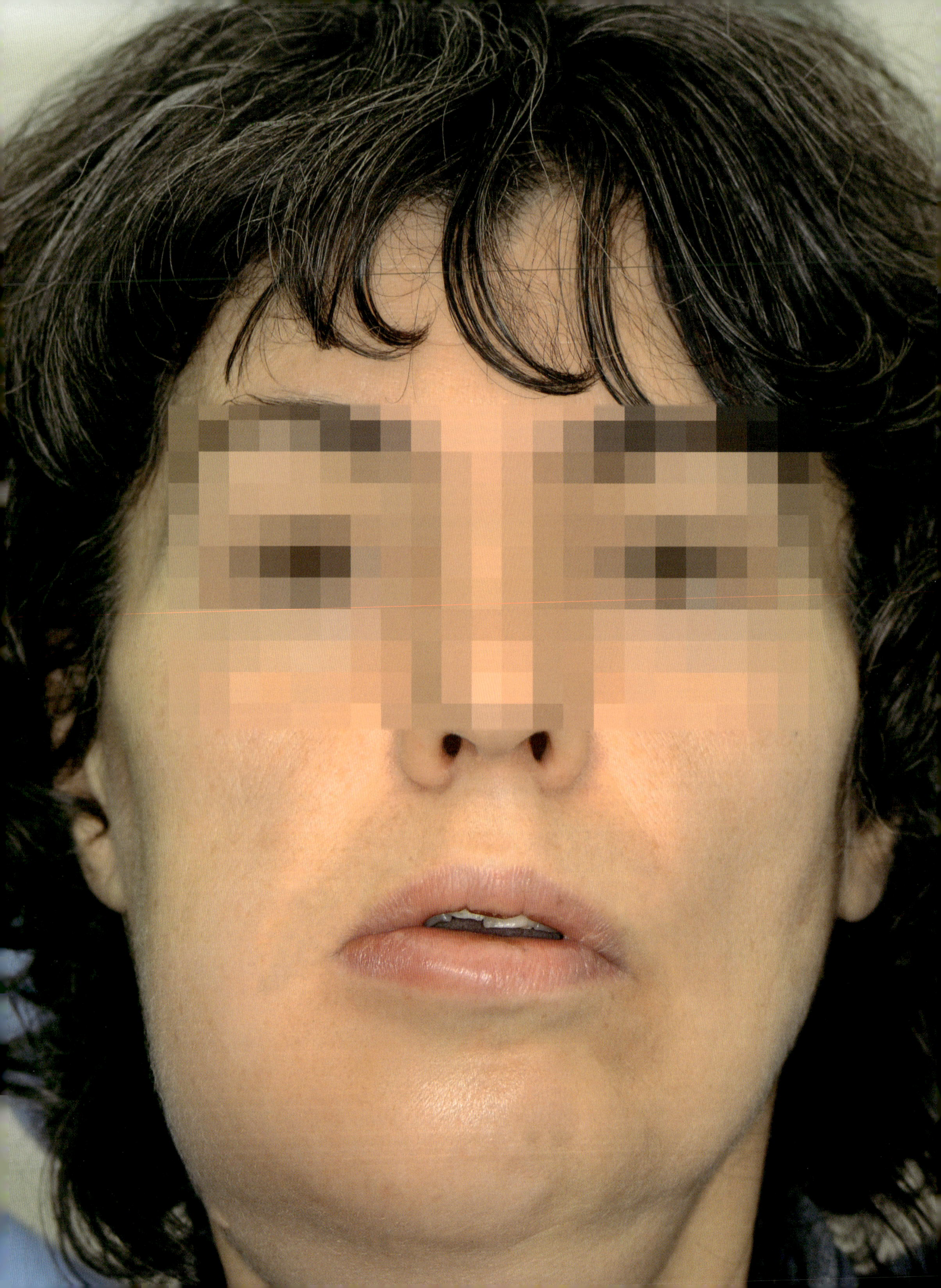

Odontogenic infections

M. Chiapasco · M. Zaniboni · P. Fusari

Introduction

Odontogenic infections include all the infectious processes originating in the teeth and periodontal tissues that can subsequently cause the possible involvement of the neighbouring anatomic structures such as the basal bone, the soft tissues and the skin of the head and neck region. Periapical periodontitis, abscesses, phlegmons, and odontogenic cellulitis are part of this category.

Removal of the primary cause of the infection, possibly associated with drainage of the purulent material and adequate antibiotic therapy, generally leads to the resolution of the problem. Conversely, a lack of treatment or an incorrect management of these infectious processes may lead to the onset of potentially severe clinical situations that may endanger the patient's life and require prompt hospitalisation.

Etiopathogenesis

Odontogenic infections are frequently caused by a combination of aerobic and anaerobic bacteria; in the majority of cases, the same bacteria that constitute the oral flora and cause caries and periodontal disease are involved, while bacteria coming from other districts such as the skin and the pharyngeal mucosa are more rarely implicated. The infectious process tends to evolve according to a predefined model in which the action of different bacterial species follows a precise chronological sequence. Aerobic bacteria play a significant role in the initial stage of the process: the proliferation of these bacteria causes a substantial modification of the ecosystem through oxygen consumption. The subsequent decrease of the redox potential and increase of carbon metabolites create a favourable environment for the development of anaerobic bacterial species, which are in fact predominant in the abscess and chronic stages of infection.

In these types of infection, the most frequently involved bacteria are aerobic Gram+ cocci, anaerobic Gram+ cocci, and anaerobic Gram- bacilli. Among aerobes, streptococci (70%) and staphylococci (5%) represent the majority of the population, while Neisseria, Corynebacterium, and Haemophilus are more rarely involved. Among anaerobes, Gram+ streptococci and pseudo-streptococci play a major role in more than one third of all odontogenic infections, while in more than half of the bacterial cultures carried out in cases of odontogenic infections Gram- anaerobes such as Prevotella, Porphyromonas, and Fusobacterium are found.

Generally, bacterial colonisation of the periapical area represents the first stage of an odontogenic infection and may occur according to different modalities.

Pulp necrosis due to caries: represents the most common contamination modality. Bacteria responsible for the carious process invade the pulp chamber and cause septic pulpitis and subsequent pulp necrosis, and then migrate along the root canals towards the apex.

Pulp necrosis due to periodontal disease: a retrograde contamination of the periapical area can occur when infection propagates apically from a deep periodontal pocket, thus involving the pulp (perio-endo lesion).

Pulp necrosis due to trauma: if any type of trauma (including bruxism sequelae) causes the interruption of the neurovascular bundle of the tooth, pulp necrosis ensues.

Retrograde contamination of the apex: infection affecting neighbouring anatomic structures (e.g. maxillary sinus) may involve the periapical region of a tooth by contiguous spread, thus causing pulp necrosis. Therefore, it is necessary to carry out a pulp vitality test on teeth that are in close proximity to a focus of suppurative infection.

Pericoronitis: the incomplete eruption of a tooth may favour bacterial proliferation in the space between the crown of the semi-impacted tooth and the surrounding soft tissues; in the most aggressive forms, infection may then spread to the oral mucosa and the soft tissues of the cheek.

Iatrogenic infections: although these cannot be defined as proper odontogenic infections, it is worth remembering that if the rules and prescription for asepsis are not thoroughly followed, any oral surgery procedure may cause infection.

When bacterial contamination occurs, the following evolution of the infectious process depends on the number of pathogens involved, their virulence, and the immune defences of the patient. If a high bacterial load and a high virulence are associated with a defective immune response, infection evolves towards acute manifestations such as phlegmon, or cellulitis, or abscess. Conversely, when the immune defences are able to thwart the infection (low bacterial load and low virulence), it evolves towards chronicisation. In the specific case of periapical infections, which are the most common among odontogenic infections, a high virulence causes the formation of an acute periapical abscess, while a low virulence causes the formation of a periapical granuloma (see Chapter 7 for details). If the periapical abscess, or acute apical periodontitis, is not treated (by means of orthograde endodontic therapy or extraction of the involved tooth), the infection may find a way through the cortical plate and periosteum and spread to the surrounding soft tissues, causing a phlegmon, cellulitis, or abscess. Fistulisation on the oral mucosa or, more rarely, on the skin, represents a frequent evolution of the periapical abscess. Conversely, osteomyelitis and dissemination in the bloodstream, which may cause severe sequelae, represent a rare (albeit serious) evolution of the phenomenon.

A periapical granuloma, instead, may not undergo visible modifications for years, or it may evolve into a radicular cyst. In both cases, a flare up of the infectious process can occur, triggering the conversion of these lesions into periapical abscess and infected radicular cyst (📷 6.1).

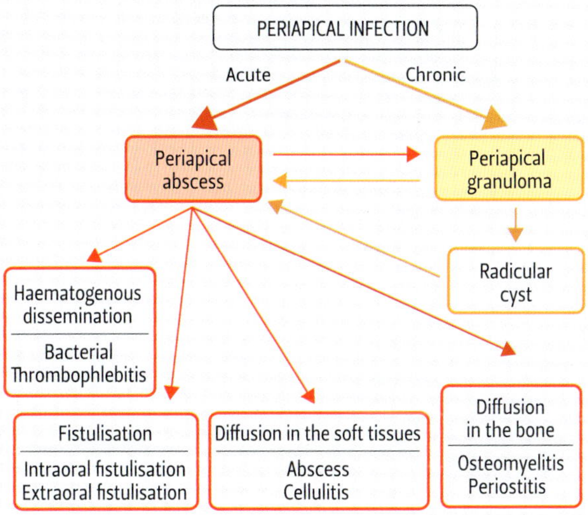

6.1 Schematisation of the evolution of a periapical infection.

Predisposing factors

As previously mentioned, the relationships between bacterial flora and immune defences are a key factor in the evolution of an infectious process.

Pathologies that are able to interfere with the chemotaxis and phagocytosis mechanisms of the leucocytes, such as diabetes, kidney disease, alcoholism, and malnutrition, favour the manifestation of the infection. The same occurs in the case of pathologies that reduce the immune response of the patient, such as leukaemia, lymphomas and others, including autoimmune diseases, immunosuppressive therapies, and the use of steroidal drugs. Finally, ineffective pharmacotherapies, when administered for long periods of time, can favour the selection of more resistant and more aggressive bacterial strains, thus exacerbating the infection or causing its diffusion.

Clinical evolution

Periapical abscess (stage 1): it is characterised by the onset of intense pain upon both biting and chewing, and upon percussion; the involved tooth does not respond to pulp vitality tests and may present an increased mobility. In the early stages of infection, radiographic exams can give negative results, while afterwards it is possible to observe an enlargement of the periodontal space associated with periapical radiolucency (6.2).

Endosteal infection (stage 2): the periapical abscess can develop into a chronic infection (periapical granuloma) or undergo a further evolution; the infection can spread from the periapical region in the cancellous bone, causing an endosteal infiltration (6.3). Radiographically, an expansion of the radiolucent area, albeit with scarcely defined margins, is observed.

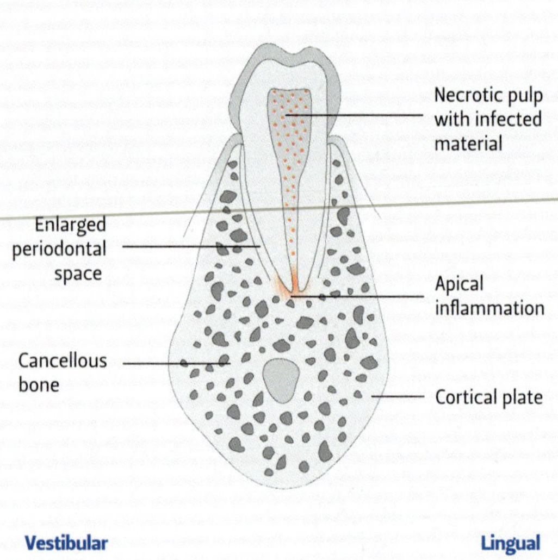

6.2 Periapical stage of the odontogenic infection.

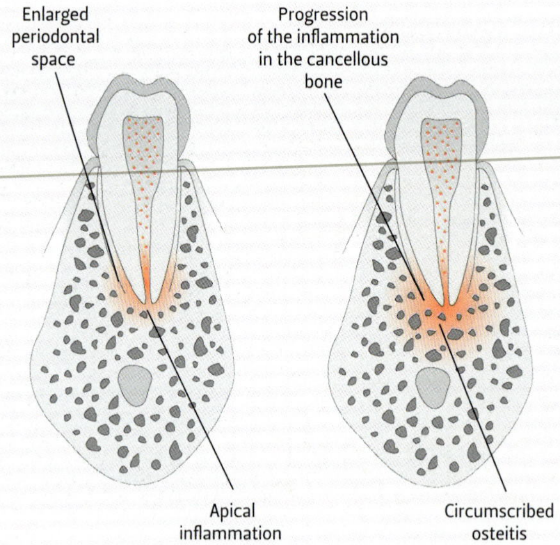

6.3 Endosteal stage of the odontogenic infection.

Subperiosteal infiltration (stage 3): it occurs after the infection has passed the cortical plate. The periosteum represents the last barrier before the diffusion of the infectious process to the surrounding soft tissues (6.4). The periosteum is put under tension by the underlying infection causing acute pain. Radiographically, no significant differences with the previous stage are visible.

Phlegmon or cellulitis (stage 4): when the infection spreads in the intraoral soft tissues, the result can be a phlegmon or cellulitis (6.5a-b), which is characterised by the diffuse infiltration of the infectious material in the submucosal or subcutaneous connective tissue, in the absence of well defined abscesses. The clinical presentation is characterised by skin or mucosa redness and hard elastic swelling of the involved area, whose margins are typically indistinct. The patient refers acute and diffuse pain, caused by the rapid and pronounced stretching of the soft tissues. Two are the possible evolutions of a phlegmon, which can form an abscess and fistulise, or evolve into diffuse infiltration.

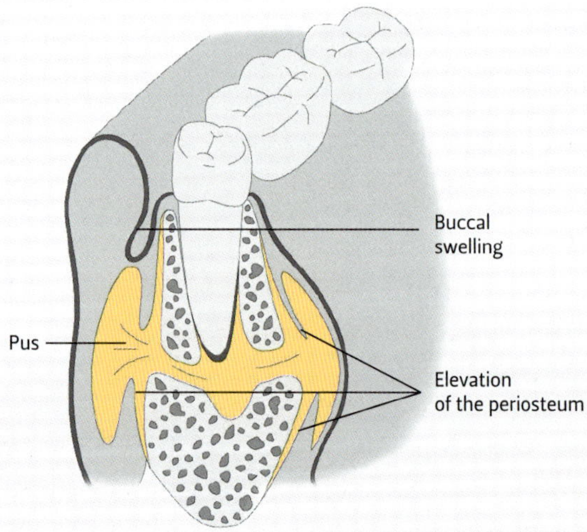

6.4 Subperiosteal stage of the odontogenic infection.

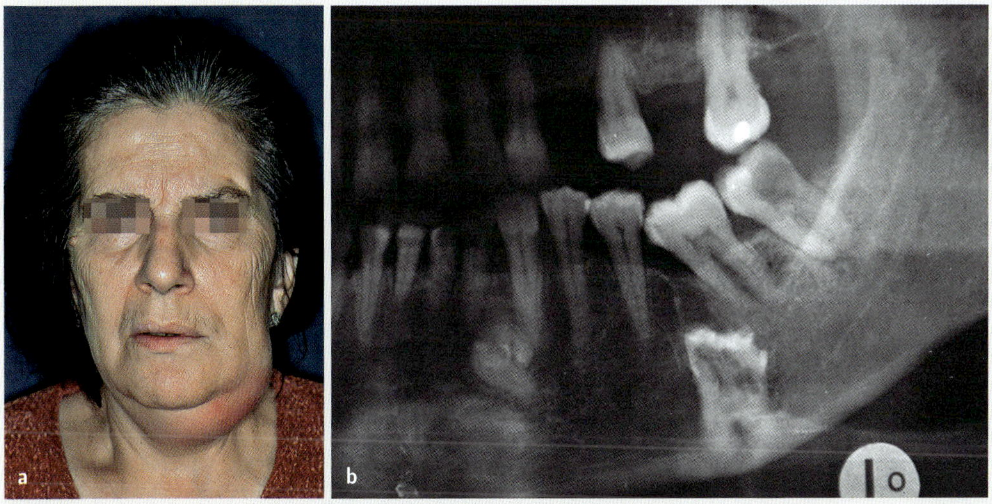

6.5 Phlegmonous (cellulitic) infiltration of the soft tissues: **a)** clinical presentation of a phlegmon of the submandibular space caused by an infection originating in a necrotic 3.8; **b)** panoramic radiograph showing an impacted 3.6 and the necrotic 3.8 (a large caries is visible).

Abscess and fistulisation (stage 5): the natural evolution of the phlegmon or cellulitis is characterised by the formation of an intraoral or extraoral abscess that can be defined as a collection of purulent material in a newly formed cavity, where the immune system tends to circumscribe the lesion (6.6a–c). For this reason, it represents a less severe evolution.

In some cases, the formation of a collection of purulent material may immediately follow the passing of the cortical plate (subperiosteal infiltration).

When an abscess is present, pain is usually circumscribed and less intense, and a well-defined fluctuating mass is clearly appreciable upon palpation. Spontaneous drainage of the abscess may occur: the interruption of the mucosal or cutaneous barrier leads to the formation of an intraoral or extraoral fistula (6.7). As the drainage of the purulent material causes the tension on the soft tissues to decrease, fistulisation is generally associated with a reduction of pain.

Diffuse infection (stage 6): a severe, albeit rare, evolution, is finally represented by an extensive diffusion of the infectious process, either in the head and neck region (e.g. Ludwig's angina) or in the bloodstream (septicaemia), with possible transfer of infected material in other organs. In cases of diffuse infection, signs of deterioration of the systemic conditions of the patient, such as hyperthermia and dehydration, are also present, and this situation may lead to septic shock if the infection is not promptly treated (see below for details).

Osteomyelitis of the jaws: it develops when the infectious process directly involves bone.

Osteomyelitis now represents a rare occurrence due to the diffusion of antibiotics; in fact, it is generally observed in immunocompromised patients. Osteomyelitis is a severe condition, and it may cause the destruction of large portions of the jawbones, with serious disabling sequelae. It develops when bacteria extensively colonise cancellous bone: the subsequent inflammation causes the compression of the intraosseous blood vessels, thus compromising the microcirculation in the medullary spaces. This mechanism leads to ischaemia, and finally to bone necrosis of the involved portion that undergoes sequestration.

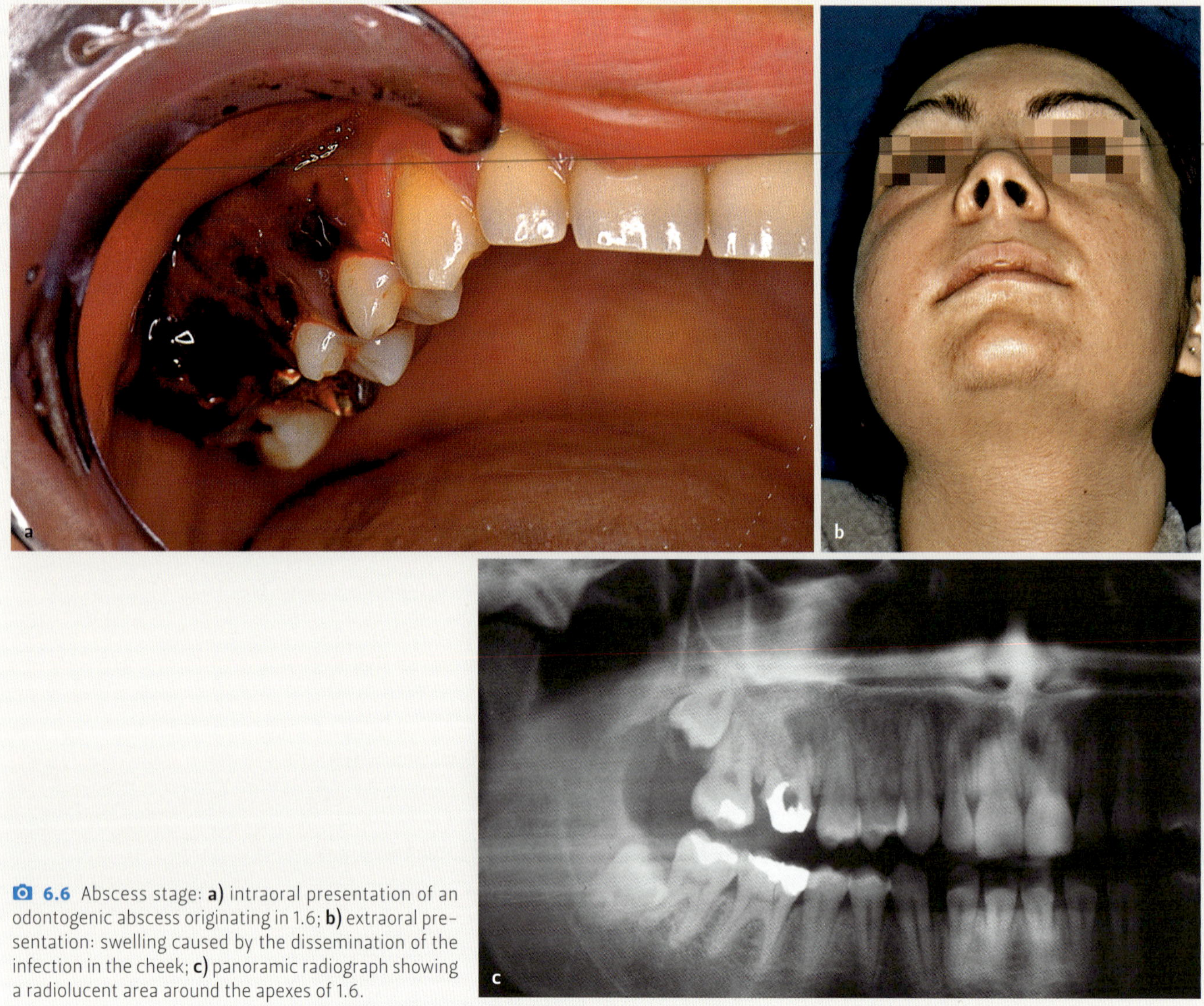

6.6 Abscess stage: **a)** intraoral presentation of an odontogenic abscess originating in 1.6; **b)** extraoral presentation: swelling caused by the dissemination of the infection in the cheek; **c)** panoramic radiograph showing a radiolucent area around the apexes of 1.6.

Ischaemia also prevents defence cells and antibiotics from reaching the area, allowing the undisturbed proliferation of the bacterial flora and the progression of the infectious process. Osteomyelitis initially involves the cancellous bone; at a later stage, it involves the cortical bone and then the periosteum, before intraoral or extraoral fistulisation occurs. In the majority of cases, osteomyelitis is observed in the mandible, as the thick cortical plates and the blood supply coming mainly from the inferior alveolar artery facilitate the onset of ischaemia.

Acute osteomyelitis generally arises shortly after the triggering event (odontogenic infection, fracture). The patient reports the onset of deep and intense pain in the affected area. Chronic osteomyelitis represents the natural evolution of the acute form when it is not treated. The clinical presentation is characterised by less pronounced symptoms: suppuration from the intraoral or extraoral fistulae that are frequently present in the chronic form may be observed. Radiographic images may not show visible alterations in cases of acute osteomyelitis, while in cases of chronic osteomyelitis, structural alterations are clearly visible and include cortical erosion, sequestra, and a characteristic mix of radiolucency and sclerosis in the involved area. The latter is caused by the alternation between areas of bone necrosis and areas of reactive sclerosis of vital bone, which represent a defensive and restorative attempt (6.8).

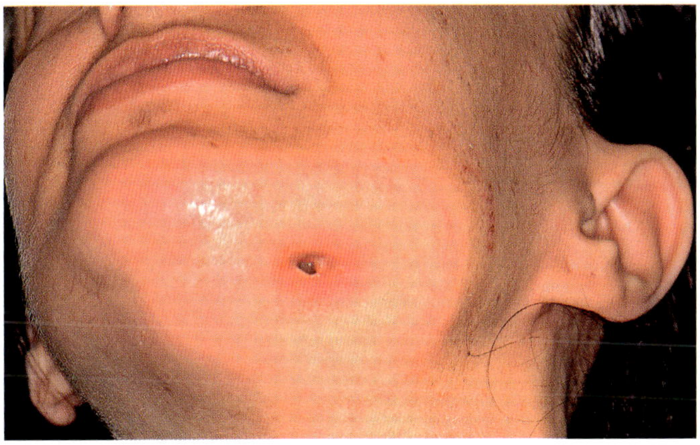

6.7 Extraoral fistulisation of an odontogenic abscess.

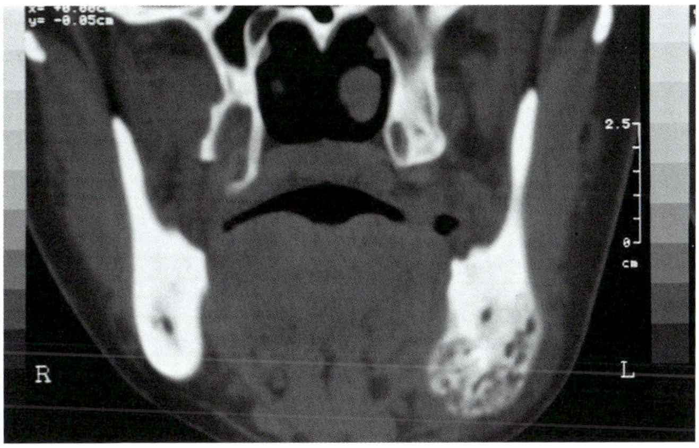

6.8 Chronic osteomyelitis in the left hemimandible: the frosted appearance of the involved bone is visible.

Clinical evolution of odontogenic infections

Stage	Type	Clinical presentation
Stage I	Periapical abscess	Intense, localised pain Pulp vitality test gives negative results Augmented tooth mobility No visible signs of infection on the radiographs, enlargement of the periodontal space
Stage II	Endosteal infiltration	Pain Negative response to pulp vitality test Periapical radiolucency with undefined margins
Stage III	Subperiosteal infiltration	Acute pain Periapical radiolucent area
Stage IV	Phlegmon or cellulitis	Intense pain Hard-elastic swelling Reddening of the skin and/or mucosa Radiographic signs similar to those of Stage III
Stage V	Abscess and fistulisation	Decreasing pain Soft swelling Presence of a fistula and purulent discharge Radiographic signs similar to those of Stage III
Stage VI	Diffuse infection	Marked pain and swelling Fever General compromission (dehydration, asthenia, etc.)

Anatomical factors influencing the diffusion of odontogenic infections

The infectious process tends to spread from the periapical region of a tooth to the adjacent areas according to predictable modalities that are mainly dependent on local anatomical factors that may be schematised as follows:

- *position of the root apex with respect to the cortical plates*: the infection tends to spread towards the cortical plate which is nearer to the root apex;
- *relationship between the point of wear on the cortical plate and muscle insertions*: once the infection has passed the cortical plate and periosteum, it tends to spread according to the anatomic planes caused by muscle insertions on the jawbones, following the path of least resistance.

A description of the areas of primary and secondary dissemination of odontogenic infections along the cervico-facial spaces is reported in the following sections.

Primary dissemination pathways

MAXILLARY INCISORS AND CANINES

Buccal position: this is the most frequent clinical presentation.

Palatal position: rarer, this is typically associated to the lateral incisor due to its root anatomy.

Canine space: the canine space is a virtual space located between the levator anguli oris muscle inferiorly and the levator labii superioris muscle superiorly. Dissemination in the canine space occurs almost exclusively as a consequence of an infectious process, involving the maxillary canine, as only this tooth has a root long enough to cause the erosion of the buccal cortical plate above the insertion of the levator anguli oris muscle. Involvement of the canine space causes a tumefaction of the infraorbital region that may cause palpebral swelling and the nasolabial fold to disappear; the clinical presentation may be similar to that of a dacryocystitis.

Perinasal and infranasal position: although a rare occurrence, infections originating in the central incisors can develop in a perinasal or infranasal position. The dissemination of the infectious process may initially involve the floor of the nasal cavity, and then extend to the paranasal cavities (paranasal sinuses empyema) and to the nasal septum (nasal septal abscess) (📷 6.9, 6.10).

Labial position: the infectious process may involve the soft tissues of the lip when the insertion of the labial muscle are low (📷 6.11).

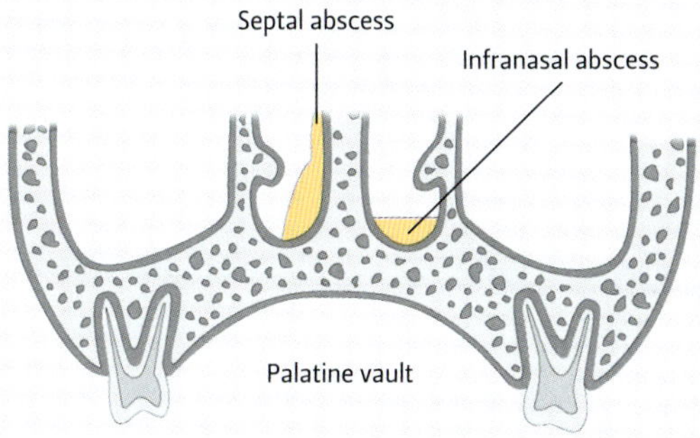

6.9 Nasal septal abscess and infranasal abscess.

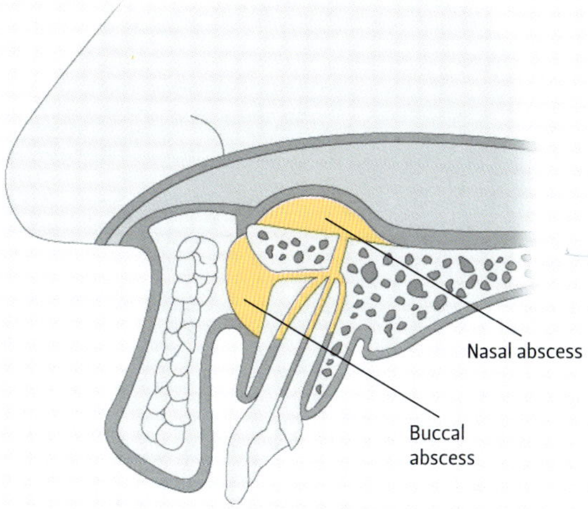

6.10 Buccal and nasal abscess.

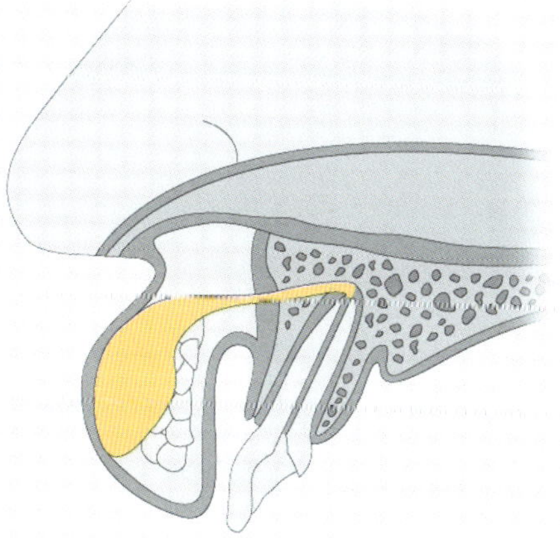

6.11 Labial abscess.

MAXILLARY PREMOLARS AND MOLARS

Buccal position: this is the most frequent clinical presentation (6.12a-b).

Palatal position: rarer, this is typically associated to infections originating in the palatal root (6.13a-b).

Cheek: dissemination in the soft tissues of the cheek may be observed when the erosion of the buccal cortical plate occurs above the insertion of the buccinator muscle: the buccal space is superficial to the buccinator muscle and deep to the platysma muscle and skin. Clinically, the patient's face is deformed by the swelling of the cheek (6.14a-b).

Dissemination in the soft tissues of the cheek may represent the evolution of an infection originating in the mandibular premolars and molars, when erosion of the buccal cortical plate occurs below the insertion of the buccinator muscle on the external oblique line of the mandible.

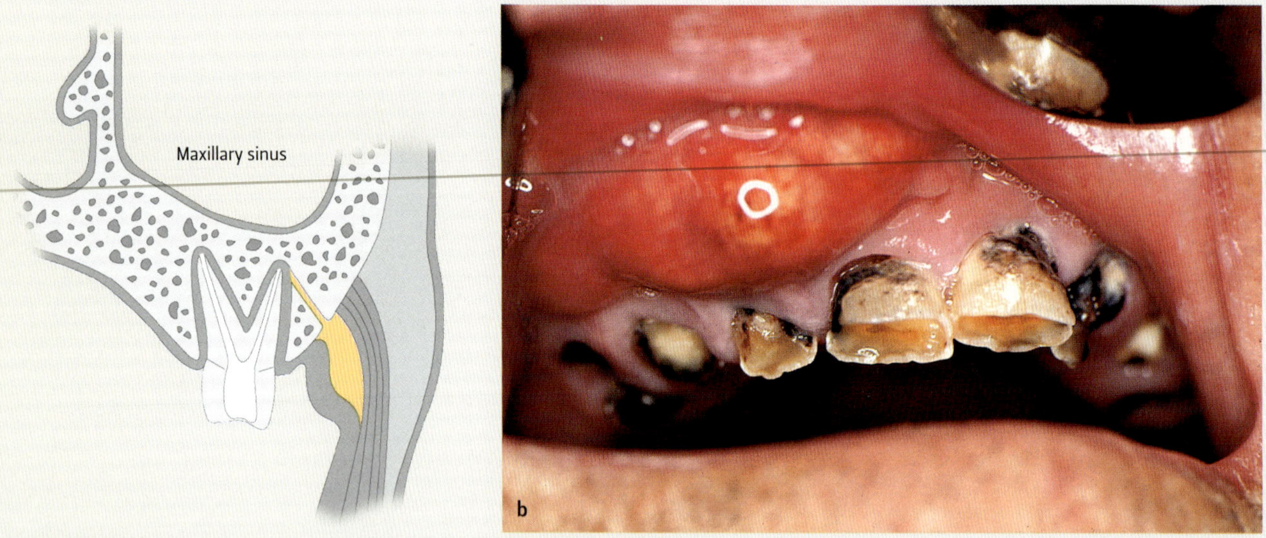

a b

6.12 **a)** Buccal abscess. **b)** Clinical presentation of a buccal abscess originating in 1.4.

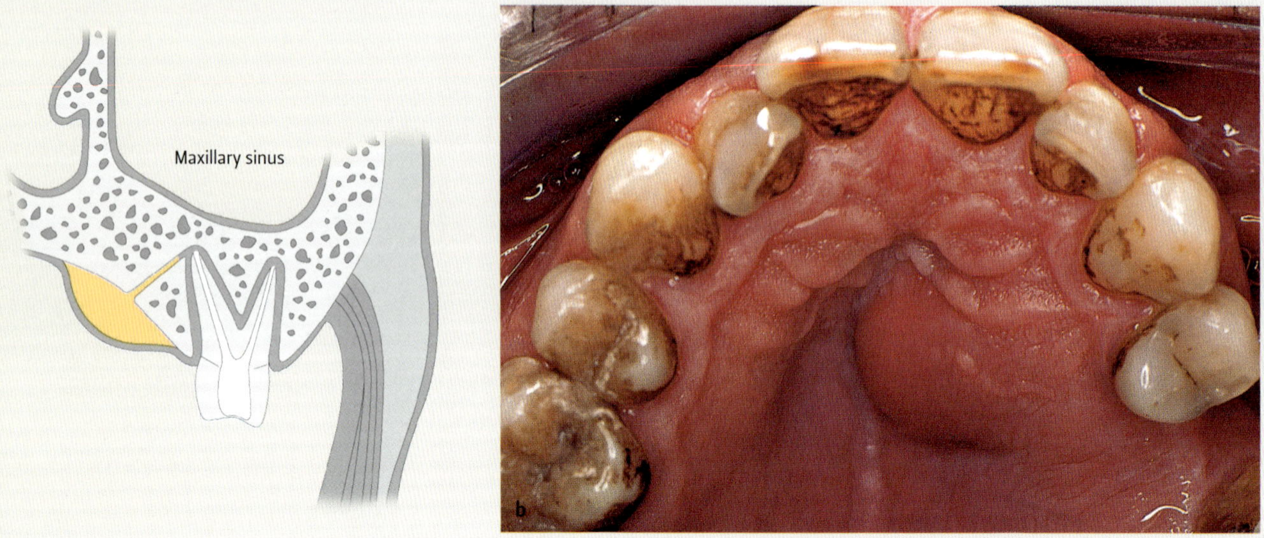

a b

6.13 **a)** Palatal abscess. **b)** Clinical presentation of a palatal abscess originating in 2.2.

Maxillary sinus: the close relationship that exists between the root apexes of the maxillary premolars and molars and the maxillary sinus is responsible for the frequent involvement of the latter in the infectious processes originating in the teeth. Periapical and periodontal infections involving the furcation of molars, as well as oroantral communications possibly associated with dislocation of tooth fragments or foreign bodies (implants, grafting materials, etc.), may contribute to the contamination of the maxillary sinus. The obstruction of the sinus ostium, typically due to reactive hyperplasia of the sinus mucosa, may initially cause the stasis and then the accumulation of mucus, thus favouring the onset of a bacterial infection. The reduced drainage of the maxillary sinus contributes to the chronicisation of the infection.

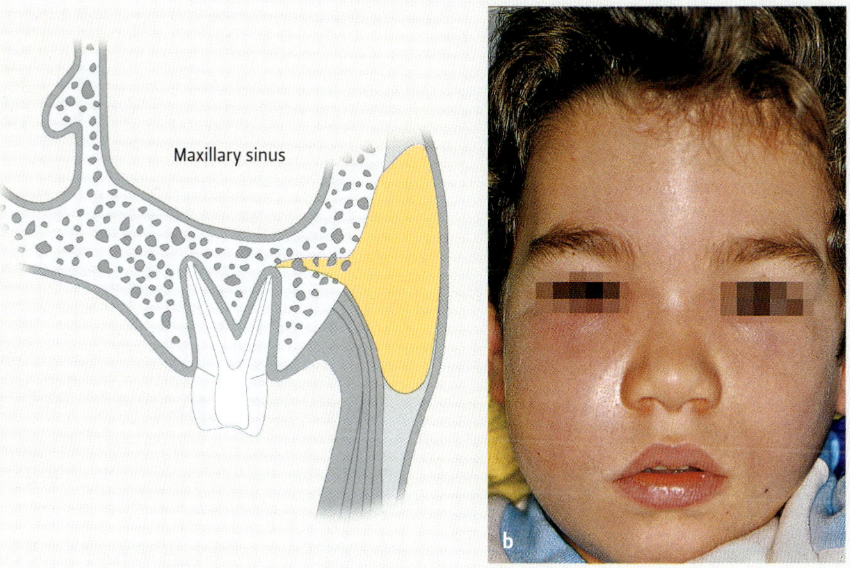

a b

6.14 **a)** Abscess involving the cheek. **b)** Clinical presentation of an abscess developing in the cheek.

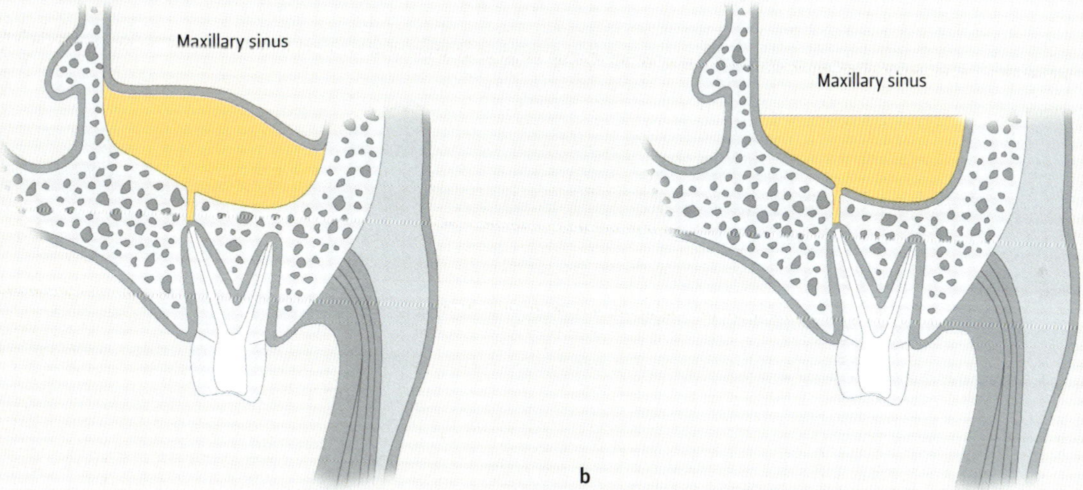

a b

6.15 Odontogenic abscess involving the maxillary sinus: **a)** if the collection of purulent material remains under the sinus mucosa and elevating it, the typical "rising sun" image can be observed; **b)** if the purulent material penetrates inside the sinus lumen, a horizontal air/fluid level can be observed.

Acute sinus infection is characterised by pain and tenderness in the area of the maxillary sinus: the pain is exacerbated by head movements and by palpation of the canine fossa. Malodorous purulent discharge from the nostril on the affected side, swelling and reddening of the skin, fever, asthenia, and nausea may be present.

Chronic sinusitis is characterised by the same signs and symptoms, albeit less intense. The alternation between the presence of symptoms and remission periods may be observed (6.15a-b).

An untreated sinus infection may result in the spread of the infectious process to the other paranasal cavities, ultimately causing a pansinusitis. The infection can also disseminate further and involve neighbouring anatomic areas such as the orbit, the base of the skull and their content, causing severe complications such as eye infections, cavernous sinus thrombosis, meningitis, encephalitis).

MANDIBULAR INCISORS, CANINES, AND PREMOLARS

Buccal position: it is the most frequent clinical presentation (6.16a).

Sublingual position: when an odontogenic infection causes the erosion of the lingual cortical plate, the insertion of the mylohyoid muscle plays an important role in causing its dissemination path.

If the infection originates in the frontal teeth (incisors and canines) or from the premolars, the erosion of the cortical plate generally occurs above the insertion of the muscle. Therefore, infection spreads in the sublingual space, which is delimited superiorly by the mucosa of the floor of the mouth, inferiorly by the mylohyoid muscle, anterolaterally by the lingual surface of the mandible, posteriorly by the geniohyoid and genioglossus muscles, and mesially by the intrinsic muscles of the tongue and genioglossus muscle that separate it in two halves (6.16b). The sublingual dissemination is characterised by the elevation of the floor of the mouth on the affected side; swelling can then involve also the contralateral side, because the intrinsic muscles of the tongue and genioglossus muscle do not completely separate the sublingual space into two independent spaces. Typically, the bilateral involvement of the sublingual space causes the tongue to be lifted towards the palate, with subsequent swallowing difficulties.

Dissemination of the infectious process along the parapharyngeal spaces may result in a severe complication, the *descending cervical cellulitis* or *Ludwig's angina* (see further for details).

Mental and submental position: infections originating in the mandibular incisors tend to erode the buccal cortical plate below the insertion of the mentalis muscle, resulting in the invasion of the space delimited by the mentalis muscle itself anteriorly, the mandibular symphysis posteriorly, the depressor labii inferioris muscles laterally, and the cutaneous plane of the chin inferiorly. The involvement of the mental area in the dissemination of an odontogenic infectious process causes swelling of the chin associated with reddening of the overlying skin.

When the infection spreads beyond the inferior margin of the mandible, below the insertion of the mylohyoid muscle (lingually) or the mentalis muscle (buccally), the submental space is involved. This fascial space is located between the mylohyoid muscle superiorly, the platysma muscle inferiorly, the inferior border of the mandible anteriorly, the hyoid bone posteriorly, and the anterior belly of the digastric muscle laterally. In this event, swelling of the submental region is observed (6.17).

MANDIBULAR MOLARS

Buccal position: when the erosion of the buccal cortical plate occurs above the insertion of the buccinator muscle, the infectious process tends to spread in a buccal and anterior direction. In fact, the insertion of this muscle on the external oblique line of the mandible dictates the path of dissemination of infections, particularly those originating in the third molars (6.18).

Cheek: when the erosion of the buccal cortical plate occurs below the insertion of the buccinator muscle, infections originating in the mandibular molars spread to the cheek (6.19).

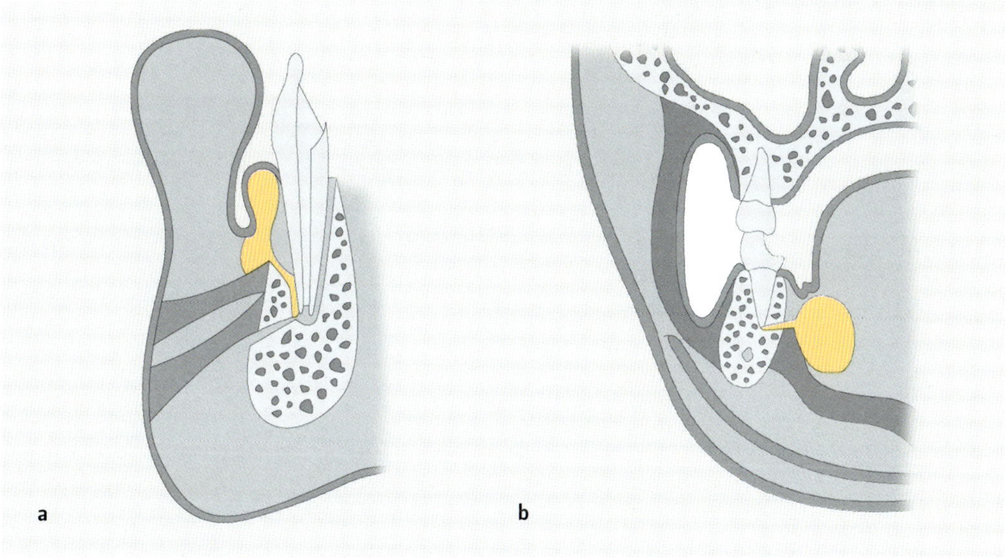

6.16 **a)** Buccal mandibular abscess. **b)** Sublingual abscess originating in the anterior mandibular teeth.

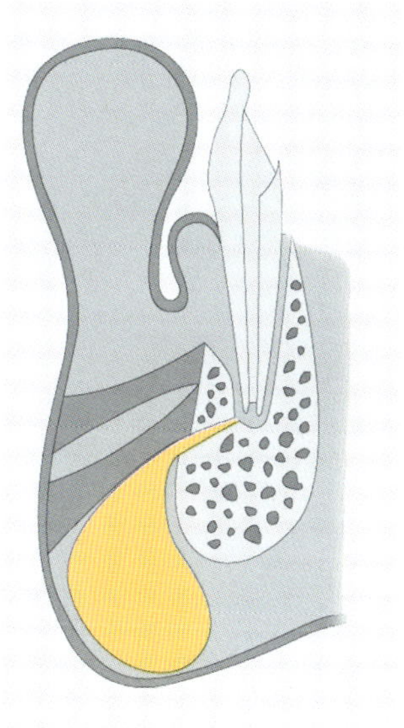

6.17 Submental abscess.

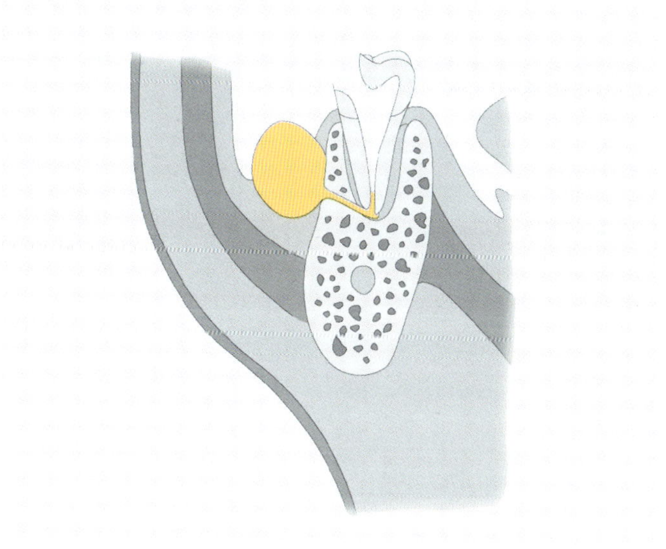

6.18 Buccal abscess originating in the mandibular molars.

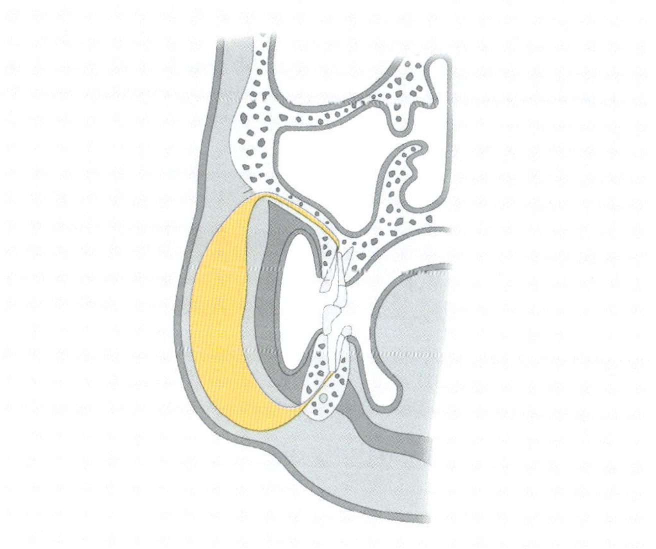

6.19 Abscess originating in the mandibular molars and involving the cheek.

Submandibular position: the involvement of the submandibular region is generally caused by the erosion of the lingual cortical plate below the mylohyoid line due to infections originating in the mandibular third molars. The relative thinness of the lingual cortical plate favours the involvement of this space which is delimited by the mylohyoid muscle superiorly, the skin, superficial fascia, and platysma muscle inferiorly and laterally, the lingual surface of the mandible anteriorly and laterally, the hyoid bone posteriorly, and the anterior belly of the digastric muscle medially. The close relationship between the submandibular space and the deep spaces of the neck is responsible for the possible secondary involvement of these latter. The spreading of infections to the submandibular space is accompanied by ipsilateral swelling that may extend up to the hyoid bone (6.20).

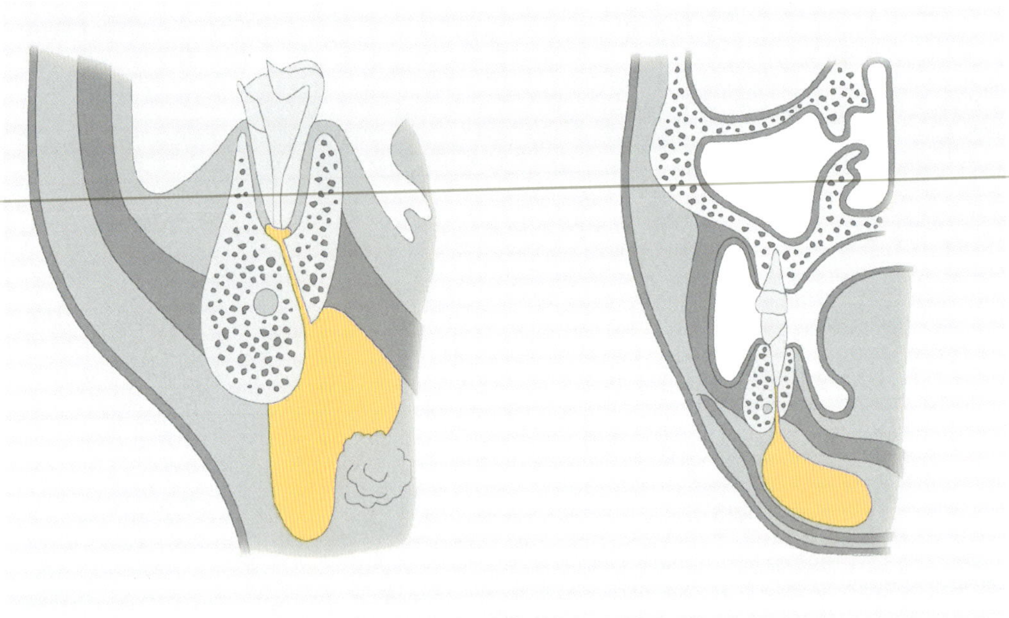

6.20 Submandibular abscess.

Secondary dissemination pathways

In cases of significant virulence or inadequate treatment, infections can spread from their area of origin to adjacent areas, but also reach distant sites, thus worsening the prognosis. Generally, infections spread along the fascial spaces following the path of least resistance, which is mainly dictated by the course of the muscle bundles and cervical fasciae. Occasionally, dissemination via the bloodstream or lymphatic system may occur; in these cases, the clinical picture may be complex with potentially severe consequences.

Dissemination by contiguity

A detailed analysis of the topographic anatomy of the muscle and fascial cavities of the head and neck is beyond the scope of this manual; however, a general description of each space is reported in the following paragraphs.

SUBMASSETERIC SPACE

The submasseteric space, together with the pterygomandibular, superficial temporal and deep temporal spaces, constitutes the masticator space. The submasseteric space is delimited by the masseter muscle laterally, and by the lateral surface of the mandibular ramus medially. It communicates with the buccal space anteriorly, with the parotid space posteriorly, with the superficial temporal space superiorly, and with the pterygomandibular space medially. The submasseteric space can be reached by an infectious process that involves the buccal space and spreads posteriorly. In some cases, infections originating in the mandibular third molars can directly involve the submasseteric space (6.21).

Symptoms associated with the involvement of the submasseteric space in an infectious process are intense pain and swelling in the area of the mandibular ramus. The masseter muscle is tender to palpation and trismus is present. Generally, no peculiar signs are visible on the skin, as the infection is contained by the masseter muscle.

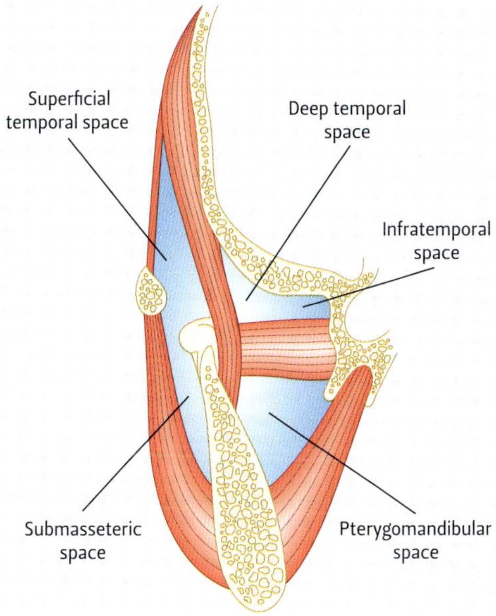

6.21 Anatomy of the masticator space.

PTERYGOMANDIBULAR SPACE

The pterygomandibular space is delimited by the medial surface of the mandibular ramus laterally, and by the internal pterygoid muscle laterally. It communicates with the infratemporal space superiorly, and with the sublingual and submandibular spaces anteriorly. Involvement of the pterygomandibular space is generally caused by the dissemination of infections developing in the sublingual and submandibular spaces. However, infections originating in the mandibular third molars may directly involve the pterygomandibular space. The symptoms associated with the involvement of the pterygomandibular space in an infectious process are intense pain in the retromolar and sublingual region, exacerbated by the palpation of the internal pterygoid muscle; severe trismus is often present, while swelling is frequently modest or absent (6.21).

The inadvertent use of a contaminated needle to perform an inferior alveolar nerve block may cause the development of an infectious process directly involving the pterygomandibular space.

TEMPORAL SPACE

The temporal space is subdivided in two parts by the temporal muscle. The superficial temporal space is delimited by the temporal fascia laterally, and by the temporal muscle medially; it communicates with the submasseteric space inferiorly. The deep temporal space, instead, is delimited by the temporal muscle laterally, and by the lateral surface of the temporal bone and the greater wing of the spehoid bone. The superficial and deep temporal spaces are rarely involved in the case of odontogenic infection; however, infection spreading from the submasseteric and pterygomandibular spaces can occasionally reach the temporal spaces. In this event, signs and symptoms include localised swelling in the temporal region (superiorly to the zygomatic arch) and intense pain exacerbated during mouth opening, due to the extension of the temporal fascia (6.21).

PAROTID SPACE

The parotid space is delimited by the superficial parotid fascia laterally, by the external auditory canal, the temporal bone and the superior portion of the digastric and sterno-cleidomastoid muscle posteriorly, by the posterior surface of the mandibular ramus and the masseter and internal pterygoid muscles anteriorly, and by the zygomatic arch superiorly. It communicates with the submandibular space inferiorly, with the lateropharyngeal space medially, and with the submasseteric and pterygomandibular spaces anteriorly. The parotid space is rarely involved in the case of odontogenic infections. However, infections developing in the submasseteric, pterygomandibular and lateropharyngeal spaces can sometimes reach this area. In this event, signs and symptoms include intense pain and swelling in the preauricular region that may extend to the areas of the zygomatic arch and mandibular ramus. The involvement of the parotid space in cases of odontogenic infection does not cause trismus per se; however, trismus is frequently present due to the concomitant involvement of the submasseteric and pterygomandibular spaces (6.22).

PARAPHARYNGEAL SPACES

Parapharyngeal spaces are rarely involved in the case of odontogenic infection. However, severe and rapidly progressive infections can reach these deep spaces and cause critical situations where even the patient's life can be at risk. The severity of these circumstances is due to the important anatomic structures that are present in the parapharyngeal spaces (particularly the internal jugular vein, carotid artery, and cranial nerves), to the possible obstruction of the upper airway, and to the possible dissemination of the infectious process to the mediastinum (mediastinitis).

Lateropharyngeal space: it is delimited by the internal pterygoid muscle and deep portion of the parotid gland laterally, the superior constrictor pharyingeal muscle medially, the skull base superiorly, the hyoid bone inferiorly, the pterygomandibular raphe anteriorly, and the prevertebral fascia posteriorly. The styloid process and the three styloid mus-

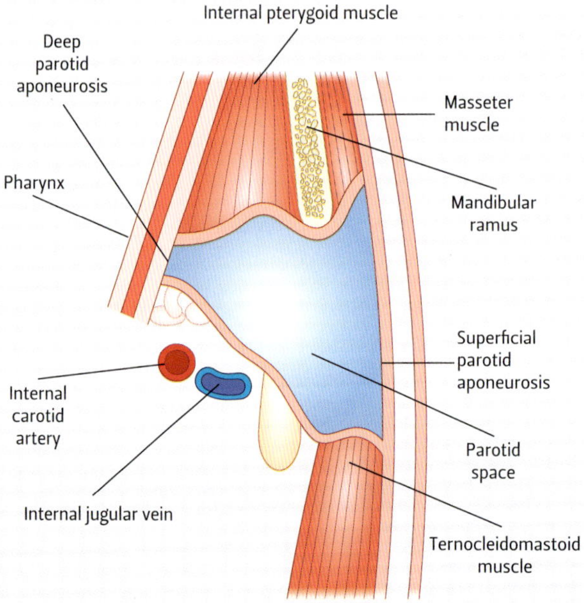

6.22 Parotid space.

cles (styloglossus, stylohyoid, and stylopharyngeous) divide the lateropharyngeal space in an anterior and a posterior part: the internal jugular vein, the carotid artery and several cranial nerves (IX, X, XI, and XII) pass through this latter. Infections developing in the pterygomandibular space may reach the lateropharyngeal space; in this event, signs and symptoms include intense pain in the area of the pharynx irradiated towards the auricular region, swelling on the ipsilateral side of the neck, dysphagia, and trismus (caused by the involvement of the internal pterygoid muscle). Moreover, in cases of severe infection, typical alterations of the vital parameters may be observed. If adequate treatment is not promptly performed, involvement of the lateropharyngeal space may lead to the onset of severe complications. The infectious process, in fact, may involve anatomic structures present in the posterior part of the lateropharyngeal space (jugular vein thrombosis, erosion of the carotid artery followed by lethal haemorrhage, involvement of the previously listed cranial nerves). A second complication is represented by the spread of the infection to the retropharyngeal space, from where it may rapidly reach the mediastinum (6.23).

Retropharyngeal space: it is delimited by the superior constrictor pharyingeal muscle and the buccopharyngeal fascia anteriorly, the alar fascia posteriorly, the base of the skull superiorly, the mediastinum inferiorly, where the alar fascia and the buccopharyngeal fascia unite (6.23). Signs and symptoms related to the spread of an infectious process to the retropharyngeal space are similar to those described for the lateropharyngeal space, which is always jointly involved. However, the situation can be worsened by the presence of dyspnea caused by the partial obstruction of the upper airway caused by the anterior dislocation of the posterior wall of the pharynx. Moreover, perforation of the pharyngeal wall may cause the penetration of purulent material inside the lungs.

Prevertebral space: it is delimited by the alar fascia anteriorly, and the prevertebral fascia posteriorly. Its involvement, generally caused by dissemination of an infectious process developing in the retropharyngeal space, may allow the infection to spread caudally quite rapidly, even below the diaphragm (6.23).

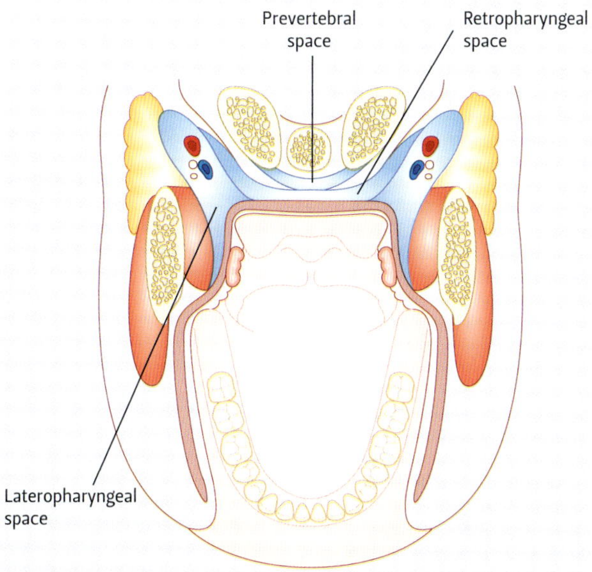

6.23 Parapharyngeal spaces.

Ludwig's angina: this is a peculiar form of dissemination of odontogenic infection: a diffuse cellulitis that involves the submandibular, sublingual and submental spaces, bilaterally.

This clinical situation, albeit rare, is still burdened by an unfavourable prognosis; therefore, the patient must be immediately referred to the hospital where adequate treatment can be provided.

The origin of Ludwig's angina is often represented by an infection originating in the second or third mandibular molars.

The bacterial flora responsible for this complication is generally formed by streptococci, particularly the streptococcus haemolyticus.

Signs and symptoms include:

- hard swelling, tender to palpation, in the submandibular and suprahyoid regions;
- elevation of the floor of the mouth and tongue protrusion;
- trismus, dysphagia, breathing difficulties, dysphonia, high fever (and subsequent dehydration).

Ludwig's angina is a rapidly progressive disease, and further complications such as its diffusion to the parapharyngeal spaces, mediastinum and thorax may cause severe consequences. Obstruction of the upper airway due to laryngeal oedema and concomitant involvement of the retropharyngeal spaces may occur, as well as dissemination of the infectious process in the bloodstream.

Cervicofacial necrotising fasciitis: this is a rare acute infection that shares the characteristics of a cellulitis and spreads predominantly in the subcutaneous tissue following the superficial myofascial planes of the neck.

Signs and symptoms include swelling of the neck, in association with the typical signs and symptoms of phlegmons that tend to extend superficially causing the necrosis of the skin.

Mediastinitis: the dissemination of odontogenic infections along the cervicofascial spaces may allow bacteria to reach the mediastinus, causing this severe complication that, still today, presents a high mortality rate.

Mediastinitis is characterised by dyspnea, acute retrosternal pain, severe alteration of the vital signs, and a high risk of septicaemia. The thoracic radiograph shows an enlargement of the mediastinus associated with the presence of air in the mediastinus itself.

Complex and diffuse complications of odontogenic infections are rarely observed today, affecting mainly debilitated patients affected by systemic diseases that compromise the immune system.

When the infectious process tends to spread, it causes systemic alterations such as:

- body temperature above 38 C° with possible dehydration;
- increased cardiac frequency;
- increased respiratory rate, in cases of partial obstruction of the upper airway secondary to the involvement of the peripharyngeal spaces;
- increased blood pressure, in cases of intense pain and anxiety;
- possible septic shock, due to the massive bacterial dissemination in the lymphatic and vascular system (see below for details).

Haematogenous dissemination

Although dissemination by contiguity is more common, the spread of odontogenic infections may also occur via the bloodstream. The peculiar configuration of the venous system in the head and neck renders the haematogenous spread of odontogenic infections possible, albeit rare; in fact, intraluminal valves are absent in these veins.

The infectious process initially causes thrombophlebitis of the veins of the involved area. Subsequently, the detachment (embolisation) of septic blood clots occurs and causing the dissemination of the infection via the bloodstream. Infections originating in the maxilla can cause thrombosis of the cavernous sinus, which can be reached via the superior and inferior ophthalmic arteries anteriorly, or via the pterygoid plexus posteriorly. The involvement of the cavernous sinus is an extremely severe complication that is difficult to treat, and it may further be complicated by the formation of a cerebral abscess.

Finally, massive dissemination of bacteria in the bloodstream may cause septicaemia, which can further evolve into septic shock.

Lymphatic dissemination

Odontogenic infections can involve the lymph nodes that are present in the involved area. The first stage is represented by reactive adenitis: the involved lymph node is swollen and hard, tender to palpation and movable. Adequate treatment of the infection causes the complete remission of the adenitis.

In cases of inadequate treatment (or absence of treatment), the following stage is represented by suppurative adenitis. At this stage, swelling increases and unsolicited pain develops; mobility of the involved lymph nodes is reduced and the margins are less defined. The most severe stage of lymphatic dissemination is represented by adenophlegmon, whereby the infection spreads to the tissues surrounding the involved lymph nodes causing the onset of cellulitis in the area.

Diagnosis of odontogenic infections

Diagnosis of odontogenic infections is based primarily on a thorough collection of the patient's medical history, followed by clinical examination and, if necessary, by additional exams (e.g. radiographs) and laboratory tests. The aim is to identify the infectious process by excluding other pathologies that can mimic its clinical presentation. The clinician must be able to identify the more severe infections that can put the patient's life at risk; in these cases, the patient must be referred to the appropriate specialist to receive adequate treatment.

Clinical examination: analysis of signs and symptoms

COLLECTION OF THE PATIENT'S MEDICAL HISTORY

The patient's medical history is the most important factor in the definition of the acute or chronic development of an infection. The patient should be asked about signs and symptoms present at the time of the evaluation (swelling, trismus, dysphagia, purulent discharge, etc.), and particularly:

- about the date of onset of the symptoms (hours, days, weeks before the examination);
- about possible variations in the intensity of the symptoms and if these variations occur slowly or rapidly;
- about the possible presence of fever.

Once these aspects are clarified, the clinician should be able to define the acute or chronic development of the disease. Some signs, such as dysphagia and dyspnoea, represent alarm bells, as they indicate the involvement of the deep spaces of the head and neck. The possible presence of pathologies or medical treatments that can negatively affect the activity of the immune system, thus favouring a more aggressive progression of the infectious process and its rapid spread, must be assessed, as this may lead to unfavourable evolutions of the infection. It is important to obtain information about previous or ongoing antibiotic therapy. Prolonged use of antibiotics, in fact, can cause antimicrobial resistance that requires specific treatments based on the results of laboratory test (culture test and antibiogram).

GENERAL CLINICAL EXAMINATION

In the first place, possible alterations of the patient's vital signs that can be present in cases of severe odontogenic infection must be identified (fever, increased cardiac frequency, increased respiratory rate, and increased blood pressure). In cases of diffuse infection, the patient is asthenic, dehydrated, and globally debilitated.

LOCAL EXTRAORAL EXAMINATION

The clinical evaluation of the patient's face allows the identification of possible asymmetry, swelling, skin erythema, or cutaneous fistulae. Palpation of the swollen area is fundamental to distinguish between a fluctuating mass (suggestive of a purulent collection) and a hard mass that is typical of cellulitis.

LOCAL INTRAORAL EXAMINATION

Intraoral examination should allow the cause of the infectious process to be identified (e.g. deep caries, pericoronitis, etc.). In the presence of intraoral swelling, palpation should help distinguish between a fluctuating mass (abscess) and a hard mass (phlegmon), thus influencing the following treatment protocol. Fistulae, when present, can be easily identified in the majority of cases. Pulp vitality tests should allow the tooth in which the infection originates to be identified. Percussion tests, when positive, indicate the presence of acute periapical periodontitis. The presence of trismus, however, is suggestive of the spread of the infectious process along the secondary dissemination pathways, thus representing an aggravating factor.

Radiographic examinations

Radiographic examinations are usually indicated to confirm the diagnosis and origin of an odontogenic infection. Periapical radiographs are usually sufficient to confirm the diagnosis of a circumscribed odontogenic infection. However, in cases of acute infections, as well as in cases of acute periapical abscess, the results of the radiographic exams can be negative. In the event of extensive infections, the recourse to a panoramic radiograph is indicated, while in severe cases of dissemination of the infectious process to the cervicofascial spaces, only a CT scan or MRI will allow adequate evaluation of the situation.

Among the possible consequences of the dissemination of an odontogenic infection, osteomyelitis and maxillary sinusitis deserve a separate description.

The radiographic appearance of acute osteomyelitis may be negative, while in the case of chronic osteomyelitis the gradual destruction of the bone can be observed as the alternation between radiolucent and radiopaque areas that give the bone a frosted appearance. Sequestra, when present, appear as normally radiopaque areas surrounded by a radiolucent halo (6.8).

Maxillary sinusitis appears on radiographs as an opacification of the involved maxillary sinus. The panoramic radiograph does not allow precise assessment of the extent of the infection and its characteristics, while a CT scan offers detailed information on these aspects and is, therefore, the exam of choice (6.24).

The traditional occipital-mental view (Water's view) has currently fallen into disuse.

Radiographic exams

	Advantages	Disadvantages
Periapical radiograph	• Chronic circumscribed infections	• Negative results in cases of acute infection
Panoramic radiograph	• Extensive infections	• Lack of definition of the radiographic image • Difficulties in assessing the actual extent of the infection
CT scan	• Complex situations with dissemination in the cervicofascial spaces	• Cost/benefit ratio • Major indication

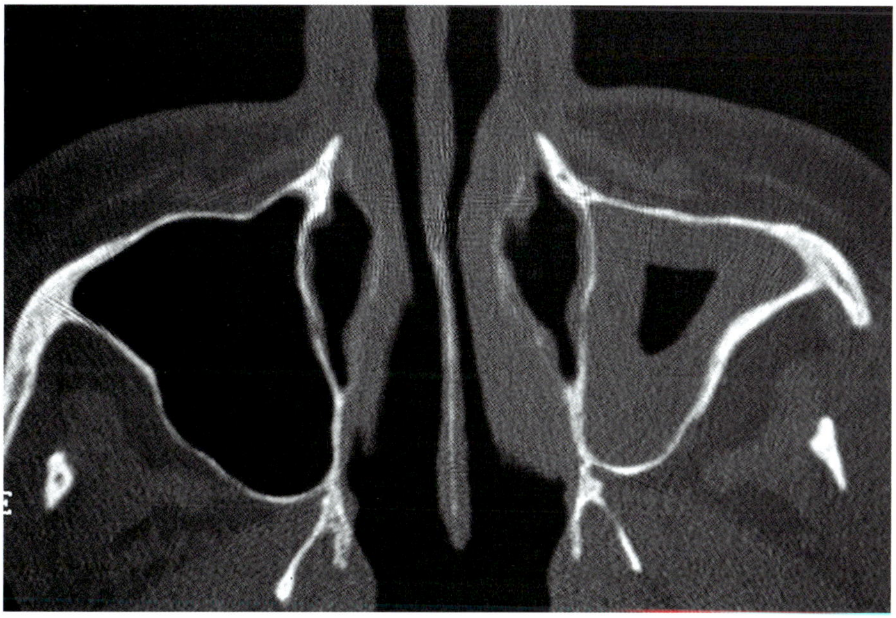

6.24 Maxillary sinusitis: CT scan showing opacification of the left maxillary sinus due to an infectious process originating in 2.6.

Differential diagnosis

The modalities of presentation, the signs and the symptoms associated with odontogenic infections, are peculiar; therefore, the diagnostic process is generally straightforward. In cases where symptoms are unclear, or when identifying the cause of infection is impossible, evaluating other possibilities is indicated. According to the area in which the infectious process develops, the differential diagnosis presents characteristic aspects.

Buccal position: bone and mucosal benign and malignant tumours must be taken into consideration.

Perinasal and infranasal position: benign and malignant tumours originating in the nasal mucosa, inflammation of the nasal cavities.

Canine fossa: benign and malignant bone tumours, local inflammation (actinomycosis), dacryocystitis.

Palatal position: benign and malignant bone tumours, tumours of the mucosa and glands (pleomorphic adenoma, adenoid cystic carcinoma, epidermoid carcinoma, mucoepidermoid carcinoma, etc.).

Cheek: benign and malignant bone tumours of the maxilla (ameloblastoma, mixoma, sarcoma, etc.), skin inflammation.

Maxillary sinus: benign and malignant tumours originating in the sinus mucosa, inflammation of the sinus (non-odontogenic sinusitis).

Temporal region: dermoid tumours, joint tumours, benign and malignant bone tumours, trauma sequelae (zygomatic trauma, trauma to the coronoid process and condyle), temporomandibular joint inflammation.

Sublingual region: inflammation of the salivary glands or obstruction of the salivary duct (sialolithiasis, sialoadenitis, ranulas, etc.), benign and malignant tumours of the salivary glands.

Mental region: local skin inflammation (actinomycosis).

Negative prognostic factors of odontogenic infections

- Immunocompromised patients
- Prolonged antibiotic therapy
- Rapidly progressive infection
- Fever, increased cardiac frequency, increased respiratory rate, debilitated patient
- Dysphagia, dyspnoea
- Trismus

Submental region: benign and malignant bone tumours, skin inflammation, dermoid cysts, thyroglossal cysts.

Pterygomandibular region: mandibular tumours, peritonsillar abscess.

Treatment

Treatment of odontogenic infections is based on the elimination of the causing agent and the drainage of the purulent material in association, if necessary, with antibiotic therapy. Elimination of the causing agent can be obtained with an endodontic treatment, whereby the involved tooth can be recovered and restored or with the extraction of the involved tooth when its recovery is not indicated or impossible (e.g. vertical fractures, severe periodontal lesions, etc.).

In cases of limited infection, the elimination of the causing agent can be sufficient to obtain complete healing. Conversely, in cases of extensive infection, and particularly when an abscess is present, the incision and drainage of the purulent collection helps reduce the bacterial load, eliminate anaerobiosis condition, prevent the dissemination of the purulent material, and reduce the tension of the soft tissues, which is responsible for the intense pain associated with these conditions.

The treatment of severe infection is more complex, although based on the same principles, and includes elimination of the causing agent, drainage of the purulent material and antibiotic therapy, but also medical treatment to restore the patient's general health: these treatments are generally performed when the patient is hospitalised.

ANTIBIOTIC TREATMENT OF ODONTOGENIC INFECTIONS

Administration of an antibiotic therapy is indicated when the infection is rapidly progressive and diffuse, when drainage is not possible (cellulitis, phlegmon), in immunocompromised patients, and when it is not possible to immediately remove the causing agent (e.g. in cases of severe trismus). Conversely, if the patient's general condition is good, the infection is limited and its causing agent can be immediately removed, the recourse to antibiotics is not necessary. In these cases, in fact, the possible side effects of antibiotic therapy (e.g. allergic and intolerance reactions, development of antimicrobial resistance, etc.) outweigh the advantages.

CHOICE OF ANTIBIOTIC

The choice of the antibiotic is generally based on empirical considerations; administered per os, it is usually directed towards the most likely causing agents. The recourse to a culture test and antibiogram to select an antibiotic for the eradication of a specific causing agent is indicated in cases of diffuse, rapidly progressive, or chronic (osteomyelitis) infections, to select the most effective antibiotic as soon as possible. In these cases, parenteral administration is generally preferred.

Penicillins represent the first choice, as their broad spectrum makes them useful against bacteria that are commonly involved in these types of infections (streptococci and anaerobic bacteria of the oral cavity). Amoxicillin has a high intestinal absorption rate (90%), rarely causes significant gastroenteric side effects, and is reasonably priced. The association between amoxicillin and clavulanate extends the spectrum of activity also to the Gram- bacteria that produce beta-lactamases. When patients are allergic to penicillins, then erythromycin or clindamycin can be used. However, it is worth noting that the use of erythromycin, which has a bacteriostatic activity, is contraindicated in cases of severe infections and for the treatment of immunocompromised patients. Clindamycin has the advantage of reaching high concentrations in the bone.

The use of cephalosporins should be limited to the treatment of severe infections (including osteomyelitis) and caused by bacteria that are resistant to other commonly used antibiotics. The administration of cephalosporins to patients with a history of allergy to penicillins should be evaluated with great care, as the risk of cross-allergy is very high. In these cases, based on the results of cultural tests and antibiogram, the administration of associations of different molecules is frequent.

In association with the medical and surgical therapy, particularly in cases of severe infection, the prescription of a liquid hypercaloric diet is indicated to compensate for the dehydration caused by fever and insufficient intake of fluids, as well as the malnutrition caused by the trismus and the general discomfort.

The use of analgetics can be effective for pain control, and the application of a warm and damp compress improves blood supply in the involved area, contributing to the action of the immune defences and the antibiotics.

The use of antibiotics should be protracted for 2-3 days after the complete remission of the infection. In the majority of cases, after an adequate surgical treatment is performed, antibiotic therapy is administered for 7 days.

Treatment of odontogenic infections according to their clinical presentation

Periapical periodontitis and endosteal stage of the infection: orthograde endodontic therapy or extraction of the involved tooth.

Abscess: endodontic therapy or extraction in association with the surgical drainage of the purulent material and antibiotic therapy (when necessary).

Cellulitis of phlegmon: endodontic therapy or extraction associated with surgical drainage of the purulent material and antibiotic therapy (when necessary).

Osteomyelitis: the treatment, particularly in cases of extensive bone destruction, is generally performed by maxillofacial surgeons under general anaesthesia, in a protected environment (hospital). Generally, it is a complex infection to treat, apart from cases of limited extension with the presence of small sequestra.

In cases of acute infection, a first approach entails the parenteral administration of an antibiotic therapy that should be chosen, if possible, based on the results of a culture test and antibiogram. However, it is worth noting that the presence of necrotic material and a compromised microcirculation have a negative influence of the local action of antibiotics.

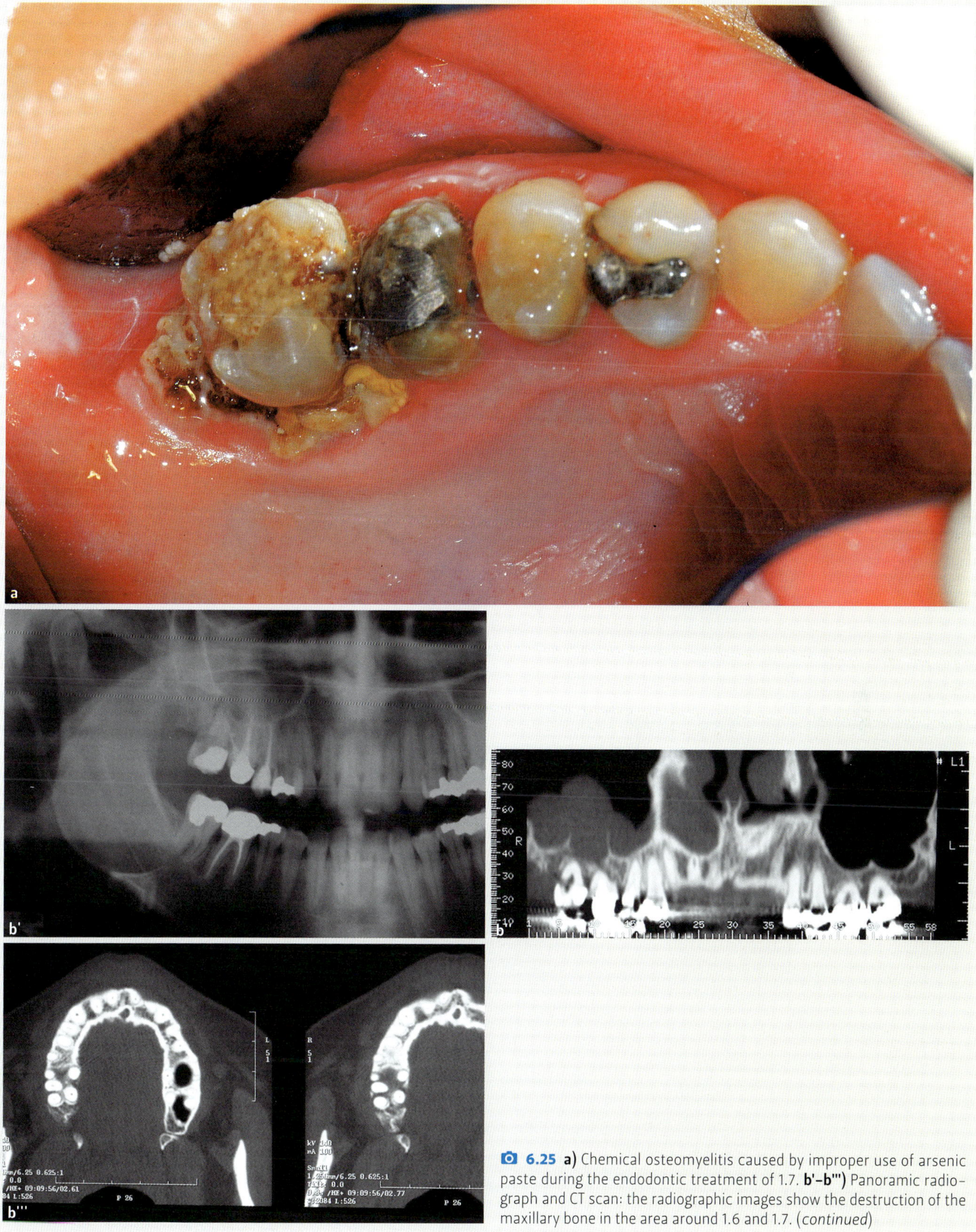

6.25 a) Chemical osteomyelitis caused by improper use of arsenic paste during the endodontic treatment of 1.7. **b'–b''')** Panoramic radiograph and CT scan: the radiographic images show the destruction of the maxillary bone in the area around 1.6 and 1.7. (*continued*)

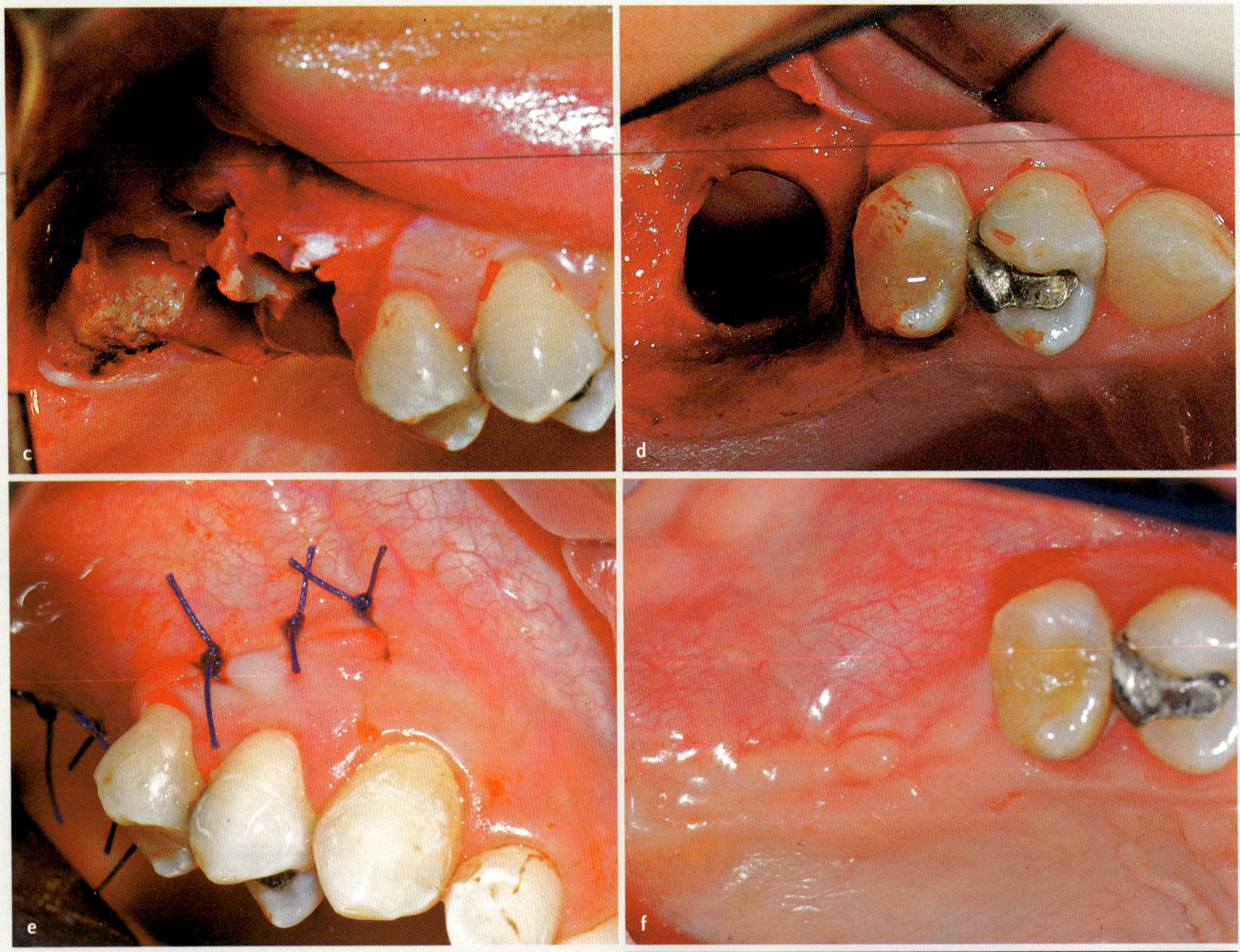

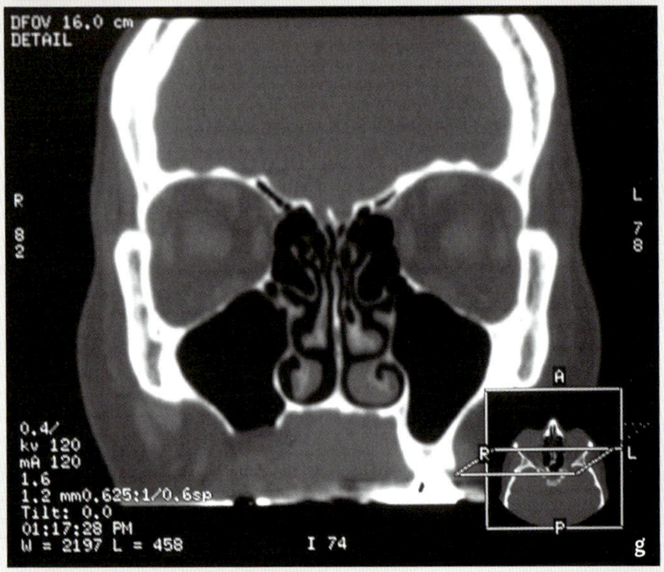

6.25 (*continued*) **c)** The necrotic alveolar ridge in the molar area of the right hemimaxilla. **d)** The surgical field after the removal of all the necrotic tissue: the inevitable oroantral communication, caused by the removal of the necrotic alveolar ridge, is visible. **e)** Suture. **f)** Clinical follow-up demonstrating complete healing of the involved area. **g)** Radiographic follow-up 12 months after surgery.

Basic techniques

Abscess

Anaesthesia

In cases of an acute infection, it is more difficult to obtain a complete anaesthesia of the involved area. When the position of the abscess allows it, it is recommended to perform a block anaesthesia. Conversely, perilesional anaesthesia is contraindicated due to the lack of effectiveness.
In the treatment of complex odontogenic infections with involvement of extraoral regions and associated with severe trismus, the recourse to general anaesthesia is recommended.

Incision

A No. 11 blade is generally used to perform a small incision in the most declivitous area of the swollen tissues to facilitate the drainage of the purulent material. The incision can be intraoral, which is always the first choice when possible, or extraoral, and its extent should be proportional to that of the abscess to favour its drainage. The incision should always be superficial, to prevent possible damage to underlying important anatomic structures. When reaching deeper areas is necessary to complete the drainage of the abscess, blunt dissection should be used exclusively: haemostatic forceps can be inserted into the incision and opened inside the cavity in different directions (📷 6.26a).
It is imperative that the clinician have adequate knowledge of local anatomy to prevent damage to important anatomic structures (see Chapter 1 for details on the regional anatomy).
In the case of extraoral drainage, the incision of the skin should be parallel to the collagen fibres in the dermis and to the muscle fibres (Langer's lines) to reduce the aesthetic impact of the resulting scar.

Drainage

Once the abscess is opened, the pus drains spontaneously; however, to obtain the complete elimination of the purulent material, the abscess is then squeezed and irrigation with sterile saline or antibiotic solutions inside the cavity is performed. The incision is kept pervious until complete drainage of the purulent material is achieved, to avoid relapses. This can be obtained by placing a rubber tube inside the abscess through the incision (📷 6.26b–d): the drain is kept in place for 3–4 days with the aid of a suture, and daily irrigations of the cavity with sterile saline are performed through the tube to quicken the healing process. In cases of intraoral placement of the drain, mouth rinses with salt water can be prescribed to favour the osmotic drainage of the abscess (📷 6.26e–h).

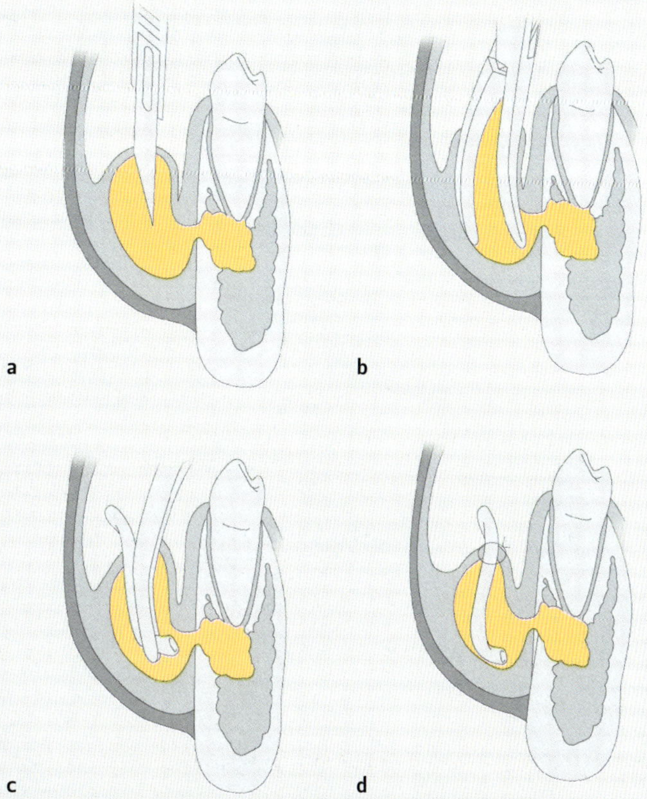

📷 **6.26** **a)** Drainage of an abscess via an intraoral approach: incision. **b)** Blunt dissection with haemostatic forceps. **c)** Placement of a surgical drain. **d)** The surgical drain is fixed in place with a suture. (*continued*)

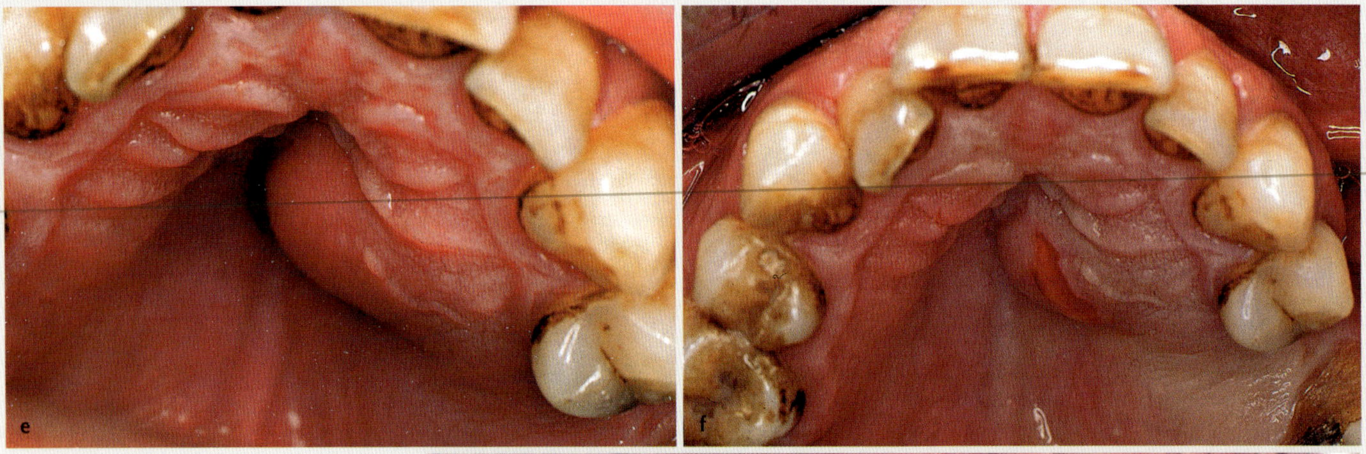

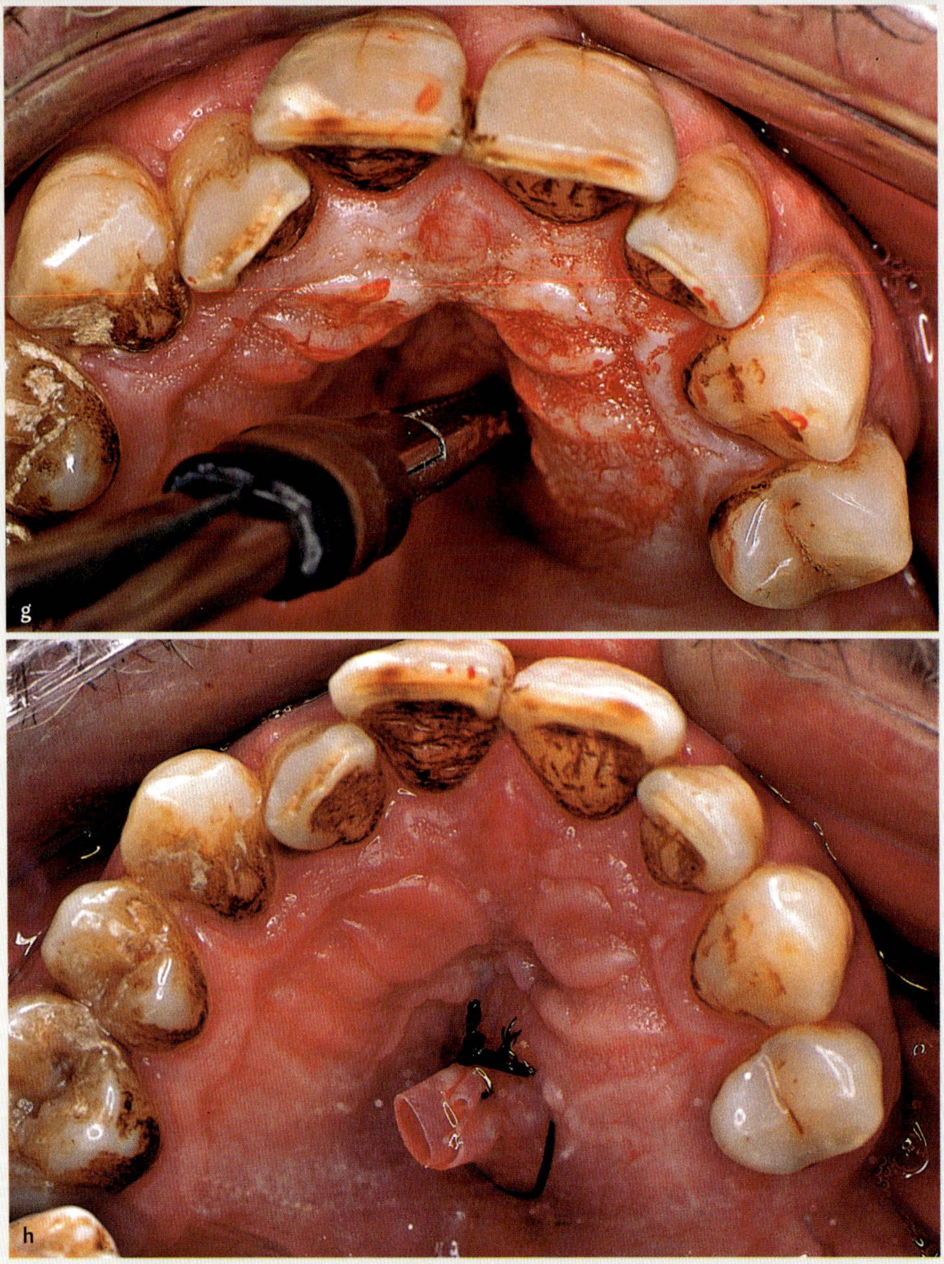

6.26 (*continued*) **e)** Palatal abscess originating in 2.2. **f)** Incision of the abscess and drainage of the purulent material. **g)** Blunt dissection with haemostatic forceps to obtain complete drainage of the abscess. **h)** A surgical drain is positioned to keep the opening pervious.

When fistulae, suppuration and sequestra are present, surgical treatment is mandatory: the infected and necrotic tissues must be removed with a thorough and vigorous curettage until well-vascularised bone is exposed, which is identifiable by active bleeding (absent in necrotic tissue). All sequestra must be removed. If healing is not achieved, more complex techniques such as extensive corticotomy associated with hyperbaric therapy can be used (6.25a-g).

In cases of phlegmon or cellulitis, a well-defined collection of purulent material is typically absent; therefore, surgical drainage is indicated only in cases of complex and diffuse infection. In the other cases, antibiotic therapy and the application of a warm damp compress favours the colliquative evolution of the infectious process: once the purulent material is liquefied, surgical drainage of the resulting abscess can be performed.

Odontogenic sinusitis: the treatment of odontogenic sinusitis follows the same principles described above, and is therefore based on the elimination of the causing agent, the drainage of possible collections of purulent material, and the administration of an antibiotic therapy. If the causing agent is a necrotic tooth, endodontic treatment or extraction allows the cause of the infection to be removed.

Drainage of the purulent material can be performed through the canine fossa, or with a transnasal approach (see Chapter 15 for details).

Two step-by-step clinical cases are presented in 6.27a-h, 6.28a-h.

Clinical case I – Phlegmon of the cheek originating in an infected cyst

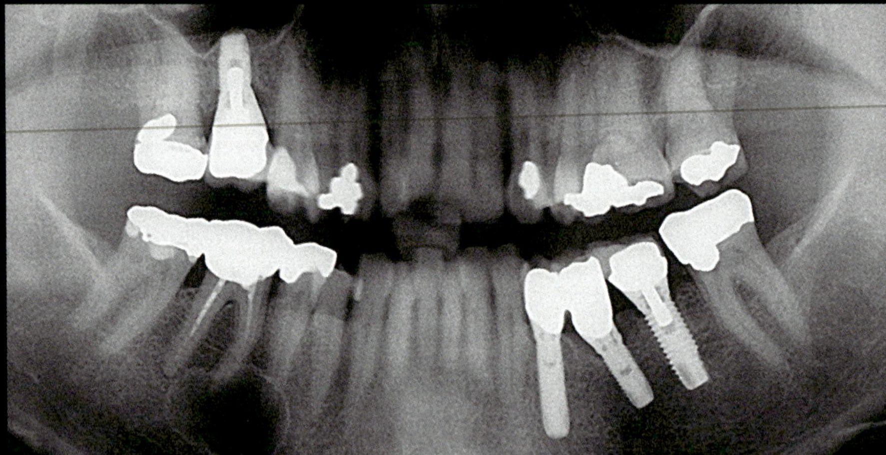

6.27a Panoramic radiograph showing a radiolucent area around the apexes of 4.5 and 4.6: this image is suggestive of odontogenic cyst.

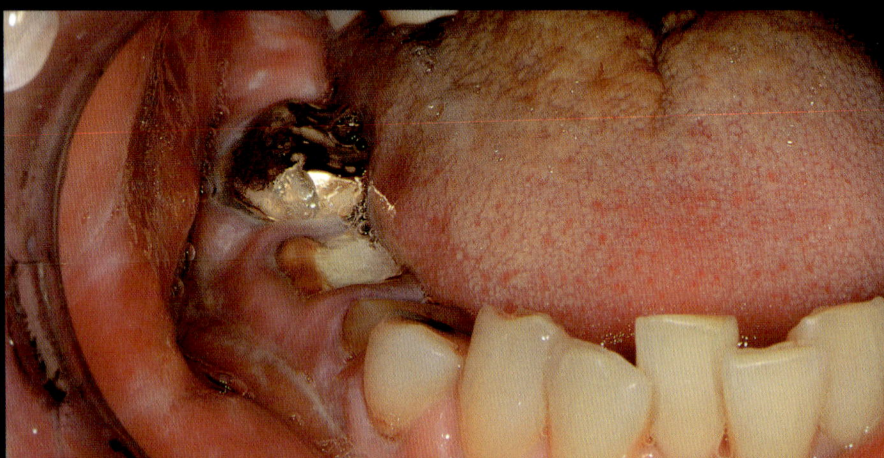

6.27b Intraoral presentation: buccal swelling due to the diffusion of the periapical infection in the buccal soft tissues.

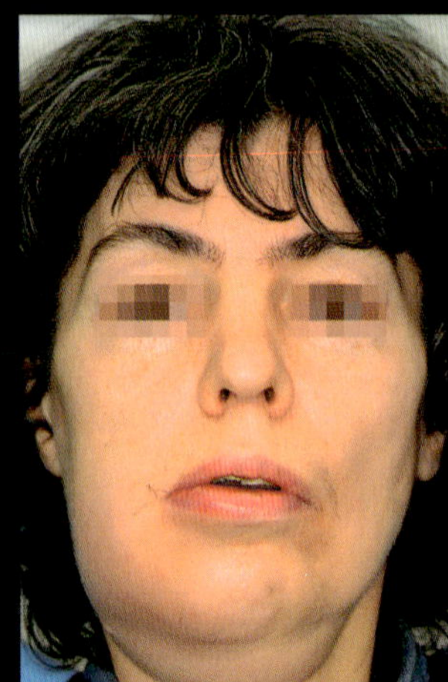

6.27c Extraoral presentation: swelling in the right submental and submandibular regions.

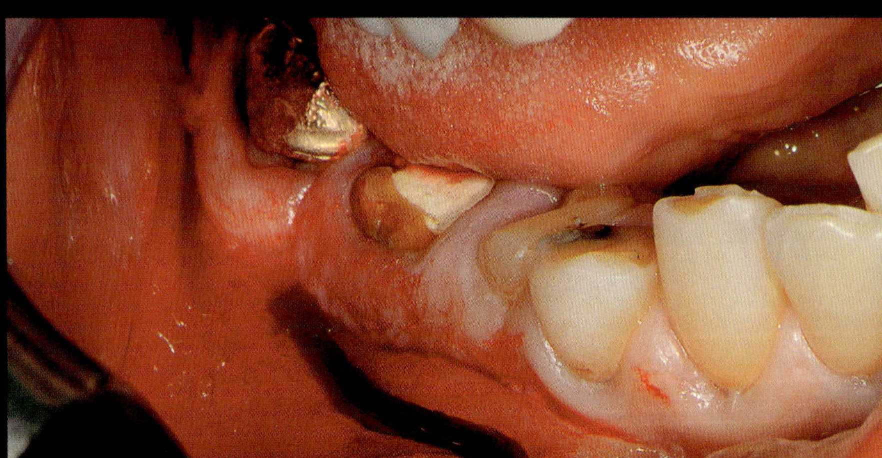

6.27d Drainage of the abscess via a submarginal incision.

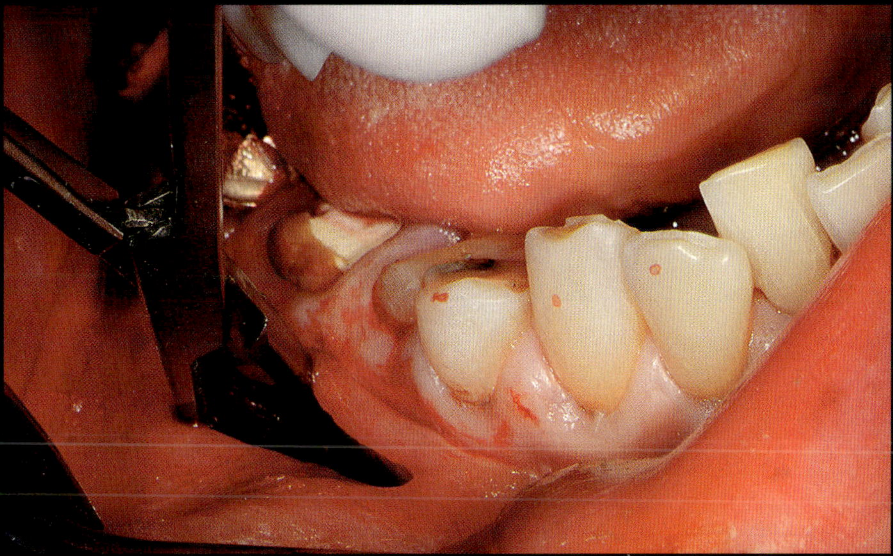

6.27e Blunt dissection with haemostatic forceps.

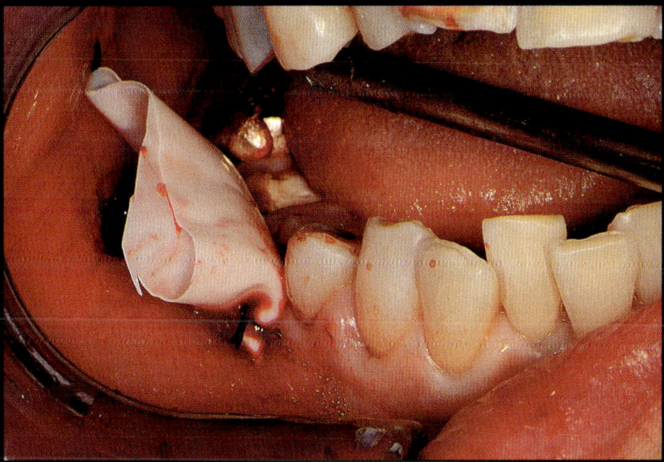

6.27f A surgical drain is fixed in place with a suture.

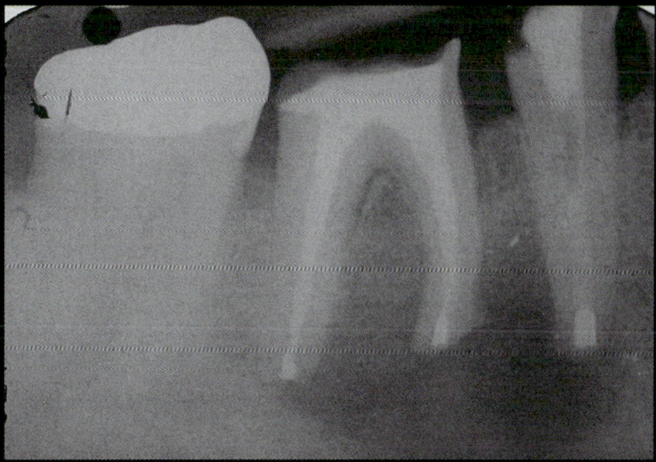

6.27g Radiographic follow-up after the removal of the periapical lesion and the endodontic retreatment and apicoectomy of 4.5 and 4.6.

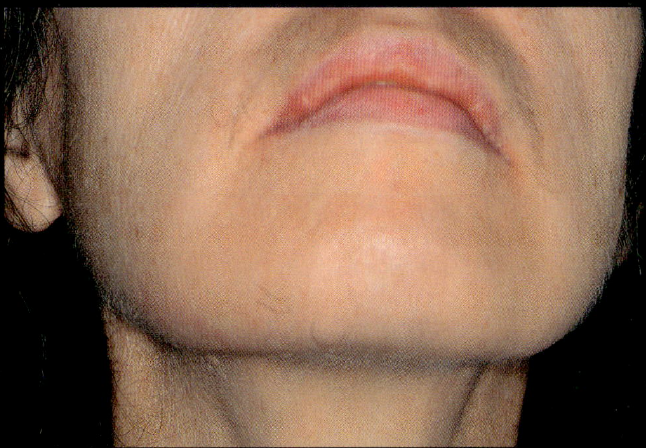

6.27h Clinical follow-up: the absence of swelling in the treated area indicates complete healing.

Clinical case 2 – Extraoral fistulisation of a periapical infection originating in 2.4 and 2.5

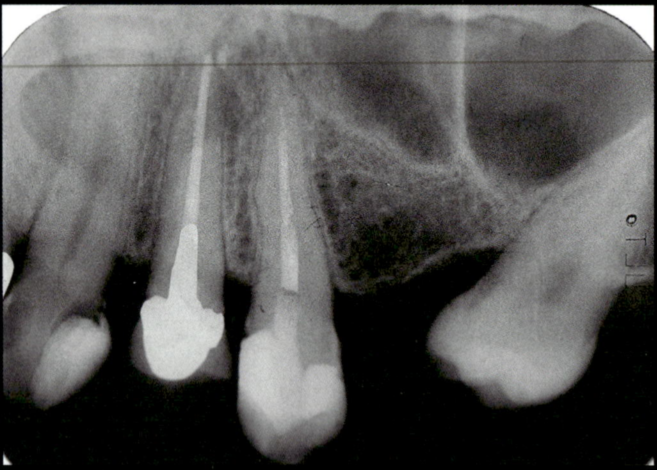

6.28a Periapical radiograph showing a radiolucent area around the apexes of 2.3, 2.4, and 2.5.

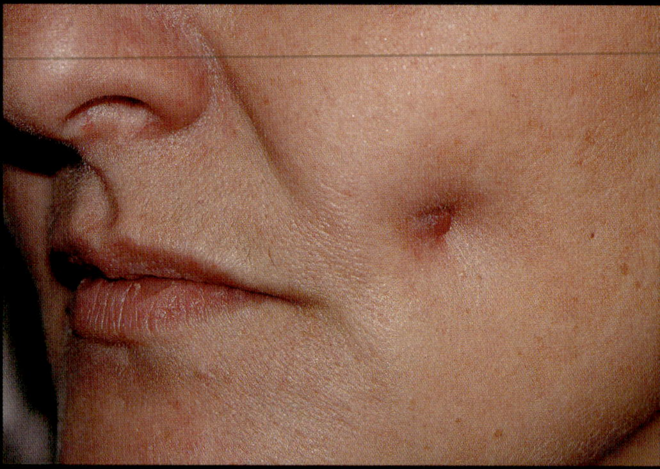

6.28b Extraoral view: presence of a fistula on the cheek.

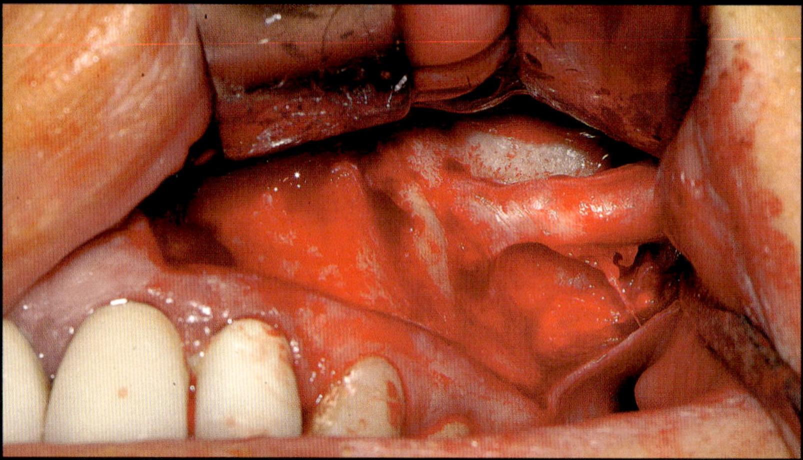

6.28c After the elevation of a full-thickness submarginal flap, the fistula is identified.

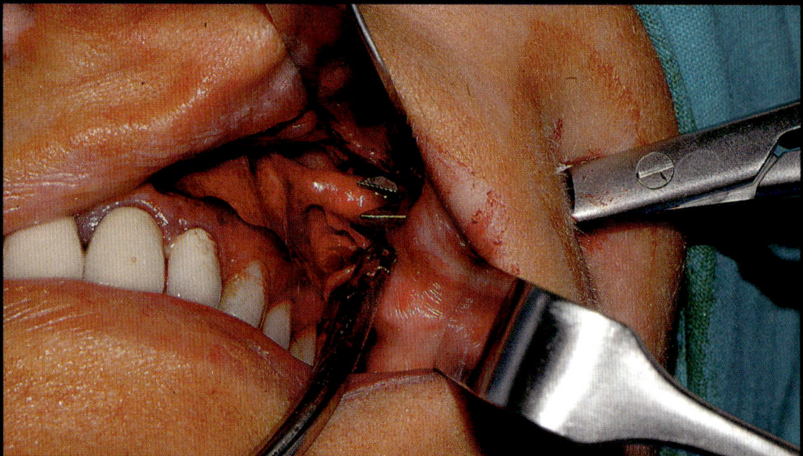

6.28d Isolation of the fistula with a percutaneous approach.

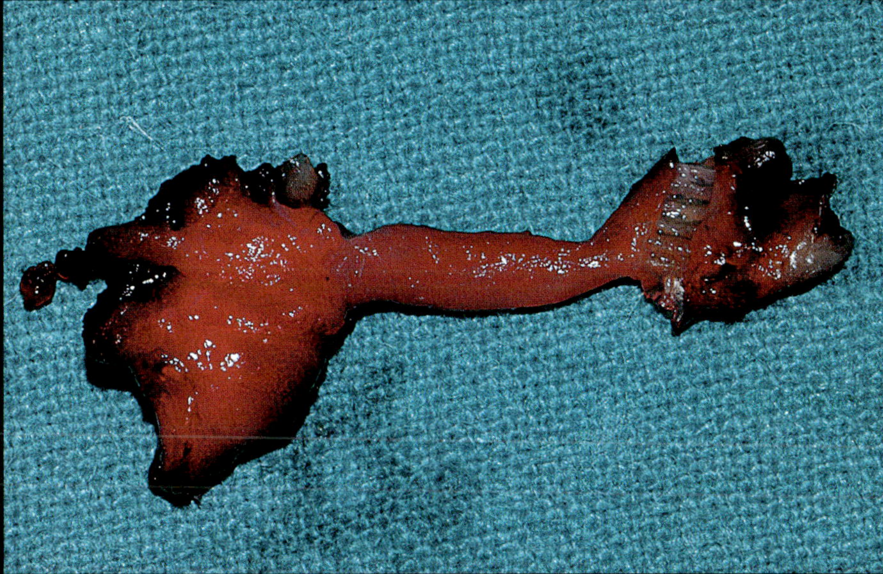

6.28e The fistula and periapical lesion removed.

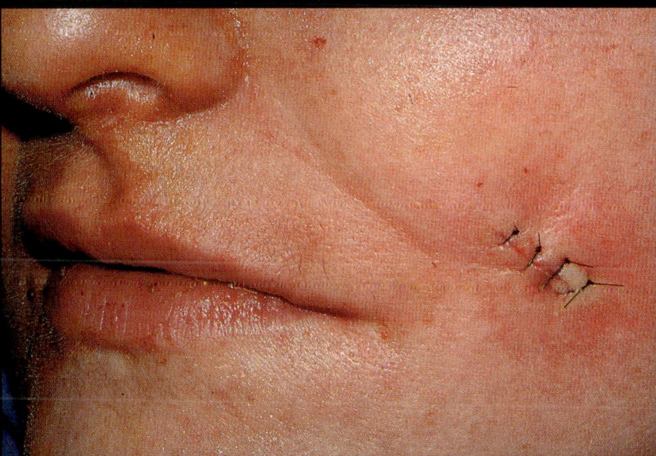

6.28f Extraoral suture.

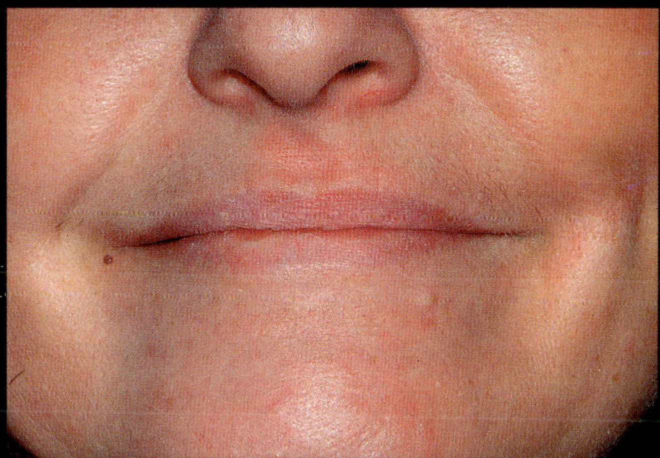

6.28g Clinical follow-up demonstrating complete healing of the facial soft tissues.

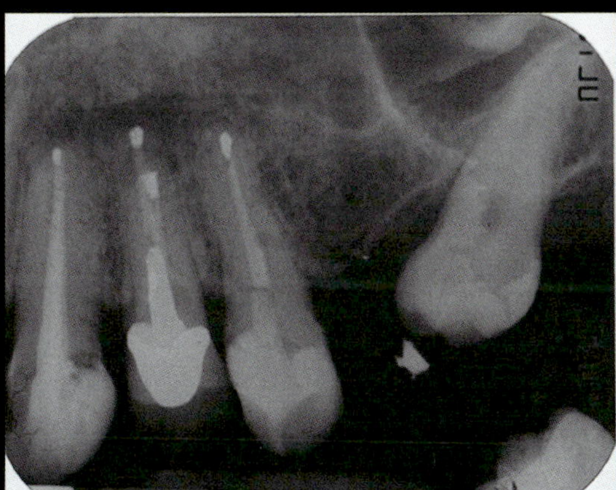

6.28h Radiographic follow-up 12 months after surgery showing ossification of the residual cavity.

REFERENCES

Aderhold L, Knothe H, Frenkel G. The bacteriology of dentogenous pyogenic infections. *Oral Surg* 1981; 52:583-7.

Bartlett JG, O'Keefe P. The bacteriology of perimandibular space infections. *J Oral Surg* 1980; 50:130.

Brusati R, Chiapasco M. Elementi di chirurgia oro-maxillo-facciale. Masson, Milano 1999.

Caccamese JF Jr, Colletti DP. Deep neck infections: clinical considerations in aggressive disease. *Oral Maxillofac Surg Clin North Am* 2008 Aug; 20(3):367-80.

Dennis MJ. Treating odontogenic infections: an update for dental professionals. *Todays FDA* 2006 Mar; 18(3):20-3, 25.

Levi ME, Eusterman VD. Oral infections and antibiotic therapy. *Otolaryngol Clin North Am* 2011 Feb; 44(1):57-78, v.

Levitt GW. Cervical fascia and deep neck infections. *Laryngoscope* 1970; 80:409-35.

Levitt GW. The surgical treatment of the deep neck infections. *Laryngoscope* 1971; 81:403-11.

Novakov IP, Safev GP, Peicheva SE. Descending necrotizing mediastinitis of odontogenic origin-personal experience and literature review. *Folia Med (Plovdiv)* 2012 Jul-Sep; 52(3):13-20.

Peterson LJ, Indresano AT, Marciani RD, Roser SM. Principles of oral and maxillofacial surgery. JB Lippincott Company, Philadelphia 1992.

Sànchez R, Mirada E, Arias J, Pano JR, Burgueno M. Severe odontogenic infections: epidemiological, microbiological and therapeutic factors. *Med Oral Patol Oral Cir Bucal* 2011 Aug 1; 16(5):e670-6.

Worthington P, Evans JR. Controversies in oral and maxillo-facial surgery. WB Saunders, Philadelphia 1994; pp. 381-96.

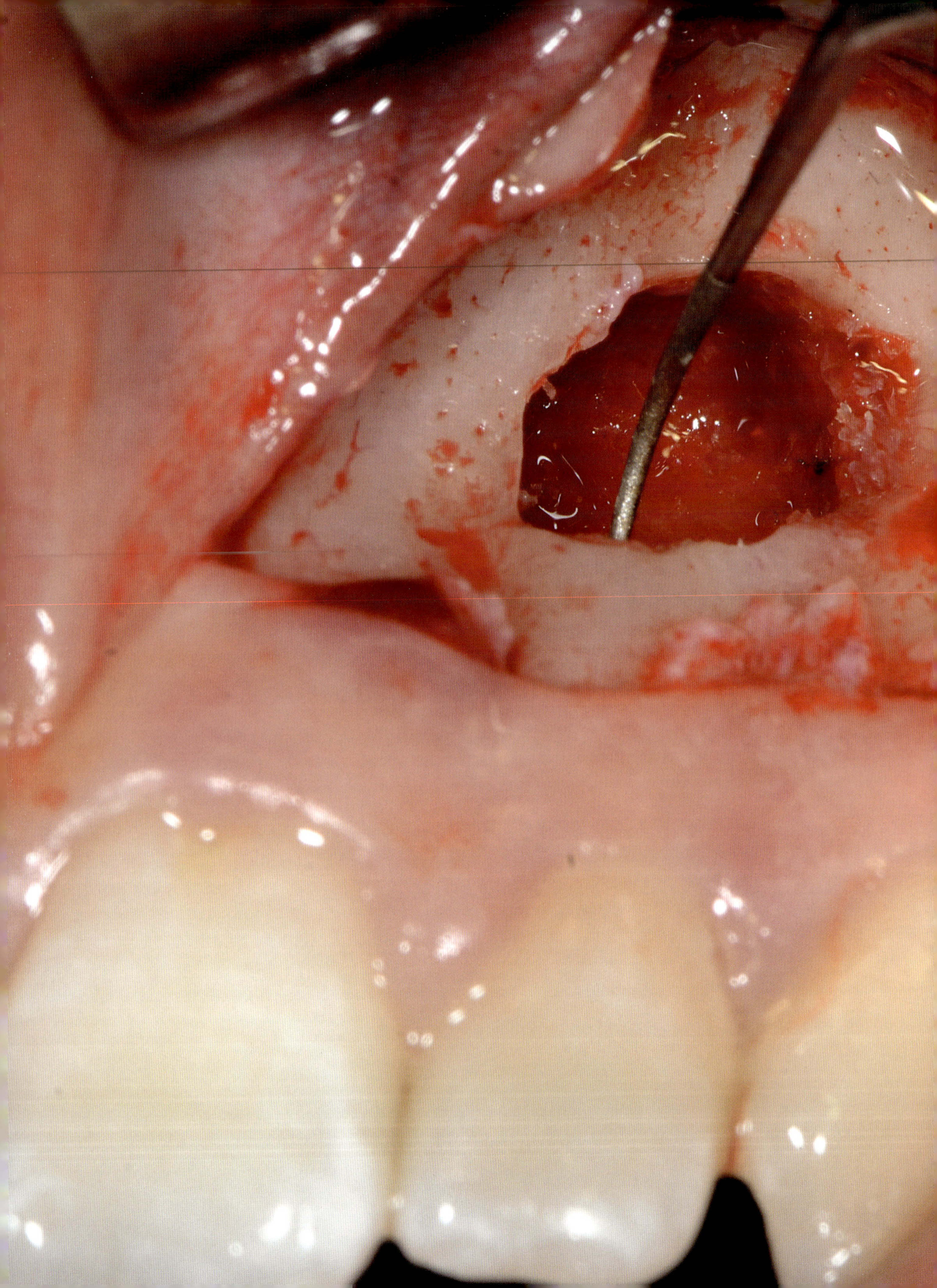

Surgical endodontics

M. Chiapasco ▪ M. Zaniboni ▪ R. Micolani ▪ A. Montinari

Introduction

When periapical and periradicular lesions are not responsive to orthograde endodontic treatment, or when orthograde endodontic treatment or retreatment is impossible (calcified root canals, presence of non-removable cemented endodontic posts or fractured instruments, etc.), surgical endodontics may represent the only treatment option to eliminate the lesion and restore the affected tooth.

Orthograde endodontic therapy, consisting in the elimination of infected and/or necrotic tissues from the root canal system, and the thorough disinfection, shaping and filling of the root canals, is the treatment of choice for pulpar and periapical disease (for details on the etiopathogenesis of these conditions, see Chapter 6 of this book). Surgical endodontics should be considered an extension of the orthograde approach, and not an alternative treatment. Therefore, the recourse to retrograde surgical/endodontic procedures should only be reserved for those cases in which the orthograde treatment, even if conducted *lege artis*, did not attain the resolution of the disease, or for cases in which the orthograde treatment is not a viable option due to the presence of impassable obstacles in the root canal system.

For these reasons, the definition "surgical endodontics" is preferable to "endodontic surgery", because the procedure must be planned and performed like an endodontic treatment performed through a surgical access.

Examination: analysis of signs and symptoms

The degenerative and/or infectious processes affecting the pulpar tissues are frequently accompanied by acute pain, which is exacerbated by pressure/percussion and by sudden temperature variations. However, these symptoms may rapidly disappear in favour of a complete absence of pain, due to the complete degeneration of the nervous structures inside the pulpar tissues. The suspension of pain and other symptoms often leads the patient to believe the episode was a random event, and that its cause found a spontaneous solution. Moreover, in the early phase of the disease, no visible sign of alteration of the bone surrounding the apex of the involved tooth may be shown by any routine radiographic examination (periapical radiograph, panoramic radiograph). Only specific and more detailed radiographic exams (e.g. CBCTs), usually requested with other indications (planning of implant therapy, visualisation of impacted teeth and surrounding structures, etc.), may show early signs of periapical bone radiolucency as a chance finding in the course of evaluations performed for other treatments.

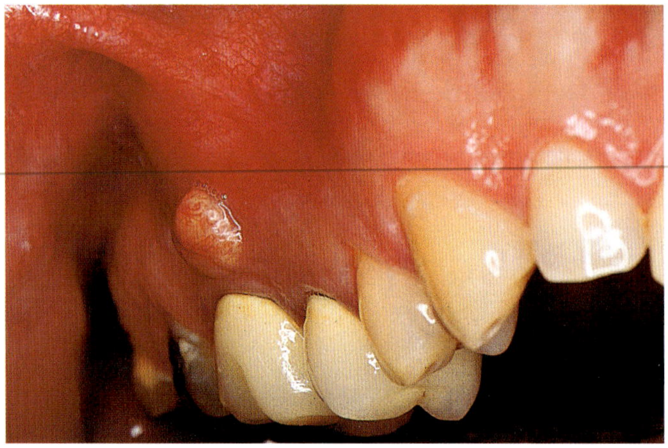

7.1 Intraoral examination shows local soft tissue swelling, in association with the presence of a buccal fistula draining purulent material.

For these reasons, endodontic lesions often have a silent evolution and reveal their presence only in the case of a new acute phase, or when the lesion deforms the cortical walls of the maxilla/mandible, thus determining a visible modification of the normal anatomy. In the latter case, inspection and palpation may lead to the identification of a defined swelling, typically located in the periapical area of the necrotic tooth from which the lesion developed. In cases of a new acute phase of the disease, the formation of a purulent exudate may lead to the resorption of the cortical wall of the maxilla/mandible, with the spontaneous formation of a fistula (see Chapter 6 for further details) (7.1).

However, all the described clinical signs are non-specific, and may also be caused by other conditions, such as a periodontal lesion or root fracture. It is therefore mandatory a thorough evaluation of the tooth and the surrounding tissues be performed: probing should aim to assess the possible involvement of the periodontal tissues in the formation of the lesion, while specific tests should aim to verify if a vertical or horizontal fracture of the root of the tooth is present.

Examination of the tooth: the presence of large restorations, prosthetic rehabilitations, and the discoloration of the tooth may suggest the presence of pulpar disease; this event can be verified with the aid of vitality and percussion tests. Generally, a tooth with periapical disease does not respond to thermal stimulation (e.g. cold test), while percussion with a rigid, blunt instrument elicits pain. Mobility of the tooth may suggest periodontal involvement in the process.

Symptoms: in the presence of a new acute phase of the periapical disease, spontaneous pain exacerbated by chewing may be present, due to the compression exerted on the infected tissue. The lesion may also fistulate on the buccal side, on the palatal side, on the lingual side, or on the skin of the cheek or neck, determining the spontaneous drainage of purulent material.

Radiographic examinations

Radiographically, periapical lesions appear as radiolucent areas (caused by the process of bone lysis and subsequent rarefaction); generally, these areas have a round or oval shape, well-defined margins, and are associated to one or more root apexes.

The routine exam for the evaluation of periapical lesions has always been the periapical radiograph, due to its superior definition compared to the panoramic radiograph (7.2).

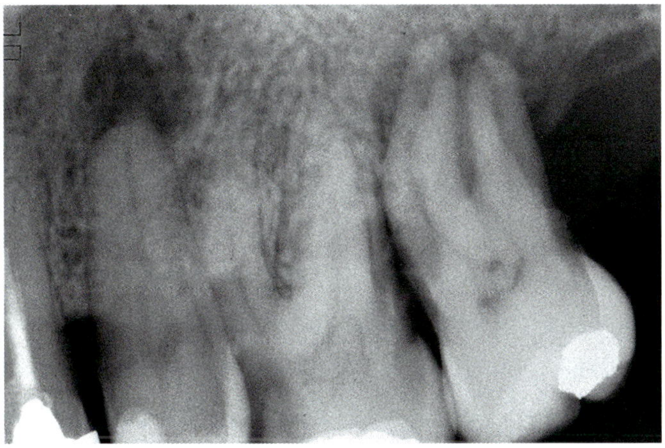

7.2 Periapical radiograph showing the presence of apical lesions caused by pulpar necrosis of 2.5 and 2.7.

However, it is worth remembering that periapical disease in its early (acute) phase may not be confirmed by standard radiographic examination because, frequently, no evident signs of radiolucency are visible in periapical radiographs. Therefore, clinical examination should guide the clinician to the correct diagnosis of the condition.

If a fistula is detected in the course of clinical examination, then a periapical radiograph can be taken with a gutta percha cone inserted into the fistula tract: the radiopaque cone can give valuable information on fistula length and course, and its relationship with the tooth from which the lesion originates.

Recent years have seen a growing recourse to the use of CBCTs for the early diagnosis of periapical lesions. This exam allows the tridimensional evaluation of the alveolar process and dental roots, thus eliminating the limitations caused by the overlaying of anatomical structures that is typical of bidimensional radiographic exams. Moreover, it offers valuable information on the dimensions, development, and tridimensional relationships of the lesion with the surrounding anatomical structures. This latter aspect is of utmost importance particularly in the presence of an evolution of the periapical lesion into a large cyst, with the involvement of neighbouring structures that must be preserved (neurovascular bundles, nasal and paranasal cavities, etc.).

Nonetheless, it is worth noting that periapical lesions, like any other neoplasm, may be detected by means of radiographs, but these exams allow only for a presumptive diagnosis, which must then be confirmed by means of a histopathological examination.

Indications

As a rule, limitations and failures of orthograde endodontic therapy represent the indications of surgical retrograde treatment. These indications can be summarised as follows:

ANATOMIC

Apical delta: the shaping and disinfection of the root canal system are fundamental phases of the orthograde endodontic therapy. Nevertheless, the mechanical action of endodontic instruments permits the shaping and cleansing of only a part of the entire root canal system, while the disinfection of lateral/accessory canals and apical delta is delegated to the action of irrigants.

One of the main causes of failure in endodontic therapy is, in fact, the presence of infected leftovers in the lateral canals, which are numerous especially in the apical third of the root. When orthograde therapy, however meticulously performed, does not lead to complete healing, a surgical approach is indicated. The procedure includes apicoectomy, which is the removal of the root apex with its apical delta; with its high density of fine accessory canals, the apical delta is the region in which the presence of bacteria and necrotic leftovers is more frequent.

Curved roots and calcifications: the wide anatomical variability of the root canal system often complicates orthograde therapy, and adequate treatment may become difficult. The root canals may present with strictures or obstructions (partial or total) of their lumen, due to the deposition of secondary dentine. In some cases, calcifications, pulpar stones, or sharp curves of the root may render the completion of a correct orthograde treatment impossible.

Root resorption and open immature apexes: both the conical shaping and the filling of the root canal system may be difficult, imprecise, or impossible in the presence of internal root resorption or open immature root apexes (📷 7.3).

IATROGENIC

Fractured instruments: an endodontic instrument, either manual or rotating, may break while used for root canal shaping, especially if the same instrument is used several times for the shaping of curved root canals. If the fractured portion of the instrument is stuck in the apical third of the root, or if it is stuck inside the root canal in such a way that it is not possible to remove it without damaging the root, the completion of an adequate orthograde treatment is not possible. In these events, the recourse to a retrograde surgical approach may allow the portion of the root apical to the fractured instrument to be treated (📷 7.4).

Ledge formation and perforation: ledge formation and perforation of the apical third of the root can, in some cases, be successfully treated with appropriate techniques and materials with the aim of sealing them. When this treatment modality is not applicable, or if it has prevented complete healing of the periapical lesion, the recourse to the surgical approach is indicated (📷 7.5).

Apical transportation: incongruous root canal shaping manoeuvres, often favoured by improper use of rotary instruments, can cause anatomical alterations of the canal, and lead either to its external transportation or to the inversion of the internal apical architecture. In these events, it may be difficult or impossible to obtain an adequate filling of the canal lumen and a competent apical seal, because a transported apex cannot guarantee any form of resistance either to the pressure of the filling material (thus determining an uncontrolled overflow) or to the reflux of fluids from the periodontal space.

Apical overflow: the extrusion of infected/necrotic or endodontic materials from the apex may cause periapical lesions. Either an infectious focus or a foreign body (e.g. gutta percha) can support an inflammatory reaction. Dispersed materials can only be removed with a surgical approach (📷 7.6).

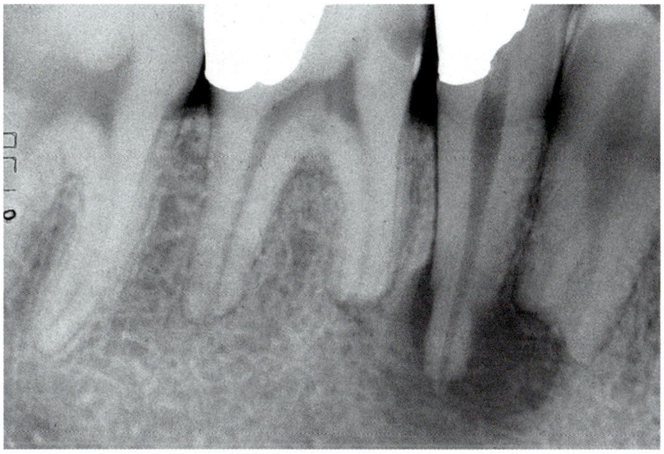

7.3 Root resorption (4.4) in association with the presence of a periapical lesion involving both 4.4 and 4.5.

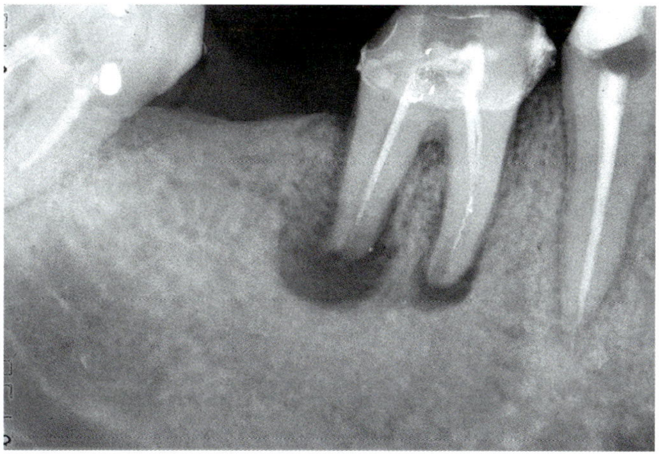

7.4 Periapical lesion (4.6) in association with the presence of a fractured endodontic instrument inside the canal of the mesial root, which hinders orthograde retreatment.

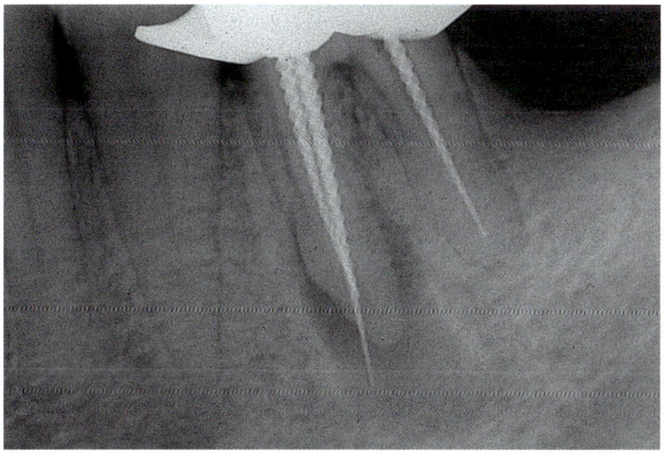

7.5 Ledge formation in the mesial root canal of 3.6.

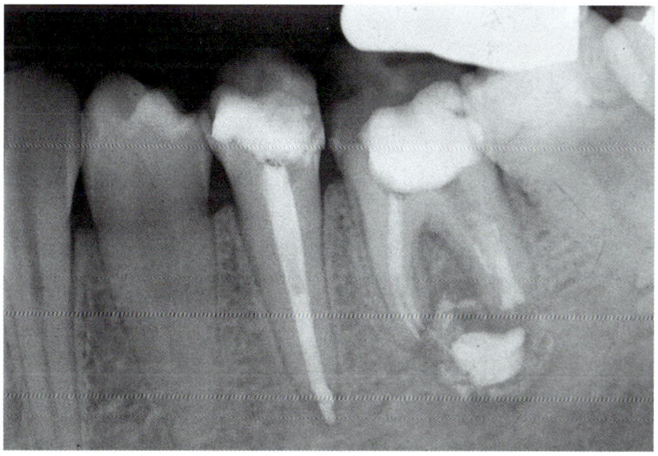

7.6 Apical extrusion of endodontic material determining chronic infection in the periapical area of 3.6.

Presence of non-removable materials inside the root canal: in cases of periapical infection, the presence of non-removable materials (e.g. insoluble cements, cemented posts) inside the root canal may render the standard orthograde treatment impossible.

PROSTHETIC

Endodontic posts: the removal of cemented endodontic posts or Richmond-type crowns, which may allow an orthograde retreatment to be performed, can be difficult and expose to a high risk of root fracture. In this case, it is safer to resort directly to the surgical retrograde approach. However, it is worth noting that the choice to perform only a retrograde treatment exposes to a non-negligible risk of failure; for this reason, it is always advisable to evaluate with great care the opportunities and the appropriate methods to safely remove endodontic posts whenever this is possible, and retreat the root canal with an orthograde approach.

Abutment teeth supporting fixed prosthetic rehabilitations: if the orthograde endodontic treatment performed before prosthetic rehabilitation appears to be radiographically congruous, radiolucent lesions associated with the abutment teeth can be treated with a surgical approach, to avoid perforation of the crown that would be necessary to perform an orthograde retreatment. On the other hand, it is worth noting that several techniques are available to remove fixed prosthetic rehabilitations without significant damage to the supporting structures, and it is currently a rare occurrence that a fixed prosthetic rehabilitation impedes the orthograde retreatment of abutment teeth.

TRAUMATIC

If a trauma has caused a fracture in the apical third of the root, it may be possible to avoid extraction by performing an orthograde treatment of the tooth, and the surgical removal of the apical (fractured) fragment. The latter, in fact, even if correctly treated via the orthograde approach, would nonetheless act as a foreign body.

RADICULAR (PERIAPICAL) CYSTS

Radicular (periapical) cysts may completely regress following orthograde endodontic treatment (or retreatment). However, the approach of choice for the treatment of these lesions, particularly the larger ones, is surgical removal (see Chapter 8 for details).

Surgical endodontics

Indications

- Anatomic
  - complex anatomy of the apical delta
  - curved roots
  - calcifications
  - root resorption and open immature apexes
- Iatrogenic
  - fractured instruments
  - ledge formation and root perforation
  - apical transportation
  - apical overflow
  - insoluble endodontic cements
- Prosthetic
  - endodontic posts
  - abutment teeth
- Traumatic
- Radicular (periapical) cysts

Contraindications

- Local
  - severe periodontal lesions
  - limited bone support
  - vertical fractures
  - unfavourable cost-benefit ratio
  - anatomic (high risk of damaging nerves/vessels)
  - difficult access to the periapical area
- Systemic
  - cardiovascular disease
  - diabetes
  - liver disease
  - pregnancy
  - alterations of the immune system

Contraindications

LOCAL

Endodontic: an evidently incongruous orthograde therapy represents a contraindication for retrograde surgery, because even if the surgical treatment is correctly performed, the outcome can be hindered by the presence of infectious/necrotic leftovers coronally to the apical seal obtained. Therefore, in these cases it is always indicated to perform an orthograde retreatment, if no insurmountable obstacles are present (anatomic, iatrogenic).

Periodontal: the presence of severe periodontal lesions associated to periapical lesions of endodontic origin significantly impairs the prognosis of the involved teeth. For this reason, deep probing, particularly when associated to tooth mobility, represents an absolute contraindication to surgical retrograde treatment.

Unfavourable crown-root ratio: apicoectomy, even when conducted in a very "conservative" way, reduces the overall support of the tooth and alters the crown-root ratio. This alteration may lead to a risk of tooth mobility and loss, in particular when the roots are relatively short and the crowns, on the other hand, are large.

Vertical fractures: the presence of a vertical fracture in a root (or tooth) is a clear indication for extraction, because no treatment of these lesions is possible. Moreover, the presence of a vertical fracture causes damage to the pulp and to the supporting periodontal tissues, which, ultimately, leads to the loss of the involved teeth (7.7a-b).

Cost-benefit ratio: the choice of a retrograde surgical approach should always be considered in the light of the possibility to obtain a more favourable cost-benefit ratio for the patient, both from a biological and from an economic point of view. Therefore, in recent years, the recourse to surgical endodontics has been primarily aimed at salvaging teeth

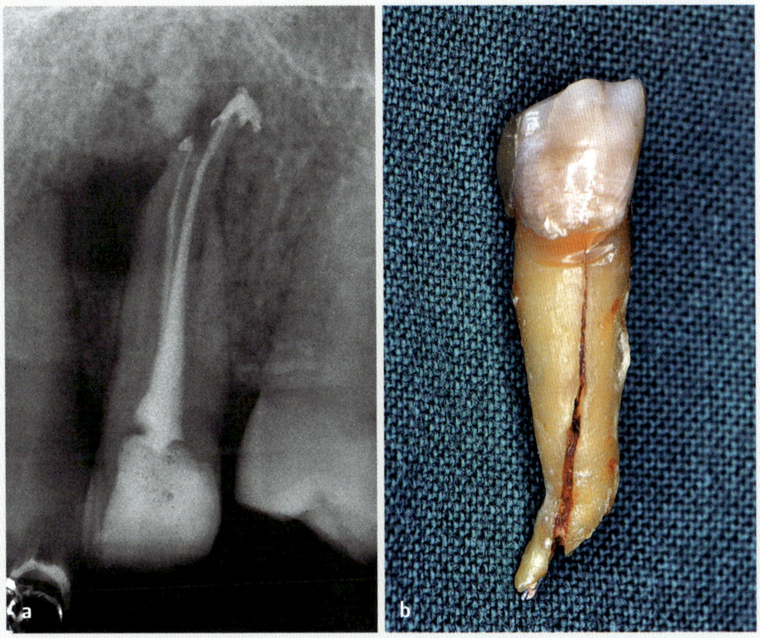

7.7 Vertical root fracture of 2.3: **a)** radiographic image; **b)** clinical view of the extracted tooth.

that have a strategic importance from the aesthetic viewpoint (incisors, cuspids). On the other hand, when the relationship between success rates, costs, and benefits is unfavourable, as it often is for posterior teeth (premolars and molars), it is preferable to extract the involved tooth and to replace it with a fixed prosthetic element supported by either natural abutments or implants.

Anatomic: the retrograde surgical approach is contraindicated whenever there is a significant risk of damage to nearby relevant anatomic structures, such as nerves and blood vessels.

Difficult access to the periapical area: the periapical area of posterior teeth (in particular, the second molar) may be difficult to reach, particularly in patients with temporomandibular joint disorders, or with a reduced mouth opening capacity. In these cases, surgical manoeuvres are more difficult and adequate control of the surgical field may be impossible. Therefore, the success rate of the procedure can be significantly lower. If this is the case, extraction of the involved tooth should be considered as a preferable option.

SYSTEMIC

Details on the systemic conditions that contraindicate surgical treatments are reported in Chapter 1.

Surgical treatment

The retrograde surgical approach can be managed in two possible ways, based on the timing of the treatment phases. It is possible to perform a retrograde surgical treatment after an orthograde endodontic treatment has been performed with success, or it is possible to perform both an orthograde and a surgical retrograde treatment in the same session.

APICOECTOMY AND RETROGRADE FILLING AFTER ORTHOGRADE ENDODONTIC THERAPY

It is the most frequently used and well-documented of the two treatment modalities. The procedure consists of the surgical removal of the periapical lesion, the resection and removal of the root apex involved in the lesion (apicoectomy), and the preparation and sealing of the apical portion of the root canal with dedicated materials (retrograde filling). Contrary to what was proposed in the past by some authors, the sole apical resection and bone curettage of the periapical cavity, with no recourse to retrograde root canal preparation and sealing, does not guarantee reliable long-term results. Indeed, the anatomic irregularity of the new apex, and the contraction of the orthograde filling material (gutta percha) during its cooling phase, may cause the presence of gaps that, if not eliminated with the retrograde preparation of the apical portion of the root canal and its retrograde filling, will be re-infiltrated after a few hours.

SIMULTANEOUS APICOECTOMY AND RETROGRADE ROOT CANAL PREPARATION AND FILLING

In this case, the orthograde endodontic treatment is performed at the same time as the surgical phase. Therefore, a full-thickness mucoperiosteal flap is elevated, an osteotomic access to the lesion is created, and the lesion is removed. Next, a complete orthograde endodontic treatment (access to the pulpal spaces, removal of the pulp, disinfection, shaping and filling of the root canals) is performed. Lastly, the resection of the apex, the retrograde preparation of the apical portion of the root canal, and the sealing of the prepared cavity are completed.

However, this treatment modality has precise indications:

- root canals for which it is impossible to obtain an adequate cleaning, drying, and sealing via the orthograde approach;
- fracture of rotary or manual endodontic instruments, when it is impossible either to retrieve or to bypass the fractured portion of the instrument;
- interruption of pulpal neurovascular bundles in the course of maxillary sinus surgery (chronic sinusitis, sinusal cysts, etc.), when the roots protrude inside the sinusal cavity;
- periapical lesions in non-cooperative patients who are to be treated under general anaesthesia (odontophobic or disabled patients).

In the past a third approach, abandoned today due to the significant failure rates, was proposed by some authors: according to this protocol, the retrograde surgical therapy represented the first phase of the treatment, while the orthograde endodontic therapy was performed at a later stage. The negative outcomes reported for this approach are due to the placement of an apical seal in root canals that still contain infectious/necrotic material, and to the possibility of damaging the apical seal during the orthograde treatment.

Surgical armamentarium

The basic surgical armamentarium for retrograde surgical endodontics is the same described for basic oral surgery interventions (for details, see specific section in Chapter 3), while some instruments are peculiar to this type of surgery:

- piezoelectric ultrasonic device (control unit and handpiece);
- diamond-coated ultrasonic tips specifically designed for retrograde cavity preparation (retrotip);
- specific carriers for the filling materials used to seal the retrograde cavity;
- specifically shaped apical pluggers and burnishers used to pack the retrograde cavity;
- micro-mirrors used to verify the cavity preparation and seal;
- carbide finishing burs used for the fine shaping of the new apex;
- paper points used for the drying of the retrograde cavity prior to the application of filling materials;
- spatulas and mixing pads used to prepare the filling materials for use;
- magnifying visual devices for medical use (medical loupes, surgical microscopes);
- coaxial light sources.

The introduction of magnifying systems (particularly in association with coaxial light sources) represents one of the most significant advancements in surgical endodontics. The use of such devices provides a detailed view of even the finest anatomic details, thus permitting greater control of the surgical field and precise verification of the apical seal. In particular, the use of light sources integrated with the magnification systems guarantees a better intraoperative visualisation of all areas by eliminating problems related to the visual interferences and to the presence of shadows in a small surgical field (7.8a–c).

However, it is worth noting that the use of magnification devices may cause an increase in operating time due to the fact that:

- magnification provides a view of the area of interest with the exclusion of all the surroundings; this causes the reduction of the field of view and the depth of the field. Therefore, the surgeon will have to be specifically trained to get used to these aspects, and the support of an expert assistant is advisable to allow the operator to always keep his/her eyes on the surgical field;

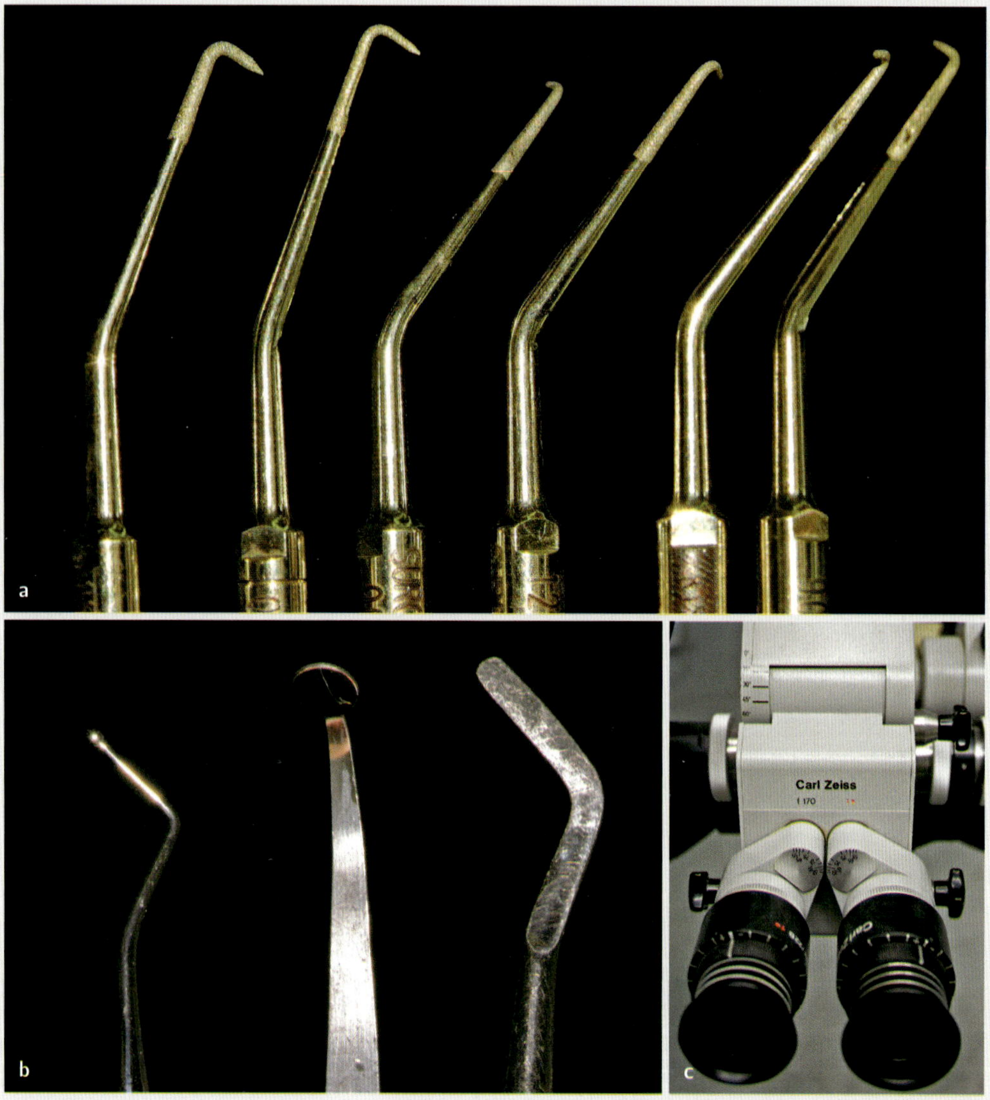

7.8 **a)** Specific surgical instruments for endodontic surgery: ultrasonic inserts. **b)** Burnisher, micro-mirror and Heidemann spatula. **c)** Operating microscope

- according to the correct technique, the microscope should be in a fixed position during the entire session, but the patient can (even involuntarily) make small movements or little adjustments to his own posture. These movements, with such a limited operating field, should be avoided as much as possible, as they disturb the operator.

Locoregional anaesthesia

Criteria regarding the anaesthesia protocols for surgical retrograde treatments are mainly based on the location of the lesion, and follow the same guidelines reported in detail in Chapter 3.

Surgical flap design

The possibility of performing a retrograde surgical treatment in a clean and controlled way, as with any other surgical specialty, relies heavily on the choice and preparation of an adequate surgical access. The flap of choice must guarantee an optimal view of the surgical field (bone, roots involved in the lesion), and must always be wider than the area of intervention. In particular, it must always be wider than the osteotomic window created to gain access to the involved roots in such a way that, once the flap is closed, the sutured incisions lie on untouched bone: this is important to avoid the risk of wound dehiscence. The choice of the type of flap (marginal, paramarginal, with or without vertical releasing incisions) depends on the clinical situation and follows the guidelines detailed in the chapter regarding the general principles in oral surgery.

However, some clarifications may be appropriate:

The surgical access is always performed on the buccal side, except in cases where apicoectomy of the palatal root of maxillary molars is needed and the buccal approach to the root is difficult or impossible. In this event, a palatal approach is indicated.

Marginal (sulcular) flaps (📷 7.9a) are particularly indicated:

- when periapical lesions have developed coronally, to avoid suturing the flap in the absence of an adequate support from the underlying bone wall;
- in the presence of frenula;
- in the presence of teeth with reduced periodontal support (due to bone resorption) or when a vertical fracture of the root is suspected, as these conditions represent an indication for extraction.

Paramarginal (submarginal) flaps may be used to avoid the involvement of the marginal periodontal tissues (keratinised mucosa, papillae) in the surgical manoeuvres, such as incision and elevation. Indications to the use of these flaps are:

- presence of teeth bearing fixed prosthetic rehabilitations (crowns, bridges), to avoid gingival retraction and exposure of the prosthetic margin;
- presence of teeth with no concomitant periodontal lesions.

Limitations to the use of paramarginal flaps are represented by the possible formation of visible scars, and by the presence of frenula in the area.

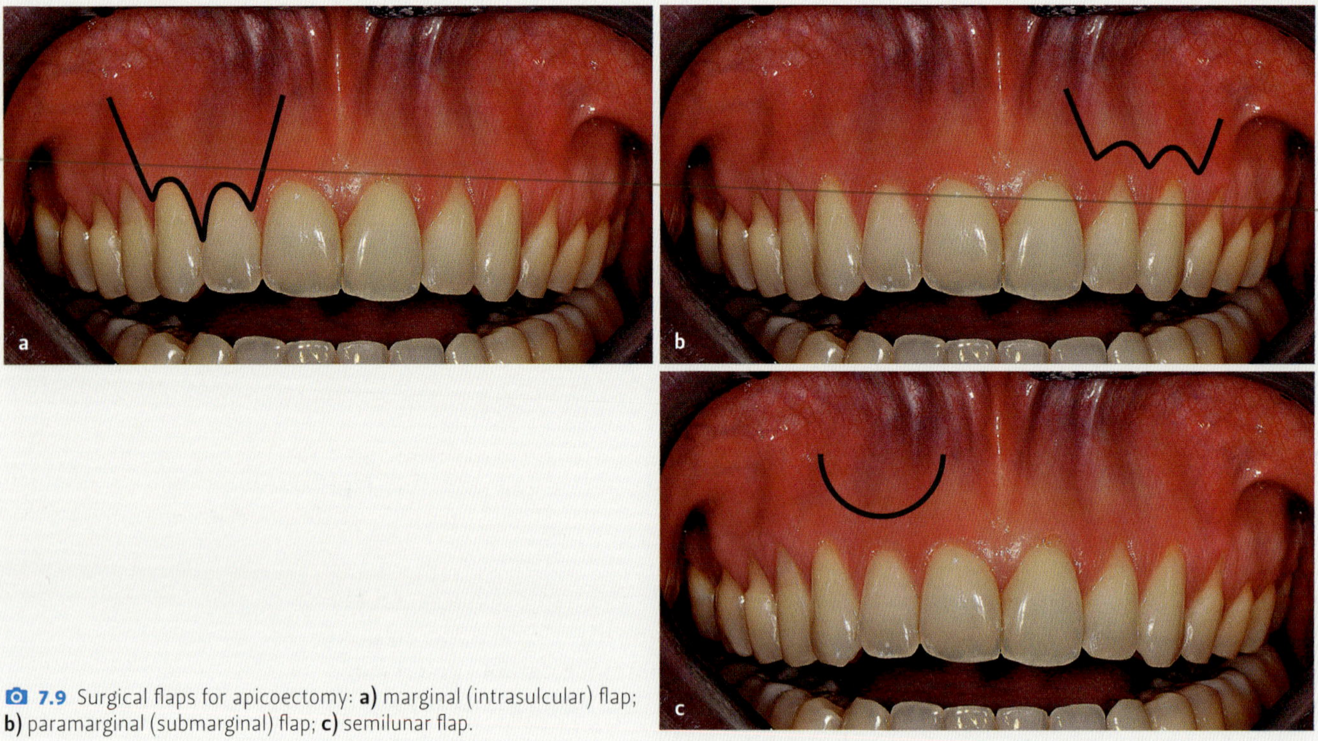

7.9 Surgical flaps for apicoectomy: **a)** marginal (intrasulcular) flap; **b)** paramarginal (submarginal) flap; **c)** semilunar flap.

The design of paramarginal flaps often requests one or two vertical releasing incisions (7.9b) but, in cases of surgical endodontics, it is possible to adopt a peculiar type of paramarginal flap called the semilunar flap. This flap, albeit outlined with a single incision, allows the creation of an adequate surgical field when a few teeth (one or two) are involved in the periapical lesion (7.9c).

Locating root apex and ostectomy

The technique used to locate the root apex is influenced by the characteristics of the bone surrounding the lesion. A possible interruption of the bony wall in the area of the periapical lesion may be identified by palpation, when complete erosion of the cortical plate has occurred. In this case, the breach created by the lesion can be extended by means of rotating instruments (burs mounted on a straight handpiece), piezoelectric instruments (dedicated inserts mounted on ultrasonic handpiece), or manual instruments (curettes, surgical spoons/curettes).

When the cortical walls are intact, preoperative and intraoperative investigations are needed to verify with due accuracy the ideal positioning of the surgical osteotomy to be made. The procedure includes:

- root length measurement based on periapical radiographs taken with the parallel rays technique;
- the measured length is then transferred on the surgical field by means of a periodontal probe or surgical callipers, and a pilot hole is drilled on the cortical wall at the measured height;
- a sterile piece of gutta percha or metal foil is placed into the pilot hole and a second periapical radiograph is taken to confirm the accuracy of the measured height.

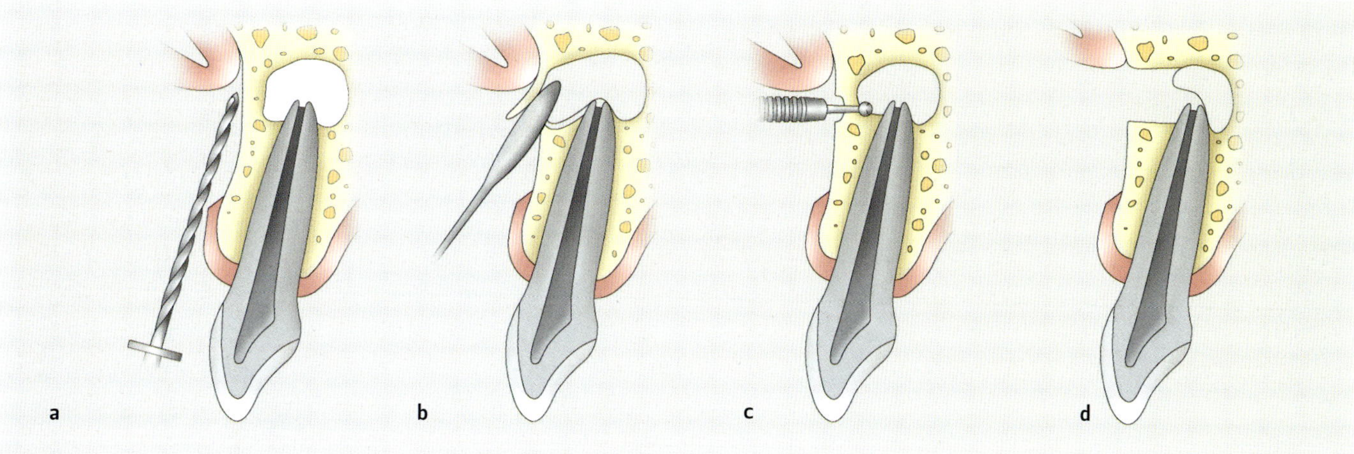

7.10 Root apex identification and ostectomy: **a)** root apex identification is obtained by measuring the length of the root on a periapical radiograph taken with the parallel rays technique and transferring it to the surgical field by means of an endodontic file; **b)** when the lesion has eroded the cortical plate, the thin layer of residual bone may be removed with manual instruments; **c)** if the cortical plate is sound, ostectomy may be performed with a round bur mounted on a straight handpiece; **d)** the root apex and the periapical lesion are identified.

Once the location of the lesion is confirmed, the pilot hole is extended with a round bur mounted on a straight handpiece or with piezoelectric instruments, under continuous irrigation of refrigerated sterile saline (7.10a-d). It is worth noting that the surgical breach on the cortical wall should be large enough to allow adequate access to the root apex and the complete removal of the lesion, but care must be taken to avoid excessive ostectomy, which may significantly reduce bone support around the involved roots.

Enucleation of the lesion and curettage of the cavity

Once the surgical access on the cortical wall is created and the lesion is exposed, it can be cleaved from the surrounding bone by means of surgical curettes and completely enucleated, to allow complete exposure of the root apex. If the lesion is firmly attached to the apex, it is indicated to completely separate the cyst wall from the surrounding bone, proceed by sectioning the apex, and remove it together with the lesion, to avoid any tearing of the cyst wall and to allow the complete removal of the lesion. A thorough curettage of the residual cavity and the portion of the root protruding into it are mandatory. In fact, healing of endodontic lesions cannot be obtained with the surgical removal of inflamed tissues alone, but a complete elimination of contaminants from the root canal system is also necessary (7.11a-d).

To obtain a competent apical seal it is paramount to keep the surgical field as dry as possible. Since the complete removal of the periapical lesion may cause bleeding from the walls of the bone cavity, it can be performed after apicoectomy and retrograde filling are completed; to access the root apex, it is sufficient to remove the exposed portion of the wall of the lesion.

Apicoectomy

The root apex is sectioned to:

- eliminate the most anatomically intricate portion of the root, in which infectious material is more frequently located;
- expose the root canal to facilitate the preparation of the retrograde cavity and its filling.

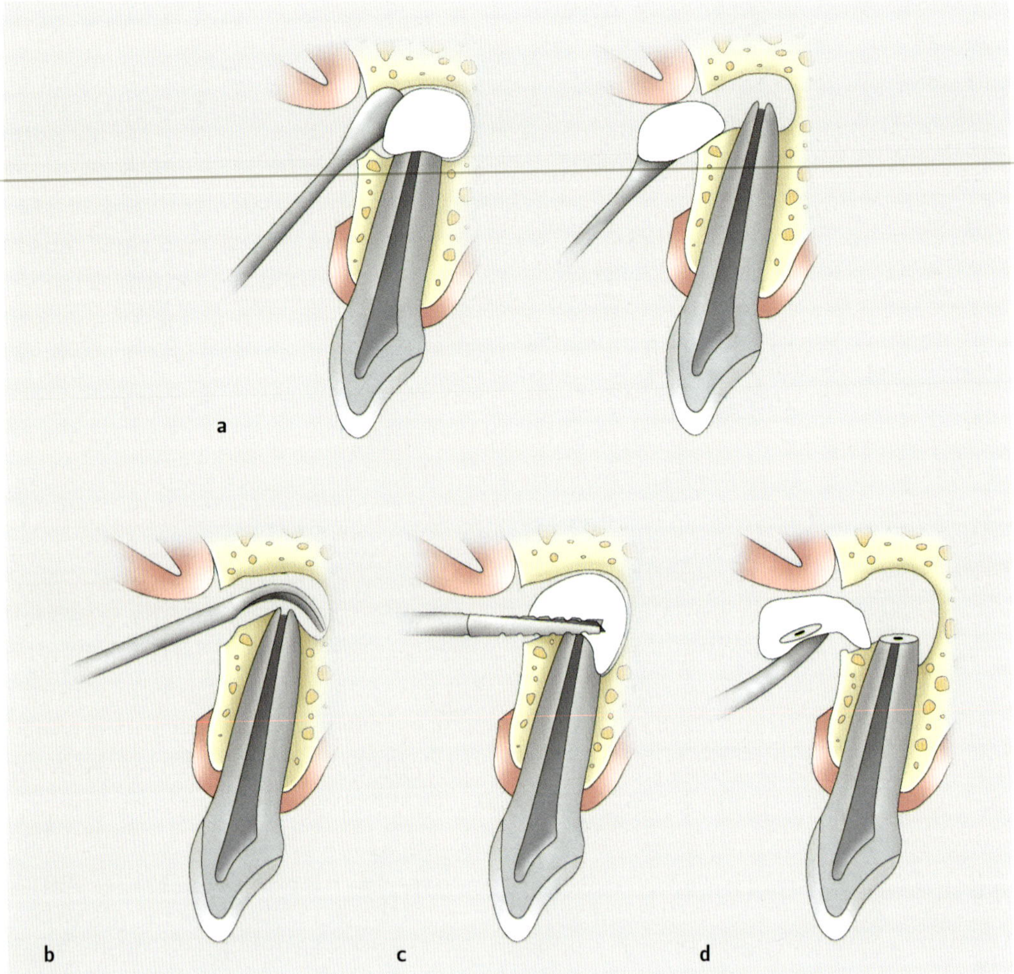

7.11 Enucleation of the periapical lesion and curettage: **a)** the lesion is cleaved from the bony walls of the cavity with the aid of surgical spoons/curettes; **b)** thorough curettage of the surrounding bone is performed; **c–d)** when the lesion is firmly attached to the apex, it may be advisable to section the apex before cleaving the lesion from the cavity walls, and remove them together.

The sectioning of the root apex may be performed with rotary (fissure bur mounted on a straight handpiece) or piezoelectric instruments (rhizotomy inserts mounted on ultrasonic handpiece) under continuous irrigation of refrigerated sterile saline. The use of round profiled burs and inserts should be avoided, because it causes a concave shape in the prepared portion of the root, which complicates the following filling phase. Apical resection may be obtained via a sharp cut of the apex or via its progressive abrasion; this latter technique is more time consuming, but it allows a better control over the quantity of removed tissue (7.12a–b).

There are two determining factors in the choice of technique used to perform apicoectomy.

PORTION OF THE ROOT TO BE REMOVED

Resection of the root must guarantee a correct visualisation of the root canal lumen, and offer a working space wide enough to allow preparation of the retrograde cavity. On the other hand, the resection should not exceed necessity, to avoid excessive loss of radicular

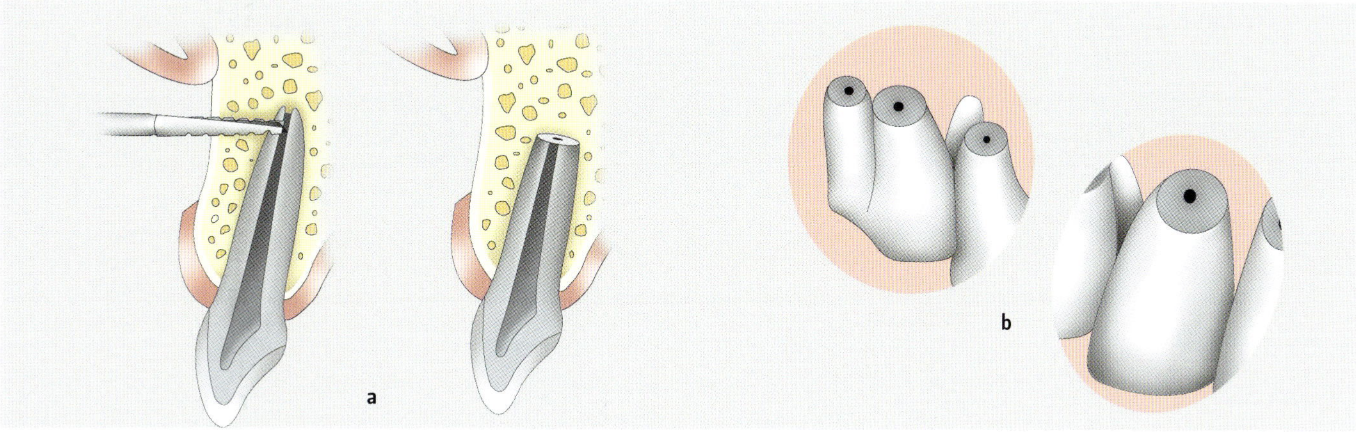

7.12 **a)** Apicoectomy conducted with a buccal approach. **b)** Apicoectomy of molars with a buccal approach.

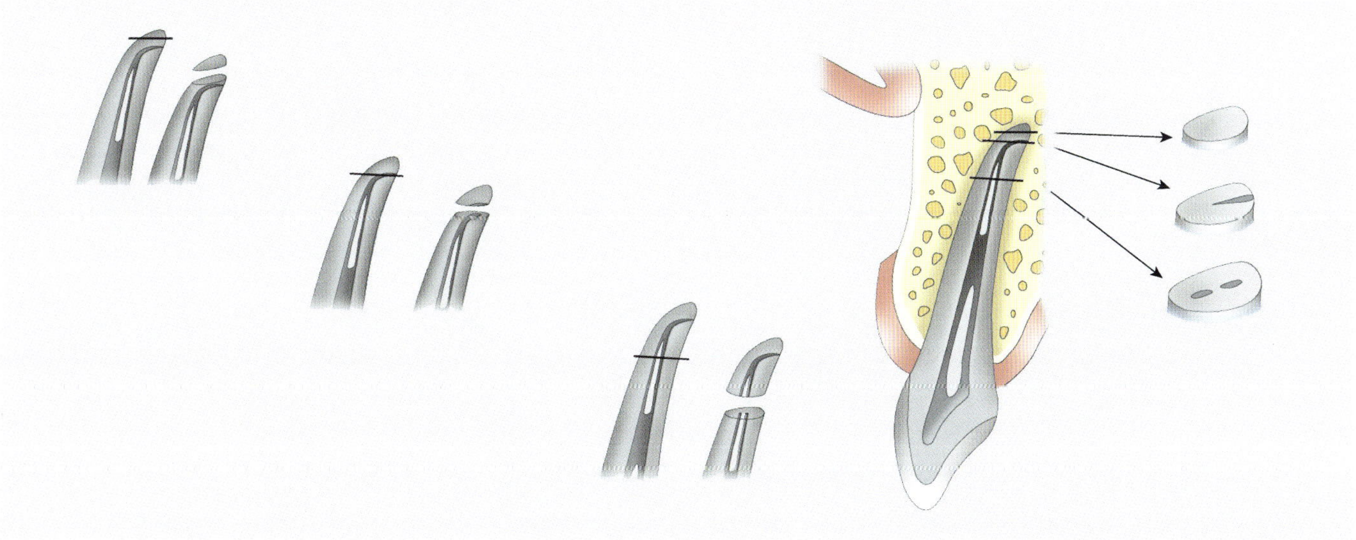

7.13 The level at which apical resection is conducted may vary: nonetheless, in cases of significant apical curvatures the choice of the wrong level for apical resection may not allow an adequate exposure of the root canal.

support. A preservative resection (1 mm) makes it possible to eliminate approximately half of the canals that are part of the apical delta, while a more extensive resection (3 mm) allows the apical delta to be eliminated. In the majority of cases, a resection ranging from 2 to 3 millimetres reduces the risk of relapse, but if other variables such as iatrogenic perforations, traumatic fractures, and apical curves are present, it may be advisable to conduct the resection more coronally (7.13).

CUTTING ANGLE

Ideally, the cutting angle should be perpendicular to the major axis of the root canal, so that the profile of its opening is round, and lies on a horizontal plain. In this manner, shaping and filling the retrograde cavity is easier, and the endodontic seal is improved. Moreover, the exposure of dentinal tubuli is reduced.

On the other hand, this approach may compel the surgeon to extend the access on the cortical wall to obtain adequate access to the cavity with the instruments used for the preparation of the retrograde cavity, particularly when maxillary molars are involved.

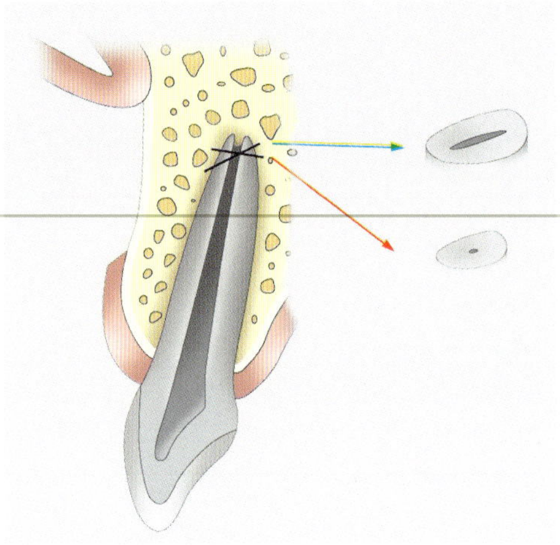

7.14 Morphology variations of the root canal profile according to different cutting angles.

Therefore, to avoid excessive bone removal while still obtaining an adequate visual control over the root canals (notably, the palatal ones), the choice of a cutting angle of 20°-30° (with respect to the major axis of the root canal) is indicated. The resulting profile of the root canal will be elliptical, thus leading to a longer perimeter of the neo-apex, and a greater number of exposed dentinal tubuli (7.14). Apicoectomy conducted with this cutting angle creates the need for a deeper retrograde cavity, to obtain a competent apical seal. In recent years, rotary instruments have been replaced by diamond-tipped ultrasonic inserts (curved micro-inserts or retrotip) for retrograde cavity preparation; the latter are smaller and easier to use at different angles, and they permit a preservative cavity preparation. Moreover, the introduction of intraoperative microscopy in surgical endodontics, bringing precise lighting (due to fibre optics and coaxial beam technologies) and a detailed view of the surgical field, has allowed the extent of surgical access to be reduced even in the most difficult areas, such as the palatal approach to the upper molar palatine roots. As far as the mandibular molars are concerned, lingual roots are still treated via a buccal approach.

Retrograde cavity preparation

In the past, the preparation of the retrograde cavity was performed with rotary instruments such as round burs mounted on specially designed mini contra-angle handpieces. Today, these have been substituted by dedicated inserts mounted on piezoelectric handpieces: the inserts have diamond-coated tips and are specifically shaped to render access to the root canal and preparation of the retrograde cavity easier. Moreover, the use of these instruments in association with magnification systems (surgical loupes or microscopes), allows for better control of the operating field, reduced trauma on the root structure, and the possibility if an extended depth of the cavity preparation. This latter aspect, in particular, is of paramount importance for the long-term success of the treatment.

Advantages

Limited extent of the surgical access on the cortical wall: the diamond-tipped inserts are much smaller than the mini contra-angle handpieces; thus, the extent of the surgical access on the cortical wall can be reduced. Moreover, the ultrasonic inserts are available in multiple shapes and angles to work on root canals that are difficult to access, eliminating the need for excessive bone removal.

Cutting angle: being available in different shapes and angles, the ultrasonic inserts are much more versatile than rotary instruments and they can follow the root canal and to prepare an adequate cavity without unnecessary sacrifice of sound dentine. Therefore, exposure of dentinal tubuli is reduced, and the perimeter of the cavity is shorter; this causes a reduction in the area of interface between the root canal walls and the filling material, with a subsequent reduction in the risk of infiltration.

Narrow and deep preparation: due to their capability of working along the major axis of the root and being relatively thin, ultrasonic inserts allow the surgeon to obtain a retrograde cavity deep enough to harbour and retain the filling material. The resulting cavity, in fact, is respectful of the original anatomy of the root canal and, thus, created with minimal sacrifice of sound dentine.

Reduced risk of perforation: using rotary instruments, such as round burs, it is very difficult to keep a working path parallel to the major axis of the root canal; in fact, the surgeon is frequently compelled to angle the head of the mini contra-angle handpiece to be able to reach the apex and create the retrograde cavity. This inclination creates a higher risk of excessive dentine removal and root stripping/perforation, insufficient retrograde cavity depth, and inadequate morphology of the retrograde cavity (typically, non-convergent cavity walls, which may cause defects in the retention of the filling material).

Cleaning and shaping of the root canal: ultrasonic inserts/tips can easily remove gutta percha and endodontic cements from the root canal, while allowing an accurate cleaning of the root canal walls with a reduced smear layer formation.

Disadvantages

Dentin fractures: an excess of power in the setting of the ultrasonic device, and incorrect movements by the surgeon during the preparation phase, may lead to cracks or dentin fractures in the area of the neo-apex. These cracks/fractures may represent a viable access point to the periapical tissues for bacteria migrating from the endodontic spaces.

Complete dentin fractures: excessive power/vibration of the ultrasonic inserts may also cause fractures and detachment of dentin portions from the neo-apex, with subsequent irregularities in the shape of the retrograde cavity perimeter, and technical difficulties in obtaining an adequate seal with the filling material. It is still under debate whether these complications may compromise the long-term results of surgical endodontics interventions. The possible presence of obstacles such as calcifications and root canal curvatures should always be considered during the preparation of the retrograde cavity.

The preparation of a deep enough retrograde cavity is a key factor not only to obtain an adequate seal of the neo-apex, but also to minimise the “dead space” between a possibly insufficient orthograde filling and the deepest portion of the retrograde filling. If the most apical portion of the root canal is left unfilled during the orthograde therapy, it may act as a reservoir for bacteria that can migrate to the periodontal spaces and cause a relapse of the periapical lesion. In fact, it is worth noting that the apical foramen, while being the main outlet of the root canal system, is rarely the only one. Therefore, a competent retrograde seal of the apical foramen is not sufficient to prevent bacterial leakage from acces-

Retrograde cavity preparation with ultrasonic instruments

Advantages

- Limited extent of the surgical access
- Versatility and choice of different cutting angles
- Narrow and deep preparation
- Reduced risk of root perforation, better shaping and cleansing of the root canal

Disadvantages

- Incomplete dentin fractures
- Complete dentin fractures

sory/lateral canals. Whenever this occurs, lesions may form along the lateral aspect of the root, and they should be put into differential diagnosis with the lateral periodontal cysts.

Apical filling

Apical filling must guarantee a watertight seal, to prevent leakage of possible bacterial left-overs from the root canal, and avoid contamination of the periapical spaces.

Materials

Ideally, the perfect material for retrograde fillings should possess all the following characteristics:

- it should be biocompatible;
- it should be insoluble;
- it should not undergo dimensional contraction (shrinking);
- it should guarantee a watertight seal by adhering to the cavity walls;
- it should not be negatively influenced by moisture;
- it should have an adequate working time;
- it should have a reasonable setting time;
- it should be radiopaque.

None of the commercially available materials for retrograde filling has all of these qualities, but many of them have been proposed and used over the years.

Cohesive gold foils: it guarantees a good seal, it is biocompatible, and it is not negatively influenced by moisture. However, the use of cohesive gold foils is time-consuming and, today, indications are lacking.

Gutta percha: it is biocompatible, insoluble, and easy to use, but it does not guarantee a watertight seal because it is negatively influenced by moisture, compaction technique, and undergoes shrinking during the cooling phase. The layer of endodontic cement used in association with gutta percha fillings is prone to infiltration over time.

Dental amalgam (silver amalgam): it has been the most widely used material for retrograde fillings for many decades. Nonetheless, it has several shortcomings:

- due to the fact that its retention is purely mechanical, the retrograde cavity must be shaped with convergent walls;
- it undergoes an initial shrinking that may hinder the periapical seal;
- until completely set, it is negatively influenced by moisture, and may cause soft tissue tattoos;
- if placed in direct contact with metal posts, galvanic currents may develop.

Composite materials: they are prone to infiltration due to polymerisation shrinkage and defective dentin adhesion. Moreover, they are negatively influenced by moisture.

ZOE (zinc oxide - eugenol) cements: initially, ZOE cements were not suitable for retrograde filling; they showed good working and setting times and guaranteed an adequate seal, but they were soluble and caused irritation of the surrounding periodontal tissues. ZOE cements of the latest generation (IRM and Super-EBA) sport good dimensional stability, sufficient biocompatibility, and good bacteriostatic properties.

IRM, which is obtained with the addition of an inert resinous filler, shows higher resistance and hardness compared to traditional ZOE cements.

Super-EBA, the latest evolution of ZOE cements, is obtained by the union of zinc dioxide and silicon with ethoxy benzoic acid (EBA). It shows high traction and compression resistance, neutral pH, a low grade of solubility, and a good dentin adhesion.

Both of these cements have demonstrated superior qualities compared to the other available filling materials.

MTA (Mineral Trioxide Aggregate): MTA is the newest addition to the retrograde filling materials category, and it is produced by mixing small hydrophilic particles of tricalcium silicate, tricalcium aluminate, tricalcium oxide, and silicium oxide. In vitro studies demonstrate that MTA guarantees a superior periapical seal compared to the aforementioned materials, shows a better adaptation to the cavity walls, activates dentinogenesis, is not affected by moisture (particularly by organic fluids such as saliva and blood), and causes a modest inflammatory response in the periodontal tissues. However, MTA may be difficult to handle, particularly when filling deep, narrow retrograde cavities. Moreover, its long setting time (3-4 hours) may be considered disadvantageous.

In light of these considerations, the latest generation ZOE-EBA cements and MTA may be considered the most reliable materials for the filling of retrograde cavities.

Management of the residual bone defect

When correctly performed, a surgical endodontics intervention leads to complete healing of the periapical lesion, and the residual bone cavity undergoes spontaneous reossification. Bone regeneration begins with blood clot organisation inside the residual cavity, and the use of any filling material (autologous bone, biomaterials) is thus unnecessary, if not contraindicated.

This result is due to the presence of intact bony walls around the area of the lesion. However, in some cases the development of the lesion leads to the erosion of both the buccal and the palatal/lingual cortical plate. In this event, the residual cavity may heal from a clinical point of view, but penetration of connective tissue from the surrounding soft tis-

Basic techniques

Retrograde cavity preparation

Choice of the piezoelectric insert

It is influenced by the position of the tooth. The selected tip must allow the surgeon to work along the major axis of the root canal; choosing the wrong insert may cause root perforations that are difficult to treat.

Choice of the power output on the piezoelectric device

Piezoelectric devices are designed to be used in a wide variety of clinical fields: prophylaxis, periodontology, prosthodontics, surgery, and endodontics. It is of the utmost importance that the appropriate power output (that is to say, ultrasound frequency) be chosen for every application; in surgical endodontics, lower frequencies are generally recommended, to avoid dentin cracks and fractures.

Apex location

It is performed with a probe. It is advisable to begin the retrograde preparation with a pilot access on the apexes (and isthmus, when present); this should be conducted with low frequency vibration and without irrigation, to establish a correct guide for the following preparation.

Retrograde cavity preparation

It is conducted with a reciprocating motion of the diamond-coated tip inside the root canal, under continuous irrigation with sterile saline, to avoid overheating and to wash away the smear layer from the cavity. It is imperative that the tip of the insert be kept parallel to the major axis of the root canal. In this phase, the direction of the preparation should be frequently checked: the retrograde cavity can be dried with paper points and verified with the aid of specifically designed micro-mirrors. The recommended depth of the retrograde preparation depends on (and is directly proportional to) the cutting angle at which the apex was resected. In the case of a 0° cutting angle, a 1-2 millimetres depth of the cavity may guarantee an adequate seal, while in the case of a 30° cutting angle a cavity depth of 3 millimetres is indicated, to obtain a reliable seal. Generally speaking, a cavity depth of at least 3 millimetres is always recommended, because it guarantees an optimal seal in all situations, irrespective of the type of filling material used. From a practical point of view, during this phase it is important to introduce in the root canal the entire diamond-coated portion of the insert.

Retrograde cavity depth

1-2 millimetres is sufficient in the case of apex resection with a 0° cutting angle, as the cavity depth is identical both on the buccal and on the palatal/lingual side of the root. A 3-millimeter depth, instead, is necessary in the case of bevelled resection of the apex, to obtain a good seal on the lower side of the bevelled root.
The choice of the ultrasonic insert (shape, dimension) should be made according to the root/canal morphology.

Apical filling

In this phase, the filling material is compacted inside the retrograde cavity to obtain a watertight apical seal. The long-term success of the treatment depends on the quality of the apical seal. Teeth presenting with a simple and easy to locate root canal system, such as teeth with a single root canal (e.g. upper central incisors), generally have a good prognosis. Conversely, the presence of multiple root canals and a complex endodontic anatomy (molars) complicates the surgical manoeuvres and may negatively affect the outcome of the treatment.

Retrograde cavity and root canal drying

The performance of filling materials is influenced by moisture. Therefore, in this phase it is fundamental to suction all fluids from the bony cavity, and to maintain an adequate haemostasis. Management of bleeding in the operating field may be obtained with fine surgical suction tips, infusion of local anaesthesia with vasoconstrictor, local application of sterile gauzes soaked in adrenaline, application of oxidised regenerated cellulose matrix or collagen sponge, and application of a concentrated solution of ferric (iron III) sulfate. Sterile paper points are inserted into the retrograde cavity until complete drying of the dentin surface is obtained. Persistent bleeding inside the retrograde cavity may suggest the presence of a root perforation (7.15).

Filling material transfer to the retrograde cavity

Sterile syringes or specifically designed carriers are used to transfer the filling material from its working plate to the retrograde cavity. If gutta percha is the material of choice, then the association with endodontic cement is recommended. If a ZOE cement or MTA is the material of choice, on the other hand, it is sufficient to mix the two components (powder and liquid) until the density of the material is suitable for compaction inside the cavity 7.16).

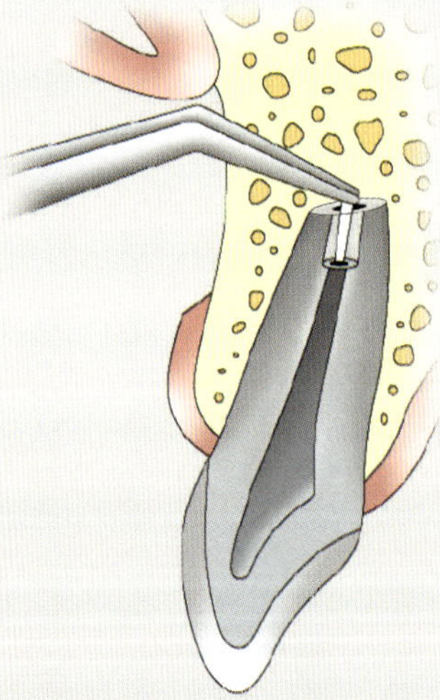

7.15 Retrograde cavity drying by means of sterile paper points.

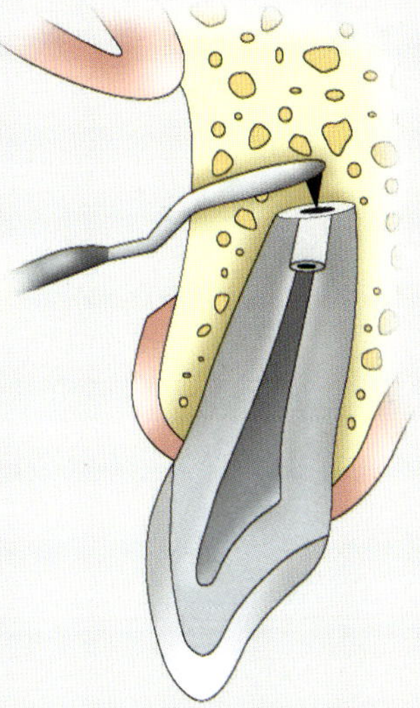

7.16 Specific carriers help transfer the filling material inside the retrograde cavity.

Compaction and burnishing

In this phase, the filling material is packed inside the retrograde cavity and condensed against the dentin walls to create a compact mass that can guarantee a watertight seal. Specifically designed obturators are used for the compaction of the filling material, and any excess of filling material is eliminated with the aid of a curette or surgical spoon. Dedicated instruments are then used to burnish the filling material around the perimeter of the cavity, to obtain the most precise adaptation of the filling at the interface between dentin and cement. When ZOE cements are used, an additional procedure can be performed to enhance the apical seal further; carbide burs mounted on straight or contra-angle low speed handpieces may be used for the finishing of the dentin-cement interface (7.17).

Irrigation, cavity revision and clinical control

Gauzes used for the management of intraoperative bleeding are removed, and irrigation with sterile saline is used to eliminate possible traces of filling materials and/or haemostatic substances. Revision of the surgical access helps to eliminate any inflamed tissue remaining, and to promote bleeding of the cortical bone.

Control radiograph

Periapical (or panoramic) radiographs taken at the end of the surgical intervention allow the outcome of the treatment to be verified, and the absence of residual traces of filling material in the periapical area.

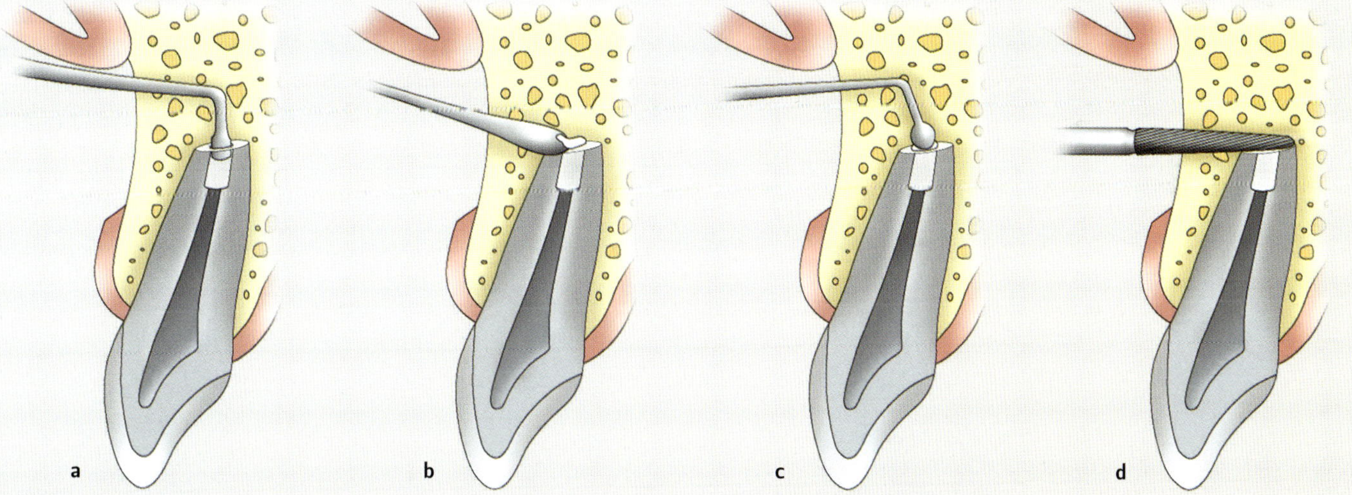

7.17 **a)** Compaction of the retrograde filling material. **b)** Excess material is removed. **c)** The filling material is burnished to assure a competent apical seal. **d)** A carbide bur is used for the finishing.

sues may occur, and reossification may be hindered. Control radiographs taken after surgery may thus show a radiolucent image (due to the connective tissue being less dense than bone), notwithstanding the complete clinical healing of the site; this renders the assessment of the outcome more difficult.

To resolve this problem, the use of regenerative techniques involving the use of semi-permeable membranes (resorbable membrane), to be placed on the buccal and palatal/lingual sides to prevent connective tissue ingrowth, has been proposed. Details on the principles and techniques of regenerative surgery are reported in Chapter 13 of this manual. However, it is worth noting that the guided bone regeneration of residual cavities after surgical endodontics treatment is still questionable, and there is still no consensus in the scientific literature on this topic.

Follow-up

Complete enucleation of the periapical lesion, a thorough curettage of the residual cavity, a watertight apical seal, and correct flap repositioning promote primary healing of the surgical wound and complete reossification of the residual cavity. The use of adequate surgical equipment and techniques, in association with intraoperative magnification that allows a better control of the operative field, may improve the prognosis of the retrograde approach.

Still, surgical endodontics cannot compensate for huge errors committed during the orthograde treatment of the root canal system. As such, prognosis of periapical lesions depends on the correct execution of the orthograde treatment, even when it represents a preparatory phase for the following retrograde surgery. It is no coincidence that teeth in which it is impossible to seal the root canals adequately via the orthograde approach are those with the worst long-term prognosis.

Success in surgical endodontics is defined by clinical and radiographic examinations. Healing of hard tissues occurs by complete reossification of residual cavities. This process, already visible on control radiographs after 6 months, generally takes 12-24 months to complete. Clinical healing implies the resolution of signs and symptoms such as swelling, pain, periodontal pockets, presence of fistulas, and tooth mobility. While persistence of these signs should be interpreted as a failure of the surgical treatment, the persistence of radiolucent areas does not always indicate a relapse of the periapical lesion; in fact, tissue healing in the residual cavity may occur by connective tissue ingrowth and scar tissue formation, as previously detailed.

Two types of healing are thus possible:

- clinical and radiographic healing;
- clinical healing without radiographic healing.

Data reported in the literature shows success rates of the retrograde surgical treatments ranging from 25% to 90%. Such a wide range is probably due to the lack of objective parameters in defining therapeutic success, to the use of a wide variety of different treatment protocols, to the analysis of different dental elements, and finally to the use of different surgical techniques. However, the key variables, which may significantly influence prognosis, are still easily detectable.

A step-by-step clinical case is presented in 7.18a-k.

Clinical case 1 – Periapical lesion around the root apexes of 2.1 and 2.2

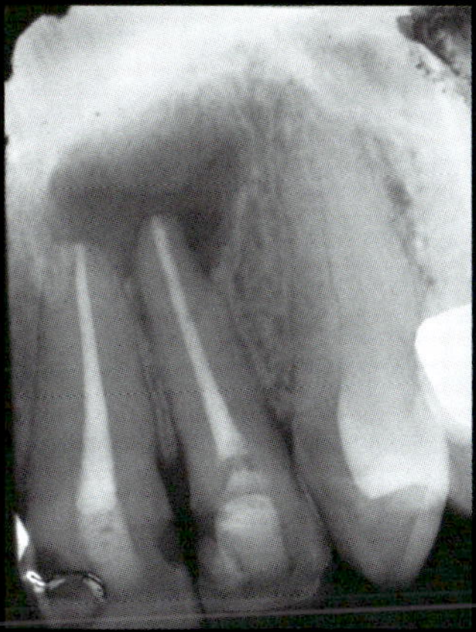

7.18a Periapical radiograph showing a radiolucent lesion around the root apexes of 2.1 and 2.2, notwithstanding the fact that both teeth underwent orthograde retreatment.

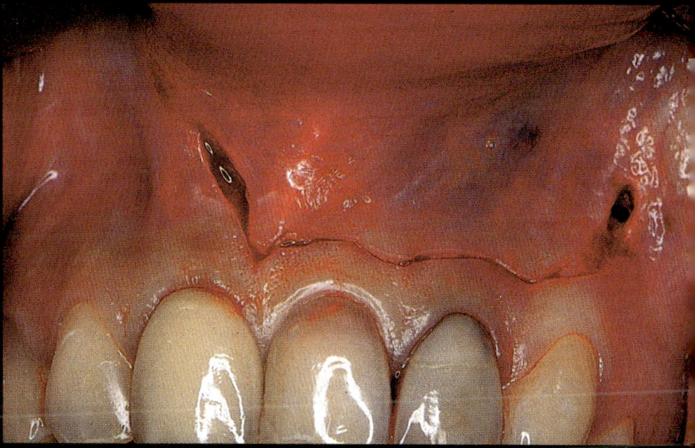

7.18b Submarginal trapezoidal flap.

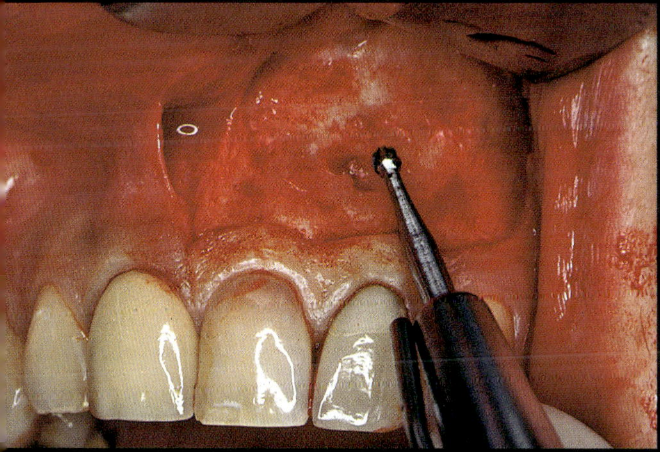

7.18c Ostectomy is performed with rotary instruments (round bur).

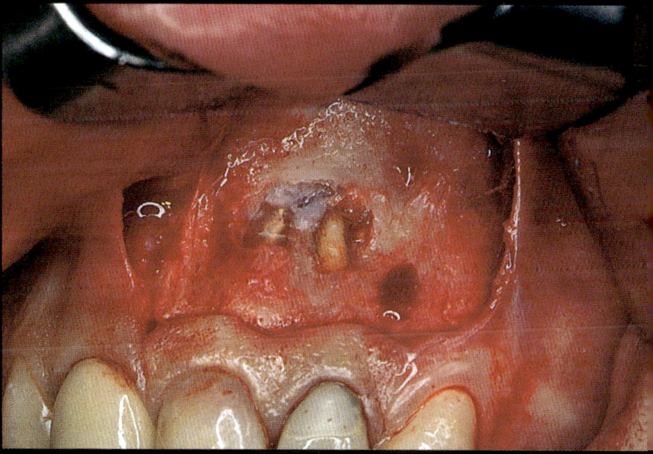

7.18d Root apexes and the lesion wall are identified.

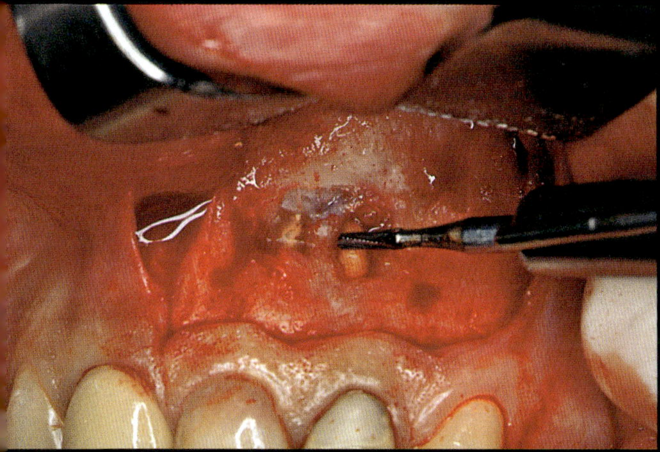

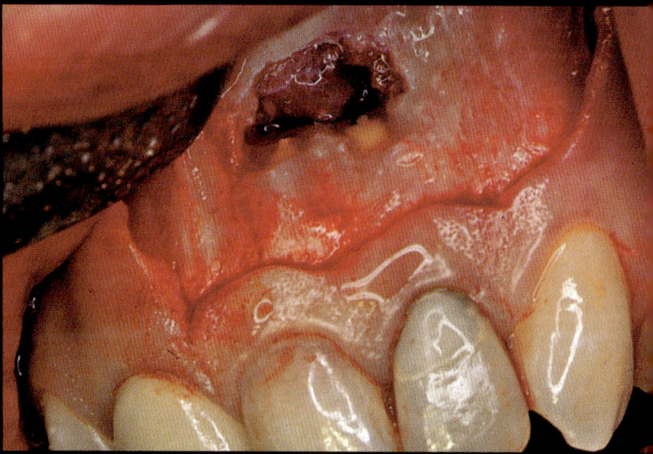

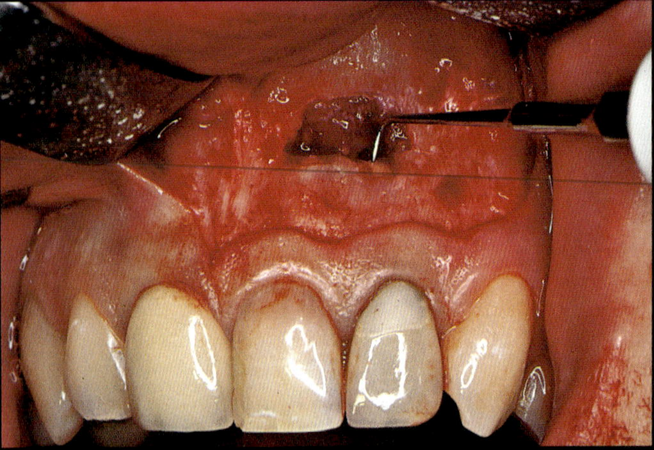

7.18g Preparation of the retrograde cavity with ultrasonic instruments.

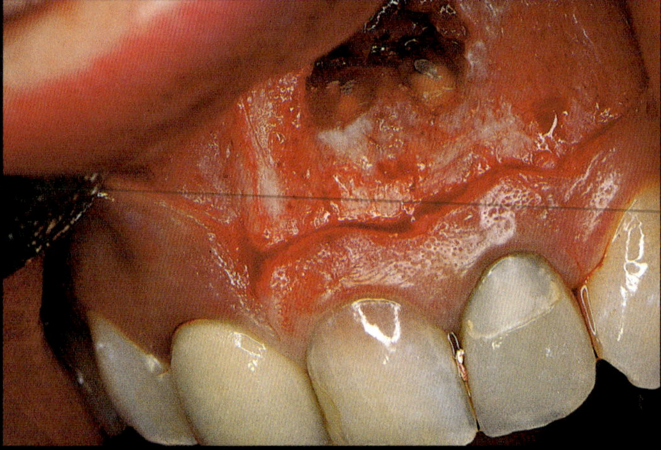

7.18h Retrograde cavity fillings are completed.

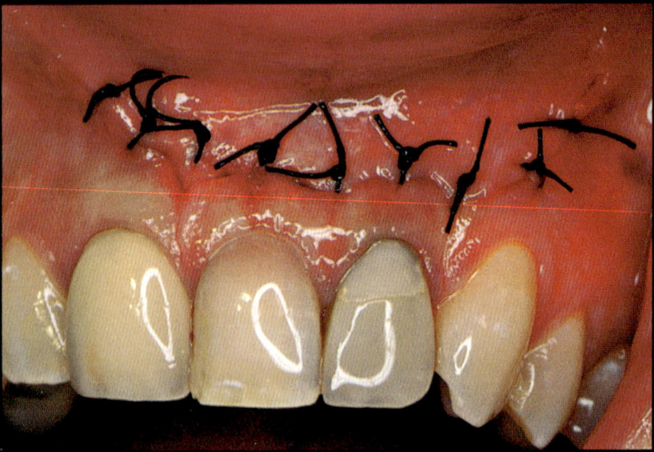

7.18i The surgical flap is sutured.

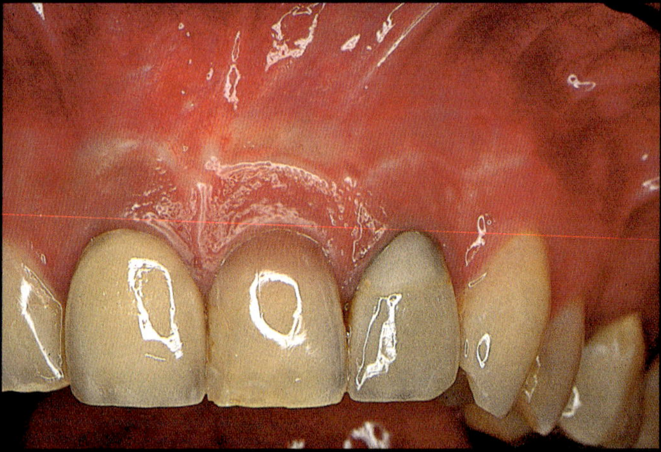

7.18j Clinical healing one month after surgery.

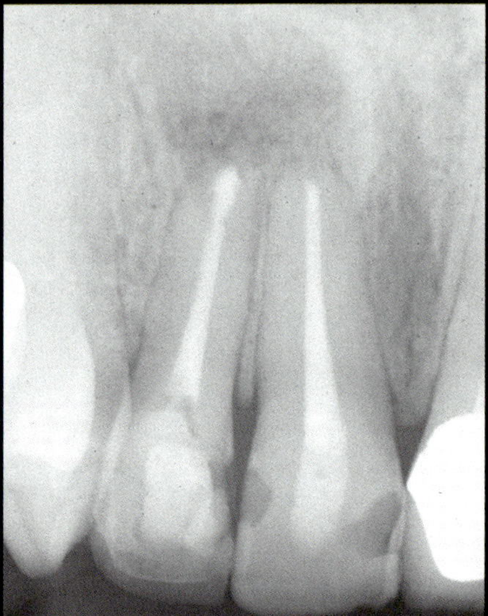

REFERENCES

ALLEN RK, NEWTON CW, BROWN CE. A statistical analysis of surgical and non-surgical endodontic retreatment cases. *J Endodon* 1989; 15:261-6.

ANDREASSEN J, RUD J. Correlation between histology and radiography in the assessment of healing after endodontic surgery in 70 cases. *Int J Oral Surg* 1972; 1:161-73.

AQRABAWI J. Sealing ability of amalgam, super EBA cement, and MTA when used as retrograde filling materials. *Br Dent J* 2000; 188(5):266-8.

CASTELLUCCI A. Progressi in endodonzia chirurgica. *L'informatore endodontico* 2002; 5(3):46-61.

CHIAPASCO M, DE CICCO L, MARRONE G, POZZI E, CRESCENTINI M, PICCOLI P. Studio longitudinale di 170 casi di apicectomia con otturazione retrograda in amalgama d'argento: risultati a distanza di tempo. *G It Endo* 1994; 1:16-21.

DE BRUYNE MA, DE MOOR RJ. SEM analysis of the integrity of resected root apices of cadaver and extracted teeth after ultrasonic root-end preparation at different intensities. *Int Endodon J* 2005 May; 38(5):310-9.

EL-SWIAH JM, WALKER RT. Reasons for apicectomies: a retrospective study. *Endodon Dent Traumatol* 1996; 12:185-91.

FRIEDMAN S. Outcome of endodontic surgery: a meta-analysis of the literature - Part 1: comparison of traditional root-end surgery and endodontic microsurgery. *J Endod* 2011 May; 37(5):577-8; author reply 578-80.

FRIEDMAN S, STABHOLZ A. Endodontic retreatment-case selection and tecnique. I, Criteria for case selection. *J Endodon* 1986; 12:28-33.

GAGLIANI MM, GORNI FG, STROHMENGER L. Periapical resurgery versus periapical surgery: a 5-year longitudinal comparison. *Int Endodon J* 2005; 38(5):320-7.

GORNI F. L'uso del microscopio operativo in endodonzia clinica e chirurgica. *Il Dentista Moderno* 1999; 11:25-50.

KHABBAZ MG, KEREZOUDIS NP, ARONI E, TSATSAS V. Evaluation of different methods for the root-end cavity preparation. *Oral Surg Oral Med Oral Pathol Oral Radiol Endodon* 2004; 98:237-42.

KIM S. Color atlas of microsurgery in endodontics. W.B. Saunders, Philadelphia 2001.

KONTAKIOTIS EG, LAGOUDAKOS TA, GEORGOPOULOS MK. The influence of root-end resection and root-end cavity preparation on microleakage of root filled teeth in vitro. *Int Endodon J* 2004 Jun; 37(6):403-7.

LLOYD A, JAUBERZINS A, DUMMER PMH, BRYANT S. Root-end cavity preparation using the Micro-Mega Sonic Retro Tip. SEM analysis. *Int Endod J* 1996; 29:295-301.

MEAD C, JAVIDAN-NEJAD S, MEGO ME, NASH B, TORABINEJAD M. Levels of evidence for the outcome of endodontic surgery. *J Endodon* 2005; 1:19-24.

SETZER FC, SHAH SB, HOHLI MR, KARABUCAK B, KIM S. Outcome of endodontic surgery: a meta-analysis of the literature - Part 1: Comparison of traditional root-end surgery and endodontic microsurgery. *J Endod* 2010 Nov; 36(11):1757-65.

SETZER FC, SHAH SB, HOHLI MR, KARABUCAK B, KIM S. Outcome of endodontic surgery: a meta-analysis of the literature - Part 2: Comparison of endodontic microsurgical techniques with and without the use of higher magnification. *J Endod* 2012 Jan; 38(1):1-10.

Taschieri S, Testori T, Francetti L, Del Fabbro M. Effects of ultrasonic root end preparation on resected root surfaces: SEM evaluation. *Oral Surg Oral Med Oral Pathol Oral Radiol Endodon* 2004; 98(5):611-8.

TASCHIERI S, DEL FABBRO M, TESTORI T, FRANCETTI L, WEINSTEIN R. Endodontic surgery with ultrasonic retrotips: one-year follow-up. *Oral Surg Oral Med Oral Pathol Oral Radiol Endodon* 2005; 100(3):380-7.

TASCHIERI S, DEL FABBRO M. Efficacy of xenogenic bone grafting with guided tissue re generation in the management on bone defects after surgical endodontics. *J Oral Maxillofac Surg* 2007; 65(6):1121-7.

TROPE M. Healing of apical periodontitis in dogs after apicoectomy and retrofilling with various filling materials. *Oral Surg Oral Med Oral Pathol Oral Radiol Endodon* 1996; 81:221-8.

VELVART P, PETERS CI. Soft tissue management in endodontic surgery. *J Endodon* 2005; 31(1):4-16.

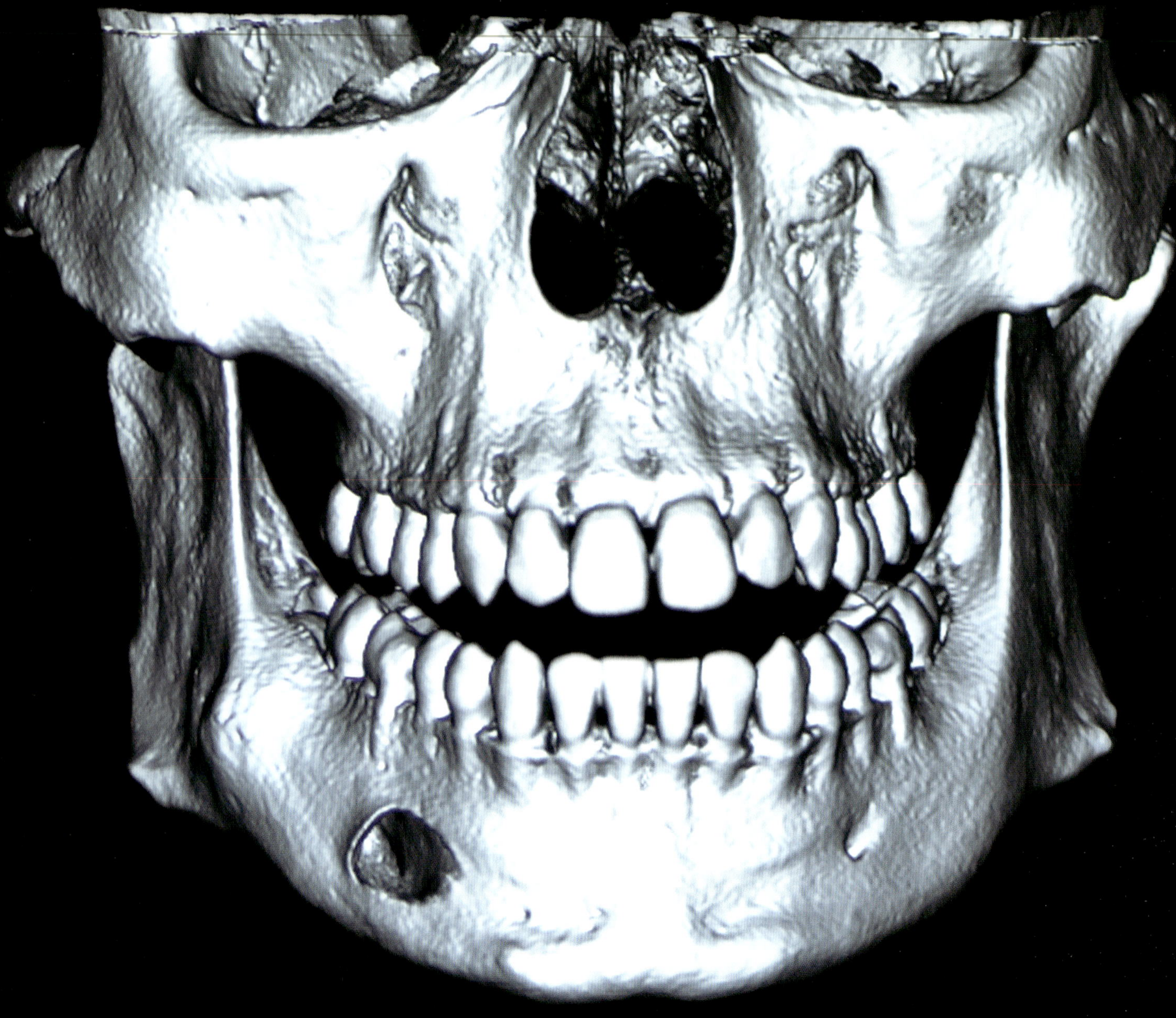

Cysts of the jaws

M. Chiapasco · M. Zaniboni · A. Rossi

Endosseous cysts of the jaws

Etiopathogenesis

Cysts of the jaws are saccate endosseous lesions: the internal side of the cyst wall is epithelial while the external side is connective, and the cavity is filled with fluid material. Etiopathogenesis of these lesions has not been completely clarified yet: the most credited hypothesis links the formation of the cyst to the degenerative activation of epithelial remnants present in the periodontal tissues.

As far as the mechanisms underlying the expansion of the cyst, the two most credited theories are the hydrostatic theory and the prostaglandin theory.

According to the *hydrostatic theory*, the secretions and by-products of degeneration of the epithelial cells, which form the internal side of the cyst wall, cause a build up of remains (dead cells, proteins, cholesterine crystals, etc.) inside the cavity. This, in turn, makes the internal osmotic pressure rise, causing fluids from the surrounding tissues to migrate through the cyst wall (which acts as a semi-permeable membrane) and inside the lesion. The resulting rise in the internal hydrostatic pressure causes an activation of osteoclast populations that are ultimately responsible for the peripheral bone resorption and the subsequent enlargement of the cavity.

According to the *prostaglandin theory*, on the other hand, both the epithelial and connective portions of the cyst wall are able to produce and release prostaglandins and prostacyclins, which can directly activate the osteoclast populations responsible for peripheral bone resorption. Details regarding the mechanisms behind cyst expansion are still unclear, and it is possible that each one of the described modalities will play a role in the process. Cysts, while not having true neoplastic characteristics, tend nonetheless to expand by causing peripheral bone resorption: the cortical plates may deform and wear thin, up to complete consumption. The behaviour may be more or less aggressive according to the histologic nature of the lesion.

Endosseous cysts of the jaws: clinical examination

Signs

Initial phase

- Normal mucosa
- No signs of dental root resorption/erosion

Advanced phase

- Erosion and/or expansion of the cortical walls
- Swelling
- Fistulisation and drainage of purulent material

Symptoms

Initial phase

- Asymptomatic

Advanced phase

- Sense of local tension or pain

Clinical examination: analysis of signs and symptoms

Clinical examination should be performed according to the principles of classic semiotics: inspection, palpation, and percussion may play a significant role in the diagnostic process.

INTRAORAL EXAMINATION

In the initial phase, when the lesion is small and has not yet caused modifications in the local anatomy, signs of its presence may be completely absent and the lesion may not be detected in the course of intraoral examination. Typically, small lesions are identified on panoramic or intraoral radiographs that have been requested to evaluate or plan different treatments. In these cases, the aspect of the overlying mucosa (colour, compactness) is frequently normal (📷 8.1a-b). Generally, cysts do not cause resorption of the roots of the involved teeth, but tend to cause root displacement, instead. On the contrary, erosion or resorption of the roots should always be considered a sign of the possible neoplastic origin (benign or malignant) of the lesion. At a later stage, the progressive expansion of the cyst may cause deformation or erosion of the cortical plates. When the cortical plate has worn thin and expanded, a typical convexity may be visible and palpable under the mucosa overlying the lesion (📷 8.2a-b); palpation, in particular, may give valuable information on the consistency of the lesion. Percussion is generally used to evaluate possible pain responses from the teeth involved in the lesion.

EXTRAORAL EXAMINATION

Extraoral examination by inspection and palpation should always be aimed at evaluating the development of a cyst when it has eroded the cortical plate and has then expanded in the soft tissues. Typical localisations are the mucobuccal fold towards the inferior border of the mandible, the buccal region, the zygomatic region and the infraorbital region. It is always important, particularly in cases of infected cysts, to evaluate the possible lymph node reaction at the submandibular and neck stations. When the cyst develops towards the floor of the mouth, it may be helpful to conduct a bimanual examination, with one hand inside the oral cavity and the other under the mandible, as in the floor of the mouth there is no bony plate that can be used as a reference point. Moreover, discomfort and pain may be elicited by palpation, particularly in the case of infected cysts.

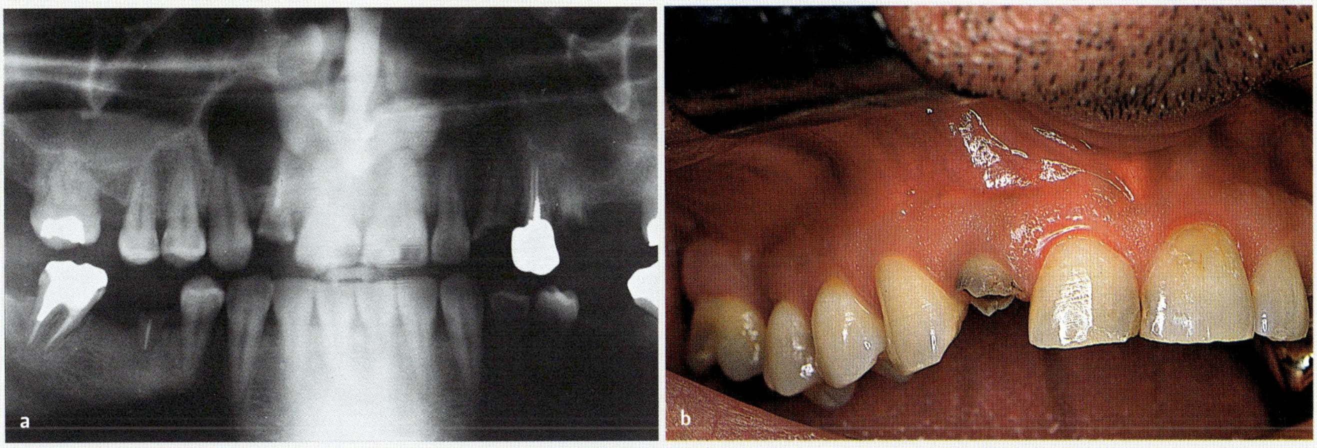

8.1 **a)** Panoramic radiograph showing a radiolucent lesion in the area of 12–13. **b)** Clinical examination shows no signs of alteration of the alveolar ridge, but only caries affecting 12.

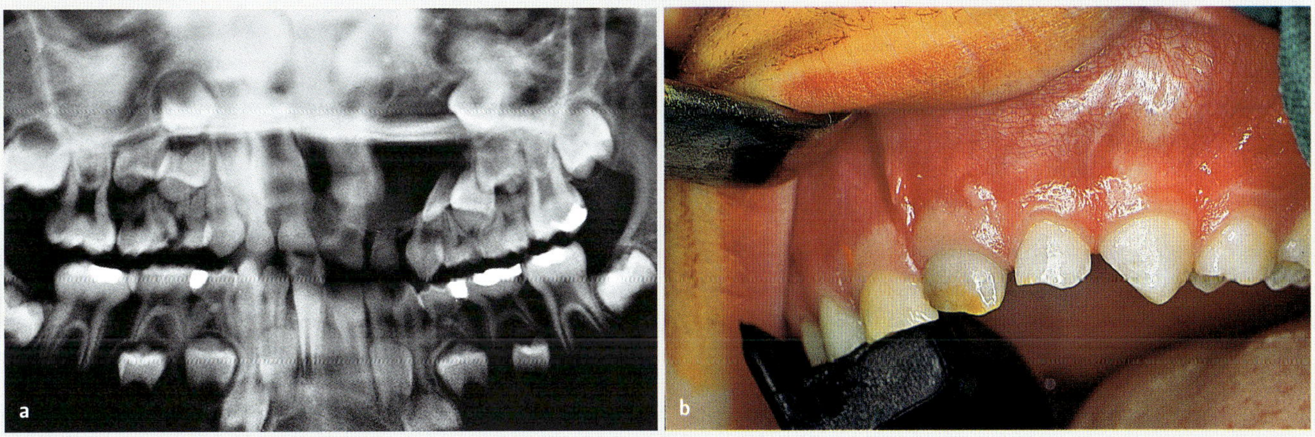

8.2 **a)** Panoramic radiograph demonstrating a large lesion in the area of 21–24. **b)** Clinical examination shows a localised swelling caused by erosion and expansion of the buccal cortical plate.

TYPICAL SYMPTOMS

In the majority of cases, particularly in the early phases, cysts are frequently asymptomatic. Infected cysts, however, may cause symptoms ranging from a localised sense of tension to pain and, in cases of cortical plate erosion, a fistula may be present and cause purulent discharge (8.3a–b). The involvement of nerves (e.g. the inferior alveolar nerve) is not generally accompanied by sensory disturbances; nerves are usually displaced by the expansion of the cyst, but not infiltrated as may happen with tumours.

The onset of sensory alteration in the areas innervated by the trigeminal nerve, although seldom caused by simple compression of the nerve by a cyst, should always raise suspicions as to possible infiltration of the nerve branch and, thus, to the neoplastic nature of the lesion.

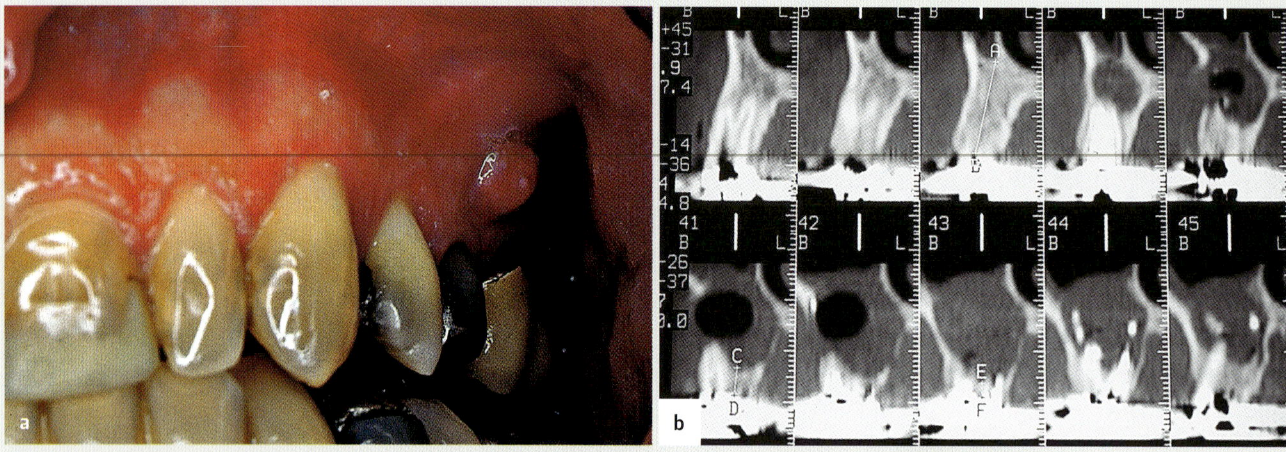

8.3 Periapical cyst associated to 26: **a)** buccal fistulisation of the lesion; **b)** CT scan (sagittal view) shows the erosion of the buccal cortical plate and the development of the lesion towards the maxillary sinus (the bottom of the sinus is cloudy).

Radiographic examination

Radiographically, cysts appear as well-defined radiolucent areas with a characteristic radiopaque border, which is due to the reactive activation of osteoblasts around the lesion. They may be unilocular or multilocular, but no pathognomonic criteria are detectable that can help distinguish between the different types of cysts. Routine radiographic examination is represented by the panoramic radiograph, as it can show the form and dimensions of even the largest lesions. Limitations to the use of panoramic radiographs for the diagnosis of cystic lesions are as follows:

- a panoramic radiograph is a bidimensional image with possible overlay of different anatomical structures, such as the nasal and paranasal cavities;
- it does not allow accurate evaluation of the following: the level of alteration in the structure of the surrounding bone, the resorption of the cortical plates, and the possible involvement of the soft tissues.

Periapical radiographs may be useful for the evaluation of small lesions, particularly in cases of periapical cysts, but are generally insufficient to conduct a complete analysis. In fact, they share with the panoramic radiograph all the limitations of a bidimensional image, and their limited dimension does not allow the visualisation of the entire lesion and surrounding structures in the majority of cases.

When panoramic and intraoral radiographs do not allow the clinician to adequately define the lesion, the radiographic exam of choice to obtain precise information on the form of the lesion and its dimensions, on the density of its content, on the erosion of the cortical plates, on its possible expansion in the soft tissues, and its relationships with the surrounding anatomical structures (neurovascular bundles, maxillary sinus, etc.) is computed tomography (CT) (8.3b) (see also Chapter 1, "Radiographic examinations" section)

On the other hand, magnetic resonance imaging (MRI) has limited indications in the evaluation of the endosseous lesions of the jaws; it is more expensive than CT, and is more suitable for the evaluation of the soft tissues. However, in selected cases it may be useful to obtain precise information on the content of the lesion (liquid or solid), and to provide valuable data on the cystic or neoplastic nature of the lesion. MRI is particularly indicated for the evaluation of lesions that develop in the soft tissues, such as dermoid cysts of the floor of the mouth.

RADIOGRAPHIC PARAMETERS

Form: The classic cyst is radiolucent, and has a rounded or oval shape (📷 8.4). Occasionally, it may appear as a multilocular lesion (📷 8.5).

Site: The site is extremely variable, but some types of cysts may have a typical localisation (e.g., the nasopalatine duct cyst is always located on the median line of the upper maxilla in the area of the nasopalatine foramen)

Number: Cysts are usually single lesions. Nevertheless, in some cases multiple lesions may be present, particularly in patients with several necrotic teeth, or patients affected by the Gorlin-Goltz syndrome (for details, see Chapter 9).

Margins: Cysts usually present with well-defined margins surrounded by a thin, radiopaque border caused by osteoblast activation and peripheral bone formation as a response to the expansion of the lesion (📷 8.4). Undefined margins should always lead the clinician to suspect the lesion may have a different origin (neoplastic). In this case, before any treatment plan is devised, it is recommended that additional examinations be performed, including an incisional biopsy of the lesion.

Homogeneity: Cystic lesions are uniformly radiolucent in the majority of cases. The presence of alternating radiopaque and radiolucent areas or bony septa inside the cavity should suggest that the lesion might not be a cyst, but rather an odontogenic or non-odontogenic neoplasm.

Alteration of adjacent structures: The expansion of cystic lesions typically causes dislocation of adjacent anatomical structures. On the contrary, erosion of the roots involved in a lesion should always lead the clinician to consider the possibility that it may have an aggressive nature (neoplasm).

Instrumental screening

	Advantages	Disadvantages
Panoramic radiograph	+ Adequate definition of the form and the extent of the lesion	+ Two-dimensional image + Anatomic structures overlay/overlap
Periapical radiograph	+ Adequate to evaluate small lesions	+ Insufficient for the evaluation of large lesions
CT scan	+ Good tridimensional definition of the form and the extent of the lesion, of the density of the cystic content, of possible cortical erosions, and involvement of the surrounding soft tissues and anatomic structures.	+ Higher economic and biological costs
MRI	+ Good definition of the lesion and its content. Indicated for the evaluation of cysts developing in the soft tissues.	+ Limited indications in cases of endosseous lesions

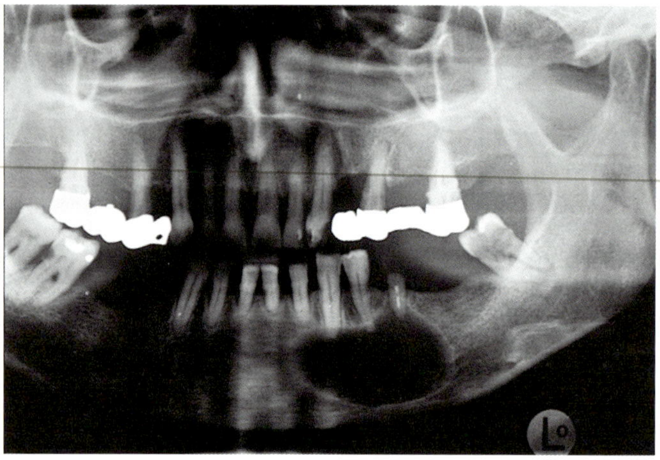

8.4 Periapical cyst involving 35: unilocular, with well-defined margins, and with the typical radiopaque margin.

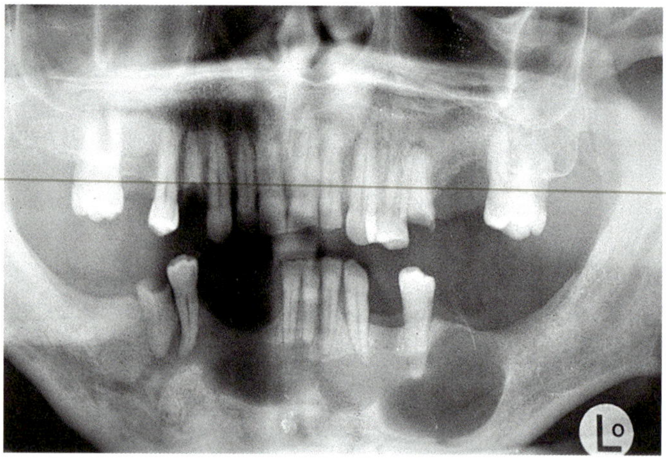

8.5 Large multilocular mandibular lesion.

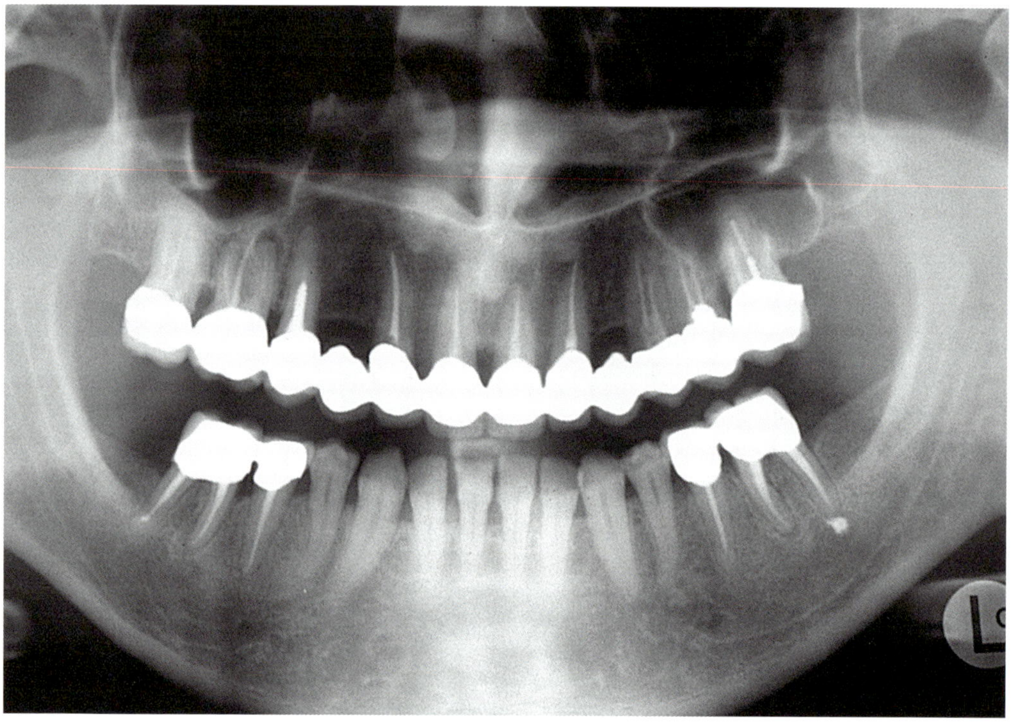

8.6 Maxillary sinus expansion mimicking the presence of an endosseous lesion.

False images and artefacts: A thorough analysis of the available radiographic images is essential; the presence of false images due to the overlaying of different anatomical structures and layers, thinness of the cortical plates, sequelae of previous surgical interventions in the area with incomplete bone healing, and the presence of pneumatised paranasal cavities such as the maxillary sinus should be excluded (8.6). A radiolucent area may also be the result of a radiographic artefact; in this case, repeating the exam may help to resolve any doubt.

Diagnosis

A precise collection of the patient's history, an accurate clinical examination, and a thorough analysis of the radiographic images should give the clinician sufficient information to give a clinical diagnosis and to plan the surgical treatment accordingly. However, it is worth stressing that clinical and radiographic diagnosis is presumptive, and should always be confirmed by means of *histological examination*.

In the majority of cases, cysts of the jaws present with peculiar symptoms and clinical signs, and have a typical radiographic appearance. In this case, the presumptive diagnosis is considered reliable enough and the histology is performed on the lesion after its surgical removal. However, should there be any suspicions that the origin of the lesion might be different (particularly, neoplastic), it is always indicated to perform additional examinations prior to the surgical removal of the lesion. *Needle aspiration* helps determine if the content of the lesion is liquid or solid and, if liquid, the type of fluid sampled. A clear, yellow fluid may generally indicate the presence of an odontogenic, non-infected cyst, while a cloudy or frankly purulent fluid may indicate the presence of an infected cyst. If a significant amount of particulate matter is present in the sampled fluid, it may indicate the presence of an odontogenic keratocyst, while if the sampled fluid is blood it may indicate the presence of an osteolytic lesion caused by vascular alterations (e.g. intraosseous angioma, high-pressure vascular malformations, etc.). In this latter case, the utmost care is advised: due to the high risk of severe haemorrhagic complications, the patient should be referred to the hospital, where trained maxillofacial surgeons may operate under general anaesthesia and controlled blood pressure with appropriate techniques, specialist support, and adequate armamentarium. If needle aspiration does not allow an adequate sample to be collected, the reason may be twofold: either the lesion is partially empty (part of the content may drain from a fistula, when present) or the content of the lesion (maybe the lesion itself) is solid. In this latter case, as solid lesions are frequently neoplasms (benign or malignant), it is imperative that an *incisional biopsy* be performed and the sample analysed histologically before planning the complete removal of the lesion. This is of the utmost importance because the simple enucleation, which is the correct treatment option in cases of cystic lesions, is absolutely insufficient in cases of neoplasms, and may expose the patient to relapse, progression of the disease and further medical and surgical treatments.

TECHNIQUE FOR NEEDLE ASPIRATION

This technique is easily applicable when the lesion has completely eroded the cortical plate and is visible just under the overlying mucosa. The softer area is detected by palpation and the needle should penetrate as far as needed to reach the content of the lesion. The gauge of the needle should be chosen with care, because a small needle may not be able to aspirate both solid materials and thick fluids, giving inaccurate or useless results. If the collected sample is liquid, it may be evaluated both visually and in vitro by bacterial culture examination (8.7a-b). If a neoplastic (solid) origin is suspected for the lesion and if the cortical plate is intact, it is possible to gain access to the lesion and perform a needle aspiration after drilling a small hole in the most easily accessible portion of the bone plate. In these cases, if the needle aspiration gives a negative result, it is possible to proceed with an incisional biopsy.

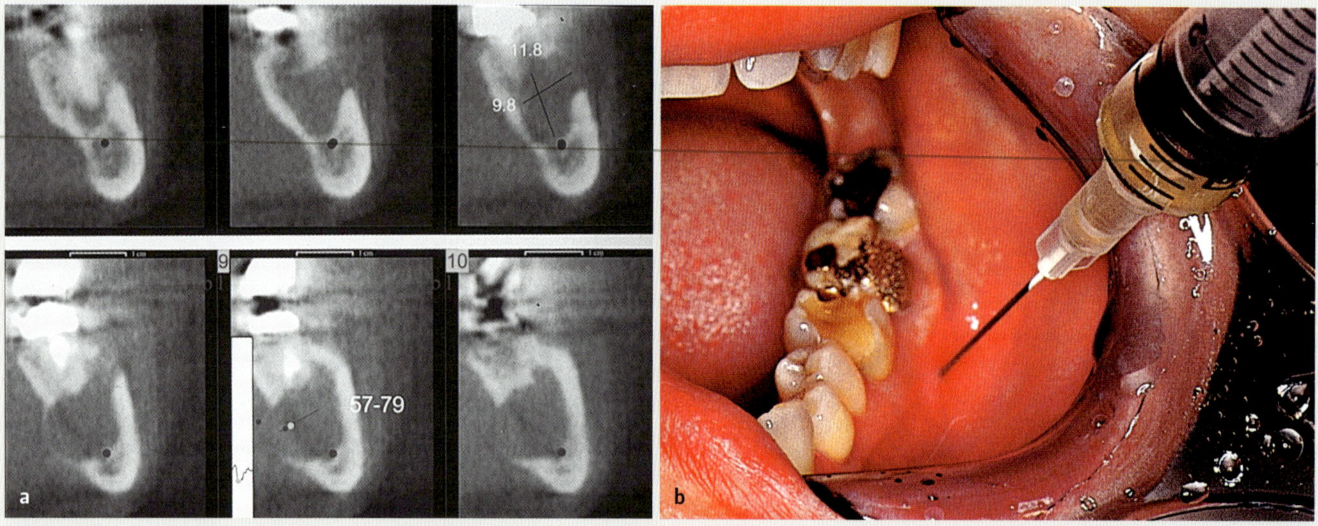

8.7 a) CT scan showing a radiolucent mandibular lesion; erosion of the buccal and lingual cortical plates, and irregular margins may suggest a neoplastic nature of the lesion. b) Needle aspiration demonstrates the presence of a clear yellow fluid content, typically found inside cystic lesions.

Tab. 8.1 WHO classification

Denomination	Incidence	Clinical aspect
Odontogenic cysts		
Gingival cyst of the newborn (Epstein's pearl)	Very rare. In the newborn, especially in the upper arch.	Small white or rosy nodules, frequently multiple; 1-5 millimetres in diameter, located on the median palatine raphe or on the alveolar mucosa.
Gingival cyst of the adult	Peak incidence between the 5th and 7th decade; originates from the dental lamina.	Asymptomatic, floating swelling, slow growth, typically located in the alveolar mucosa of the premolar and molar area, typically less than 1 centimetre in diameter.
Dentigerous (follicular) cyst	The second most frequent odontogenic cyst, the first being the periapical cyst. More frequent in the area of the third mandibular molars and maxillary canine, followed by the mandibular premolars and maxillary molars.	Slow growth, asymptomatic except in cases of superinfection. It originates after the formation of the crown of the tooth is complete due to the accumulation of fluid between the epithelial layer of the enamel organ of the follicle and the enamel layer of the tooth.
Lateral periodontal cyst	Peak incidence between the 3rd and 8th decade. Frequently observed in the mandible (more than 90% of cases). Represents less than 1% of all odontogenic cysts.	It is located along the side of a dental root. Generally asymptomatic, associated to a vital tooth.
Eruption cyst	Typically observed in children under 10. Frequently associated with the maxillary incisors and permanent first molars.	Associated with deciduous or permanent erupting teeth, it is capped with soft tissue accompanied by blood extravasation that causes the floating consistency and the red-bluish colour.
Glandular odontogenic (sialo-odontogenic) cyst	Peak incidence between the 2nd and 6th decade, frequently observed in the anterior region of the mandible (85% of cases).	
Inflammatory cysts		
Periapical cyst	The most frequent odontogenic cyst (50% of all odontogenic lesions).	
Residual cyst	No age predilection.	
Paradental cyst	Peak incidence between the 1st and 4th decade, typically located in the area of the first molar. Frequently located in the mandible, in 23% of cases it develops bilaterally.	
Non-odontogenic cysts		
Nasopalatine cyst	Peak incidence between the 4th and 6th decade, with a predilection for males and the anterior region of the maxilla.	Hard elastic (or floating, if the bony wall is eroded) swelling located in the anterior portion of the palate. Advanced phase: swelling on the buccal side.
Nasoalveolar and nasolabial cyst	Peak incidence between the 4th and 6th decade, with a significant predilection for females.	Unilateral swelling of the upper lip that causes rising and dislocation of the nasolabial fold. The lesion remains confined in the soft tissues. If large, it can cause nasal obstruction.
Pseudocysts		
Stafne's bone cavity	Peak incidence between the 4th and 6th decade, with a predilection for males.	

TECHNIQUE FOR INCISIONAL BIOPSY

Biopsy follows the general principles presented in the dedicated section of this manual (see Chapter 9 for details). Generally, the surgical flap is elevated in a convenient position where the lesion is more easily accessible and a sample of adequate dimension can be collected. If the lesion has eroded the cortical plate, the sample can be collected with the aid of a scalpel and surgical tweezers, thus minimising the surgical trauma and avoiding the creation of artefacts, which would render the histologic interpretation more difficult. However, if the cortical plate is intact, a small osteotomic window is created with rotating or piezoelectric instruments to expose the lesion and collect the sample as previously described. The sample is immediately stored in a sealed container filled with formaline solution (10%, neutral buffered), which is then sent to the pathologist.

Classification

Despite having several characteristics in common, cysts of the jaws present different peculiarities from etiopathogenetic, clinical, therapeutic, and prognostic point of views. For this reason, over the years several classifications have been proposed to frame them, the most credited of which is the WHO (*World Health Organization*) classification, which also includes the neoplasms of the jaws, and is based on embryological and histological criteria (tab. 8.1).

Radiographic aspect	Differential diagnosis	Treatment
No visible signs on standard radiographs (periapical radiograph, panoramic radiograph).		No treatment needed. Spontaneous regression is generally observed in the first 3 months after birth.
No visible signs on standard radiographs (periapical radiograph, panoramic radiograph).	Gingival mucocele, Fordyce's granules, peripheral odontogenic tumors, lateral periodontal cyst.	Surgical excision. No tendency to relapse.
Well-defined unilocular radiolucency (variable dimensions) with radiopaque margins surrounding the crown of an impacted tooth.	Keratocystic odontogenic tumour, ameloblastoma.	Surgical enucleation. Third molars, if involved, are extracted. When functionally important teeth are involved, orthodontic repositioning can be attempted.
Well-defined, round or oval small radiolucent area along the side of a dental root.	Keratocystic odontogenic tumour, gingival cyst of the adult, periapical cyst originating from a lateral canal.	Surgical enucleation. Relapse is rare.
Unilocular radiolucency surrounding the crown of an erupting tooth.	Dentigerous (follicular) cyst.	No treatment is needed; it generally disappears once the eruption of the tooth is completed. In cases of persistence, surgical excision is indicated.
Unilocular or multilocular radiolucency, honeycomb appearance, well-defined margins.	Ameloblastoma, keratocystic odontogenic tumour, intraosseous mucoepidermoid carcinoma.	Surgical excision and curettage of the residual cavity. Due to the high relapse rate (30%), some aAuthors suggest the en bloc resection of the affected segment.
Well-defined, round radiolucency surrounding a root apex or associated with a lateral root canal.	Lateral periodontal cyst.	Surgical excision associated with apicoectomy and retrograde filling of the root canal.
Well-defined, round unilocular radiolucency not associated with a dental root.	All osteolytic lesions.	Surgical excision.
Well-defined, round radiolucency associated with a tooth.	Periapical cyst.	Surgical excision.
Round, oval or heart-shaped radiolucency in the area of the nasopalatine foramen.		Surgical excision. Relapse is rare.
No visible signs on standard radiographs (periapical radiograph, panoramic radiograph).		Surgical excision. Relapse is rare.
Radiographically, it appears as an elliptic or round radiolucency located in the posterior mandible, below the inferior alveolar canal.	All radiolucent lesions located in the posterior mandible, below the inferior alveolar canal.	No treatment is needed.

In the last revision of this classification some lesions, which were previously considered cysts, have been framed differently:

- the keratocyst has been placed among the odontogenic tumours due to its locally aggressive behaviour and its high relapse rate in cases of conservative treatment (simple enucleation): it has been accordingly renamed *keratocystic odontogenic tumour*;
- the calcifying odontogenic cyst has been placed among the odontogenic tumours due to its high relapse rate in cases of conservative treatment, and has been renamed *calcifying odontogenic tumour*;
- the aneurysmal bone cyst and the simple bone cyst have been framed as *bone related lesions* due to the complete lack of the epithelial-connective wall that is typical of the cystic lesions.

Therefore, these lesions will be described in Chapter 9 together with other neoplasms of the jaws.

The actual cystic lesions have a very low relapse rate after complete removal of the epithelial-connective wall and the elimination of the cause that caused them in the first place. Details regarding the treatment of these lesions are described in the next sections of this chapter.

ODONTOGENIC NON-INFLAMMATORY CYSTS

Gingival cyst of the newborn (Epstein's pearl)

These cysts are frequently multiple, and appear as small white or pinkish nodules measuring 1-5 millimetres in diameter. The most frequent localisation is the palatal midline and, less frequently, on the alveolar mucosa of the maxilla and mandible. Generally, they undergo spontaneous regression weeks after birth, and therefore no treatment is necessary.

Gingival cyst of the adult

These gingival cysts have their peak of incidence between the 5th and the 7th decade, and probably originate from remnants of the dental lamina.

They are typically located in the premolar area of the mandible, and appear as a painless, fluctuating swelling with a very slow growth (📷 8.8).

Dentigerous (follicular) cyst

The dentigerous (or follicular) cyst, as its name implies, originates from the dental follicle when degenerative phenomena cause the accumulation of fluids between the enamel organ and the crown of the impacted tooth. It has a slow growth rate and is generally asymptomatic. It is the second most frequent odontogenic cyst after the periapical (or periradicular) cyst. The dental follicles more prone to develop a dentigerous cyst are those of the lower third molars and upper canines, followed by those of the lower premolars and the upper third molars, with a higher cumulative incidence for mandibular localisation. Since the lower third molars and upper canines have the highest incidence of impaction, there seems to be a direct correlation between delayed eruption and the probability of degenerations occurring to the dental follicle. Dentigerous cysts may also develop during eruption; in esethese cases, they cause a localised, translucent swelling of the alveolar mucosa known as *eruption cyst*.

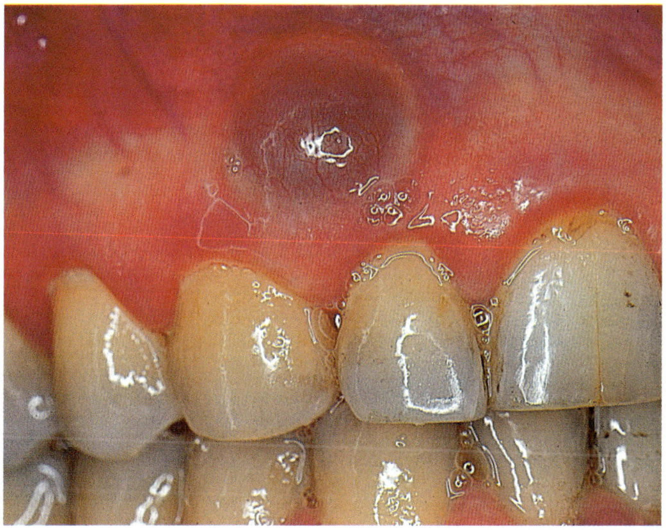

8.8 Gingival cyst of the adult.

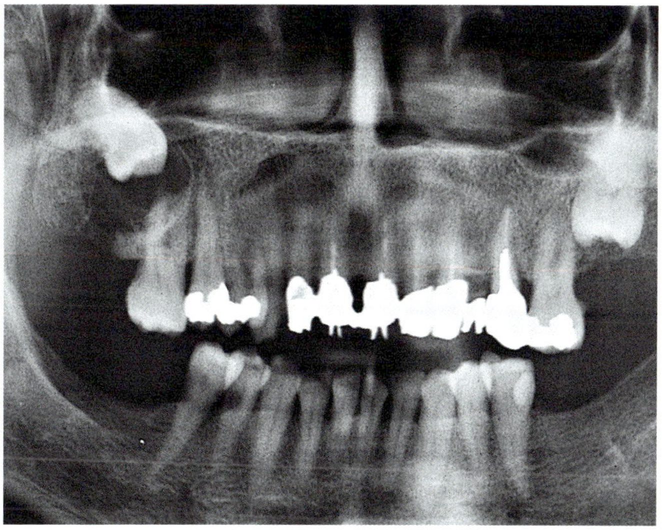

8.9 Dentigerous (follicular) cyst associated with 18, impacted.

Radiographically, the dentigerous cyst appears as a unilocular lesion of variable dimensions (from a small enlargement of the follicle to a very large lesion, involving adjacent anatomical structures such as the mandibular ramus and body, and the inferior alveolar nerve): the lesion is surrounded by a thin radiopaque border, and it develops around the crown of an impacted tooth (8.9).

Lateral periodontal cyst

Radiographically, the lateral periodontal cyst appears as a small, radiolucent intraosseous lesion, rounded or oval, with well-defined margins, always associated with a dental root. The lesion is visible on the mesial or distal side of the root, coronal to the apex, and is more frequently associated with lower canines and premolars. It does not have an inflammatory origin; therefore, the associated tooth is vital and, as it is typically asymptomatic, it is usually discovered on radiographs taken in the course of other treatments. According to the most credited theory on the etiopathogenesis of the lateral periodontal cyst, this lesion originates from the dental lamina.

INFLAMMATORY CYSTS

Periapical (radicular) cyst

It is the most frequent cystic lesion of the oral cavity, accounting for 50% of all odontogenic cysts. It originates from the apex of an erupted, non-vital tooth; deep caries determining pulpar necrosis and incongruous endodontic treatments are the main causes for infection to spread inside the root canal system and reach the apex. The chronic irritative stimulus exerted by bacteria and toxins migrating from the root canal to the periapical bone causes a hyperplastic response on the epithelial cell rests of Malassez, which are part of the periodontal ligament. In rare cases, it can develop on one side of the apex and, in this event, a differential diagnosis with the lateral periodontal cyst is necessary; if pulp vitality tests are positive and the pulp is vital, the lesion is not a periapical cyst.

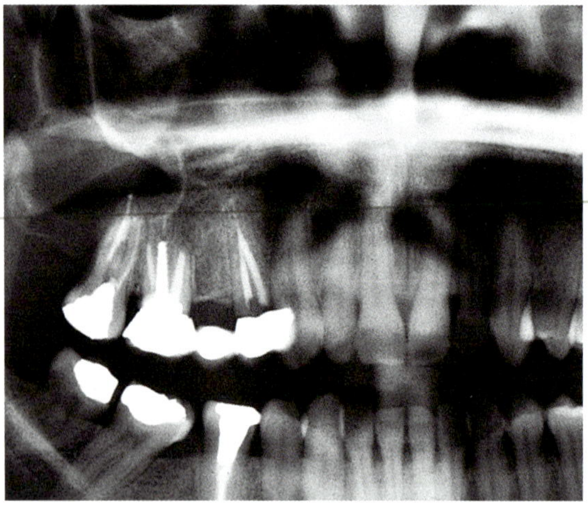

8.10 Periapical cyst associated with 17.

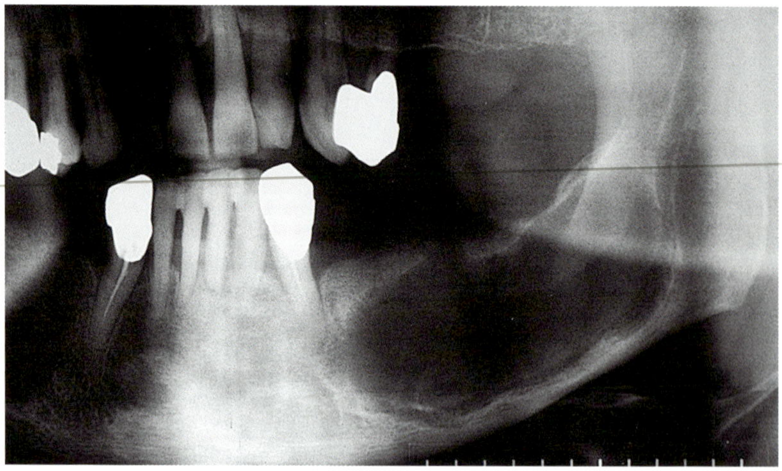

8.11 Large residual cyst involving the left hemimandible.

The periapical cyst is generally asymptomatic and is usually discovered on radiographs taken in the course of other treatments. Radiographically, it appears as a radiolucent area with a rounded shape developing around a root apex (8.10); histologically, the external side of the cyst wall is a non-keratinised stratified squamous epithelium.

Residual cyst

The residual cyst develops from an undiagnosed and untreated periapical or dentigerous cyst. When those cysts are not identified and the associated teeth are extracted, the surrounding soft and hard tissues may heal while the lesion is still present and may continue to develop (8.11). Therefore, they do not have any peculiar characteristics, except for the fact that their growth continues even after the cause (the associated tooth) is removed.

Paradental cyst

It develops around the crown of partially impacted lower third molars after recurrent pericoronitis. It has no peculiar characteristics or behaviour.

NON-ODONTOGENIC CYSTS

Non-odontogenic cysts derive from the proliferation of non-odontogenic epithelial remnants that may remain trapped along the fusion lines of osseous processes during embryogenesis. For this reason, they are also defined as "fissural cysts". These lesions may develop in relative proximity to teeth but, when this is the case, they do not cause the loss of vitality of the dental element. The cyst wall has a typical stratified epithelium layer, while a layer of respiratory epithelium may be found in the lesions developing in the upper maxilla.

Nasopalatine cyst

This is the most common among fissural cysts and develops in the anterior portion of the upper maxilla (premaxilla), in the area of the nasopalatine foramen. Clinically, it appears as a fibro-elastic or fluctuant (if the cortical plate is eroded) swelling, located in the an-

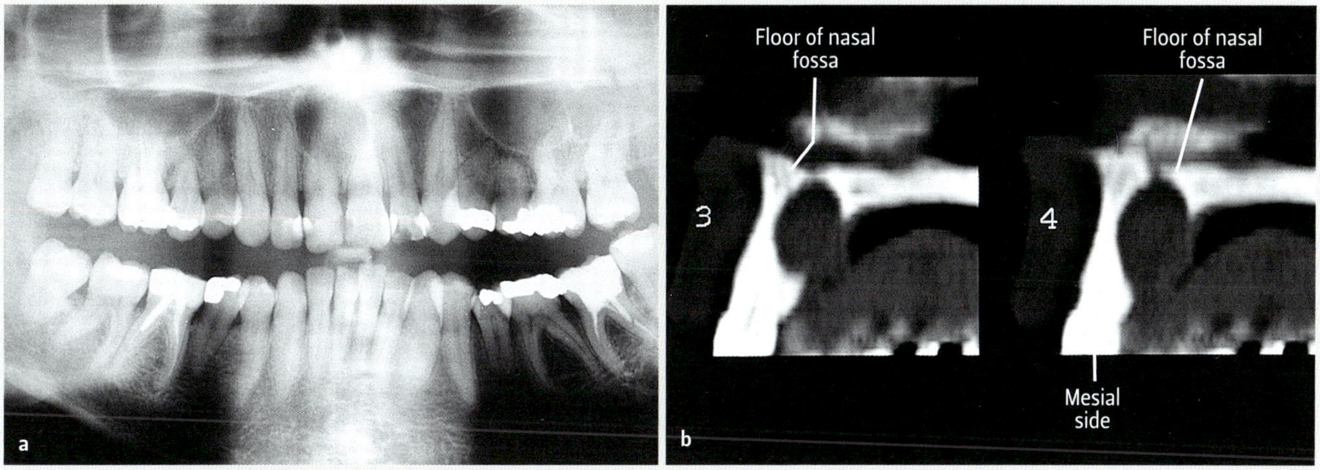

8.12 Nasopalatine cyst: **a)** panoramic radiograph; **b)** CT scan.

terior region of the hard palate. A buccal swelling may be appreciated, but only at a later stage. Radiographically, the lesion appears as a rounded or oval radiolucent area in the interincisive region and, in the early phase, it may appear as a normal, albeit wide, nasopalatine canal. When the anterior nasal spine overlays the lesion, this latter may appear as an inverted heart shape (8.12a-b).

Nasoalveolar and nasolabial cyst

They develop in the soft tissues laterally to the nasal pyramid and adjacent to the upper lip. Resorption of the buccal cortical plate of the upper maxilla is rare.

PSEUDOCYSTS

While showing radiographic and/or clinical features similar to those of actual cysts, the pseudocysts do not have an epithelial wall. In the past, lesions such as the simple bone cyst and the aneurysmal bone cyst were included in this category but, as reported above, they have been reclassified among the bone lesions and will therefore be described in detail in Chapter 9. Thus, the only nosological entity still classified as a pseudocyst is Stafne's bone cavity.

Stafne's bone cavity (bone defect)

Radiographically, Stafne's bone cavity appears as a rounded or elliptic lesion typically located in the posterior mandible under the inferior alveolar canal. It is not a cyst, but a depression of the lingual cortical plate of the mandible that typically harbours an accessory lobe of the submandibular gland. It generally represents a casual finding on panoramic radiographs taken in the course of dental treatments, and a cone beam CT may easily clarify its non-cystic nature (8.13a-b). Obviously, no treatment is necessary.

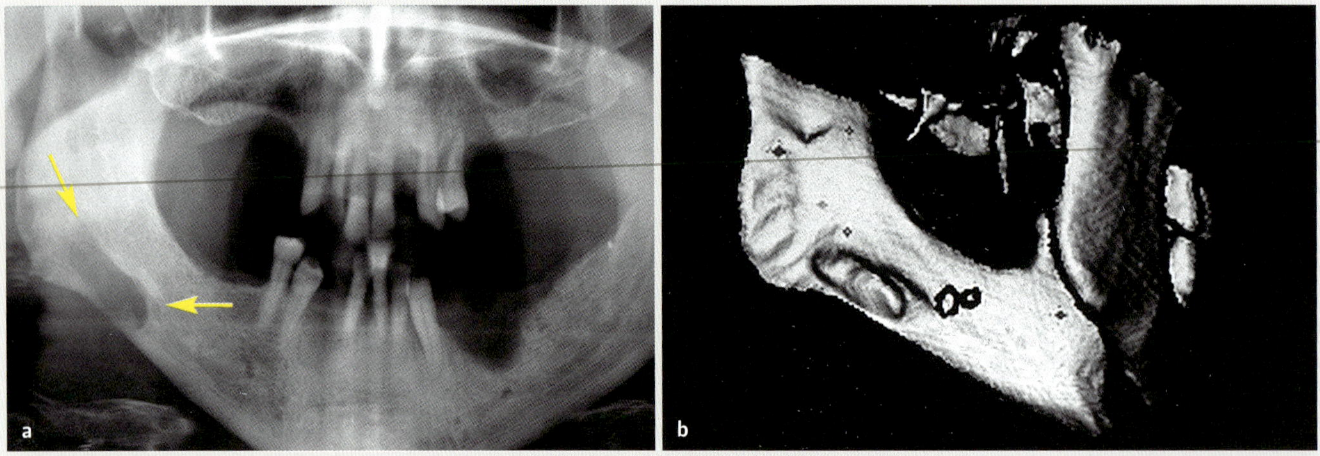

8.13 Stafne's bone cavity: **a)** the radiolucent area is located below the mandibular canal (arrows); **b)** CT scan confirms that the radiolucent area is not a cyst.

Differential diagnosis

There are numerous endosseous lesions that may resemble a cyst, either clinically and/or radiographically. The most frequently found are:

- simple bone cyst;
- aneurysmal bone cyst;
- ameloblastoma;
- odontogenic mixoma;
- calcifying epithelial odontogenic tumour (Pindborg tumour);
- odontogenic fibroma;
- primitive malignant tumours and metastases.

The systematic analysis of the non-cystic lesions is beyond the scope of this chapter: details on these lesions are reported in Chapter 9.

Surgical treatment

The first choice for treatment of cystic lesions of the jaws is enucleation, while the second choice is represented by *marsupialisation*. Finally, a third option is to perform a marsupialisation of the lesion initially, followed by complete enucleation at a later time.

ENUCLEATION

It consists in the complete removal of the lesion in a single surgical session. The residual bone cavity typically undergoes spontaneous reossification due to a bone regeneration process that begins with the organisation of the primitive blood clot that forms inside the cavity soon after the removal of the cyst.

The main advantage of this approach is represented by the shortening of the healing time. Disadvantages, however, are more significant in cases of large lesions developing in close proximity to relevant anatomic structures (nerves, vessels, maxillary sinus etc.),

Basic techniques – Enucleation of endosseous cysts of the jaws

Access flaps

The choice of the flap to be elevated for access to a cystic lesion follows the general principles of flap design described in the dedicated chapter. The location of the lesion, its development towards the margin of the alveolar crest, and the periodontal condition of the involved teeth are additional factors to be considered in the choice of flap design, as are the number of releasing incisions to be made and the position of the primary incision (marginal or submarginal, crestal).

Access flaps: envelope flap (no releasing incisions)

This is mainly indicated in cases of mandibular cysts with a predominant lingual development, particularly in the anterior region of the mandible, where the favourable curvature (convexity) allows good visibility of the surgical field. This flap may also be chosen in cases of buccal approach for the enucleation of lesions situated in posterior or anterior areas of the mandible, to avoid the recourse to releasing incisions in proximity to anatomic structures such as the mental foramen. Finally, the envelope flap is indicated for the enucleation of cysts developing on the palatal side of the maxilla (8.14, 8.15).

Access flaps: three-corner flap (one releasing incision)

This provides better visibility of the surgical field compared to the envelope flap, as retraction is easier and exposes a wider area due to the releasing incision. Whenever possible, the releasing incision should be made on the opposite side with respect to the dominant direction of the blood vessels that vascularise the flap; for this reason, generally, the releasing incision should be conducted mesially. This flap is typically indicated when a buccal approach to the lesion is advised (8.16).

Access flaps: four-corner flap (two releasing incisions)

This offers the best visualisation of the surgical field, as the two releasing incisions allow for a better retraction and ample exposure of the area. However, because the two releasing incisions limit the blood supply to the flap, it is imperative that the rules described in Chapter 3 regarding the general principles of flap design be followed (8.17).

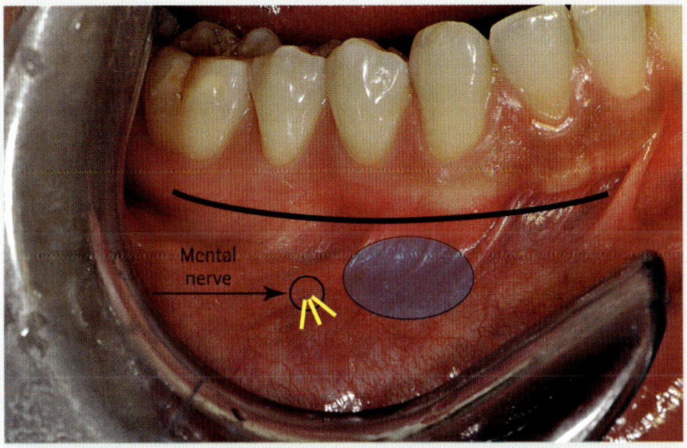

8.14 Envelope flap on the buccal side of the right hemimandible.

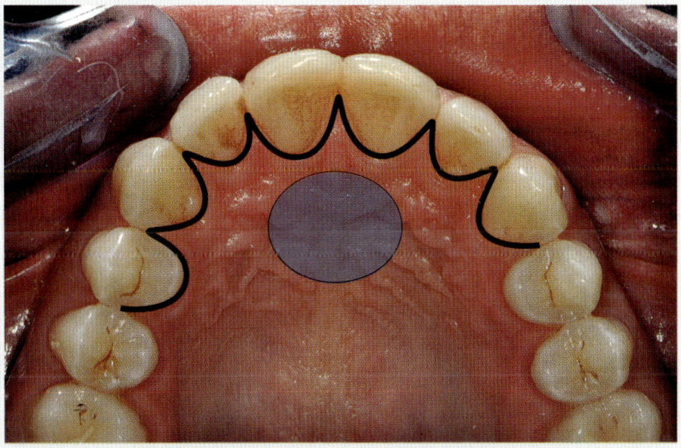

8.15 Palatal flap (no releasing incisions).

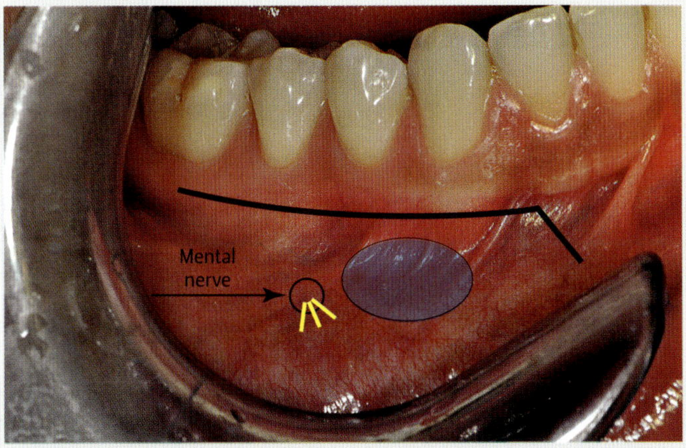

8.16 Three-corner flap.

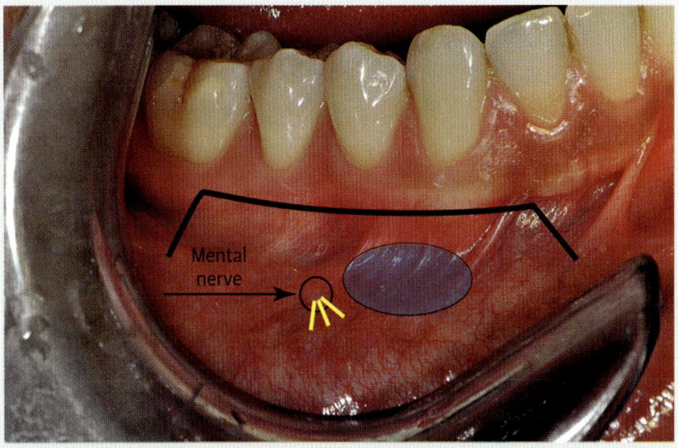

8.17 Four-corner flap.

Access flaps: marginal (sulcular) and submarginal

The marginal flap is indicated when:

- the cyst develops towards the crestal margin of the alveolar ridge;
- there are periodontally compromised teeth in the area;
- there is a possibility that one or more teeth may be extracted as part of the intervention.

In the first event, the marginal incision is indicated to allow the margin of the flap to be sutured above sound bone at the end of the intervention, thus guaranteeing the flap adequate support and avoiding dehiscence (see the general principles in Chapter 3 for details).

In the second event, the marginal incision makes it possible to evaluate the periodontal conditions of the involved teeth and to intervene both on the cyst and on the periodontal tissues if deemed necessary. In the third event, should the extraction of one or more teeth be performed in conjunction with the enucleation of the cyst, the marginal incision allows an adequate repositioning of the flap, while a submarginal incision would leave a band of marginal gingiva comprised between the post-extractive sockets and the surgical incision with inadequate blood supply.

The submarginal flap is indicated whenever the clinical conditions described above are not present. It is worth restating, however, that care must be taken to guarantee that the margins of the flap may be sutured above sound, well-vascularised bone (8.18a-b).

Access flaps: crestal flap

The crestal flap is indicated in edentulous areas, whenever the cyst develops towards the crestal margin of the alveolar ridge. The objectives are: a) to maximise visibility in the surgical field; and b): to allow the sutured flap to rest on sound bone (8.19).

Flap elevation and exposure of the cortical plate

After a full-thickness incision of the soft tissues is performed, the flap is elevated with the aid of specifically designed elevators. If the cyst has not eroded the cortical plate, this procedure may result rather easily, as a thick layer of intact bone is a valuable aid in the cleavage of the surgical flap. If, on the contrary, the lesion has completely eroded the cortical plate, the cystic wall is in direct contact with the periosteum.

In this event, the elevation of the surgical flap must be performed with great care, as the lack of a well-preserved bone plate renders the identification of the correct cleavage plane more difficult and the separation of the cystic wall from the periosteal layer of the flap necessary. Whenever this is the case, it is advisable to begin the elevation of the surgical flap from the peripheral areas, where the cortical plate is intact, and keep the identified cleavage plain as a guide when the area in which the cortical plate is eroded is reached (8.20).

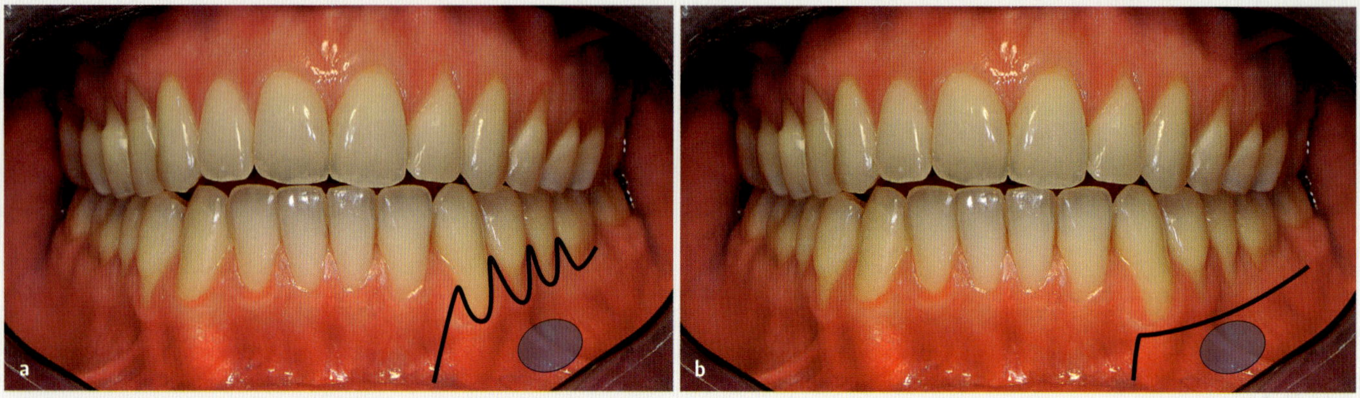

8.18 **a)** Marginal (sulcular) flap. **b)** Submarginal flap.

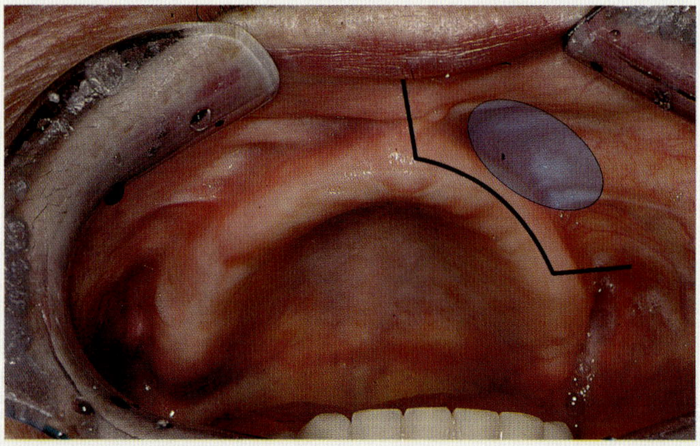

8.19 Crestal incision in the edentulous ridge.

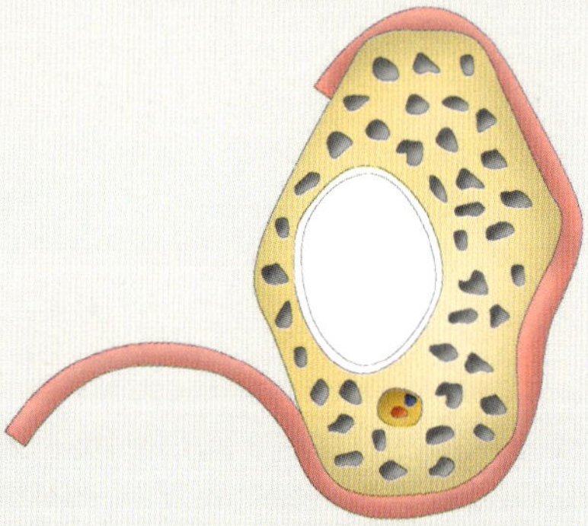

8.20 Flap elevation.

Access osteotomy

This is performed with a round bur mounted on a straight handpiece or with piezoelectric instruments. It is imperative that sthe relationship between adequate visibility and the preservation of the cortical bone be optimised, while the border of the access osteotomy must be kept at a safe distance from the margins of the flap, to guarantee that they can be sutured on sound bone at the end of the procedure (8.21).

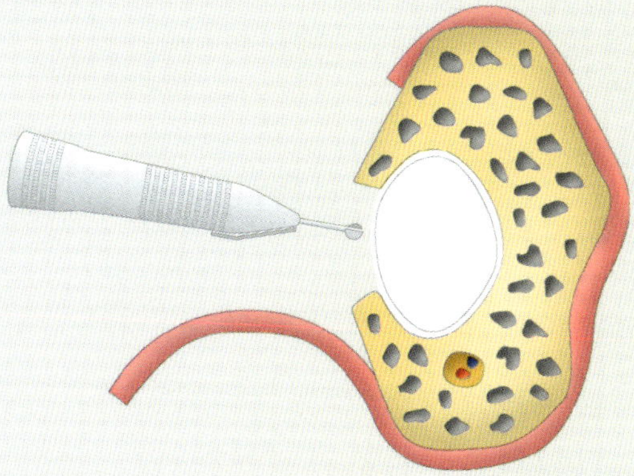

8.21 Access osteotomy.

Cyst cleavage and enucleation

Once the cystic wall is identified, its cleavage from the bone cavity (or from the soft tissues, if the lesion has eroded the cortical plate) begins with the aid of a surgical curette or specifically designed elevators; the latter may be straight or angled, according to specific needs. This operation may also be performed by means of piezoelectric instruments. However, it is important that all instruments be kept in contact with the bony walls, to avoid any early damage of the cystic wall. If the tension of the cystic wall impedes the enucleation manoeuvres, part of the content of the lesion may be drained with a syringe. The cyst is kept in tension with Allis or haemostatic forceps to complete its cleavage from the cavity walls until enucleation is completed. The removal of the entire lesion in one piece may be useful to avoid the risk of incomplete excision, but it is not always possible, particularly in cases of lesions with a thin cystic wall firmly adherent to the root of the involved teeth or to the cavity walls. Even if it is removed piece by piece, the treatment may be successful if a thorough revision of the residual cavity is performed (8.22).

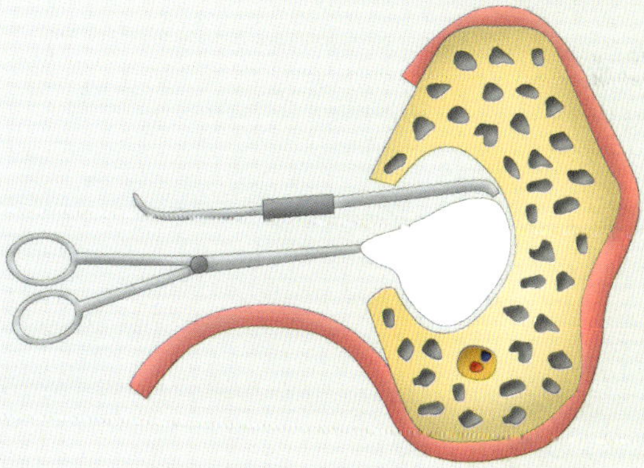

8.22 Cleavage of the cyst from the walls of the bone cavity.

Revision of the residual cavity

The revision of the residual cavity is performed with surgical curettes or surgical spoons with the aim of removing possible epithelial-connective tissue remains. Profuse irrigation inside the cavity allows the removal of debris and the careful inspection of the bony walls to verify the absence of any cystic wall leftovers.

Haemostasis

Technical details on the techniques to obtain an adequate haemostasis are reported in Chapter 3. However, it is worth remembering that blood clot formation is the basis for bone regeneration; the recourse to techniques and devices, such as bipolar coagulation, with the aim of obtaining a completely bloodless surgical field is thus contraindicated.

Suture

A competent suture is always indicated, except when an infectious cyst is removed; in this event, it may be indicated to place a surgical drain or folded iodoform gauze inside the cavity to allow spontaneous healing by secondary intention (8.23).

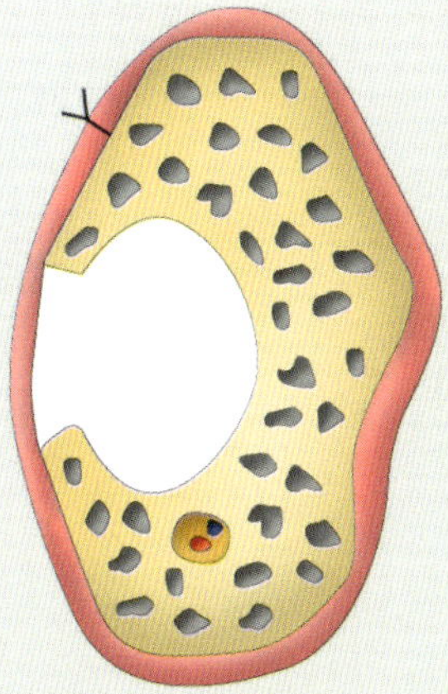

8.23 Suture.

Enucleation of the lesion

Advantages

- Resolution in a single surgical session
- Shorter recovery time

Disadvantages

- High biologic cost in cases of very large lesions
- Possible need for endodontic treatment of vital teeth involved in the lesion
- Risk of iatrogenic fracture of the mandible in cases of very large lesions

Marsupialisation

Advantages

- Simple to perform
- Reduced risk of iatrogenic fracture and nerve/vessel damage
- No loss of vitality of the involved teeth

Disadvantages

- Slow resolution of the pathology
- Difficult hygiene of the accessory cavity
- Halitosis

and are mainly represented by the risk of damage to such structures (neurovascular lesions, oroantral communications, mandibular fracture, etc.). In these cases, or when a dentigerous cyst is associated with an impacted tooth that is important from a functional viewpoint (e.g. cuspids), marsupialisation is indicated and should be considered the treatment of choice (for details on surgical exposure and orthodontic repositioning of impacted teeth, see further in this chapter).

It is worth remembering that the complete treatment of periapical cysts includes the removal of the lesion, and *the removal of its cause*. These cysts are always associated to a non-vital, infected tooth that must be treated to avoid relapse. The treatment options for the associated tooth are:

- orthograde endodontic therapy;
- surgical retrograde endodontic therapy;
- extraction. If the extent of the lesion is limited, orthograde endodontic therapy alone may cause the complete resorption of the lesion.

MARSUPIALISATION

Marsupialisation is based on the principle of creating ample communication between the cyst and the oral cavity, such as to eliminate the internal pressure of the cyst. The absence of any internal pressure will cause the interruption of osteoclast activity and the stimulation of bone repair mechanisms by activation of osteoblasts; these processes lead to peripheral bone regeneration and, thus, reduction of the extent of the lesion. Moreover, marsupialisation allows histopathological examination of the portion of the cystic wall that is removed.

The chief indications for marsupialisation are twofold:

- cases in which the extent of the lesion is significant and exposes to high intraoperative risks (mandibular fracture, neurovascular lesions, lesions to vital teeth, etc.);

Basic techniques – Marsupialisation

Access flaps

As far as marsupialisation is concerned, surgical access to the lesion is not obtained with a proper flap: an excision of soft tissues and of a portion of the cystic wall is performed, to create an ample communication between the lesion and the oral cavity. If the cyst is not associated to an impacted tooth, the location of the surgical access should be chosen considering the ease of reach, because the patient will have to perform a daily cleansing of the cystic cavity (8.24a).

On the contrary, when marsupialisation is aimed at exposing an impacted tooth to be repositioned with an orthodontic treatment, the location of surgical access should be chosen considering the need for an adequate access to the tooth crown (for brace positioning), and the repositioning path programmed by the orthodontist (8.24b).

Access osteotomy and cyst opening

In the event that the cyst has not eroded the cortical plate, controlled ostectomy is performed with rotating or piezoelectric instruments; the extent of the access should be decided considering the need for an ample communication to facilitate cleansing manoeuvres. If one or more teeth involved in the lesion are extracted, the communication between the cyst and the oral cavity may be created following the post-extractive sockets. Once the lesion is exposed, a portion of the cystic wall is removed and the content is drained; this phase represents the basis for the healing process, because it causes the interruption of osteoclast activation by eliminating the hydrostatic pressure inside the cystic cavity (8.25a-b).

Communication maintenance

It is imperative that an ample communication be maintained to avoid its spontaneous closure. For this reason, the cystic wall is sutured to the bloody margin of the surrounding soft tissues. The patency of the surgically created communication is maintained either by packing the cystic cavity with iodoform gauze or by using a specifically designed acrylic obturator. The iodoform gauze should be accurately folded inside the cystic cavity to maximise the quantity of material used and thus its absorbent capability, while one of the ends should be left protruding out of the cavity about an inch (it may be kept in place with a single stitch) to maintain the patency of the communication. The iodoform gauze must be replaced weekly, and it should be used for several weeks (3 - 8), according to specific needs (8.26a-b). Peripheral bone regeneration, in cases of complete spontaneous healing, may take several months. Alternatively, once the extent of the lesion is decreased to the point where the risk of damage to neighbouring anatomic structures is eliminated, the treatment can be completed in a second surgical session by enucleating the residual cyst (combined technique).

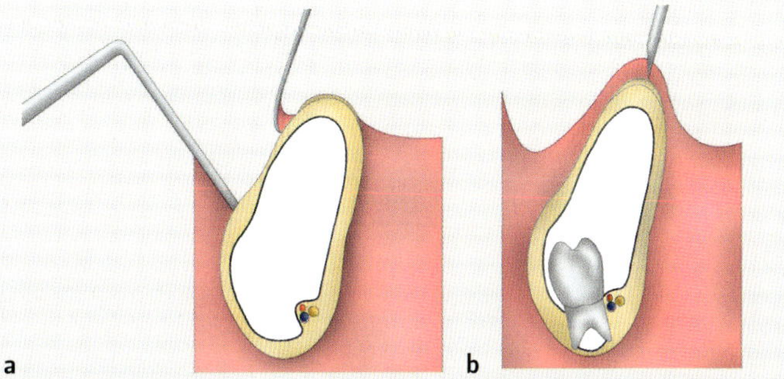

8.24 a) Incision of the soft tissues above the lesion. **b)** Crestal incision in cases of a cystic lesion associated with an impacted tooth to be retrieved.

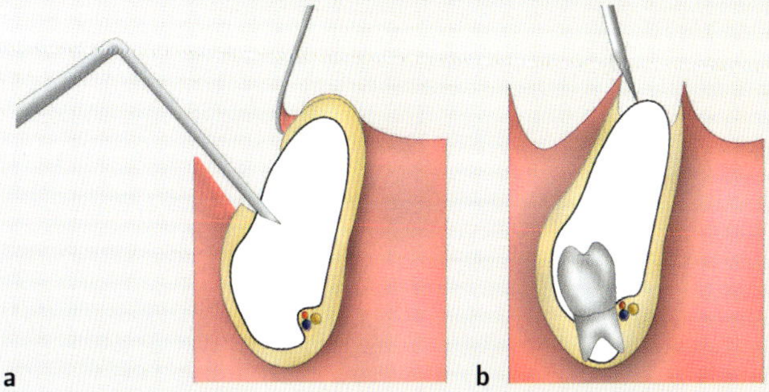

8.25 a) Access osteotomy and opening of the cystic wall. **b)** Crestal opening of the cystic wall in cases of impacted tooth retrieval.

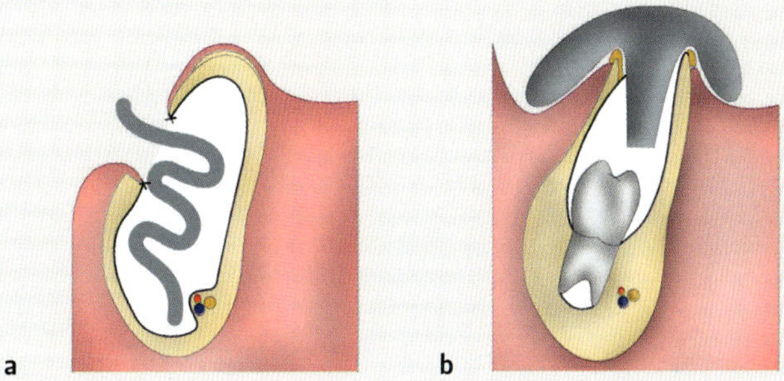

8.26 a) Access maintenance: iodoform gauze packing. **b)** Custom acrylic obturator used in cases of orthodontic repositioning of an impacted tooth.

- dentigerous (follicular) cysts developing around an impacted tooth that is important from a functional point of view and should be uncovered and repositioned, such as a cuspid or premolar.

Advantages of this technique are represented by its relatively easy application (it is possible to treat even large lesions under local anaesthesia), the reduced risk of iatrogenic fractures and neurovascular lesions, and the elimination of the risk that vital teeth involved in the lesions may lose their vitality.

Disadvantages of marsupialisation are mainly represented by a slower resolution of the pathology, with greater discomfort for the patient; since an "accessory cavity" is created inside the oral cavity, oral hygiene manoeuvres are more difficult and food debris may stagnate inside the opened lesion and cause halitosis.

COMBINED TECHNIQUE

A combined technique may represent an acceptable compromise between the two techniques previously described. In the first surgical session, a marsupialisation of the cyst is performed, followed after time by the complete enucleation of the lesion in a second surgical session, when the extent of the lesion and the intraoperative risks are reduced. Moreover, the initial marsupialisation frequently causes a thickening of the cystic wall, which renders the removal of the lesion easier and reduces the risk of leaving small portions of the cystic wall attached to the surrounding bone, which may cause a relapse.

Surgical protocol for cyst enucleation

Specific surgical armamentarium

The surgical armamentarium used for cyst enucleation is the same as that described for basic oral surgery interventions, though some instruments are peculiar to this type of surgery:

- round and/or fissure burs for the access osteotomy, when the cyst has not completely eroded the cortical plate;
- surgical curettes and elevators for the cleavage of the cystic wall from the surrounding bone and/or soft tissues;
- when treating a periapical cyst, if a retrograde endodontic therapy is to be performed the specific surgical instruments are needed (see Chapter 7 for details).

Both the access osteotomy and the cleavage of the cystic wall may also be performed also with piezoelectric instruments.

Locoregional anaesthesia

Criteria regarding anaesthesia protocols for the treatment of cysts are mainly based on the location of the lesion and follow the same guidelines as those reported in detail in Chapter 3. A step-by-step clinical case illustrating the enucleation of a residual cyst is presented (🔍 8.27a-h).

Surgical protocol for cyst marsupialisation

To carry out the marsupialisation of a cyst, no specific instruments are needed, except for materials that allow the maintaining of an ample communication between the lesion and the oral cavity, such as surgical drains or custom made acrylic obturators with a wedge protruding inside the cystic cavity.

For a better understanding of the procedure, see the step-by-step clinical case (8.28a-e).

Marsupialisation associated to orthodontic repositioning of an impacted tooth

In some cases, marsupialisation of a dentigerous cyst may be sufficient to allow spontaneous eruption of the associated impacted tooth. When spontaneous eruption is impeded, specifically designed dental braces can be applied to the tooth to associate orthodontic traction to marsupialisation, with the aim of repositioning the tooth in the planned position.

A step-by-step clinical case is presented (8.29a-e).

Clinical case 1 – Enucleation of a residual cyst

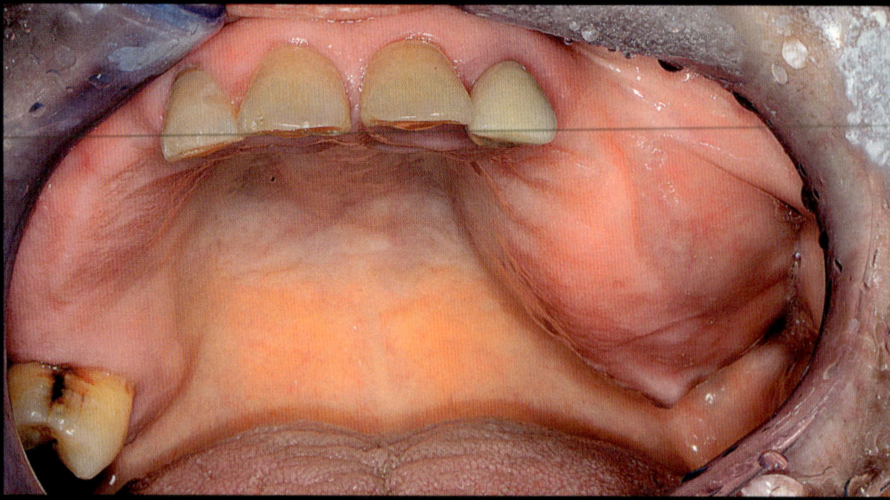

8.27a Preoperative clinical situation: pronounced swelling of the buccal and palatal side of the edentulous alveolar ridge in the left hemimaxilla.

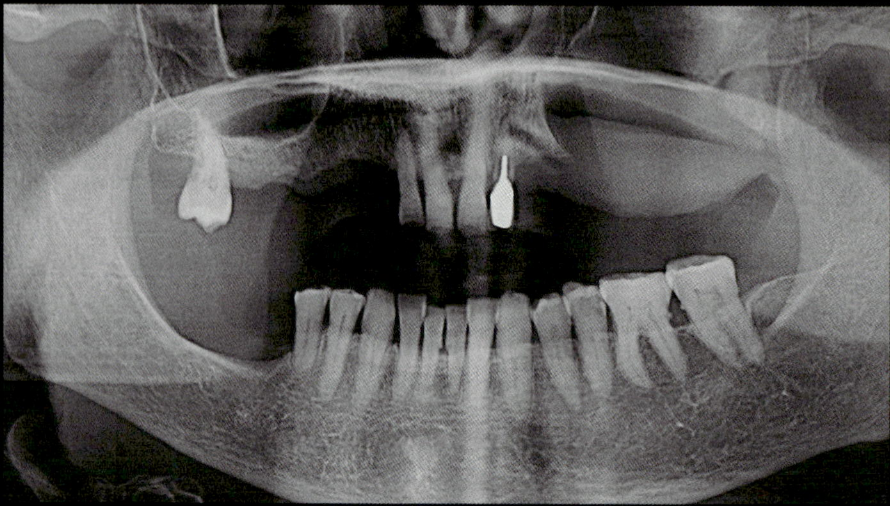

8.27b Preoperative panoramic radiograph showing a large osteolytic lesion (residual cyst) extending from the canine region to the molar region.

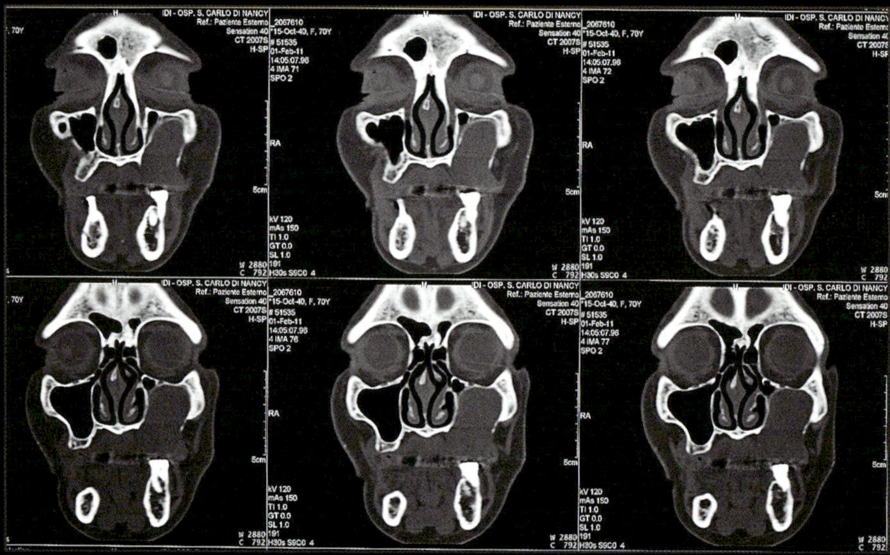

8.27c CT scan showing that the lesion has eroded the buccal and palatal cortical plate of the maxilla, and has dislocated the floor of the maxillary sinus against the orbital floor.

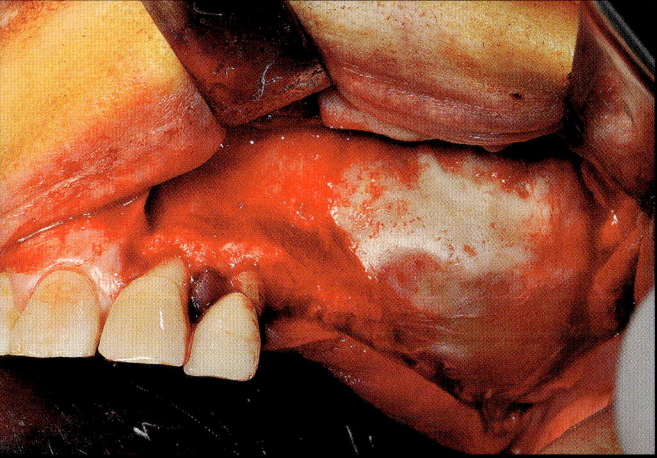

8.27d Incision and elevation of a four-corner, full-thickness flap, and identification of the cyst wall.

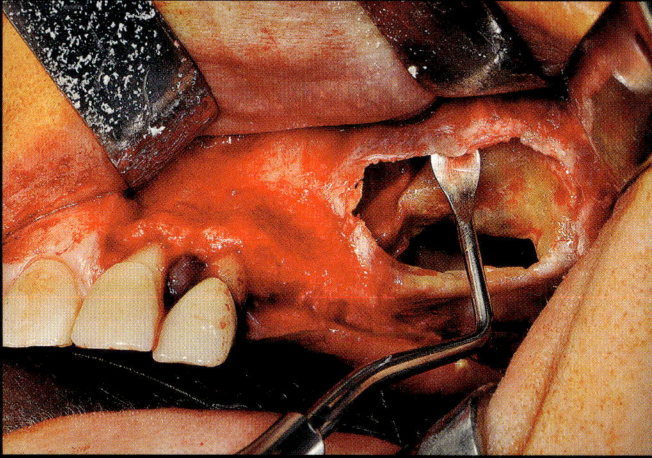

8.27e Cleavage of the cyst from the bony walls of the cavity.

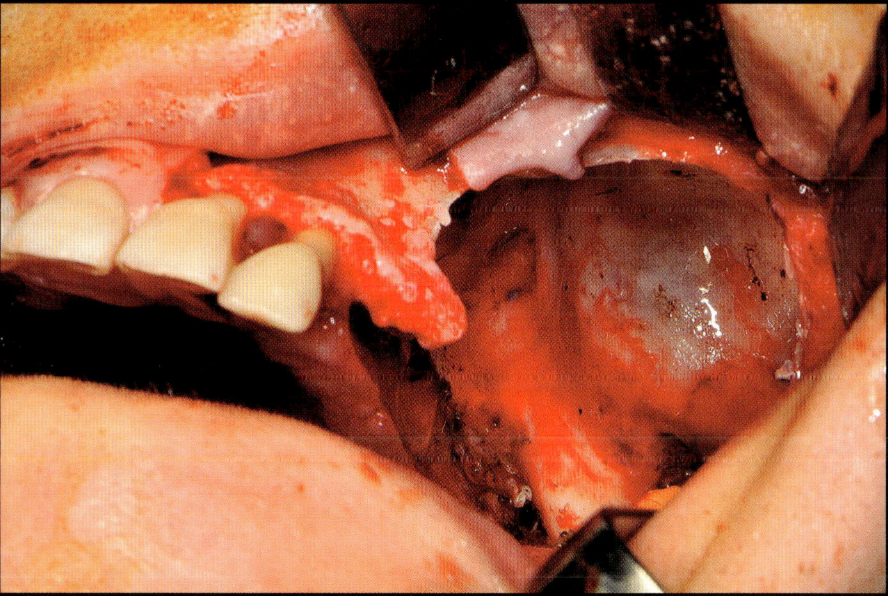

8.27f Residual cavity after the enucleation of the lesion.

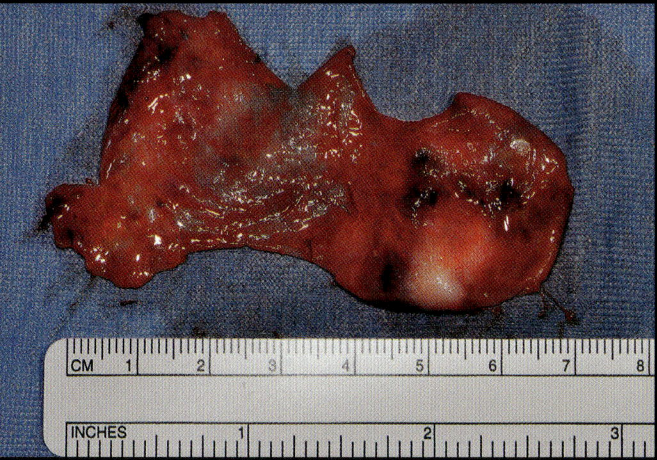

8.27g The removed lesion.

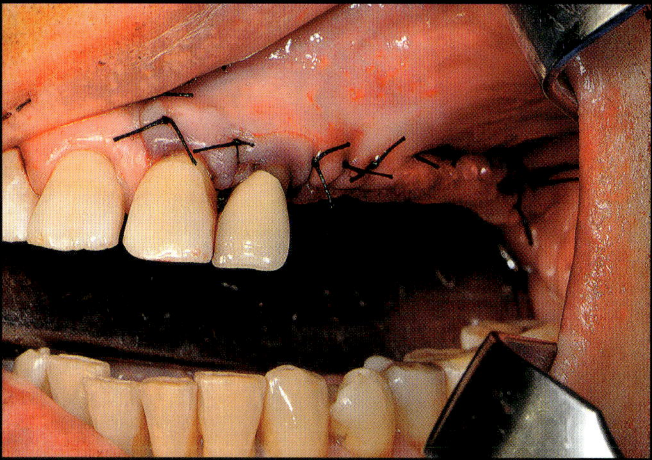

8.27h Suture.

Clinical case 2 – Marsupialisation of a mandibular cyst

8.28 Marsupialisation of a mandibular cyst: **a)** panoramic radiograph showing a large multilocular lesion extending from 35 to 44: all teeth, except from 34 and 45, are vital; **b)** opening of the cyst wall and drainage of the fluid content; **c)** the cyst wall is sutured to the oral mucosa; **d)** the access is kept open with the aid of a custom made acrylic obturator; **e)** radiographic follow-up 12 months after surgery showing the complete reossification of the residual cavity.

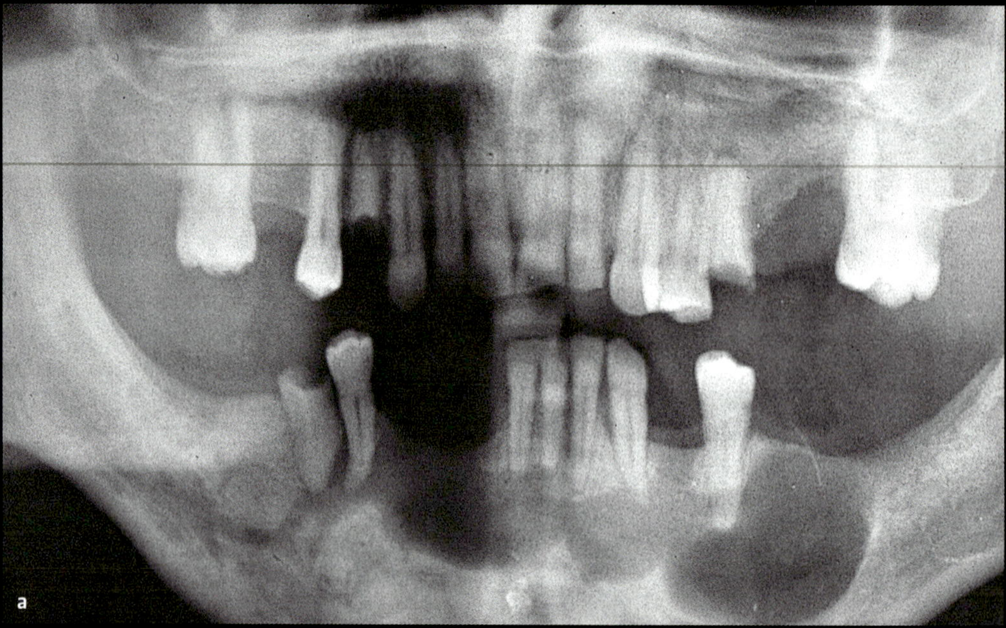

a

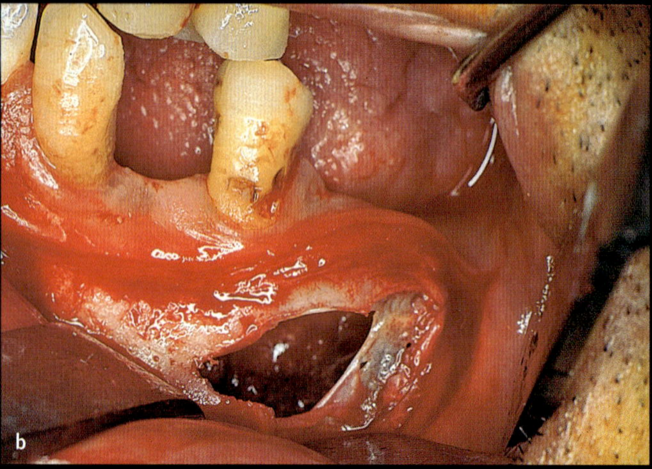

b

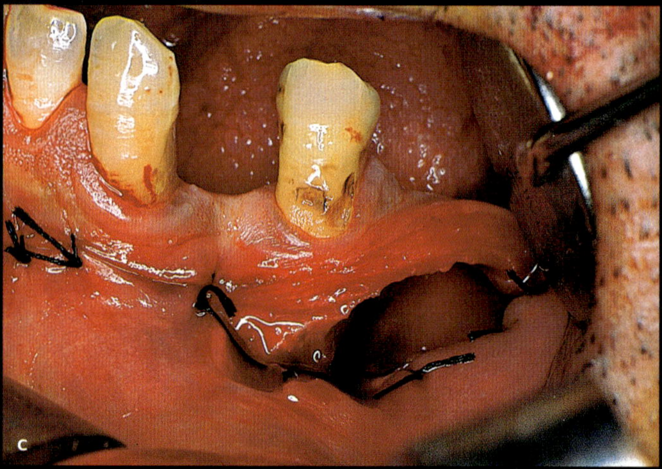

c

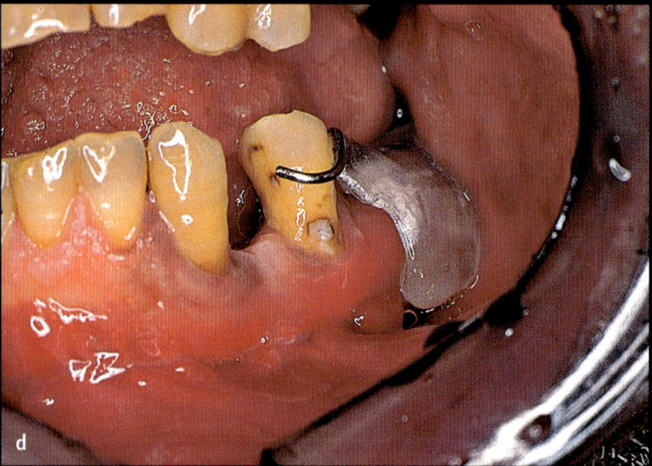

d

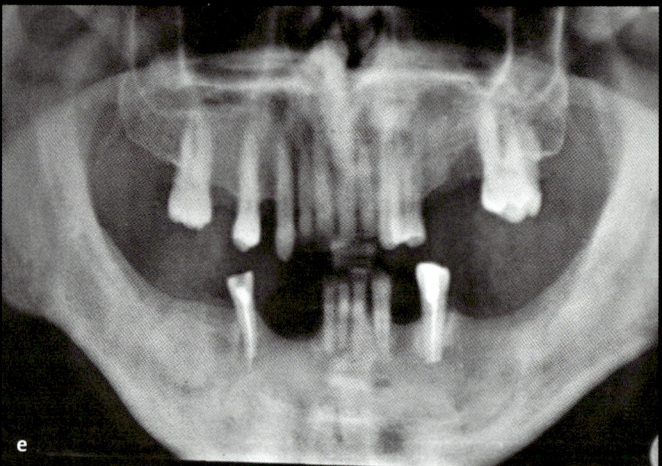

e

Clinical case 3 – Marsupialisation of a dentigerous cyst for the orthodontic repositioning of impacted 3.3

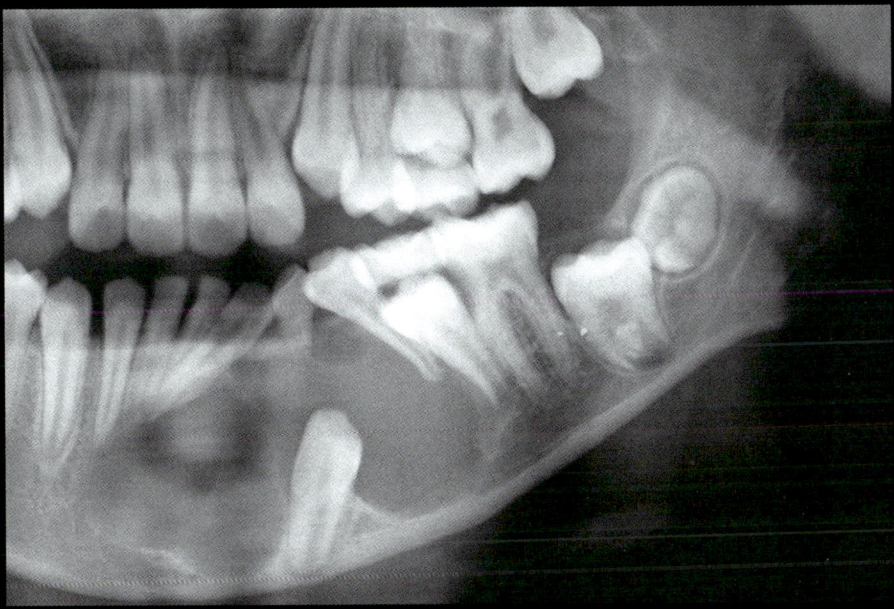

8.29a Large osteolytic lesion (dentigerous cyst) associated with 3.3, deeply impacted. Given the functional importance of the tooth, marsupialisation in association with orthodontic repositioning of 3.3 is planned.

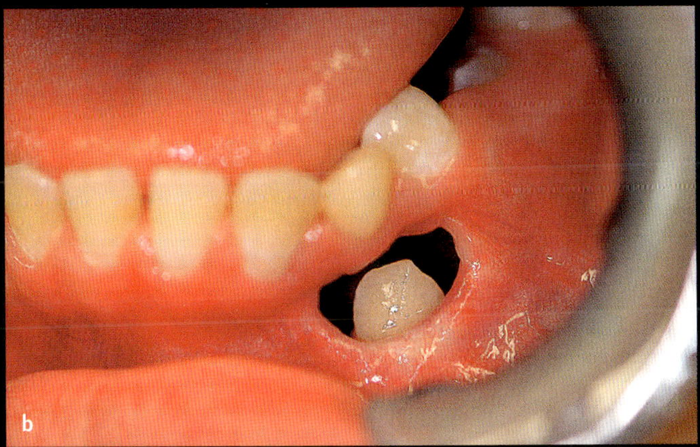

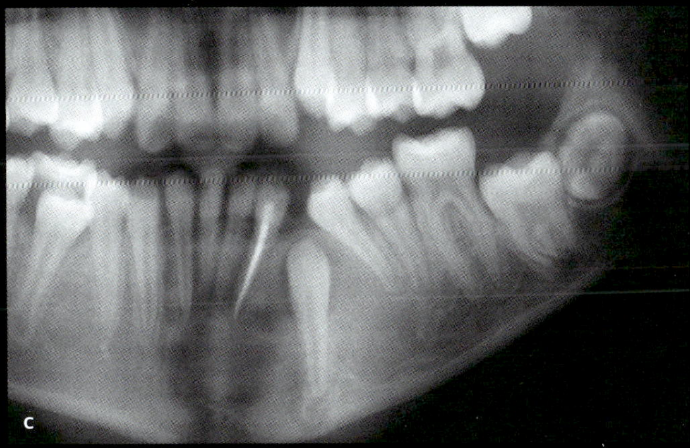

8.29b–c After marsupialisation the impacted tooth begins to erupt, and the cystic cavity starts to shrink.

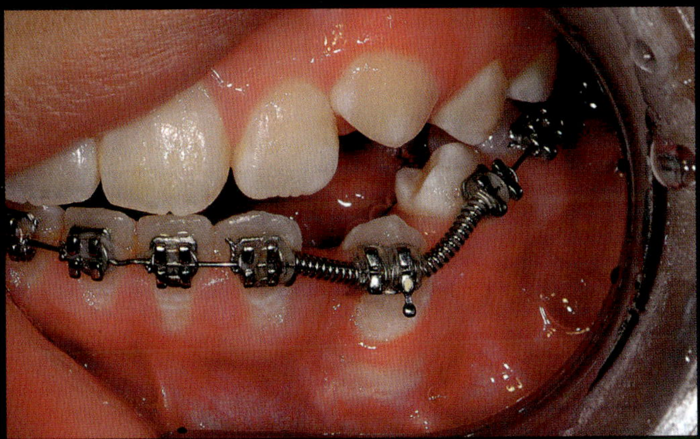

8.29d Orthodontic treatment to accelerate and guide the eruption of 3.3.

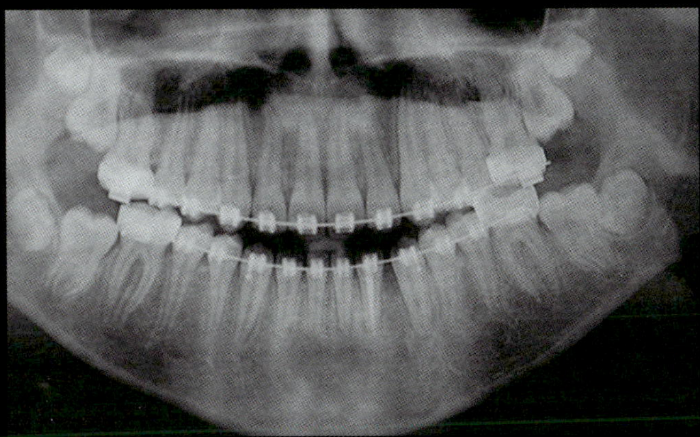

8.29e Panoramic radiograph showing the correct dental alignment, and complete healing of the residual cavity.

Surgical approach according to different areas of the jaws

CYSTS IN THE ANTERIOR MAXILLA

Anaesthesia

When a palatal approach is indicated, local anaesthesia should target the nasopalatine nerves, while in cases of a buccal approach it is performed in the buccal vestibule.

If the cyst develops towards the nasal cavities, the use of topical anaesthetics in the form of sprays or creams may be indicated, as a direct injection of local anaesthetics in the nasal mucosa can be very painful. In cases of large lesions that develop towards the canine fossa or the medial portion of the maxillary sinus, infraorbital nerve block may be indicated (see Chapter 3 for details).

Relevant anatomic structures

Nasopalatine nerves - *Surgical implications*
Section of the nasopalatine nerves, whether accidental or planned if they represent an obstacle to the treatment, does not generally cause relevant long-term sequelae.

Nasal cavities - *Surgical implications*
In the event that a cyst has eroded the nasal floor, the nasal cavities should be identified and the nasal mucosa should be adequately protected to prevent its perforation. If laceration of the mucosa occurs, it must be repaired with resorbable sutures to avoid contamination of the residual cavity by the endonasal bacterial flora.

CYSTS IN THE POSTERIOR MAXILLA

Anaesthesia

When a buccal approach is indicated (the most frequent circumstance), local anaesthesia should target the posterior alveolar nerves in association with infusion in the vestibular fornix. If the cyst develops towards the maxillary sinus, an infraorbital nerve block is indicated, either with an intraoral approach or, better still, with a percutaneous approach (see Chapter 3 for details). If the cyst develops towards the palate, however, and a palatal approach is indicated, anaesthesia should target the greater palatine nerve.

Relevant anatomic structures

Greater palatine neurovascular bundle - *Surgical implications*
Subperiosteal flap elevation effectively prevents significant bleeding from the greater palatine artery as well as possible damage to the greater palatine nerve. The only danger zone is the area of the palatine foramen: it is recommended this area be identified and protected if the cyst develops in its proximity.

Maxillary sinus - *Surgical implications*
Generally, endosseous cysts that develop in the lateral-posterior area of the maxilla tend to displace the floor of the maxillary sinus cranially and gradually, without eroding it. For this reason, a favourable cleavage plane is usually present between the cystic wall and the

sinusal floor. However, in some cases the cyst can erode the floor of the sinus (particularly if the content is infectious), and the cystic wall may adhere to the Schneiderian membrane; this renders cleavage between the two planes more difficult. In the event of a perforation or tear of the sinusal membranes, it is not recommended that its closure be attempted with sutures, due to the thinness of the membrane itself. To avoid a possible residual oroantral communication, it is sufficient to reposition the access flap with an airtight suture.

CYSTS IN THE ANTERIOR MANDIBLE

Anaesthesia

Frequently, cysts in the anterior mandible require a buccal approach; thus, anaesthesia of the mental nerve in association with infiltration of anaesthetic in the vestibular fornix is indicated. In cases of large lesions, anaesthesia of the inferior alveolar nerve is recommended. In case a lingual approach is necessary (a rare occurrence), or in case of cysts developing towards the floor of the mouth, anaesthesia of the lingual nerve or plexus anaesthesia of the floor of the mouth is indicated.

Relevant anatomic structures

Mental nerve - *Surgical implications*
The nerve should always be identified and protected to avoid any accidental lesion, particularly when rotary instruments are used.

Incisive nerve - *Surgical implications*
The incisive nerve is the thinnest terminal branch of the inferior alveolar nerve (the thickest one being the mental nerve) and, due to its small diameter, it is not always possible to identify it and avoid its section. In this event, however, functional sequelae are frequently negligible.

Blood vessels in the floor of the mouth - *Surgical implications*
Branches of the sublingual and submental arteries may be involved in the surgical manoeuvres in cases of a lingual approach to the cyst, or when a lesion developing towards the floor of the mouth has eroded the lingual cortical plate. Subperiosteal dissection generally prevents damage to these vessels but, in the event that profuse bleeding occurs, adequate haemostasis is essential to avoiding the development of a related haematoma in the floor of the mouth.

CYSTS IN THE POSTERIOR MANDIBLE

Anaesthesia

Local anaesthetic blocks of the inferior alveolar nerve, buccal nerve, and lingual nerve are indicated to obtain adequate anaesthesia in this area. Integration with plexus anaesthesia in the buccal vestibule may be indicated to reduce bleeding.

Relevant anatomic structures

Inferior alveolar neurovascular bundle - *Surgical implications*
As regards cysts developing in the posterior mandible, the neurovascular bundle is frequently in proximity to the lesion, or in direct contact with the cystic wall. Non-infec-

tious lesions with a thick cystic wall may render cleavage from the neurovascular bundle and the preservation of its integrity easier, even if sensory alterations, albeit transient, may result from the manipulation of the nerve during the surgical manoeuvres. In cases of bleeding from the inferior alveolar artery, haemostasis must be obtained without the recourse to bipolar coagulation, because the heat generated by the bipolar pliers may cause irreversible damage to the nerve.

Lingual nerve - *Surgical implications*
The risk of damage to the lingual nerve is higher in cases of cysts developing towards the lingual cortical plate, particularly in the area of the mandibular ramus and the retromolar trigone. A subperiosteal elevation of the surgical flap and an adequate protection of its lingual aspect with specific retractors prevent possible damage to the lingual nerve.

Mental nerve - *Surgical implications*
Damage to the mental nerve may be prevented by positioning the releasing incisions of the access flap mesially or distally to the mental foramen, and by identifying and protecting the foramen itself during the surgical manoeuvres.

Facial artery - *Surgical implications*
Lesions of the facial artery result in a profuse and dangerous bleeding, which is generally not manageable in a private practice under local anaesthesia. It is thus imperative that a strictly subperiosteal elevation of the surgical flap be performed and that the buccal and caudal sides of the flap be protected with specific retractors, particularly when rotary instruments are used. If a laceration of the facial artery occurs, compression and bipolar coagulation do not generally help control the profuse bleeding, and the ligature of the artery with an extraoral approach (in the neck) may be necessary.

Branches of the mylohyoid artery - *Surgical implications*
Branches of the mylohyoid artery may be encountered if a lingual approach to a cyst is indicated, or if the cyst has eroded the lingual cortical plate. A careful subperiosteal dissection is generally sufficient to avoid any lesion to these vessels.

Follow-up

As previously mentioned, cysts have a negligible relapse tendency once they are completely removed, with the only exception being the case in which a periapical lesion is enucleated, but the associated tooth (the original cause) is not extracted. The group of cyst-like endosseous lesions that showed a high relapse tendency (keratocyst, odontogenic calcifying cyst, etc.) have, significantly, been reclassified as benign neoplasms; their treatment and follow-up are described in detail in the dedicated chapter.

Once the cyst is enucleated, the residual bone cavity undergoes spontaneous and progressive reossification due to the early organisation of the blood clot that forms inside it. Therefore, it is not indicated to fill the residual cavity with autogenous bone or biomaterials; these, in fact, increase postoperative morbidity and delay complete healing. The recourse to bone regeneration techniques is indicated only if the lesion has eroded both the buccal and the lingual/palatal cortical plate, as previously described with regard to surgical endodontic treatments. In fact, in these cases the residual cavity could be invaded by connective tissue originating from the surrounding soft tissues; the interposition of connective tissue jeopardises organisation of the blood clot, thus preventing reossification. As a result, some a complete clinical healing can be observed some time after surgery, while radiographs may show an unmodified cavity is still present, thus raising doubts regarding the possibility of an incomplete healing or relapse of the lesion. Resorbable membranes, however, may be used to isolate the residual cavity by preventing connective tissue ingrowth, leaving enough time for the blood clot to organise and for spontaneous reossification to take place.

Complete reossification of the residual cavity usually takes between 6 and 24 months, according to the extent of the lesion, the number of intact bone walls, and the patient's age (healing periods are shorter in younger patients).

Therefore, the follow-up period should last no less than 1 to 2 years, during which regular clinical and radiographic examinations should be performed to verify that postoperative recovery and complete healing have been achieved.

Standard radiographic examination, in these cases, is represented by the panoramic radiograph; if the lesion was relatively small and located near the crestal margin of the alveolar ridge, a periapical radiograph may be sufficient to visualise the entire area of interest. In cases of large cysts that have been originally evaluated with CT scans, it may be indicated to perform the same exam some time after surgery.

The step-by-step clinical case (8.30a-h) illustrates the procedure described for the enucleation of an odontogenic cyst and demonstrates the spontaneous reossification of the residual cavity after its removal.

Clinical case 4 – Enucleation of an odontogenic cyst

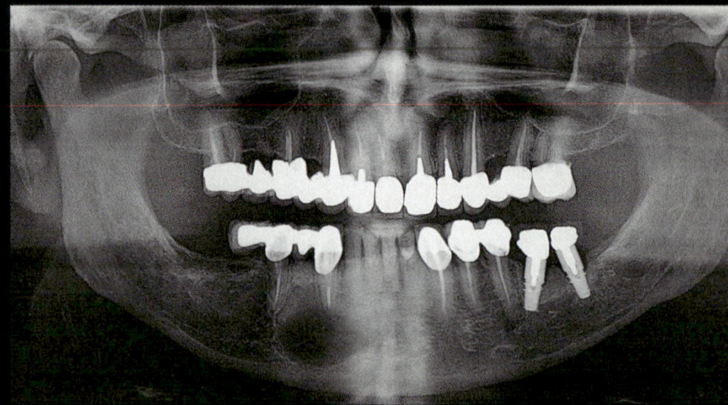

8.30a Panoramic radiograph showing an odontogenic radiolucent lesion associated with 4.3.

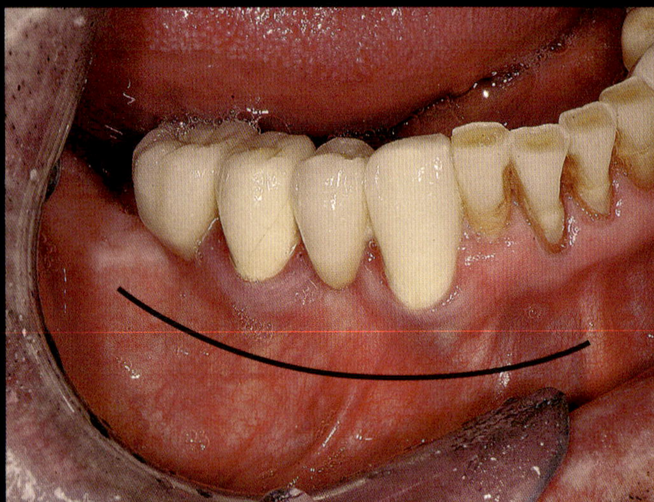

8.30b Preoperative clinical situation and flap outline.

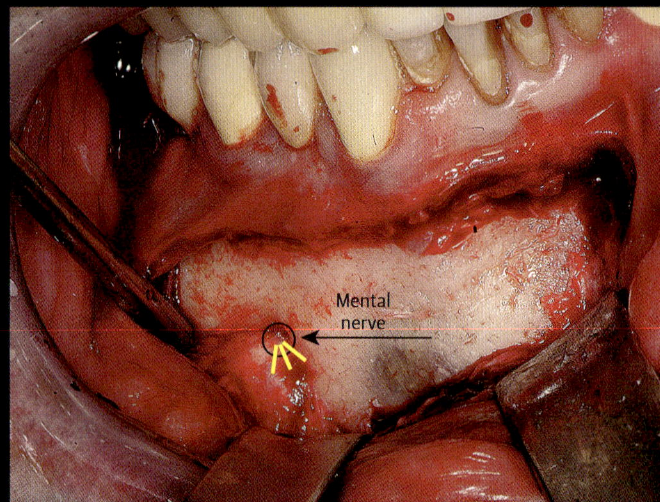

8.30c Flap elevation and identification of the mental neurovascular bundle.

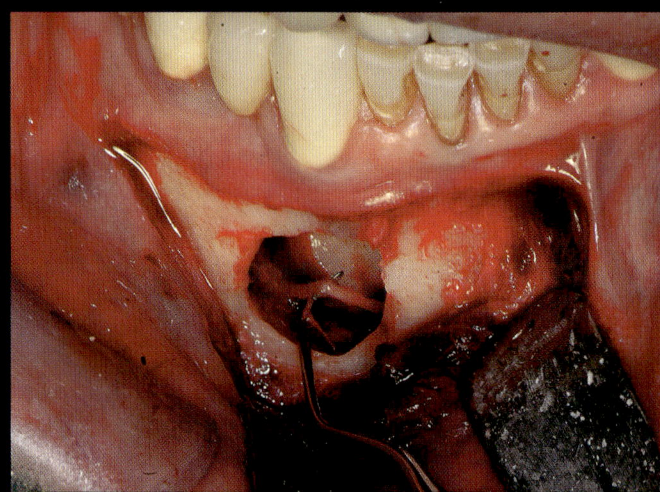

8.30d Operating field after the enucleation of the lesion: notice the preservation of the inferior alveolar nerve and its incisive branch.

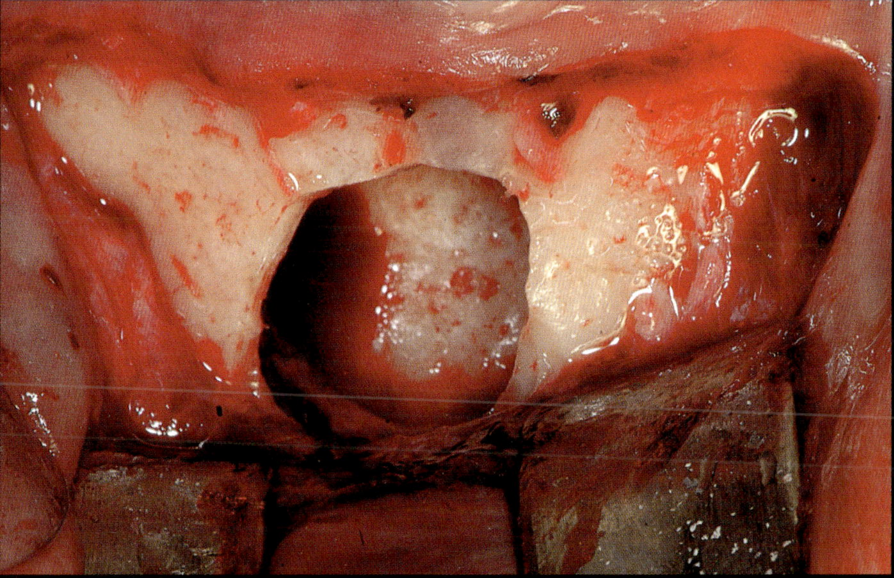

8.30e Operating field after the enucleation of the lesion.

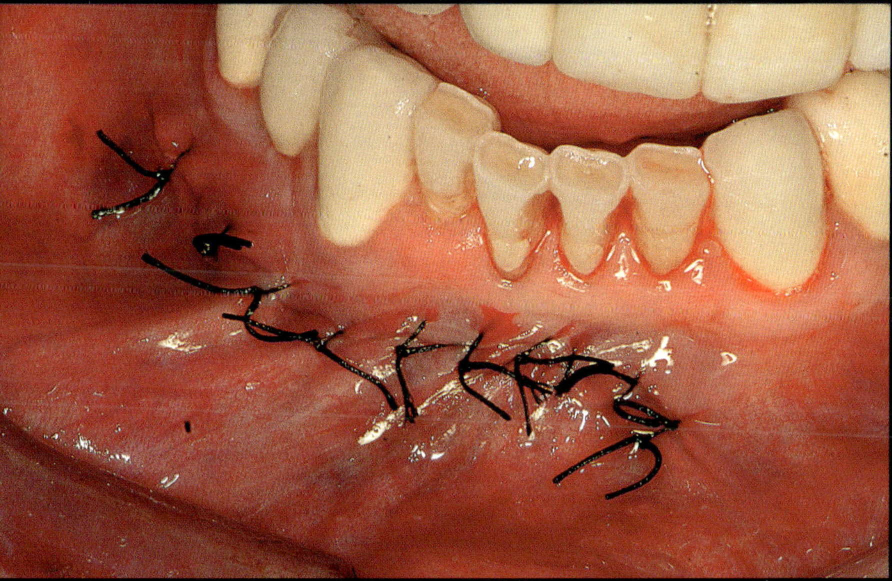

8.30f Suture.

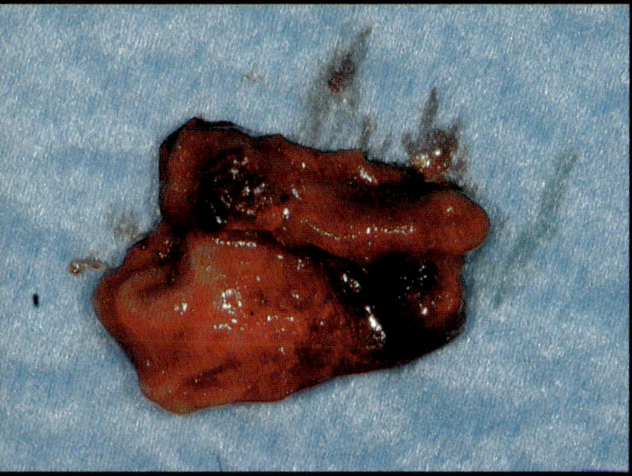

8.30g The removed lesion.

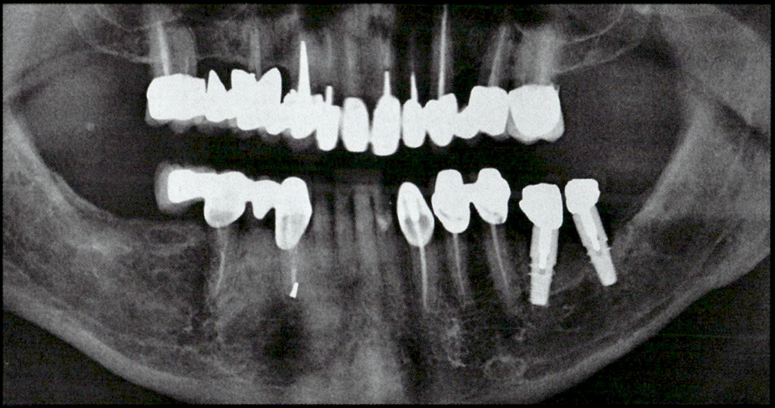

8.30h Radiographic follow-up showing the reossification of the residual cavity, and

Cysts of the maxillary sinus

Etiopathogenesis

These cysts develop inside the maxillary sinus: the etiopathogenesis is still unclear, and this accounts for the different classifications proposed for these lesions. However, two main types are identified: a secretory form and a non-secretory form.

The secretory cyst (a proper cyst) is caused by the obstruction of the excretory duct of a tubuloacinar gland. This is typically due to allergic oedema or infection; however, there seems to be no correlation between endodontic/periapical disease and the formation of these lesions, as the wide consensus in the scientific community on this topic would confirm.

The non-secretory cyst forms inside an oedematous sinusal membrane, because of infection or allergy. The exudate, with its high protein content, causes a rise in the osmotic pressure that, ultimately, draws fluids inside this subepithelial space to the point in which a single space is lined with a layer of flattened fibroblasts (interstitial pseudocyst or antral pseudocysts).

It is incorrect to define these cysts as "mucoceles", as these latter are tumour-like lesions with an aggressive behaviour that more frequently affects the frontal and sphenoid sinus, and only rarely the maxillary sinus.

Clinical examination: analysis of typical signs and symptoms

Cysts of the maxillary sinus are generally asymptomatic, and their presence is often a casual finding in the course of radiographic examinations performed with different indications (e.g. dental treatments). Unlike endosseous lesions, a sinusal cyst may undergo relevant dimensional variations and, in some cases, it can spontaneously regress. Sometimes the patient reports sensations such as teeth-related pain, facial neuralgia, a sense of endosinusal or endorbitary tension, and ocular disturbances; these symptoms generally appear if the cyst occupies the entire sinusal lumen, thus occluding the ostium and determining a certain degree of pressure towards the orbital floor.

Occasionally, spontaneous rupture of the cyst inside the maxillary sinus and drainage of its liquid content in the middle meatus may occur, thus determining a spontaneous regression of the lesion and the associated clinical symptoms and radiographic evidence.

Instrumental screening

The most common exam used for the diagnosis of maxillary sinus cysts is the panoramic radiograph: the lesion appears as a slightly radiopaque area, with well-defined margins and an upper convexity (the so-called "rising sun" image). If doubts remain on the presence or nature of the lesion, the recourse to a CT is indicated.

Differential diagnosis

Differential diagnosis should be made with:

- proper mucoceles (rarely involving the maxillary sinus);
- maxillary sinusitis (it causes clouding of the sinusal lumen but the "rising sun" image is lacking);
- benign and malignant intrasinusal tumors.

Treatment

Generally, surgical treatment is not necessary, particularly if the cyst is asymptomatic; conversely, if the patient refers relevant symptoms, surgical treatment consisting in the removal of the lesion via an endoscopic (FESS - Functional Endoscopic Sinus Surgery) or intraoral approach is indicated. In this latter case, the cyst is reached through a window osteotomy created on the anterior-lateral wall of the sinus: the bone lid should be kept pedicled to the Schneiderian membrane and repositioned with resorbable sutures once the lesion is enucleated, as described by Biglioli and Goisis (2002).

Surgical protocol

Specific surgical armamentarium

Surgical armamentarium is the same as that described for the enucleation of endosseous cysts.

Locoregional anaesthesia

Buccal plexus anaesthesia in the area of the sinus may be sufficient, but infraorbital nerve block with an intraoral or percutaneous approach is recommended.

Access flaps

A marginal or submarginal buccal flap is indicated: if a three-corner flap is chosen, the releasing incision should be performed mesially to better expose the anterior-lateral wall of the sinus.

Osteotomy and enucleation

A bony window is designed by means of rotary or piezoelectric instruments, taking care to keep the bone lid pedicled to the sinusal membrane on the superior margin of the osteotomy. The bone lid is then reflected buccally or towards the sinusal lumen to reach the cyst and enucleate it. Once the lesion is removed, the bone lid is repositioned and stabilised in place with resorbable sutures.

Suture

It is recommended that the suture be airtight, to prevent the formation of an oroantral communication.

A step-by-step clinical case illustrating the surgical treatment of a secretory cyst of the maxillary sinus is presented (8.31a-f).

Follow-up

The probability of relapse after enucleation of a sinusal cyst is very low, but other cysts may develop from different tubuloacinar glands of the Schneiderian membrane. Radiographic examination 6 to 12 months after surgery may be indicated, although it is not mandatory, to ascertain complete healing.

Clinical case 5 – Secretory cyst of the maxillary sinus

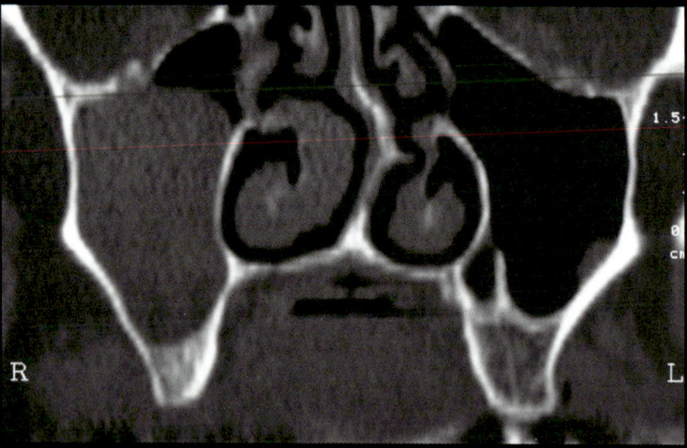

8.31a Large secretory cyst of the right maxillary sinus.

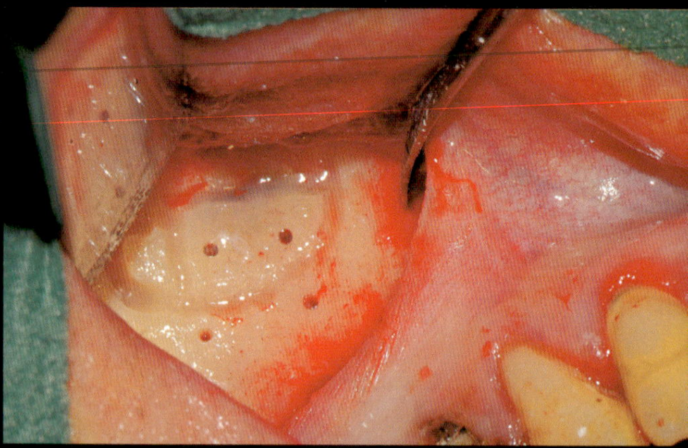

8.31b Exposure of the anterior-lateral wall of the maxillary sinus.

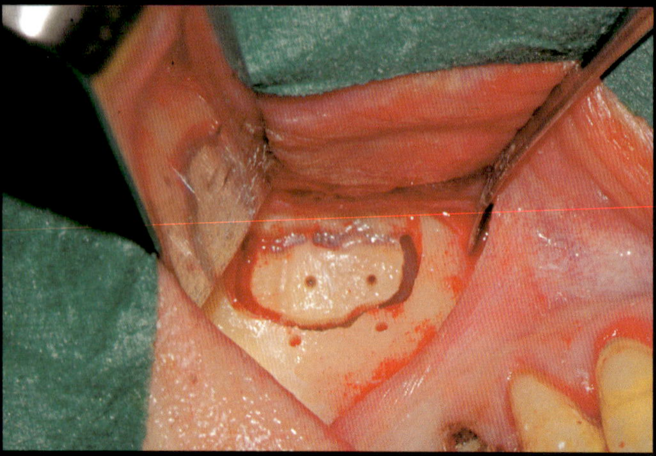

8.31c Pre-drilled holes are created for the ensuing fixation of the bone lid.

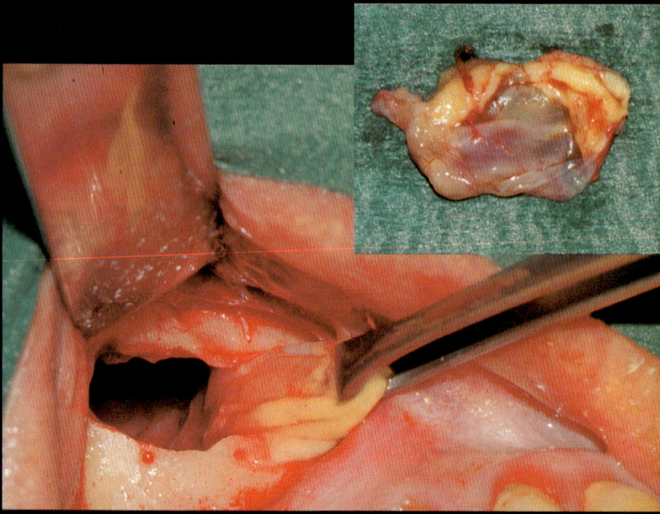

8.31d Removal of the cyst and, in the box, the enucleated lesion.

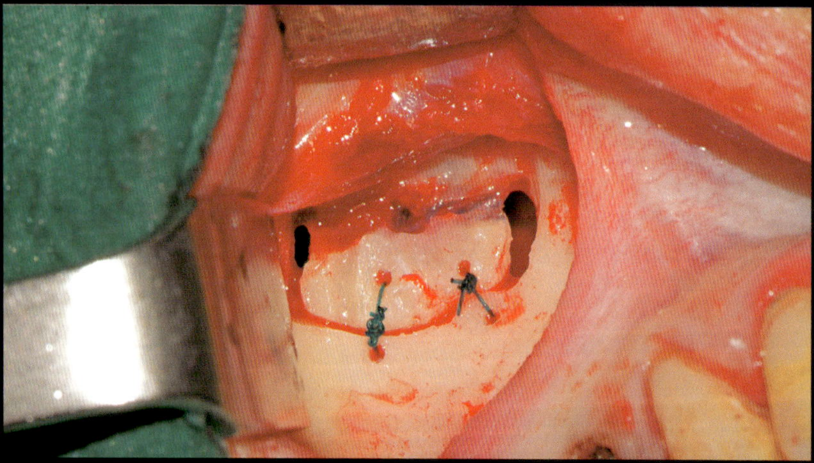

8.31e Repositioning and stabilisation of the access bone lid.

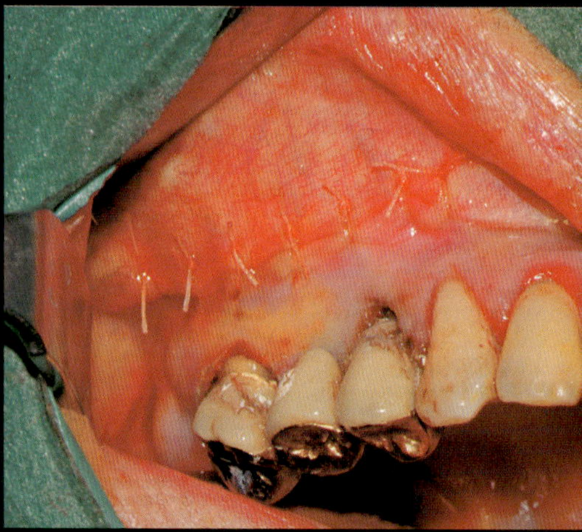

8.31f Suture of the access flap.

Dysembryogenic cysts of the floor of the mouth

Etiopathogenesis

The dysembryogenic cysts of the floor of the mouth (also known as dermoid and epidermoid cysts) derive from the proliferation of epithelial remnants that are caught in the midline during the fusion of the first and second pharyngeal arches, or from remnants of the tuberculum impar (His' tuberculum). Some of these cells are totipotent blastomers that can generate not only ectodermal, but also mesodermal and endodermal tissues. Acquired forms are also described, deriving from traumatic or iatrogenic events that lead to the incarceration of cutaneous tissue and its annexes. Dermoid cysts of the head and neck district account for 6%-7% of the total; of these, 25% are located in the floor of the mouth.

Classification

Dysembryogenic cysts of the floor of the mouth may be classified according to histologic or topographic-anatomic criteria.

Histologic criteria divide these cysts as follows:

- *epidermoid type*: stratified squamous epithelium lines a connective cyst wall; no cutaneous annexes are present (hair, sebaceous glands, sweat glands);
- *dermoid type*: mainly lined with stratified squamous epithelium that, in some areas, may show a cuboidal aspect; the connective cystic wall contains cutaneous annexes;
- *teratoid type*: in the same cyst, the epithelial layer may vary from simple, to stratified squamous, to pseudostratified, to ciliated or columnar. Inside the connective cystic wall, epithelial annexes may be found, together with mesoderm and endoderm derived tissues such as bone, muscle, gastric or respiratory mucosa, blood vessels.

The two latter types contain a caseous-like material composed of keratin, sebaceous material or both, demonstrating the presence of sebaceous glands, hair follicles and sweat glands inside the cystic wall. Moreover, it is worth noting that the presence of three different histologic types could support the hypothesis that the epidermoid type may be a fissural cyst deriving from the inclusion of epithelial cells, while the dermoid and teratoid types derive from totipotent cells that remained included during the early embryonic development.

Classification of dysembryogenic cyst of the floor of the mouth

Histologic	Anatomic-topographic
Epidermoid	Median genioglossal
Dermoid	Median geniohyoid
Teratoid	Lateral

According to the anatomic-topographic classification, these cysts are divided as follows:

- *median genioglossal cyst*: located under the tongue, along the midline, between the genioglossus and mylohyoid muscles;
- *median geniohyoid cyst*: located along the midline in the submental space, between the skin and the geniohyoid muscles, the clinical manifestation includes the typical "double chin" aspect;
- *lateral cyst*: located in the submandibular space, it usually develops caudally towards the hyoid bone and laterally, determining a dislocation of the tongue on the opposite side. The lateral cysts are very rare, and some authors do not consider them as independent nosologic entities but, instead, as laterally dislocated median cysts.

Clinical examination: analysis of signs and symptoms

Generally, the evolution of these lesions is slow and progressive; in the majority of cases no symptoms are present until the cyst becomes very large or infection of the content ensues. In this latter case, the cyst may rapidly enlarge. For these reasons, these lesions are rarely diagnosed in children and teenagers, as they typically manifest between the second and fourth decade of life. Clinical examination is based on traditional semeiotics, particularly on inspection and palpation.

Median genioglossal cyst: it appears as a dome-shaped swelling along the midline of the floor of the mouth; the overlying mucosa has a normal appearance, while the tongue is dislocated upwards and backwards (8.32). The patient may report a feeling of endoral encumbrance, dysphonia, and impaired swallowing, but in complete absence of pain.

Median geniohyoid cyst: it presents with the characteristic "double chin" appearance, while signs of its presence inside the oral cavity are often barely visible or absent. As for the median genioglossal cyst, the patient refers no pain, while for very large median geniohyoid cysts both the typical "double chin" and the symptoms described for the median genioglossal cyst (feeling of endoral encumbrance, dysphonia, and impaired swallowing) may be present at the same time (8.33).

Clinical examination

Signs

Median genioglossal cyst

- Swelling located in the floor of the mouth

Median geniohyoid cyst

- Swelling in the submental region ("double chin")

Symptoms

Median genioglossal cyst

- Absence of pain
- Feeling of endoral encumbrance
- Dysphonia
- Impaired swallowing

Median geniohyoid cyst

- Absence of pain
- Feeling of submental encumbrance

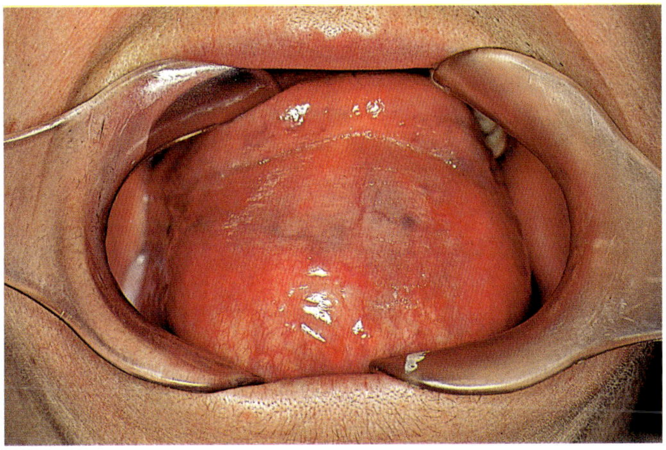

8.32 Large dermoid cyst of the floor of the mouth determining the typical tongue dislocation.

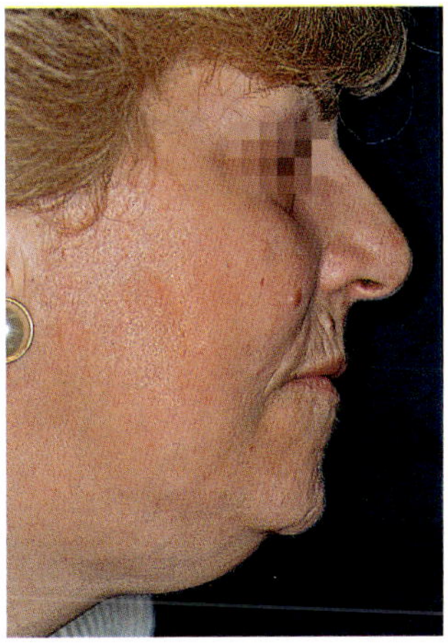

8.33 Same patient: the distinctive "double chin" appearance is caused by the development of the lesion in the submental space.

Palpation is very useful for evaluating the extent and consistency of the lesion. Since the floor of the mouth and the submandibular space are entirely made of soft tissues, the recourse to bimanual palpation is recommended: one hand is placed under the chin in the area of the submandibular space, while the fingers of the other hand are used to palpate the floor of the mouth. The cyst feels soft to the touch and well-delimited with respect to the surrounding tissues.

Instrumental screening

Since dysembryogenic cysts are lesions of the soft tissues, standard radiographic exams such as orthopantomography are not indicated. Ecography may give valuable information on the extent and type of content of the lesion, but precise interpretation of the resulting images can be difficult for the clinician.

Magnetic resonance imaging (MRI) is surely the most specific exam, as it can define with the highest precision the morphology, extent, and type of content of the cyst, and also its relationships with the muscles of the floor of the mouth (8.34).

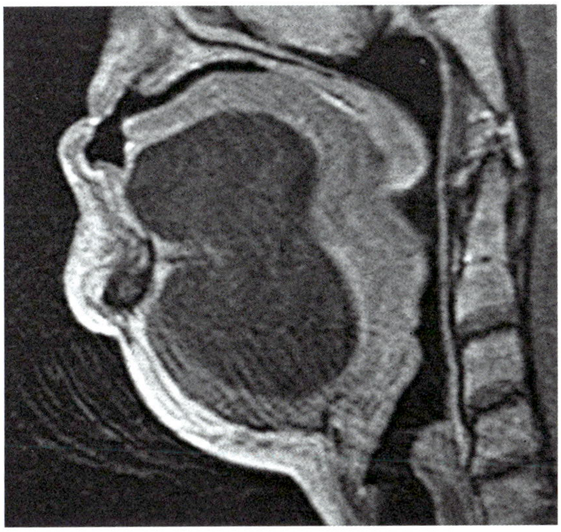

8.34 MRI of the same patient showing a large dermoid cyst that involves both the floor of the mouth and the submental space.

Needle aspiration of the cystic content should instead be avoided due to the risk of infection resulting from the diffusion of the material in the soft tissue of the floor of the mouth, which may render the following treatment more difficult.

Differential diagnosis

Differential diagnosis is performed typically with neoplastic and cystic lesions such as the following: ranula, thyroglossal duct cyst, cystic hygroma, lipoma, fibroma, haemangioma, cystic lymphangioma, neurofibroma, pleomorphic adenoma, cystic adenolymphoma, Hodgkin and non-Hodgkin lymphomas. Definitive diagnosis can only be obtained by histopathological examination of the lesion.

Treatment

These cysts are treated with a surgical approach consisting in the complete enucleation of the lesion, preferably via an intraoral access.

Surgical protocol

Specific surgical armamentarium

Since this type of surgery involves only soft tissues, the surgical armamentarium is very simple and includes:

- scalpel;
- dissecting scissors;
- haemostatic forceps;
- retractors;
- bipolar coagulation system;
- suturing materials.

Locoregional anaesthesia

Median genioglossal cysts of limited extent may be treated under local anesthesia in cooperative patients: block anaesthesia of both lingual nerves associated with perilesional anaesthesia is indicated. Conversely, for the treatment of large median genioglossal cysts or median geniohyoid cysts, the recourse to general anaesthesia with nasotracheal intubation is recommended.

Surgical techniques

In the past, the intraoral approach was destined to the treatment of small to medium sized cysts located above the geniohyoid muscles, while the extraoral approach was chosen in cases of large lesions, or cysts located below the geniohyoid muscles. Today, the intraoral approach is used also to treat large lesions, with the access incision performed along the midline. This type of incision does not cause any unfavourable functional sequelae on the tongue, while allowing the surgeon to operate in an almost bloodless operating field, due to the paucity of blood vessels in the midline of the floor of the mouth. Moreover, the absence of extraoral incisions allows avoiding any risk of unaesthetic scars in the submental region.

Relevant anatomic structures

Submandibular duct (Wharton's duct), lingual nerve, sublingual gland, sublingual blood vessels, and muscles of the floor of the mouth. Keeping the incision strictly along the midline and separating the cyst from the surrounding soft tissues by blunt dissection prevents damage to these structures.

Follow-up

Relapse of dysembryogenic cysts of the floor of the mouth after surgical removal is very rare. However, a 12-month clinical follow-up is advisable; MRI can be performed to verify complete healing.

A step-by-step clinical case illustrating the enucleation of a large dysembryogenic cyst is presented (8.35a-g).

Clinical case 6 – Enucleation of a dysembryogenic cyst of the floor of the mouth

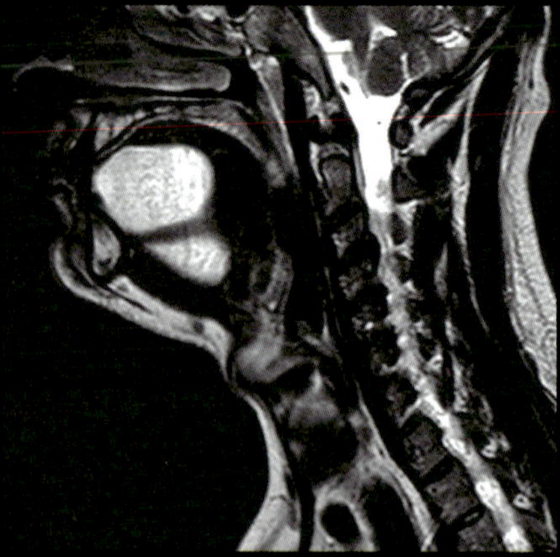

8.35a Preoperative MRI (sagittal view) showing a large dysembryogenic cyst occupying the anterior portion of the floor of the mouth, and extending below the mylohyoid muscles.

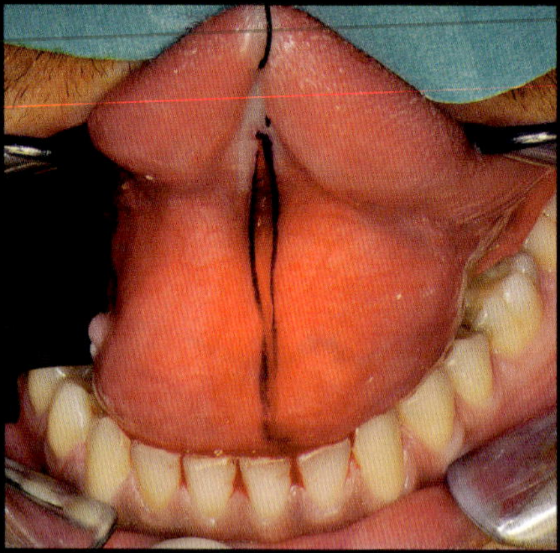

8.35b The incision of the mucosa is performed along the midline of the floor of the mouth and the lower surface of the tongue.

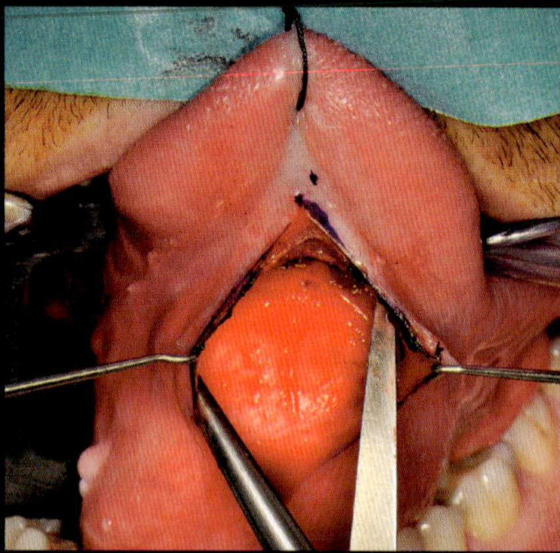

8.35c The lesion is exposed and separated from the surrounding soft tissues by blunt dissection.

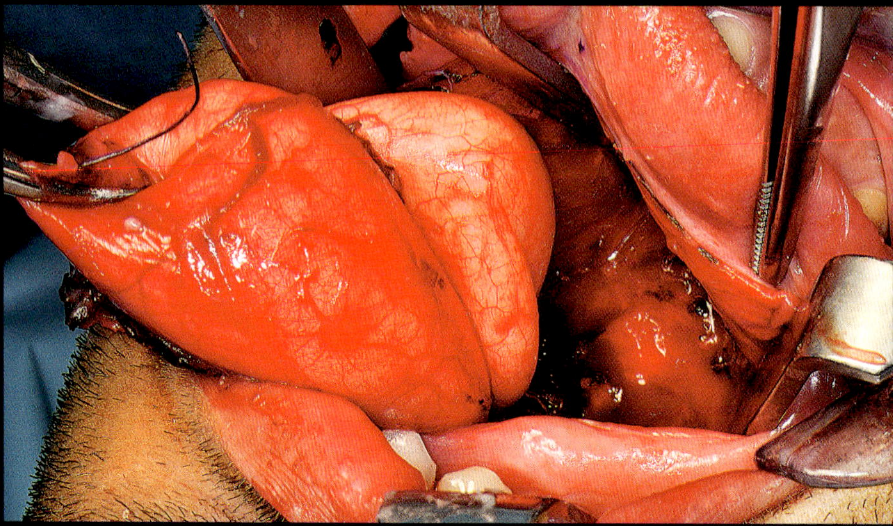

8.35d Enucleation of the lesion.

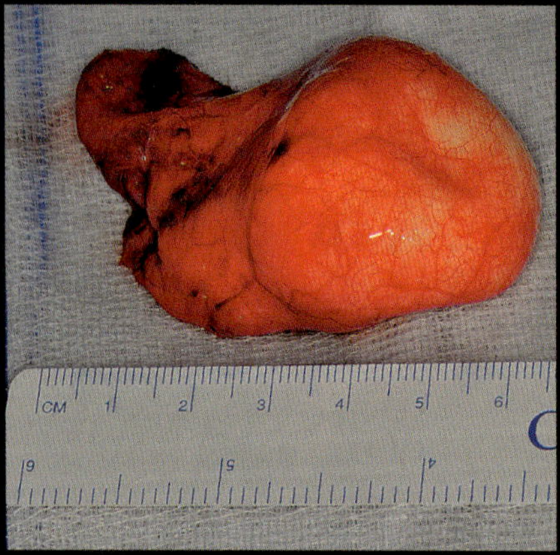

8.35e The removed lesion.

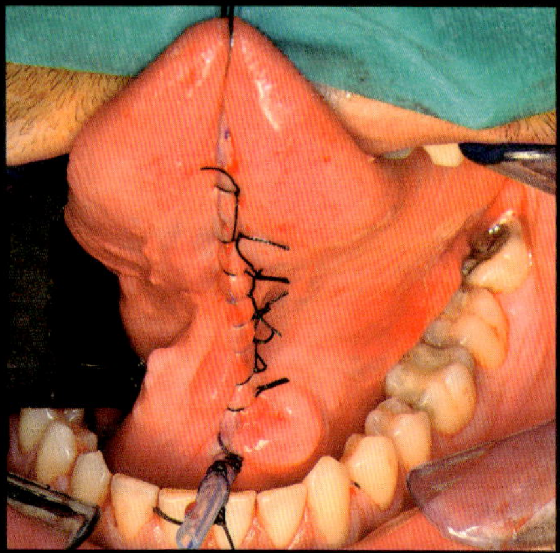

8.35f The incision is sutured and a surgical drain is fixed in place.

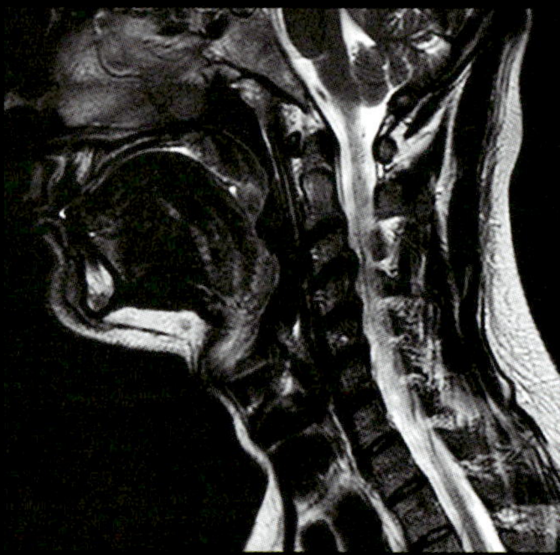

8.35g Follow-up: MRI showing the restoration of the normal anatomy of the region.

REFERENCES

BIGLIOLI F, GOISIS M. Access to the maxillary sinus using a bone flap on a mucosal pedicle: preliminary report. *J Cranio Maxillofac Surg* 2002; 30:255-9.

BODNER L. Effect of decalcified freeze-dried bone allograft on the healing of jaw defects after cyst enucleation. *J Oral Maxillofac Surg* 1996; 54(11):1282-6.

BRUSATI R, CHIAPASCO M. Elementi di chirurgia oro-maxillo-facciale. Masson, Milano 1999.

BRUSATI R, GALIOTO S, TULLIO A, MOSCATO G. The midline sagittal glossotomy for treatment of dermoid cysts of the mouth floor. *J Oral Maxillofac Surg* 1991; 49:875-8.

DEVENNEY-CAKIR B, SUBRAMANIAM RM, REDDY SM, IMSANDE H, GOHEL A, SAKAI O. Cystic and cystic-appearing lesions of the mandible: review. *AJR Am J Roentgenol* 2011 Jun; 196(6 Suppl):WS66-77.

MACDONALD-JANKOWSKI DS. Orthokeratinized odontogenic cyst: a systematic review. *Dentomaxillofac Radiol* 2010 Dec; 39(8):455-67.

NEW GB, ERICH JB. Dermoid cysts of the head and neck. *Surg Gynecol Obstet* 1937; 65:48-55.

PETERSON LJ, INDRESANO AT, MARCIANI RD, ROSER SM. Principles of oral and maxillofacial surgery. JB Lippincott Company, Philadelphia 1992.

PINDBORG JJ, KRAMER IRH, TORLONI H. Histological typing of odontogenic tumors, jaw cysts and allied lesions. World Health Organization, Geneva, 1971; pp. 15-23.

SUMMERS GW. Jaw cysts: diagnosis and treatment. *Head & Neck* 1979; 1(3):243-58.

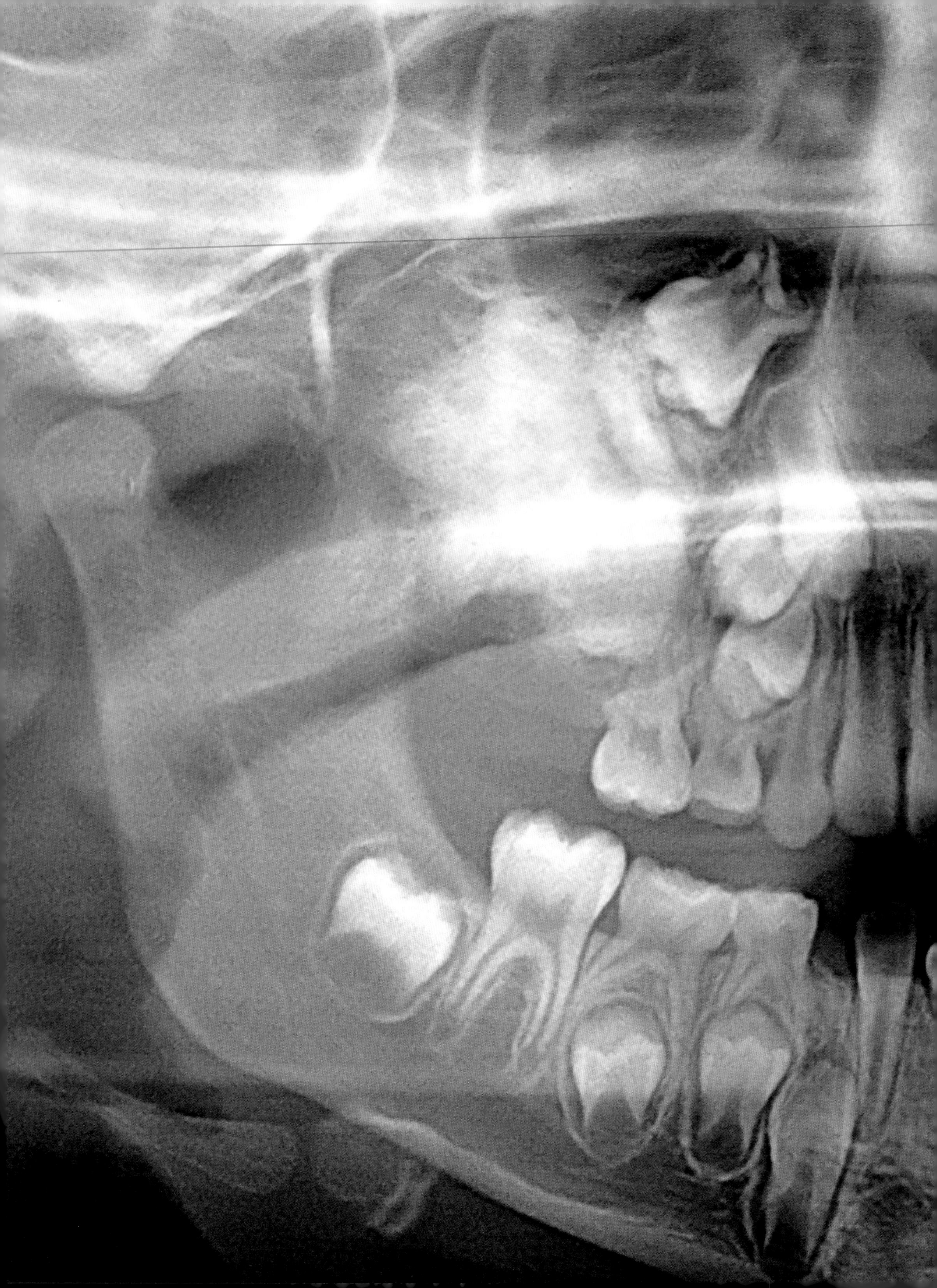

Benign tumours of the oral cavity

M. Chiapasco ▪ M. Zaniboni

Introduction

The management of malignant tumours of the oral cavity falls within the scope of maxillofacial surgery; therefore, details on this subject are not treated in this manual. However, diagnosis and treatment of benign tumours, despite requiring in some cases a specific training in maxillofacial oncology, fall within the scope of oral surgery. Accordingly, this chapter contains details on benign tumours affecting the hard and soft tissues of the oral cavity to give the surgeon all the basic elements for adequate management of these lesions, in particular regarding etiopathogenesis, clinical and radiographic diagnostic elements, differential diagnosis, and prognosis, including the basic principles of surgical treatment.

Summary tables containing the essential data of all the lesions treated will be presented, to give the clinician an easy to use and particularly useful tool for the differential diagnosis process. A systematic treatise of all neoplasms of the head and neck district can be found in specialty textbooks of maxillofacial surgery.

From a general point of view, neoplastic and pseudoneoplastic lesions of the jaws can be divided into two distinct groups: the *odontogenic* forms and the *non-odontogenic* forms. Depending on the localisation, however, these lesions can affect the hard tissues (jawbones) or the soft tissues of the oral cavity.

Because the clinical and/or radiographic features of some neoplasms, both benign and malignant, may present similarities, special care will be dedicated to outlining simple guidelines that may help the clinician in the process of differential diagnosis. However, it is worth noting that a definitive diagnosis is impossible based on signs, symptoms and instrumental screening. For this reason, the first section of this chapter is dedicated to a diagnostic procedure that is fundamental for a correct diagnosis and a precise preoperative planning: the biopsy.

Biopsy – General principles

Even if they are not frequently involved in the treatment of neoplastic lesions of the jaws for the aforementioned reasons, the dentist and the oral surgeon nonetheless play a fundamental role in early identification of the lesions, because affected patients initially turn to dental practice. Therefore, the oral surgeon must attain the correct diagnosis by means of clinical examination, instrumental screening, and biopsy; the latter is the only exam that allows a definitive diagnosis to be made, after histopathological examination of the sampled tissue. According to the result of histology and the specific training of each clinician, the adequate treatment modality and the best-suited specialist to perform will be chosen.

Incisional biopsy

The term "incisional biopsy" refers to the partial removal of a lesion in association with a portion of apparently normal surrounding tissue, with the aim of obtaining a preoperative histopathological diagnosis. This type of biopsy is indicated whenever the presumptive clinical diagnosis is uncertain, particularly in cases where a precise diagnosis is fundamental for choosing the appropriate therapy. It is worth remembering that whenever an erosive/ulcerative lesion of the oral mucosa that does not heal spontaneously within 2 - 3 weeks is observed, an incisional biopsy is mandatory for the early diagnosis of lesions such as the squamous cell carcinoma. The latter, in fact, initially appears as a small ulcerative lesion on the mucosa, and is refractory to any treatment with topical medications; if left untreated, it may develop into a large lesion which can be difficult to treat and cause an unfavourable "*quoad vitam*" prognosis.

Specific surgical armamentarium

- Scalpel.
- Scissors.
- Atraumatic surgical pliers.
- Bone rongeurs and rotary or piezoelectric instrumentation for bone biopsy.
- Leak-resistant containers prefilled with 10% neutral buffered formaline.

TECHNIQUE

Two are the possible situations:
- biopsy of the superficial soft tissues;
- biopsy of the deep tissues.

Biopsy of the superficial soft tissues

After adequate perilesional anaesthesia, partial excision of the lesion is performed by removing a lozenge of mucosa comprising both a portion of pathologic tissue and a portion of apparently normal surrounding tissue. The pathologic tissue must be manipulated with great care, using atraumatic surgical pliers to avoid possible artefacts caused by mechanical trauma. Once the portion of tissue to be removed is delimited by means of an incision, the cleavage can be completed either with scissors or with a scalpel (📷 9.1). Generally, no sutures penetrating the lesion are applied, and the area is left to heal by secondary intention (📷 9.2a-d).

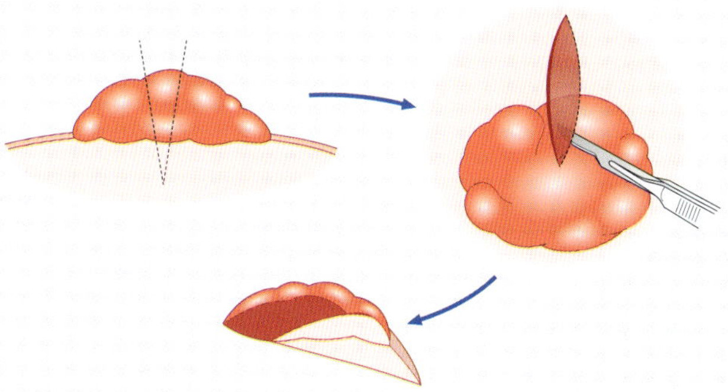

9.1 Basic technique for incisional biopsy: a lozenge-shaped sample is harvested, comprising a portion of the lesion together with a portion of apparently normal tissue.

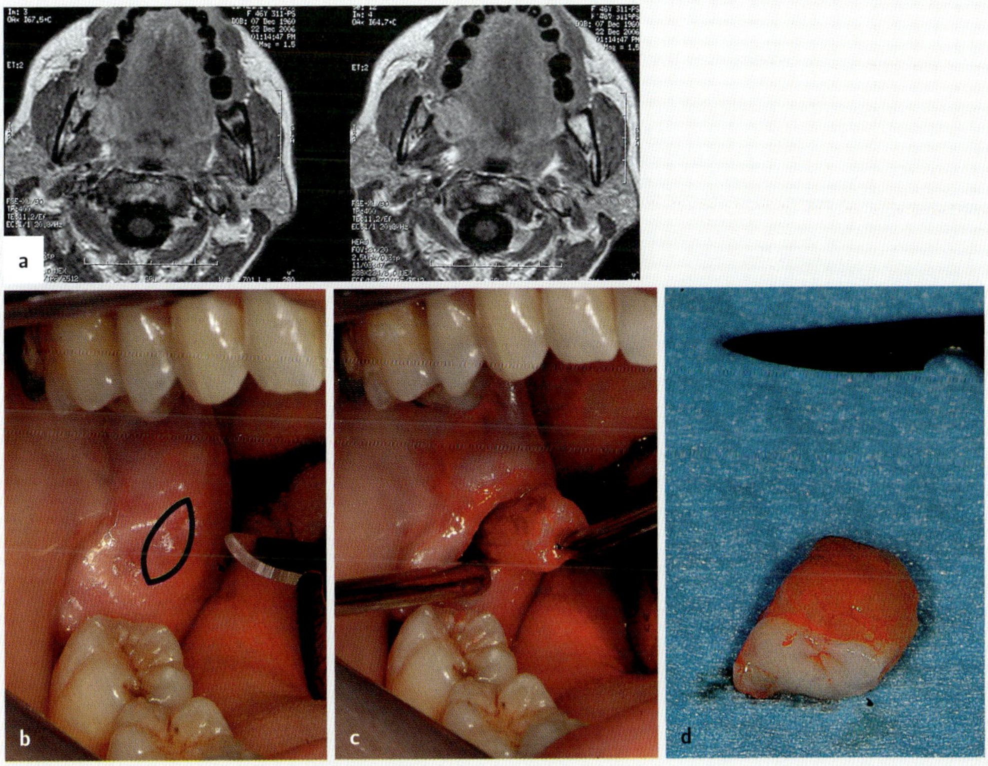

9.2 a) MRI axial slice showing an apparently solid round mass located mesially to the right mandibular ramus: these elements are suggestive of a neoplasm. **b)** Incisional biopsy of the lesion. **c)** Sample taken from the lesion after incision of the superficial soft tissues. **d)** The tissue sample.

The tissue sample is immediately placed inside a leak-resistant container filled with 10% neutral buffered formaline; the patient's details are written on the outside label of the container, a specific form reporting details regarding the lesion, the sampling procedure and the presumptive diagnosis is filled out, and everything is sent to the histology laboratory.

Biopsy of the deep tissues

Lesions developing in the deep tissues may involve either the submucosal soft tissues or the hard tissues (osseous or endosseous lesions).

When a biopsy of the submucosal soft tissues is performed, incision of the mucosal layer is performed with a scalpel, the lesion is identified, and a sample is collected with the aforementioned modalities.

In the event of a bone biopsy, once the incision of the mucosal layer and the full-thickness elevation of the soft tissues are performed, the collection of the sample can be performed. In the event of an endosseous lesion, an access osteotomy must be created; once the lesion is exposed, a sample can be collected with a scalpel (soft tissue) or chisels, rotary instruments, or piezoelectric instruments (hard tissue) (9.3a–f).

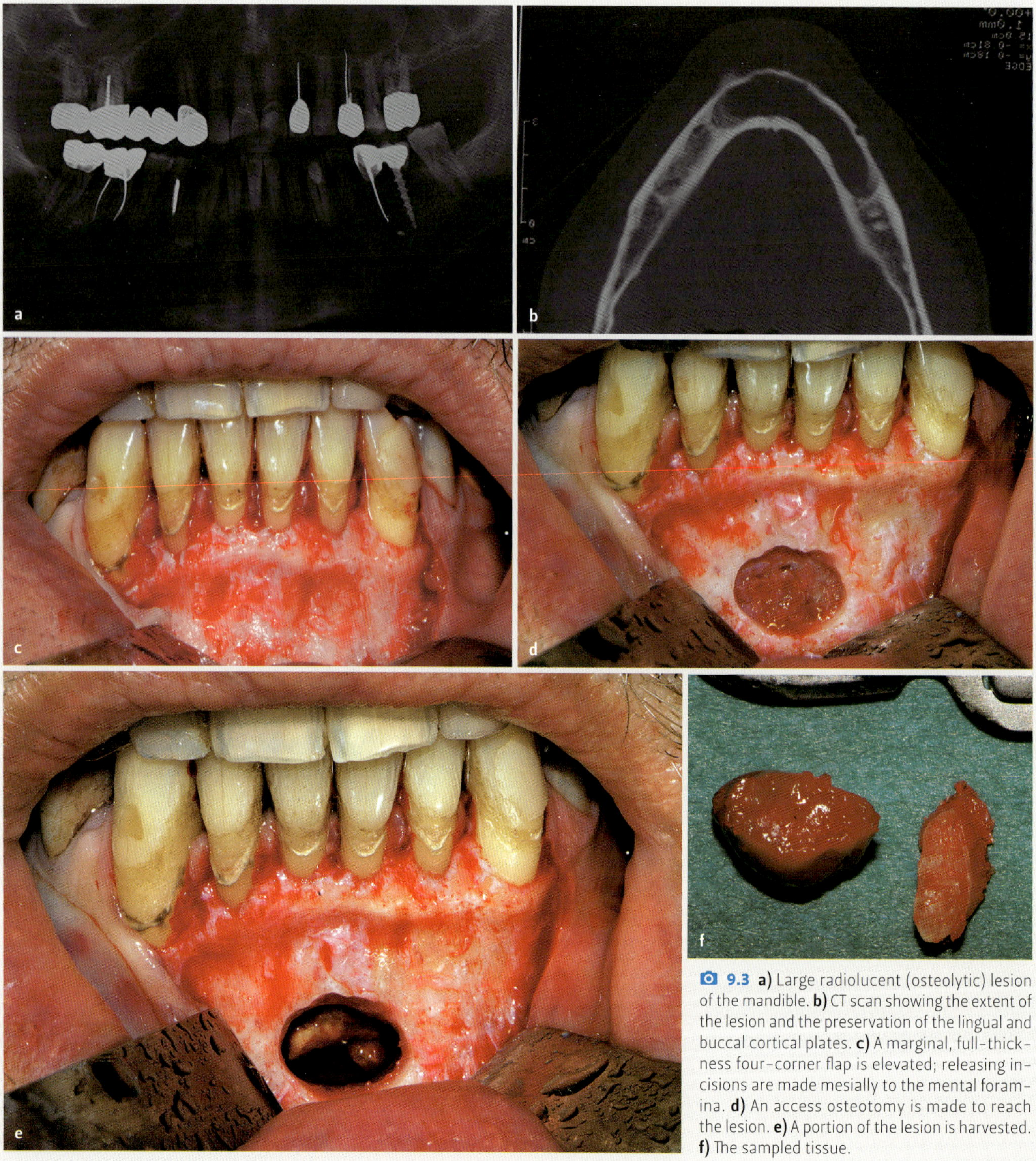

9.3 **a)** Large radiolucent (osteolytic) lesion of the mandible. **b)** CT scan showing the extent of the lesion and the preservation of the lingual and buccal cortical plates. **c)** A marginal, full-thickness four-corner flap is elevated; releasing incisions are made mesially to the mental foramina. **d)** An access osteotomy is made to reach the lesion. **e)** A portion of the lesion is harvested. **f)** The sampled tissue.

Excisional biopsy

Excisional biopsy, contrary to incisional biopsy, implies the complete removal of the lesion together with a portion of apparently normal surrounding tissue. This type of biopsy is indicated for manifestly benign lesions, and is thus useful to confirm the presumptive diagnosis. In the same way as for the incisional biopsy, excisional biopsy can be performed on lesions of the superficial soft tissues, or of the deep soft and hard tissues; therefore, the same basic principles apply.

TECHNIQUE

Excisional biopsy of the superficial soft tissues

With the aid of a sterile dermographic pencil, the area to be sampled is outlined, including some millimetres of apparently normal tissue around the lesion to be reasonably sure that all the pathologic tissue is removed, and to provide the pathologist with a peripheral band of normal tissue as a reference. The most common shape used for tissue excision is the lozenge, as the residual wound is easier to suture. However, the shape of the excision may vary according to the morphology of the lesion (9.4a–c).

An incision along the line traced with a dermographic pencil is made and, while tensioning the margin of the lesion with atraumatic tissue pliers, excision is completed with the aid of dissecting scissors or the scalpel blade. Whenever possible, a cleavage of the surrounding tissues from the muscle layer is performed, to facilitate a tension-free suture of the wound. That said, if suturing and healing of the wound by primary intention is not possible or indicated, sutures can be avoided and the wound is left to heal by secondary intention. In this latter case, to reduce postoperative discomfort it may be indicated to place a haemostatic dressing on the wound: oxidised regenerated cellulose gauze and iodoform gauze may be placed inside the wound and fixed in place with sutures (9.5a–d).

Excisional biopsy of the deep tissues

The same principles described for the incisional biopsy of the deep tissues apply.

Histologic examination for benign tumours

Type	Indication
Incisional biopsy	Uncertain clinical diagnosis Presumptive diagnosis confirmation Preliminary diagnosis of non-cystic radiolucent endosseous lesions
Excisional biopsy	Frankly benign lesions
Needle aspiration biopsy	Lesions of the deep tissues

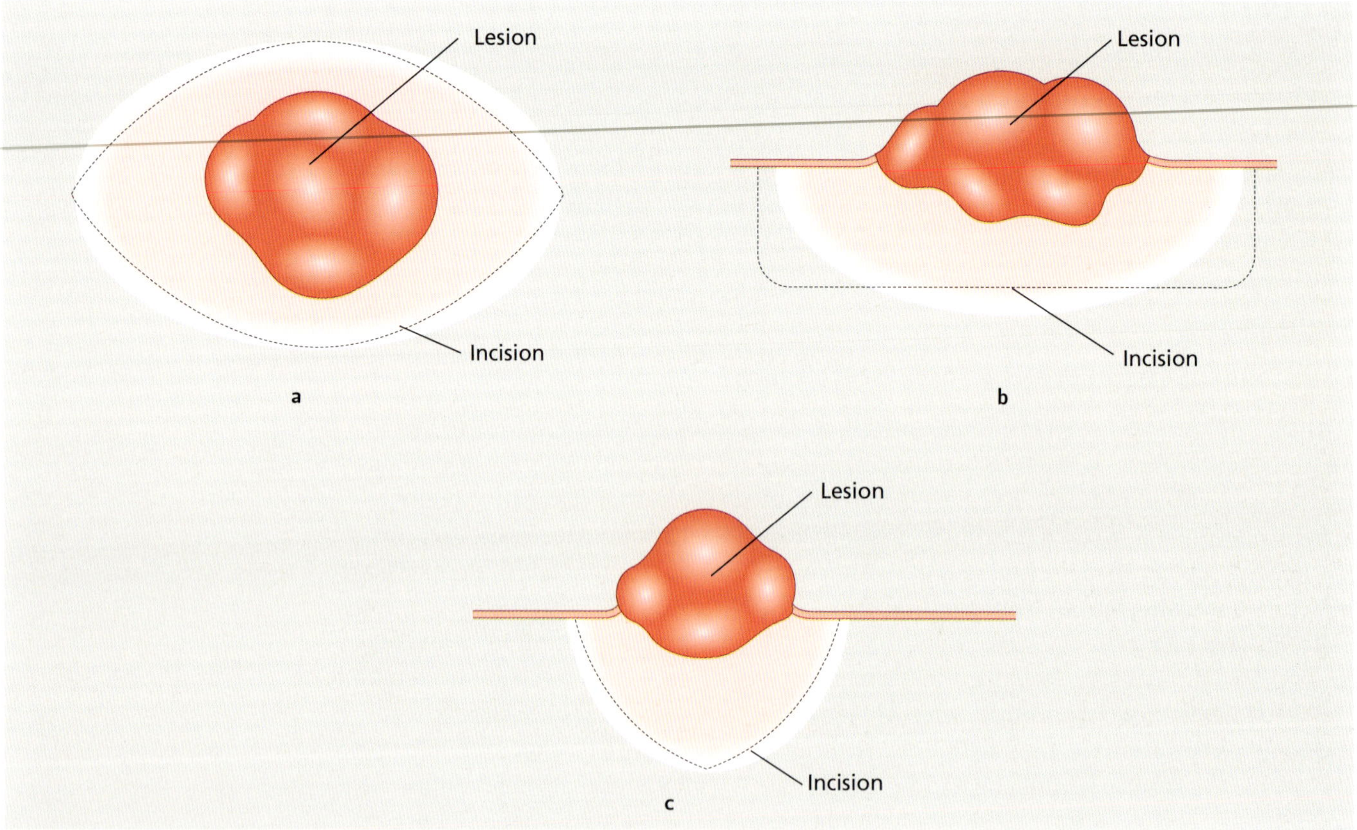

9.4 Basic technique for excisional biopsy of the superficial soft tissues.

Needle aspiration biopsy

Percutaneous core biopsy is indicated whenever an incisional biopsy is difficult to perform, or exposes to the risk of damaging relevant anatomic structures that must be preserved. It is indicated for solid lesions of the deep soft tissues (neck, major salivary glands, floor of the mouth, etc.), where extensive incision and elevation would otherwise be necessary to reach the lesion and perform an incisional biopsy. Although this type of biopsy is not frequently used in oral surgery, it is worth remembering that the objective of any sampling technique is to obtain a significant portion of the lesion. Therefore, the gauge of the needles used in this procedure is larger than that of other needles commonly used in oral surgery for other applications (anaesthesia, irrigation, etc.). Generally, 18-16-14 gauge needles are used and, if indicated, a relatively new procedure called "vacuum assisted" biopsy can be performed using an 11 gauge needle coupled with a vacuum-assisted device (VAD).

Needle aspiration biopsy consists of three phases: precise localisation of the lesion, penetration of the needle through the overlying tissues and into the lesion, and aspiration of the sample. While being a relatively simple and minimally invasive procedure to perform, it does not always provide completely reliable results due to the possibility that the sample is harvested outside of the lesion, thus giving a false negative.

Besides being useful for collecting tissue samples for histopathologic examination, needle aspiration may represent a practical preliminary diagnostic tool for cases of radiolucent endosseous lesions. It can clarify whether a lesion is solid or has a fluid content and, in this latter case, if the liquid is clear, cloudy, purulent, or haematic.

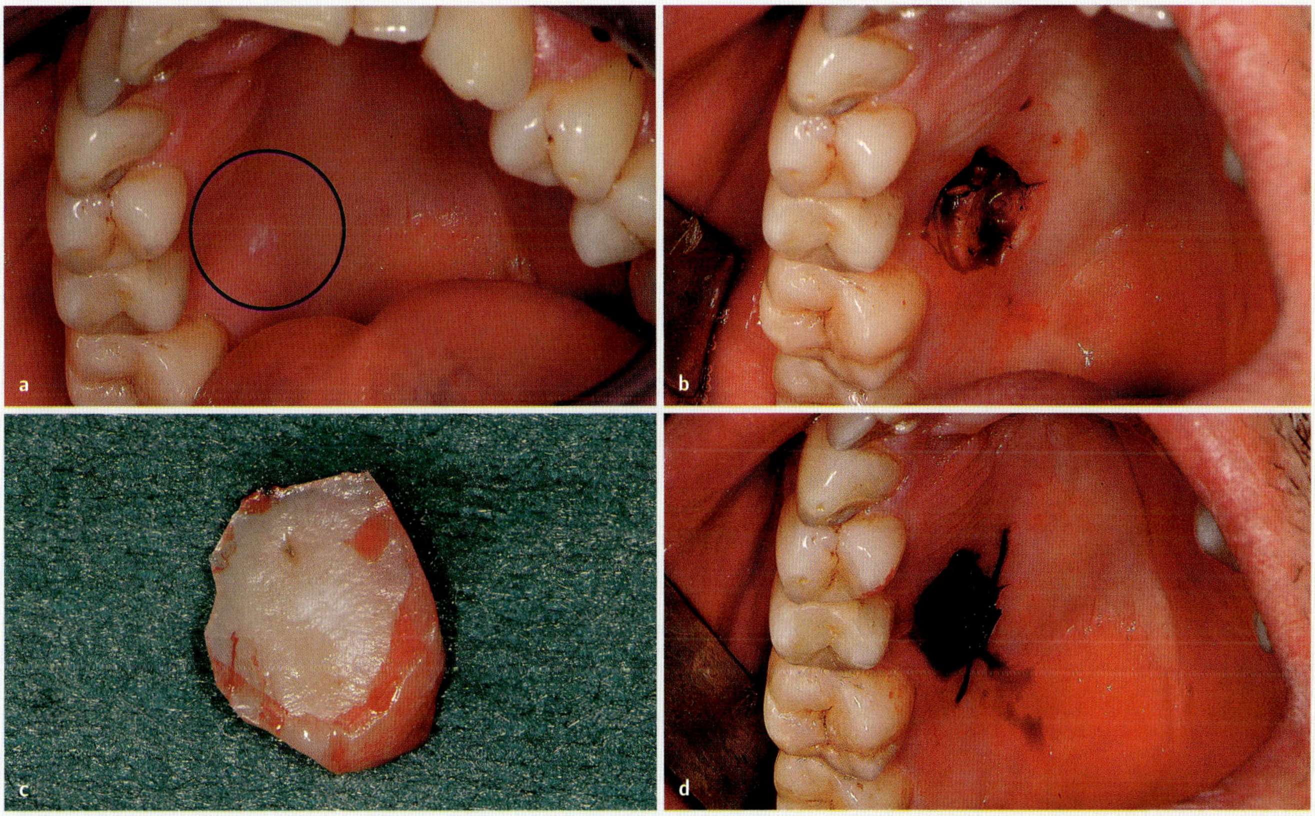

9.5 **a)** Leucoplastic lesion on the hard palate (right premolar area). **b)** Excisional biopsy of the lesion. **c)** The removed lesion. **d)** Application of oxidised regenerated cellulose gauze stabilised with sutures.

Benign odontogenic tumours

Benign odontogenic tumours are a heterogeneous group of lesions, and it is therefore difficult to classify them in a simple way due to the great variability of their histologic, clinical and radiographic features, and their behaviour. These neoplasms originate in the two most superficial germ layers, the ectoderm and the mesoderm. The most credited classification (WHO 2005) divides benign odontogenic tumours according to their histological characteristics:

- odontogenic epithelium with mature, fibrous stroma without odontogenic ectomesenchyme;
- odontogenic epithelium with odontogenic ectomesenchyme, with or without hard tissue formation;
- mesenchyme and/or odontogenic ectomesenchyme, with or without odontogenic epithelium;
- bone-related lesions.

A systematic description of all benign tumours of the oral cavity lies beyond the scope of this manual. Therefore, the most peculiar aspects of the more common benign neoplasms will be summarised together with the general principles for diagnosis, prognosis, and treatment (see tab. 9.1); a detailed description of the histologic features of these lesions is available in anatomic pathology textbooks.

Tab. 9.1 WHO classification (2005) of benign tumours of the oral cavity

Denomination	Incidence	Clinical features
Odontogenic tumours		
Odontogenic epithelium with mature, fibrous stroma without odontogenic ectomesenchyme		
Ameloblastoma (or adamantinoma)	Although rare, it is the second most common odontogenic tumour. It mainly occurs in the 3rd, 4th and 5th decades and shows no gender predilection. Mandibular localisation is more frequent (80%), with a marked predilection for the area of the third molar and mandibular angle.	Variants: · solid/multicystic · desmoplastic · unicystic. Initial stage: endosseous development without cortical plate involvement, typically asymptomatic. Intraoral and extraoral examination is generally negative. Advanced stage: progressive swelling of the affected osseous segment due to erosion or dislocation of the cortical plates in absence of pain. Involved teeth can show mobility and malocclusion; perforations of the mucosa may be present, and paraesthesia can occur with the compression of sensory nerves.
Squamous odontogenic tumour	Very rare, it shows the same incidence in the mandible and maxilla, with a predilection for the anterior areas.	Fibrous connective tissue mass covered by squamous epithelium.
Calcifying epithelial odontogenic tumour (Pindborg tumour)	It represents 1% of all odontogenic tumours; it exhibits no gender or age predilection. In two thirds of the cases, it is localised in the mandible, particularly in the molar region. It is frequently associated with an impacted tooth.	Two forms: endosseous and peripheral. It is a slow growing mass, normally asymptomatic. In the advanced stages, deformation of the involved bone segment and a sense of tension may be present.
Adenomatoid odontogenic tumour	It represents 3% of all odontogenic tumours. It mainly occurs in the 2nd and 3rd decades; the incidence in males is almost twice of that found in females. It generally involves the anterior region of the maxilla, and is often associated with unerupted teeth.	Slow growing, asymptomatic swelling.
Keratocystic odontogenic tumour	Peak incidence between the 2nd and 3rd decade. More frequently localised in the mandible (65%-83%), in the majority of cases in the area of the mandibular angle.	Multiple, very aggressive. The patient often refers pain, swelling and exudate drainage. It may erode the cortical plates and compromise the adjacent structures.
Odontogenic epithelium with odontogenic ectomesenchyme, with or without hard tissue formation		
Ameloblastic fibroma	It represents 2% of all odontogenic tumours. It occurs in young subjects with a peak incidence in the 2nd decade, does not exhibit any gender predilection, and is more frequently localised in the mandible.	Often mistaken for an ameloblastoma. Painless swelling that frequently interferes with tooth eruption. No tendency to actively infiltrate bone.
Ameloblastic fibroma/ fibrodentinoma	Frequent in the 2nd decade. It mainly occurs in the posterior mandible.	In the majority of cases, it appears as an asymptomatic swelling associated with eruption disturbances.
Compound and complex odontoma	It occurs in the 2nd to 4th decades. Compound odontomas are more frequent in the anterior maxilla, while complex odontomas are more frequent in the posterior mandible.	Localised swelling, developing typically on the buccal side.
Odontoameloblastoma		Locally aggressive tumour, similar to the ameloblastoma.
Ameloblastic fibro-odontoma	Young subjects, peak incidence in the 2nd decade.	Simultaneous presence of two types of tissue: one is similar to that of the ameloblastic fibroma while the other is similar to that of the odontoma (enamel and dentin). Slow growing, painless swelling.
Calcifying cystic odontogenic tumour	Peak incidence in the 2nd decade, more frequent in females and in the maxilla.	It exhibits features of both cysts and solid tumors.
Mesenchyme and/or odontogenic ectomesenchyme with or without odontogenic epithelium		
Odontogenic fibroma	It exhibits no gender or age predilection.	Slow growing mass that causes expansion and resorption of the cortical plates.
Odontogenic mixoma/ mixofibroma	It occurs in the 2nd and 3rd decades; it shows a slight predilection for the posterior region of the mandible.	Slow growing tumour, locally aggressive. Initial stage: clinically asymptomatic. Advanced stage: expansion of the cortical plates, teeth mobility and migration.
Benign cementoblastoma	It generally occurs in young patients, peak incidence is in the 3rd decade, and there is no distinct gender preference. The most common localisation is the area of the first mandibular molar.	Mandibular swelling associated with pain.

Radiographic feature	Differential diagnosis	Therapy
Well-defined radiolucent area. If unilocular, it cannot be distinguished from an endosseous cyst; if multilocular, it may be a single lesion divided by osseous septa. When associated with an impacted tooth it cannot be distinguished from a dentigerous cyst. Suggested exams: panoramic radiograph and CT scan.	Residual cyst Dentigerous (follicular) cyst Keratocystic odontogenic tumour Odontogenic mixoma Odontogenic fibroma N.B. no osteolithic lesion can be excluded until histopathologic examination is performed.	Surgical excision. It exhibits a significant relapse frequency, particularly after conservative treatment: the patient must be followed for a long time to diagnose possible relapses and, in this latter event, should be treated with a radical approach.
	Ameloblastoma	Less aggressive than ameloblastoma, with a lower tendency to relapse after excision.
It can present in different ways according to the evolutive stage: radiolucent with well-defined margins, radiopaque, radiolucent with radiopaque areas, and floccular appearance associated with an unerupted tooth.	Odontogenic mixoma, ameloblastoma.	Surgical excision. Low relapse frequency. As it exhibits a locally invasive behaviour, if the cortical plates are eroded, it must be treated with a radical approach (as with an ameloblastoma).
Unilocular radiolucent area surrounding an unerupted tooth (similar to a dentigerous cyst).	Dentigerous (follicular) cyst.	Enucleation of the lesion. No tendency to relapse.
It may appear as small, round or oval unilocular radiolucent areas, or as a multilocular radiolucent lesion with irregular margins. Radiolucency can involve the mandibular body, angle, and ramus. The lesion may cause tooth dislocation and, rarely, root resorption.	Dentigerous cyst, ameloblastoma, odontogenic mixoma, adenomatoid odontogenic tumour, ameloblastic fibroma, central giant cell lesion, aneurysmal cyst.	Enucleation associated with bone curettage and local application of Carnoy's solution. It shows a high relapse frequency, particularly after conservative treatment (5%-62.5%). In case of relapse, "en bloc" resection of the affected area with 1-centimetre safety margins is the treatment of choice.
Radiolucent area with well defined margins and a typical radiopaque border (sclerotic reactive bone).	Ameloblastoma, residual cyst, dentigerous (follicular) cyst, keratocystic odontogenic tumour, odontogenic mixoma, odontogenic fibroma, central giant cell lesion, histiocytosis.	Surgical excision.
Well-defined radiolucency associated with malposition of teeth.	Adenomatoid odontogenic tumour, osteoblastoma, keratocystic odontogenic tumour.	Enucleation associated with bone curettage. Malignant degeneration is rare (ameloblastic fibrosarcoma).
Radiopaque masses with irregular margins, always separated from the surrounding bone by a radiolucent rim. Complex odontomas appear as a uniformly radiopaque mass, while compound odontomas contain incompletely developed dental structures that appear as small malformed teeth.	Sclerosing osteomyelitis, osteoma, periapical cemental dysplasia, ossifying fibroma, cementoblastoma.	Surgical removal of the lesion, which is generally straightforward due to the presence of an easily identifiable cleavage plane. These lesions show no tendency to relapse.
Radiolucent area with randomly dispersed masses of radiopaque material inside.	Ameloblastoma Odontogenic mixoma Dentigerous cyst Keratocystic odontogenic tumour Central giant cell lesion Histiocytosis.	Surgical excision associated with bone curettage.
Well-delimited area with peripheral radiolucent border and radiopaque masses inside.	Ameloblastoma, residual cyst, dentigerous cyst, keratocystic odontogenic tumour, odontogenic mixoma, odontogenic fibroma, central giant cell lesion, histiocytosis.	Enucleation of the lesion, no tendency to relapse.
Well-defined unilocular or multilocular radiolucency. Presence of interspersed calcified areas.	Dentigerous cyst, keratocystic odontogenic tumour, ameloblastoma.	Enucleation may prove insufficient, and vigorous curettage is necessary as it has a tendency to relapse.
Multilocular radiolucent area possibly associated with unerupted or dislocated teeth.	Differential diagnosis with all radiolucent lesions of the jaws.	Surgical excision, no tendency to relapse.
Unilocular or multilocular radiolucent lesion; in this event, it may not be distinguished from endosseous cysts or ameloblastomas. Sometimes it is more radiopaque, showing the so-called "frosted glass" appearance.	Residual cyst, dentigerous cyst, keratocystic odontogenic tumour, odontogenic mixoma, odontogenic fibroma, ameloblastoma.	Surgical excision. However, due to the relative local aggressiveness and the friability of the mass, the resection of the affected segment with safety margins may be indicated, particularly with respect to large lesions. Relapse rate ranges from 10% to 30%.
Round radiopaque mass with peripheral radiolucent rim, fused to the roots of a single tooth (frequently the first mandibular molar); root resorption may occur.	Odontoma, osteoblastoma, focal sclerosing osteomyelitis, hypercementosis.	Enucleation of the lesion. Low tendency to relapse.

(continued)

Tab. 9.1 WHO classification (2005) of benign tumours of the oral cavity (*continued*)

Denomination	Incidence	Clinical features
Bone-related lesions		
Ossifying fibroma	It exhibits a predilection for young females; peak incidence is between the 3rd and 4th decade.	It is mostly seen in the posterior mandible; it causes a painless swelling and facial asymmetry in the advanced stage.
Fibrous dysplasia	The monostotic form is equally distributed in both genders, and it is six times more common than the polyostotic. The polyostotic form is more frequent in females. Both forms occur mainly in children. It is frequently located in the maxilla, and it may involve adjacent bones.	Asymptomatic swelling causes facial asymmetry. It may cause tooth displacement, malocclusion, and root resorption.
Osseous dysplasia	It exhibits a predilection for females; peak incidence is between the 4th and 5th decade. It frequently involves the mandibular alveolar ridge.	Numerous clinical presentations, such as periapical osseous dysplasia and focal osseous dysplasia.
Central giant cell lesion	It generally occurs in females, peak incidence is between the 2nd and 3rd decade, and shows a predilection for the mandible, particularly the premolar and molar areas.	Generally asymptomatic, it may rarely cause pain and paraesthesia, swelling and loosening of teeth.
Cherubism	It exhibits a predilection for young males. The mandible is more frequently involved than the maxilla.	Symmetric, painless swelling. It may cause tooth displacement and delayed tooth eruption.
Aneurysmal bone cyst	It generally occurs in the 3rd decade, it rarely involves the jaws.	Osteolytic lesion filled with blood. It may present with marked swelling, malocclusion, tooth displacement and tooth loosening. Root resorption may occur.
Simple bone cyst	Peak incidence in the 2nd decade, with no gender predilection. Almost exclusive mandibular localisation, generally in the anterior region.	Mild pain, tooth dislocation or pathological fractures are rare. Teeth are frequently vital.
Non-odontogenic tumours		
Papilloma or inverted papilloma	It represents 2.5% of all lesions of the oral cavity. Peak incidence in the 5th decade, with a predilection for males. HPV is the correlated etiologic factor. The most frequent localisations are palate, vermilion border, and uvula.	Two forms: • exophytic or papillomatous (well-defined elevated small mass, hard-elastic, painless); • inverted (invagination and growth towards the underlying stroma).Pink or white exophytic lesions, soft tissue alterations cause a granular or cauliflower appearance. Generally, it is a single, asymptomatic lesion. It may undergo spontaneous regression, but also degenerate into epidermoid carcinoma.
Schwannoma (neurilemmoma)	Peak incidence between the 2nd and 4th decade, with no gender predilection. In the oral cavity, the most frequent localisation is the tongue, but it can also affect the palate and mucosa of the cheeks, lips, and gums.	Slow growth mass, elastic consistency. White-grey colour, well-defined margins, encapsulated, asymptomatic. Pain ensues only with compression of the surrounding tissues.
Ossifying fibroma	It frequently occurs in young females, peak incidence in the 3rd and 4th decade.	It develops almost exclusively in the jaws in proximity of teeth, determining a painless swelling and, in the advanced stage, facial asymmetry.
Desmoplastic fibroma	It occurs more frequently in young females, and exhibits a predilection for the mandibular angle and ramus.	Dense greyish tissue mass; asymptomatic in the initial stage, painful swelling in the advanced stage.
Osteoblastoma	Extremely rare, it generally occurs in young males and develops in the molar and premolar areas.	Fast growth, with a tendency to erode the cortical plates. Soft consistency; it tends to cause erythema of the overlying mucosa. Involved teeth may show mobility.
Osteoid osteoma	It rarely affects the jaws. It occurs more frequently in young subjects, and exhibits no gender predilection.	Slow growth, well-defined (usually small) lesion.
Osteoma	It generally occurs in young subjects, exhibits no gender predilection, and it frequently affects the mandible. Osteomas of the head and neck are rare.	Slow growth. It is formed by newly formed mature bone, both cancellous and cortical.
Lipoma	Rare in the oral cavity. Most frequent localisations: mucosa of the cheeks, tongue, and floor of the mouth.	Asymptomatic submucosal yellowish mass with intact overlying mucosa.
Haemangioma	Congenital benign neoplasm caused by proliferation of endothelial cells.	Clinically it is not possible to distinguish it from a vascular malformation. It appears as an irregular red-brownish or bluish mass.

Radiographic feature	Differential diagnosis	Therapy
Variable presentation: radiolucent areas alternated with radiopaque foci.	Fibrous dysplasia, osteoblastoma.	Surgical excision with ample safety margins is indicated.
Three different radiographic patterns are described: cystic, sclerotic, and mixed radiolucent/radiopaque.	Ossifying fibroma.	It frequently seems to stabilise with skeletal maturation. The surgical approach is indicated for functional alterations or disfigurement.
Radiolucent or radiopaque areas, or alternation of the two.	Fibrous dysplasia Ossifying fibroma	Generally, no treatment is needed, with the exception of those cases in which complications following infections or facial deformities arise.
Radiolucent multilocular (more frequent) or unilocular lesions, with scalloped, well-defined but non-sclerotic borders. Intralesional wavy bony septa are a typical feature.	Ameloblastoma, odontogenic mixoma, keratocystic odontogenic tumour, adenomatoid odontogenic tumour, ossifying fibroma, ameloblastic fibroma.	Enucleation. In cases of relapse, radical treatment is indicated.
Well-defined multilocular radiolucent lesions showing the typical "soap bubble" appearance.	Central giant cell lesion.	Lesions generally regress after puberty. Before puberty, a surgical approach should be chosen only in cases of severe functional disturbances.
Unilocular or multilocular radiolucent lesions.	Keratocystic odontogenic tumour, central giant cell lesion, ameloblastic fibroma, ameloblastoma, odontogenic mixoma.	Curettage. If the lesion extends to the soft tissue, the risk of relapse is higher.
Unilocular radiolucency without expansion of the cortical plates. The upper margin of the lesion may extend between the roots of the teeth, gaining the typical scalloped appearance.	All the radiolucent lesions of the jaws.	Surgical excision.
Negative, except in cases of endonasal or endosinusal development.	Papillary hyperplasia, condyloma acuminatum, verruciform xanthoma.	Surgical excision with ample safety margins, due to the high frequency of relapse.
Negative.	Neurofibroma.	Enucleation of the lesion, no tendency of relapse.
Various presentations: radiolucent areas alternated with radiopaque foci.	Fibrous dysplasia, osteoblastoma.	Surgical excision with ample safety margins is indicated.
Well-defined radiolucent area.	Fibrosarcoma.	"En bloc" resection with safety margins.
Radiolucent area that may rarely present calcified radiopaque foci.	Osteoma Osteoid osteoma Osteosarcoma Cementoblastoma Ossifying fibroma Fibrous dysplasia.	Curettage or surgical excision with safety margins, no tendency to relapse.
Small radiolucent area with a peripheral sclerotic rim.	Osteoma Osteoblastoma Osteosarcoma Cementoblastoma Ossifying fibroma Fibrous dysplasia.	Enucleation and curettage, or "en bloc" resection of the affected segment.
Radiopaque area; in some cases a radiolucent margin separating it from the surrounding bone may be visible.	Osteoblastoma Osteoid osteoma Exostosis.	If small and asymptomatic, periodical radiographic and clinical examination may be sufficient. In cases of large lesions, surgical removal may be indicated. It has no tendency to relapse.
Lobulated, well-defined mass formed by mature adipocytes.	Granular cell tumour Neurofibroma Traumatic fibroma Mucocele.	Surgical enucleation; low tendency to relapse.
Negative, except in cases of endosseous development.		Surgical excision.

However, it is worth remembering that the following lesions, previously considered endosseous cysts, have now been reclassified as benign tumours:

- the keratocyst, now renamed keratocystic odontogenic tumour;
- the calcifying odontogenic cyst, now renamed calcifying cystic odontogenic tumour;
- the aneurysmal bone cyst (the name was left unchanged but the term is a misnomer, as the lesion is neither an aneurysm nor a cyst);
- the simple bone cyst (same as above).

Except for the simple bone cyst, the main reason that led to the reclassification of these lesions as benign tumours is the significant incidence of relapse in cases of conservative treatment (simple enucleation) compared to odontogenic cysts.

The general aspects of the surgical treatment of benign neoplasms will be described further on in this chapter, and for every approach, the lesions that more frequently request it will be specified.

Although the most common benign tumours are not singularly described in detail to simplify the reading of this textbook, an exception is made for the lesion known until a few years ago (and still known by many) as keratocyst, which has been reclassified in 2005 by the WHO as *keratocystic odontogenic tumour*. This lesion is relatively frequent, and can also present as multiple endosseous lesions associated to other defects in different body systems such as the skin, endocrine system, eyes, and nervous system, thus representing an autosomal dominant condition that bears the name of the first clinicians who described it: *the Gorlin-Goltz syndrome*.

The main simil-cystic lesion is frequently located in the mandible and, typically, in the posterior region of the mandibular body and the inferior portion of the ramus; the posterior areas are the most frequently involved even when the lesion is located in the upper maxilla.

Multiple lesions are present in 7% of patients, and the Gorlin-Goltz syndrome affects half of these. This syndrome is characterised by the presence of basal-cell carcinomas of the skin (although 10% of the affected patients do not show evidence of these tumours), multiple or multilocular keratocystic odontogenic tumours (75% of the patients), palmar and plantar pits, bifid ribs, vertebrae anomalies, kyphoscoliosis, frontal and temporoparietal bossing, hypertelorism, mandibular prognathism, and calcification of the falx cerebri.

The tumour has a locally aggressive behaviour, as it tends to infiltrate bone and, when bone is eroded, the surrounding soft tissues. Therefore, relapse after conservative treatment is frequent (over 50%), because early infiltration exposes to the risk of incomplete excision.

Diagnosis

Generally speaking, as mentioned in Chapter 1 of this manual, the correct collection of the patient's medical history and a thorough clinical examination are always extremely useful for evaluating the different clinical features of the lesion, thus leading to a presumptive diagnosis. Aspects such as the speed at which the lesion grows, its consistency (soft, elastic soft, elastic hard, hard, and bone-like hard), its mobility in relation to the superficial and deep plane, spontaneous or compression-induced tenderness, chromatic alterations of the intraoral and extraoral superficial tissues are all important elements to evaluate (📷 9.6, 9.7). However, imaging tests (described in Chapter 1) play a fundamental role in the early presumptive diagnosis of tumours. In this respect, it is worth remembering that in cases of neoplastic lesions, radiographic examinations such as the panoramic radiograph may be insufficient, with the exception of small endosseous lesions such as odontomas (9.8a-b).

Although it is not possible to make generalisations, it is safe to say that Computed Tomography is generally indicated for the evaluation of lesions involving the hard tissues of the jaws (9.9a-b), while Magnetic Resonance is particularly effective in showing details of the lesions involving the soft tissues (9.10a-b).

Nonetheless, it should be always emphasised that a definitive diagnosis can only be obtained with the histopathologic examination of a tissue sample taken from the lesion. Frequently, in fact, different pathologies may show similar signs and symptoms, and they cannot be distinguished solely based on clinical and/or radiographic examinations.

However, symptoms and clinical signs exist that can suggest a more or less aggressive behaviour of a neoplasm. The malignant nature of the lesion should always be suspected when one or more of the following signs is present:

- rapid growth associated with pain;
- ulceration of the superficial soft tissues that does not spontaneously heal in a short time span;

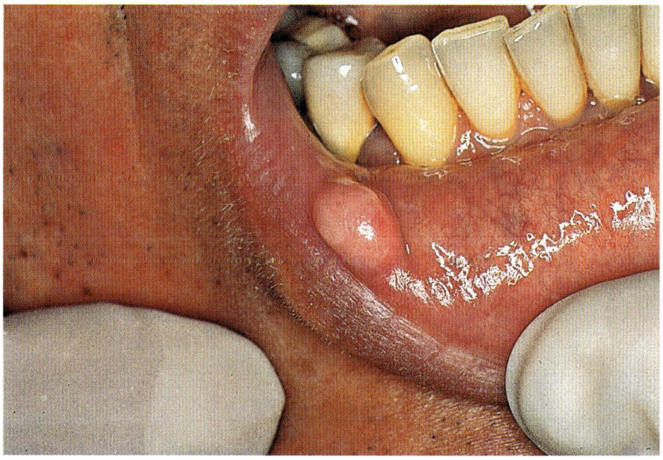

9.6 Papilloma of the inferior lip.

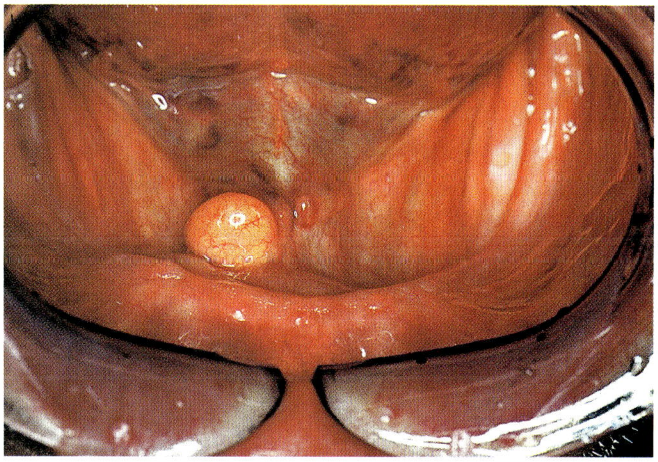

9.7 Lipoma of the floor of the mouth.

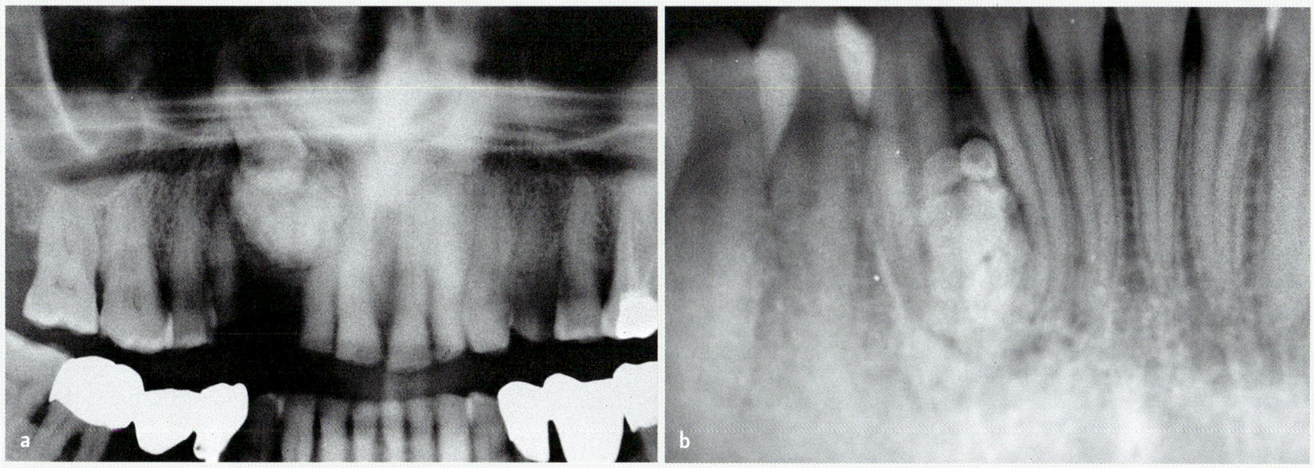

9.8 **a)** Complex odontoma of the maxilla (left canine region). **b)** Compound odontoma of the mandible (right canine region).

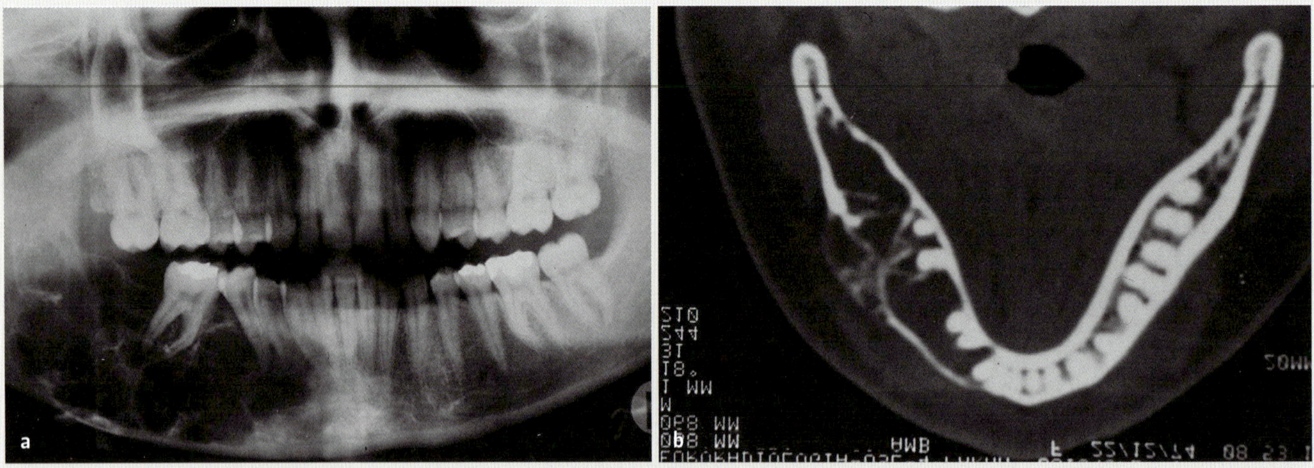

9.9 **a)** Panoramic radiograph showing a large radiolucent lesion with radiopaque areas ("soap bubbles" or "honeycomb" appearance) in the posterior region of the right hemimandible (odontogenic mixoma). **b)** CT scan showing erosion of the buccal cortical plate.

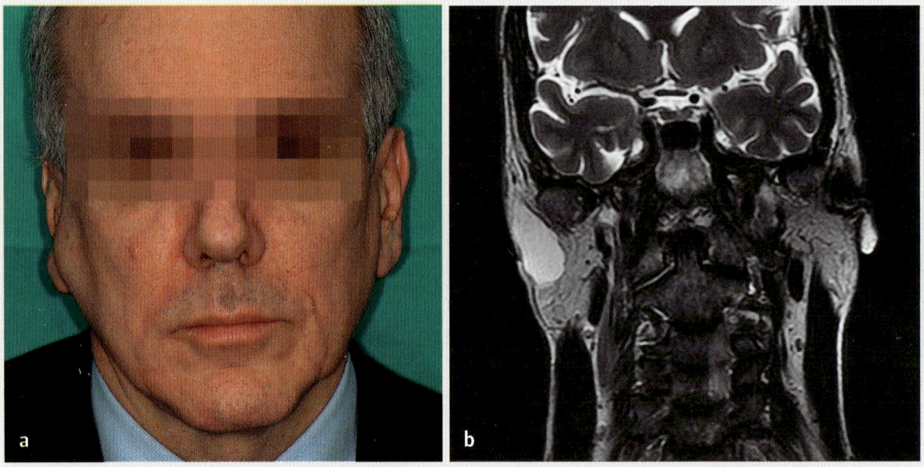

9.10 **a)** Extraoral examination: asymmetry on the frontal plane due to swelling in the right parotid region. **b)** MRI (coronal plane) showing a lesion located between the skin and the parotid gland (definitive diagnosis after histopathologic examination: lipoma).

- insurgence of functional impairment of a nerve bundle in direct contact with the lesion;
- irregular margins;
- bone erosion and infiltration of the surrounding soft tissues;
- erosion of dental roots;
- impairment of the general health condition of the patient.

In these cases, the clinician must resort to every diagnostic means necessary to obtain a definitive diagnosis as soon as possible and, should the malignancy of the lesion be confirmed, immediately refer the patient to an oncology and/or maxillofacial surgery unit.

Treatment

Benign odontogenic tumours

The common objective is to remove the entire lesion to avoid the possibility of relapse. The type of surgical treatment and the extent of the excision mainly depend on the type of tumour and, in particular, on its aggressiveness (capability to infiltrate the soft tissues, frequency of relapse, presence or absence of a cleavage plane, location of the lesion).

Although it is not possible to generalise, the typical treatment options for benign odontogenic lesions of the jaws are:

- *enucleation*;
- *enucleation associated with bone curettage* (with or without the local application of cytotoxic solutions);
- *"en bloc" resection* with safety margins determined according to the type of lesion, followed by immediate or delayed bone reconstruction.

In cases of "*low aggressiveness*" odontogenic tumors, well-defined and with a low frequency of relapse (e.g. odontomas), a conservative treatment may be indicated (enucleation) in association with periodic radiographic and clinical examinations.

In cases of "*locally aggressive*" tumours (e.g. ameloblastoma and keratocystic odontogenic tumour), simple enucleation frequently leads to a relapse of the lesion. Consensus on the treatment modalities is not yet unanimous; however, according to the histologic type, localisation, and the development pattern of the lesion, current orientations indicate the following surgical protocols:

- in cases of *unilocular* lesions developing in the mandible without infiltrating the surrounding soft tissues, the first approach is represented by enucleation associated with thorough curettage of the residual cavity with manual and rotary instruments, and local application of cytotoxic substances such as Carnoy's solution. This approach eliminates small clusters of neoplastic cells which, due to the tendency towards local infiltration of these tumours, may remain after the enucleation of the main lesion, representing potential sources of relapse;
- in cases of *multilocular* lesions developing in the mandible, the previous treatment modality can still be chosen, bearing in mind that it may expose the patient to a higher risk of relapse. Should a relapse of the lesion occur, a more radical approach will be necessary in the second surgical treatment;
- in cases of *multilocular* lesions developing in the mandible that *have eroded the cortical plates* and infiltrated the surrounding soft tissues, simple enucleation and curettage are insufficient to remove all the neoplastic cells. Therefore, the treatment of choice is frequently an "en bloc" resection with ample safety margins, followed by immediate or delayed reconstruction of the resected tissues. Technical details regarding this treatment modality are not described in this textbook as they lie outside the tasks of the oral surgeon;
- as far as the upper maxilla is concerned, *benign but locally aggressive* lesions should be treated from the beginning with a more radical approach than mandibular lesions. In fact, all things being equal (extent of the lesion, morphology, and histologic type), due to the local anatomy of the maxillary region which is characterised by thin cortical plates that are easily eroded, pneumatised spaces that offer no resistance to the growth of the lesion, and proximity to the basicranium and to the infratemporal fossa, the lesion may grow rapidly and relapses are more frequent and more complex to treat.

Four step-by-step clinical cases are presented (9.11-9.14).

Clinical case 1 – Odontoma of the right mandibular ramus

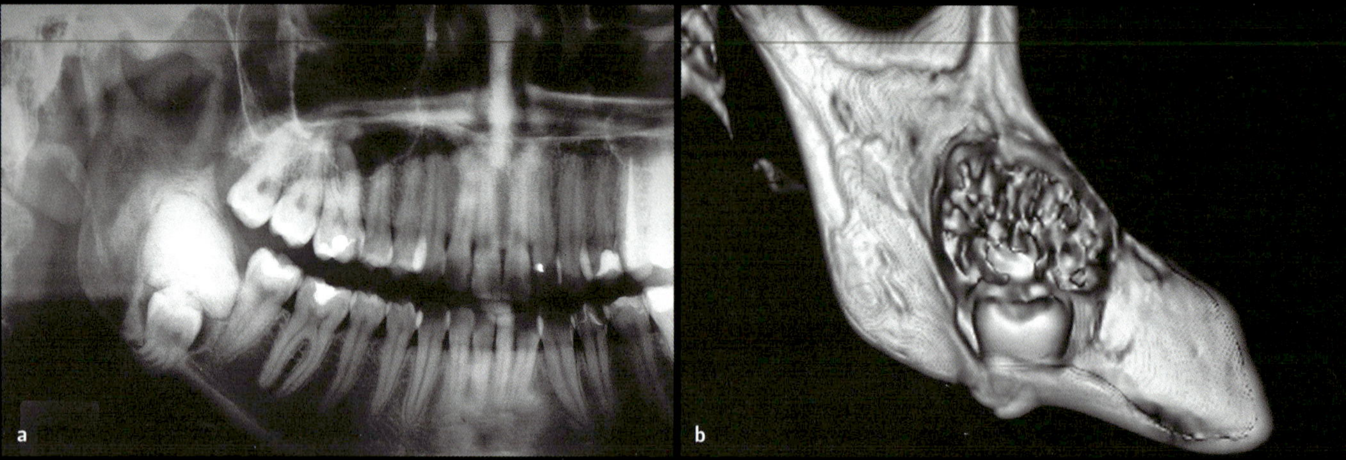

9.11a-b Radiographic exams show a radiopaque lesion of the right mandibular ramus that prevents eruption of the third molar.

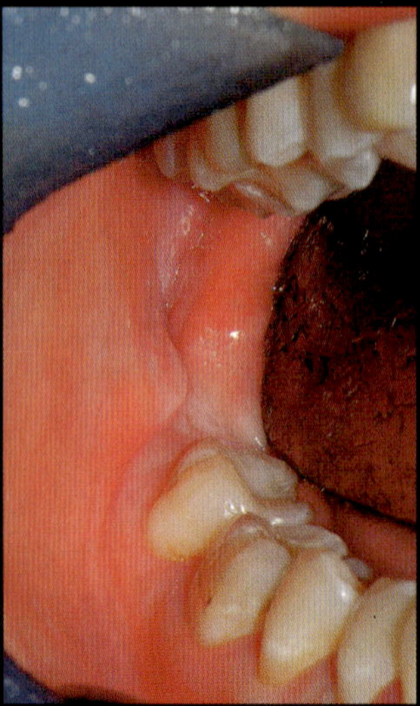

9.11c Preoperative intraoral situation.

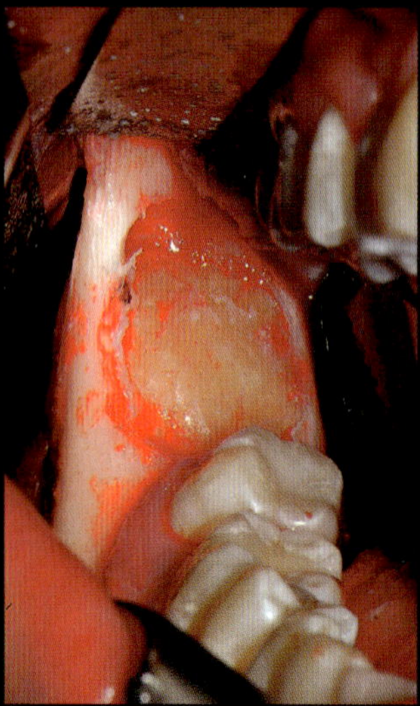

9.11d Full-thickness elevation of the surgical flap and exposure of the lesion.

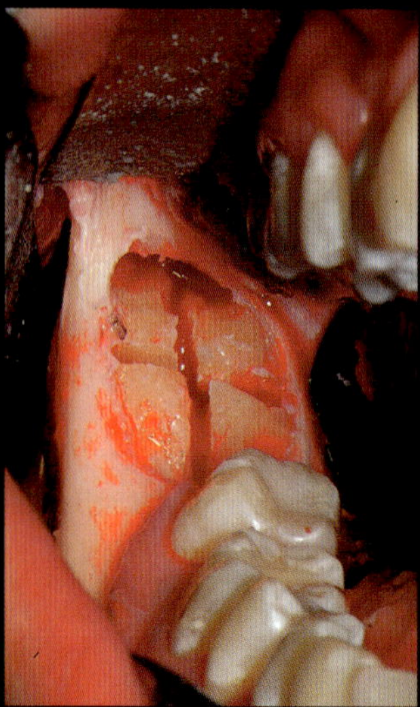

9.11e The lesion is divided into four parts for easier removal.

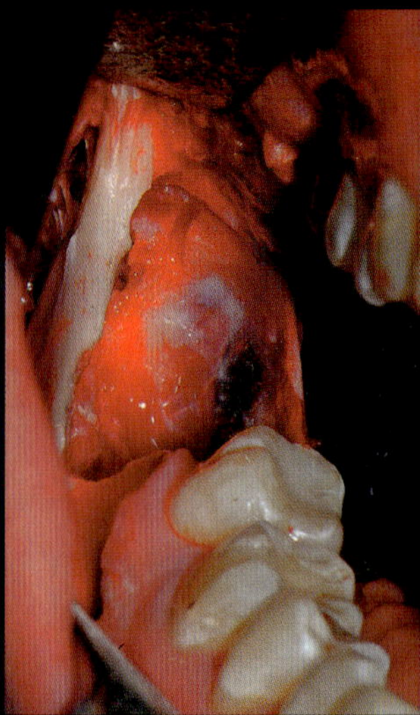

9.11f The residual cavity after complete enucleation of the lesion.

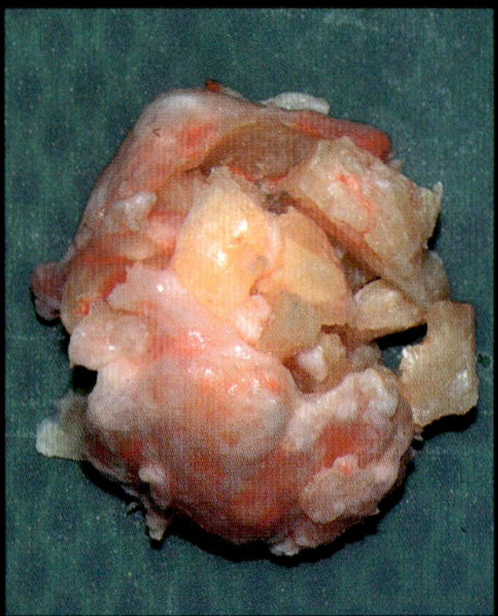

9.11g The removed lesion (odontoma).

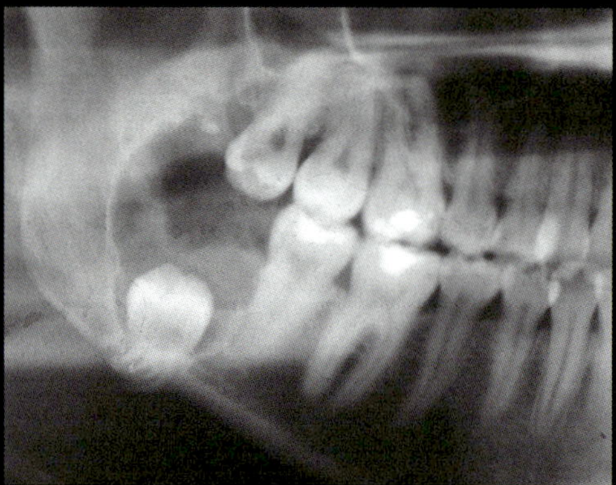

9.11h Postoperative radiographic follow-up.

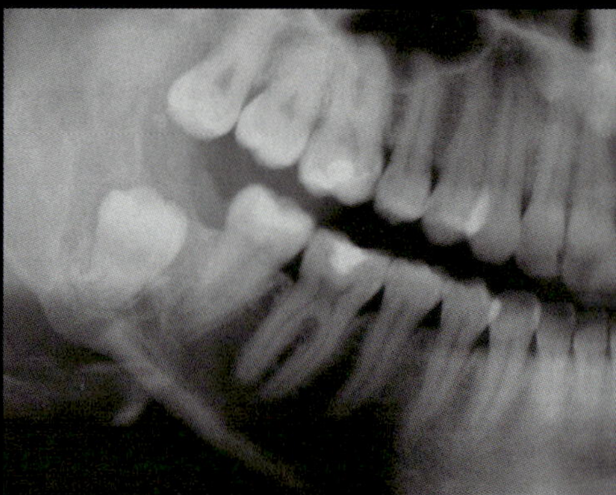

9.11i Radiographic follow-up some time after surgery: reossification of the residual cavity and coronal migration of the third molar are visible.

Clinical case 2 – Keratocystic odontogenic tumour of the mandible

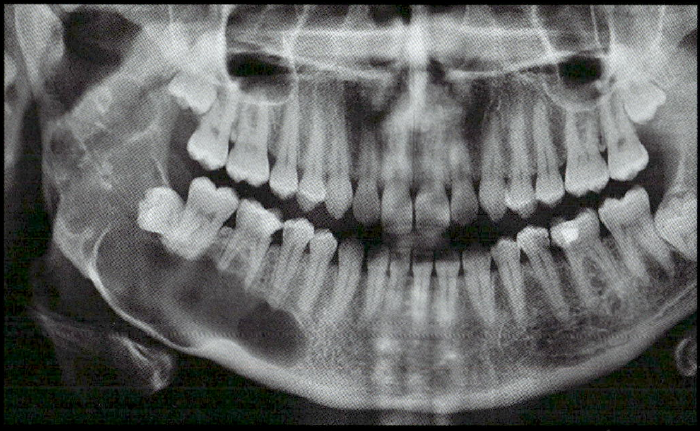

9.12a Panoramic radiograph showing a large, radiolucent mandibular lesion extending from the area of the first premolar to the coronoid process and the mandibular notch (keratocystic odontogenic tumour).

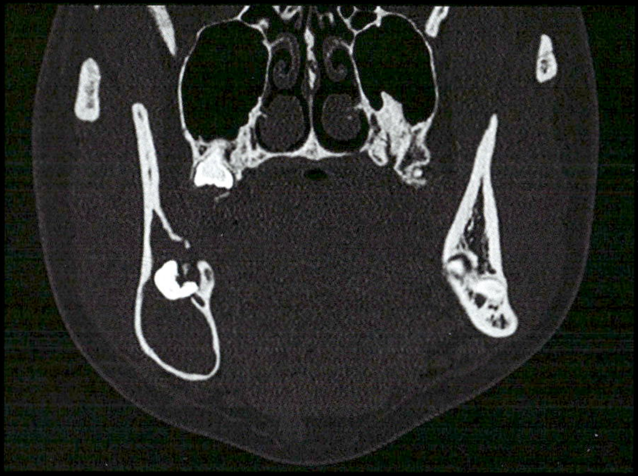

9.12b CT scan (coronal slice) showing the development of the lesion inside the mandible: the cortical plates are not eroded.

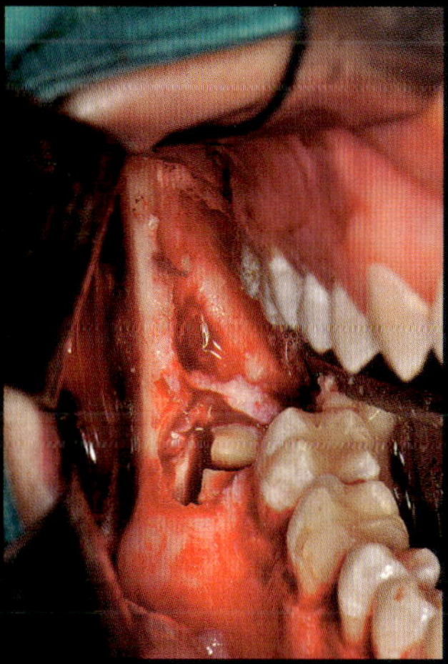

9.12c Skeletonisation of the mandible, access osteotomy and odontotomy of the impacted third molar.

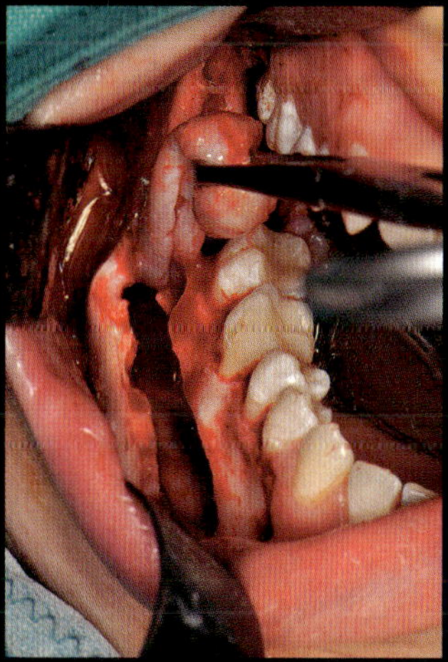

9.12d Enucleation of the lesion associated with thorough curettage of the bony walls of the residual cavity and local application of Carnoy's solution.

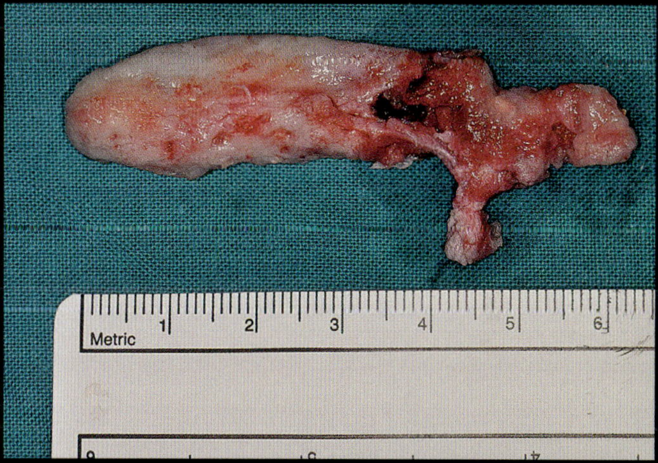

9.12e The excised lesion.

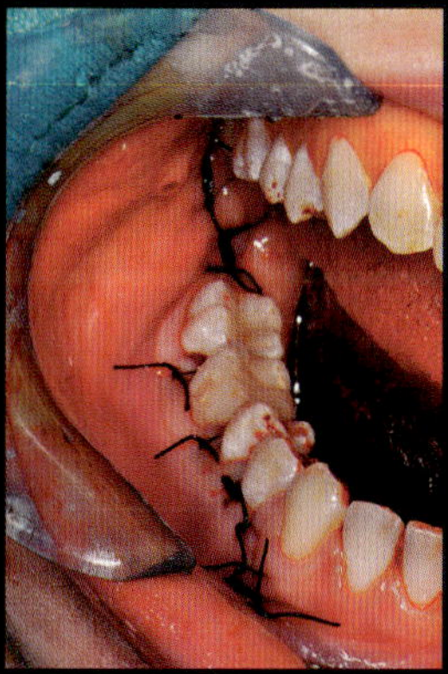

9.12f The access flap is sutured.

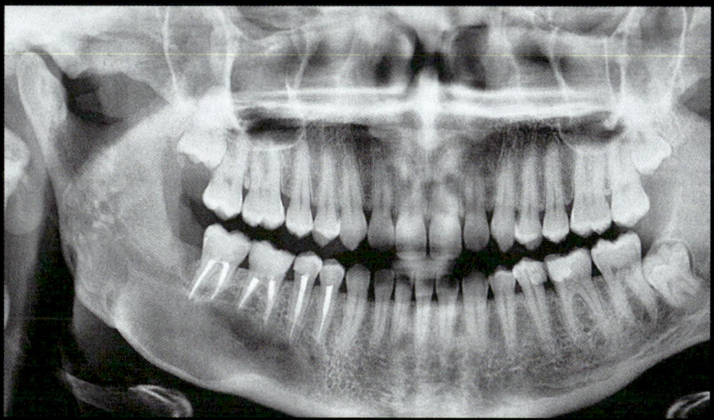

9.12g Radiographic postoperative follow-up examination showing the almost complete reossification of the mandible (the molars and premolars were endodontically treated prior to surgery due to their relationships with the lesion).

Clinical case 3 – Ameloblastoma of the right mandibular ramus

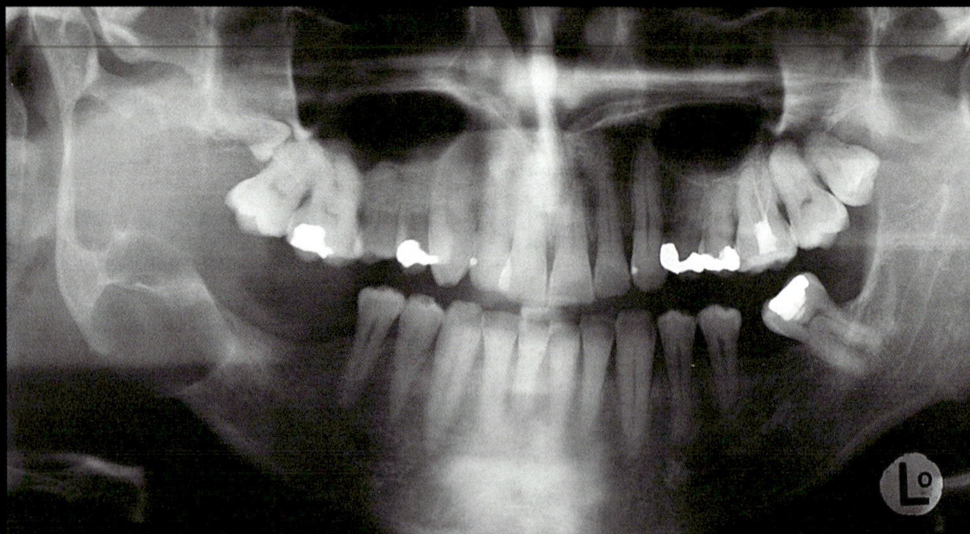

9.13a Panoramic radiograph showing a radiolucent, multilocular lesion of the right mandibular ramus.

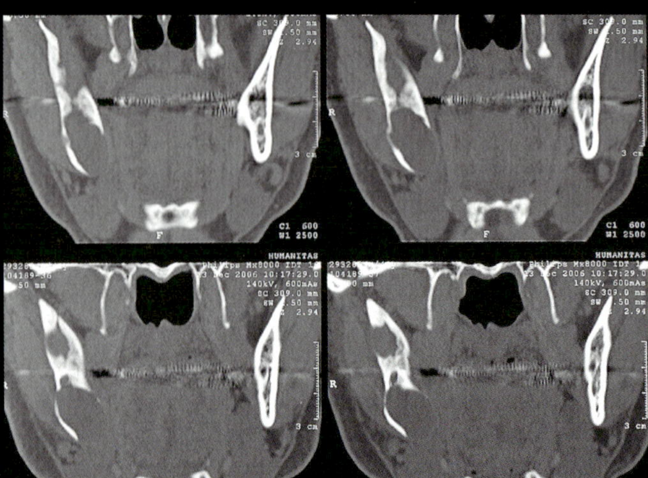

9.13b CT scan showing erosion of the cortical plates and infiltration of the surrounding soft tissues (ameloblastoma).

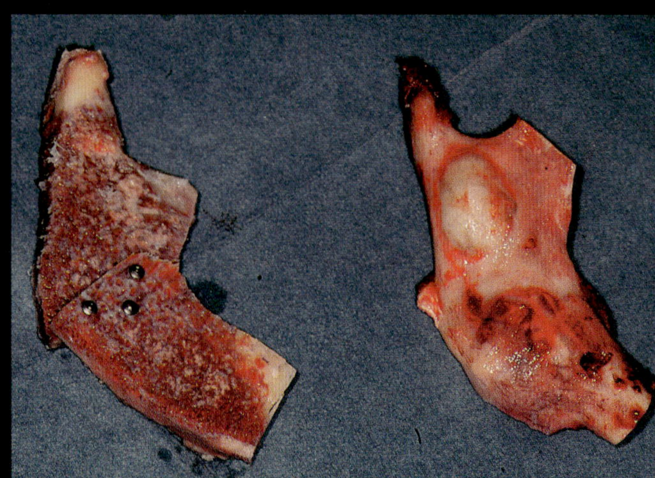

9.13c Complete resection of the mandibular ramus (left) and bone graft harvested from the ilium and modelled to substitute the mandibular ramus (right) (surgery in cooperation with Prof. Roberto Brusati).

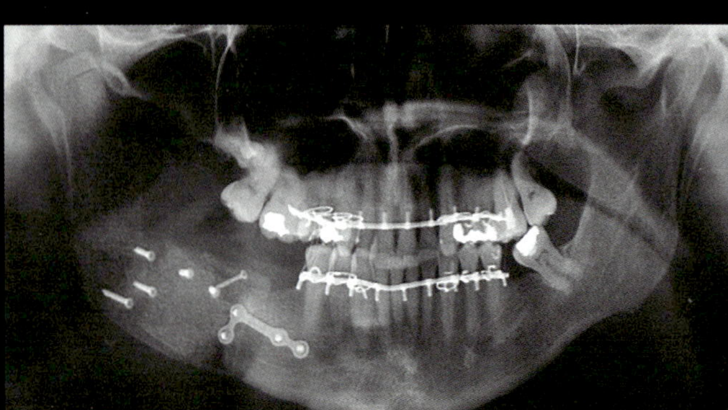

9.13d Postoperative panoramic radiograph showing the complete restoration of the mandibular morphology.

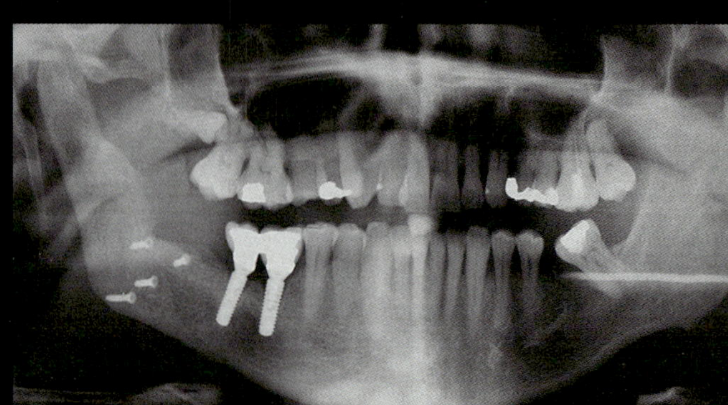

9.13e Follow-up panoramic radiograph two years after surgery, and after implant-supported rehabilitation of the edentulous area.

Clinical case 4 – Ameloblastoma of the maxilla

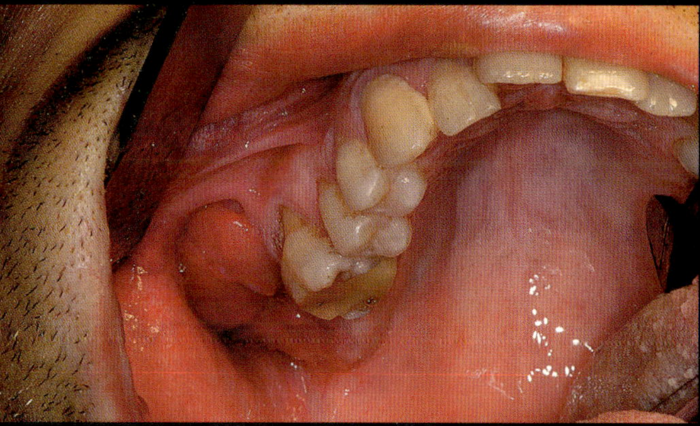

9.14a Intraoral examination: a sessile mass is visible in the molar and retromolar region of the right posterior maxilla (ameloblastoma).

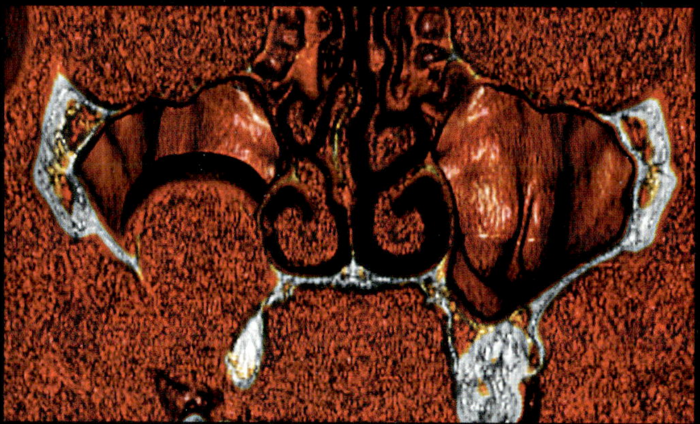

9.14b CT scan (coronal view, 3D reconstruction) showing an apparently solid mass that has completely eroded the alveolar ridge of the posterior maxilla and occupies part of the lumen of the right maxillary sinus.

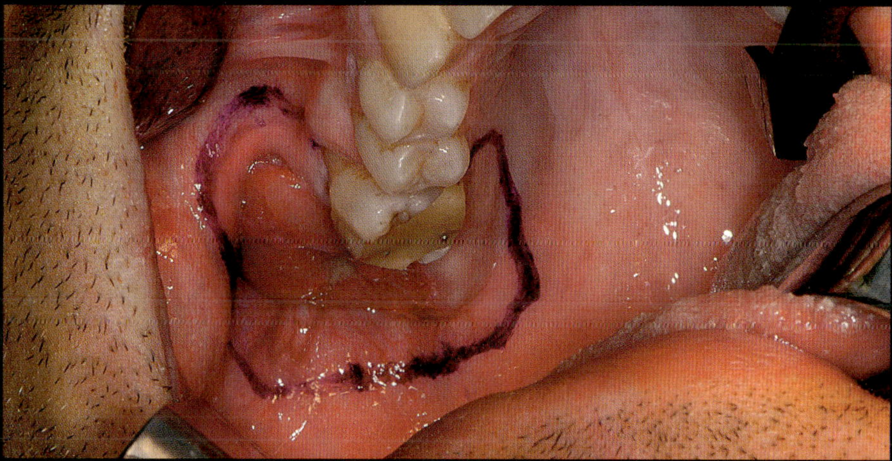

9.14c The area to be removed is outlined with a sterile dermographic pencil, keeping adequate safety margins.

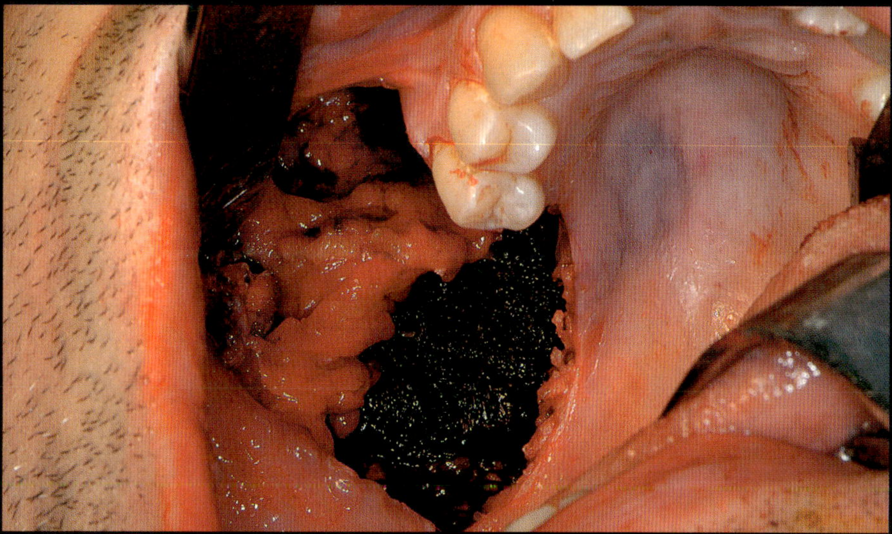

9.14d The residual defect after excision of the lesion.

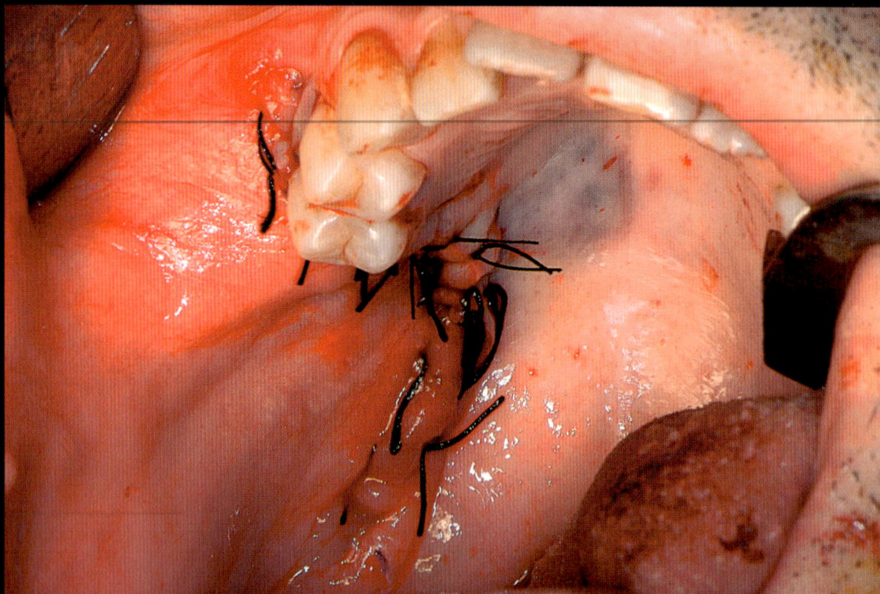

9.14e Closure of the large breach by means of a buccal fat pad flap covered with a local flap (buccal mucosa) (surgery in cooperation with Dr. Giacomo Colletti).

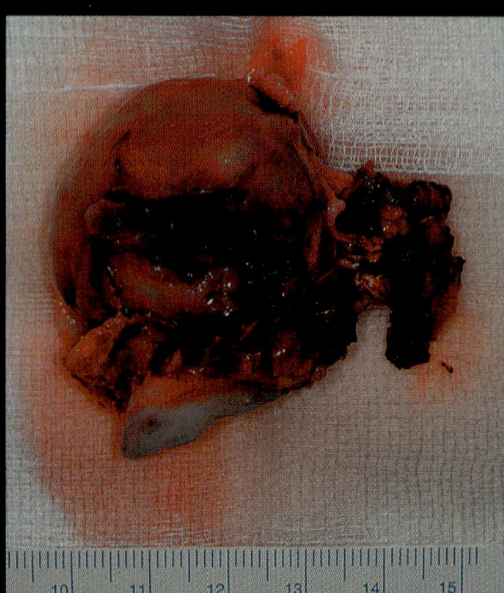

9.14f The excised lesion.

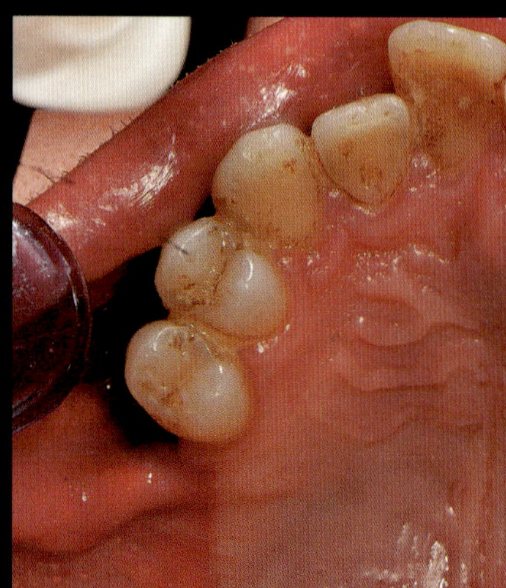

9.14g Healing of the surgical wound (intraoral view).

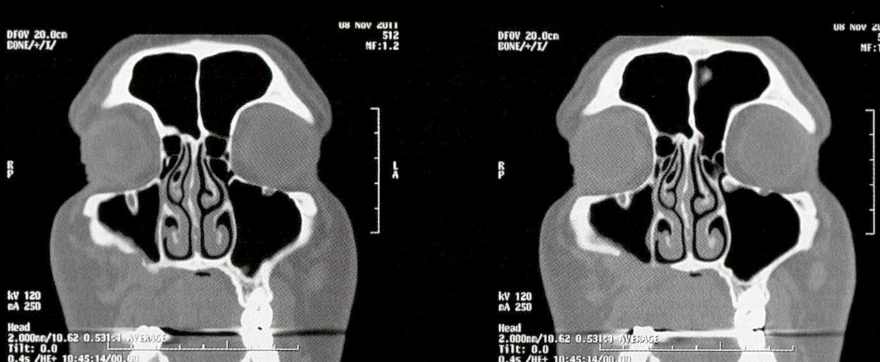

9.14h Maxillofacial CT scan showing complete removal of the mass, and healing of the surrounding tissues.

Non-odontogenic benign tumours

This definition includes neoplasms originating both from the epithelial tissues (e.g. papillomas) and from the connective tissues (e.g. angiomas, osteomas, fibromas, lipomas, etc.) (see tab. 9.1 for details). For the sake of clarity, these lesions can be divided according to their localisation; therefore, they are described as *tumours of the hard tissues* and *tumours of the soft tissues*.

The treatment, largely variable depending on the type of lesion, its localisation, and its local aggressiveness, follows the same principles previously described for the treatment of odontogenic tumours.

As far as tumours of the soft tissues are concerned, some appear as a well-defined, encapsulated mass (e.g. lipomas); in this event, the cleavage and removal of the lesion is easier, and it is not necessary to perform a resection with safety margins (9.15a-h). Conversely, some tumours of the soft tissues are not encapsulated (e.g. angiomas) and the excision must be performed with safety margins, to be reasonably sure that the entire lesion has been removed (9.16a-g).

Tumours of the hard tissues usually show frankly benign characteristics, such as slow growth and limited local aggressiveness (e.g. osteomas); in these events, simple excision is the treatment of choice (9.17a-g). Conversely, some of them may exhibit the tendency to infiltrate not only the hard tissues from which they originate, but also the surrounding soft tissues (e.g. ossifying fibroma); in these cases, an "en bloc" resection with ample safety margins in association with immediate or delayed reconstruction of the removed tissues is indicated, to avoid a high relapse rate.

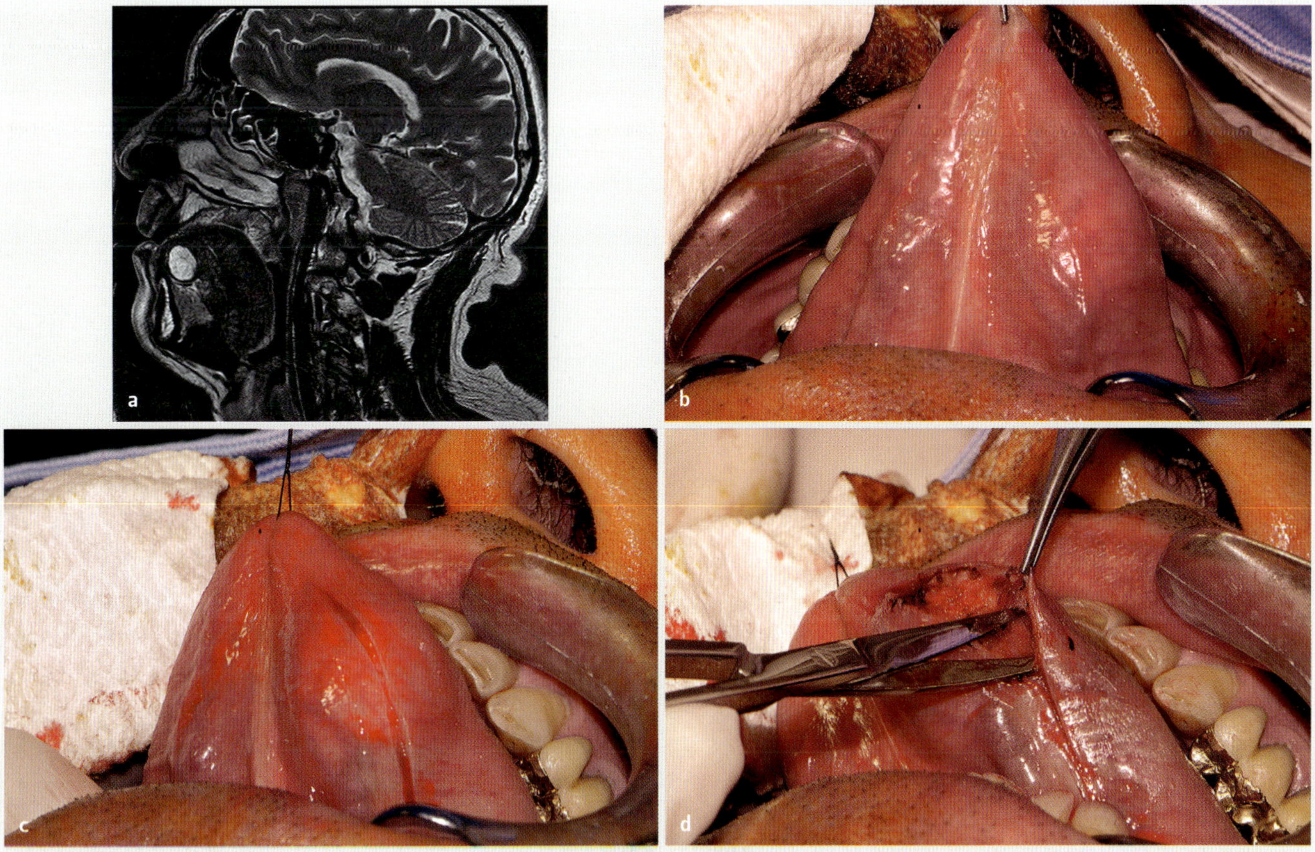

9.15 **a)** MRI (sagittal view) showing the presence of a round, well-defined mass inside the tongue. **b)** Preoperative image showing a localised swelling in the left hemitongue. **c)** Incision of the lingual mucosa. **d)** Blunt dissection of the lingual mucosa. (*continued*)

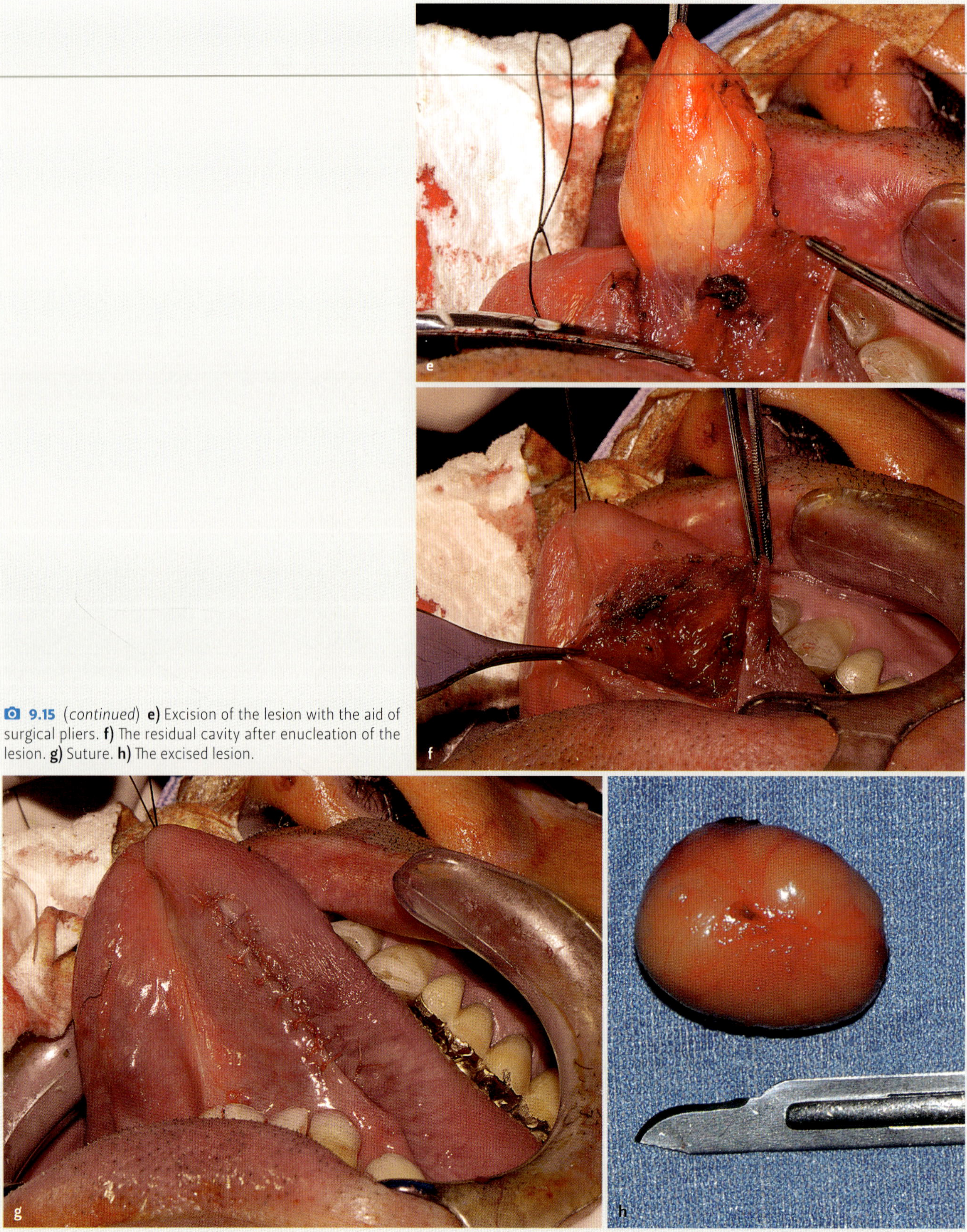

9.15 (*continued*) **e)** Excision of the lesion with the aid of surgical pliers. **f)** The residual cavity after enucleation of the lesion. **g)** Suture. **h)** The excised lesion.

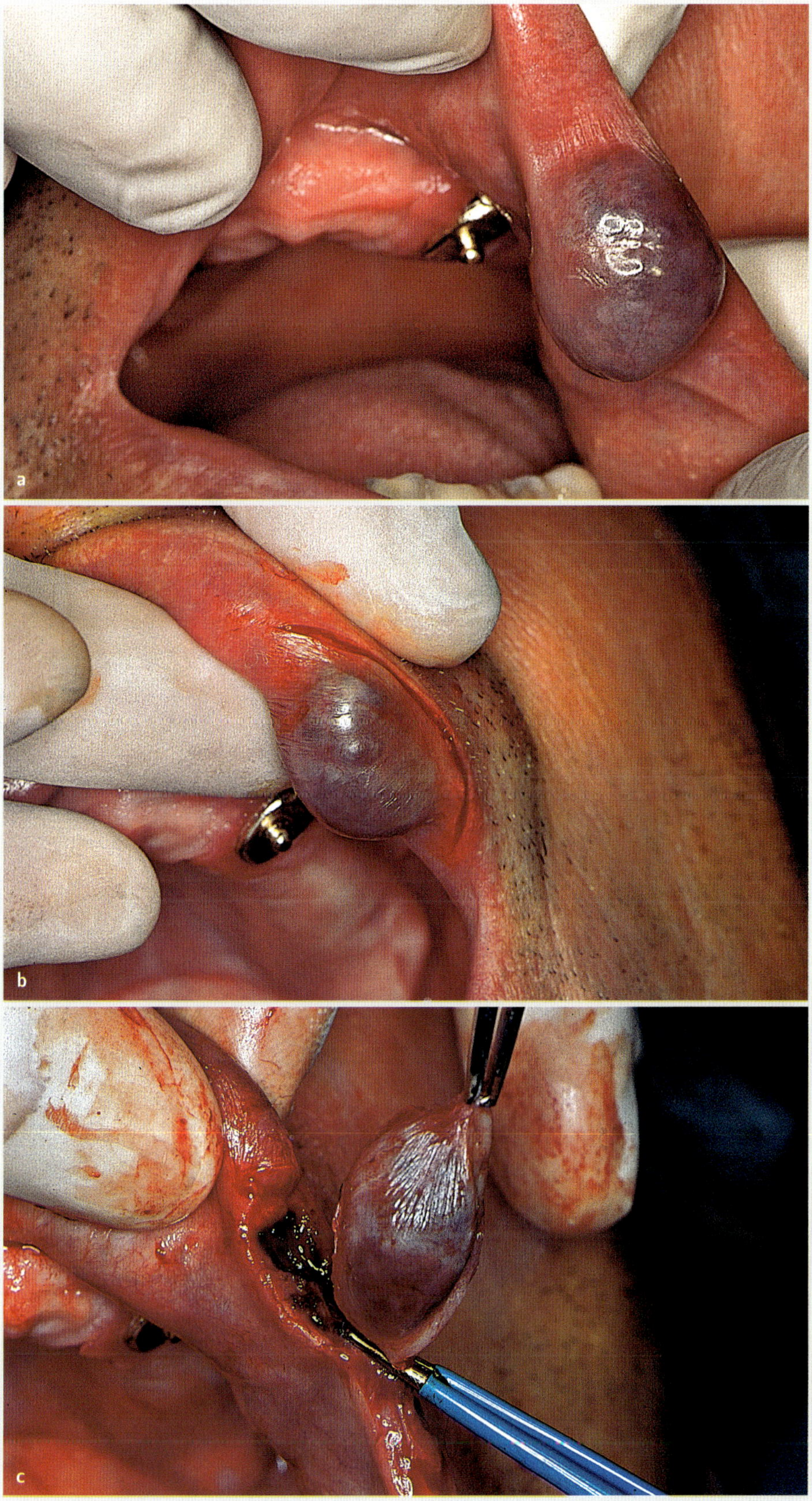

9.16 **a)** Haemangioma of the upper lip. **b)** Lozenge-shaped incision (3-millimetre safety margins). **c)** Excision of the lesion: the combined and alternated use of surgical scissors and bipolar coagulation prevents profuse bleeding. (*continued*)

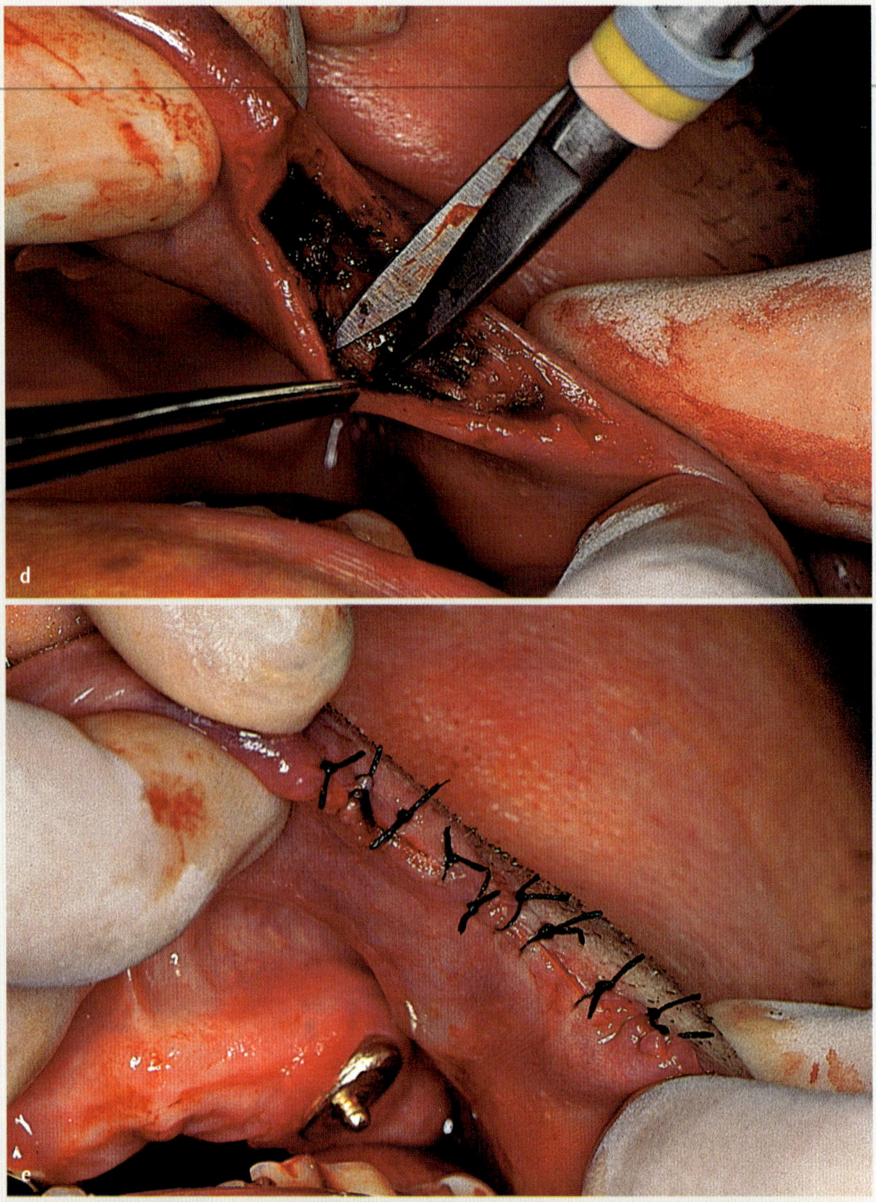

9.16 (*continued*) **d)** Blunt dissection of the mucosa to facilitate tension-free suture and primary intention healing of the surgical wound. **e)** Suture. **f)** Clinical examination 12 months after surgery. **g)** Adequate restoration of the labial morphology.

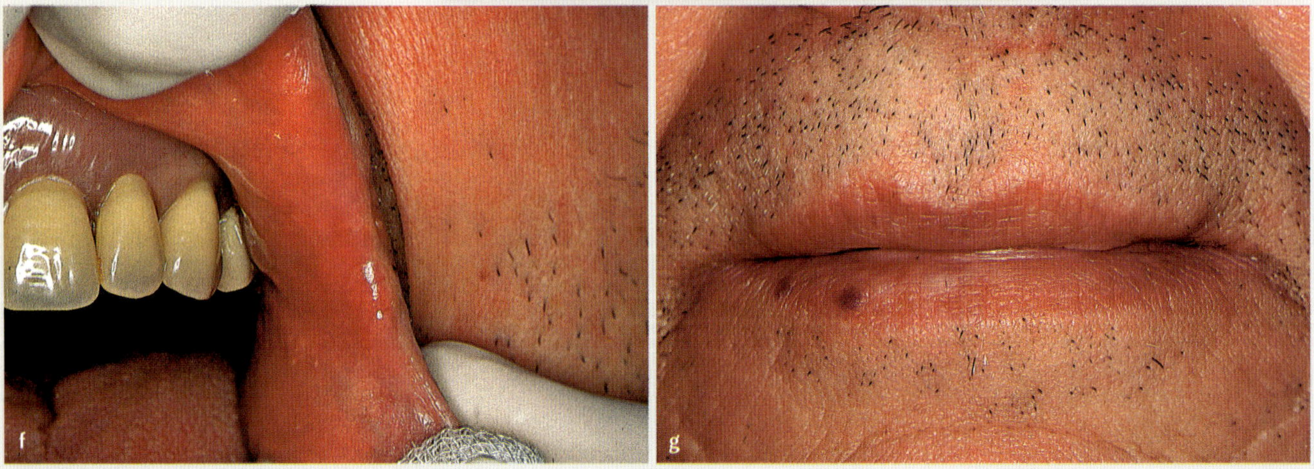

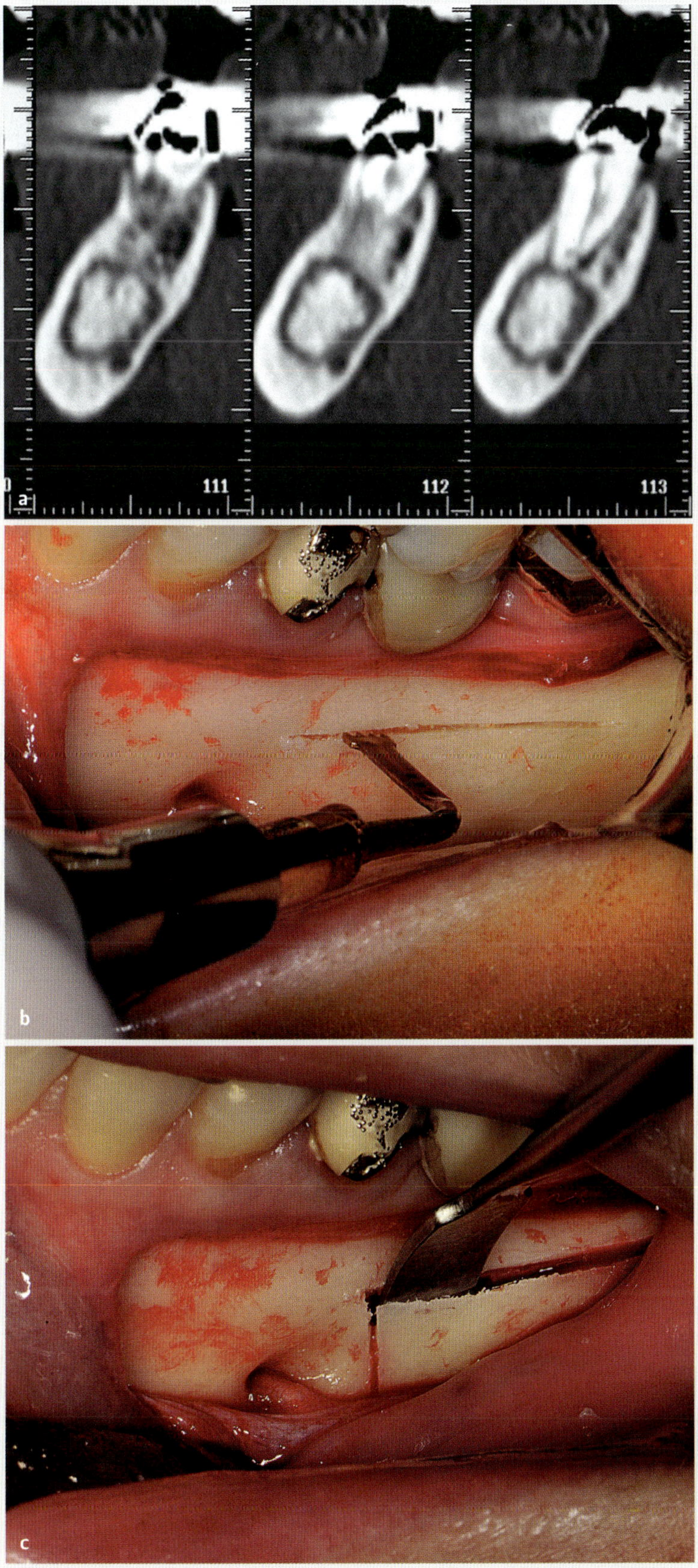

9.17 a) CT scan showing a well-defined radiopaque lesion developing inside the mandible, in close proximity to the inferior alveolar neurovascular bundle (osteoma). **b–c)** After elevation of a submarginal, full-thickness flap, piezoelectric instruments are used to create a bone lid which is then removed with the aid of surgical chisels. (*continued*)

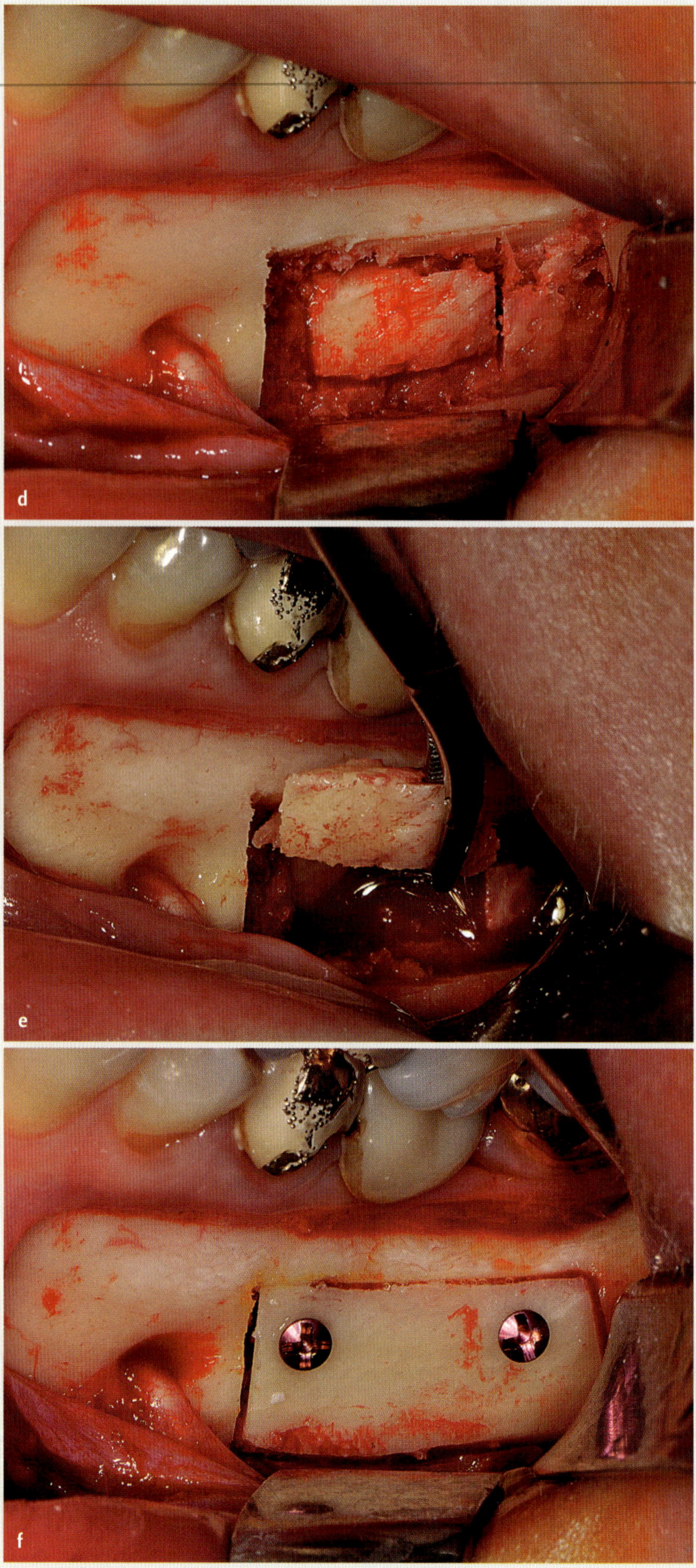

9.17 (*continued*) **d)** Once the bone lid is removed the lesion can be reached and delimited. **e)** The lesion is removed. **f)** The bone lid removed to access the lesion is repositioned and fixed in place with titanium microscrews. (*continued*)

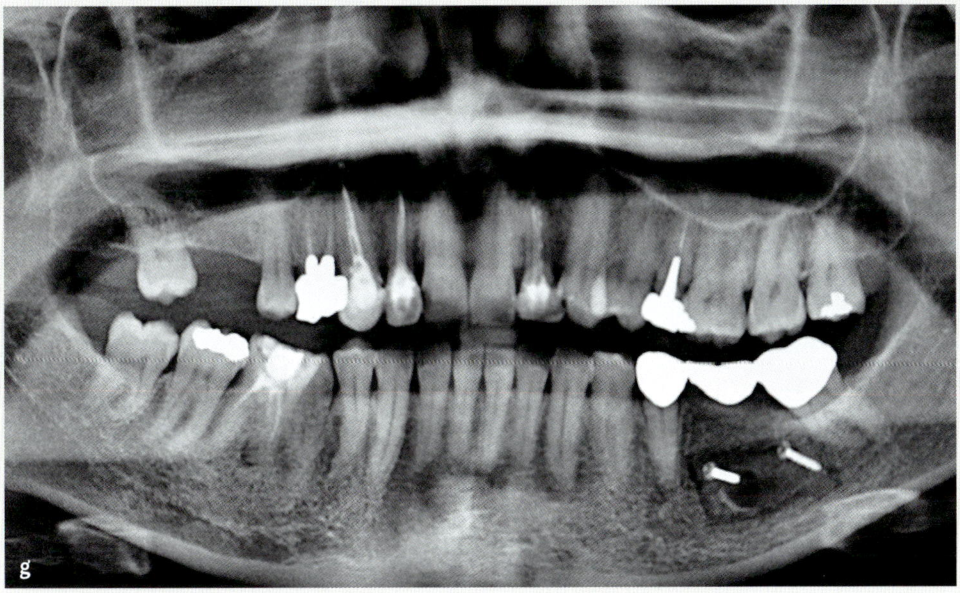

9.17 (*continued*) **g)** Postoperative radiographic follow-up examination.

REFERENCES

BATSAKIS JG. Tumours of the head and neck. Clinical and pathological considerations. 2nd ed. *Williams & Wilkins*, Baltimore, 1979; pp. 226-9.

BRUSATI R, CHIAPASCO M. Elementi di chirurgia oro-maxillo-facciale. Masson, Milano 1999.

KRAMER IRH, PATH FRC, PINDBORG JJ, MERVYN S. The WHO Histological Typing of Odontogenic Tumours. A Commentary on the Second Edition. *Cancer* 1992 Dec; 70(12):2988-93.

MORGAN PR. Odontogenic tumors: a review. *Periodontol 2000*. 2011 Oct; 57(1):160-7.

PHILIPSEN HP, REICHART PA. Classification of odontogenic tumours. A historical review. *J Oral Pathol Med* 2006 Oct; 35(9):525-9.

PINDBORG JJ, KRAMER IRH, TORLONI H. Histological typing of odontogenic tumors, jaw cysts and allied lesions. World Health Organization, Geneva, 1971; pp. 15-23.

SLOOTWEG PJ. Lesion of the jaws. *Histopathology* 2009 Mar; 54(4):401-18

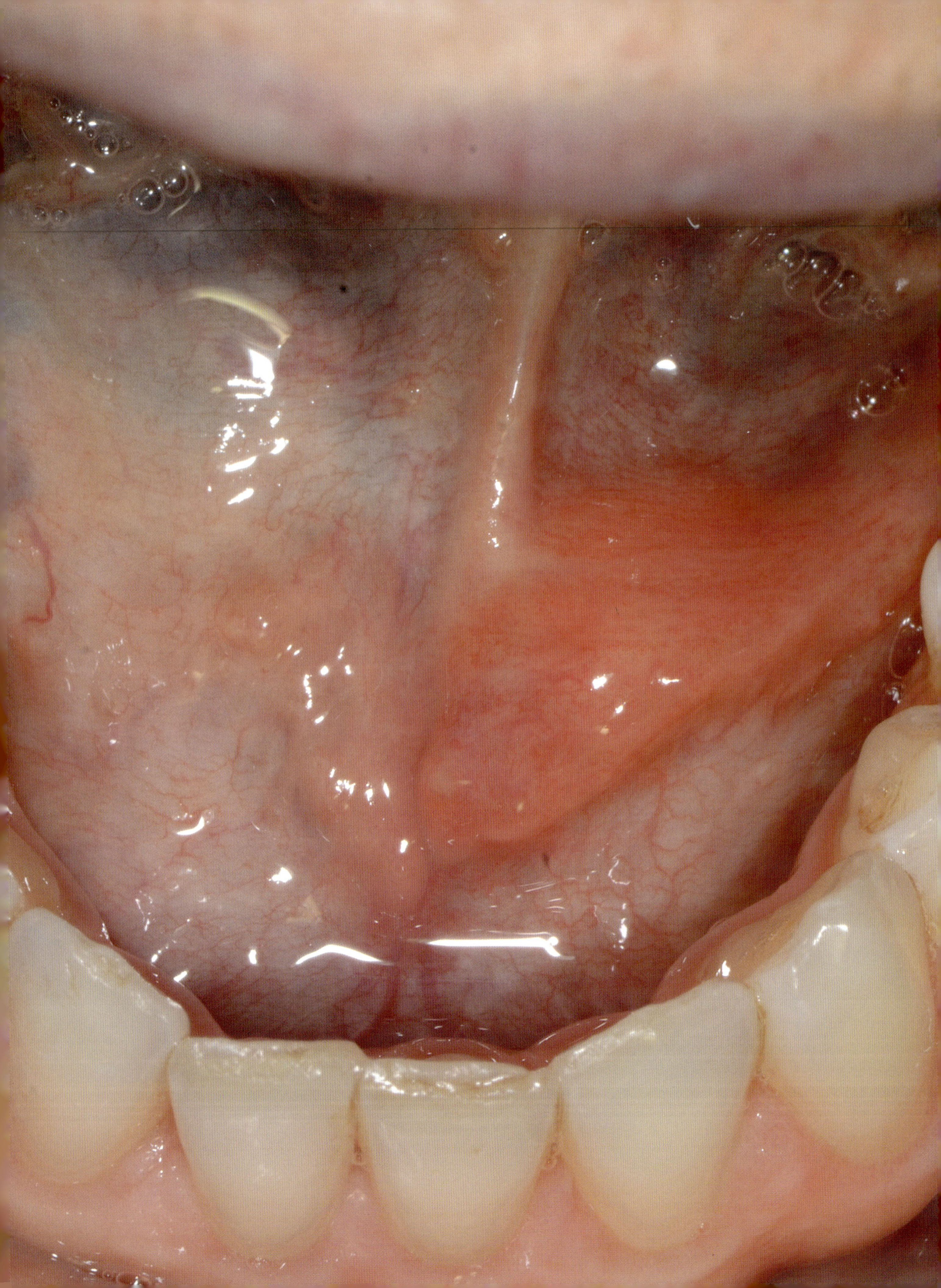

Surgical pathology of the salivary glands

M. Chiapasco · M. Zaniboni · A. Rossi · L. Maccarini

Introduction

The majority of pathologies affecting the salivary glands, such as acute and chronic sialoadenitis and tumours, are generally treated by maxillofacial surgeons and ENT surgeons.

Therefore, this chapter focuses only on those conditions that can be treated by the oral surgeon in a private practice environment, such as sialolithiasis of the major salivary glands, and cysts or pseudocysts of the minor salivary glands.

Sialolithiasis of the salivary glands

Epidemiology and etiopathogenesis

The formation of salivary gland stones, or sialolithiasis, is one of the most common pathologies affecting the salivary glands, and it may occur inside the glandular parenchyma or in the salivary ducts.

The major salivary glands are more frequently affected, with the submandibular gland involved in 80%-90% of cases, the parotid gland in 5%-20% of cases, and the sublingual gland in just 0.5%-2% of cases. Conversely, the minor salivary glands are rarely affected (< 1% of cases).

Sialolithiasis affects both male and female patients, but exhibits a slight gender predilection for the former, with peak incidence occurring between the 2nd and 6th decade of life.

The dimension of salivary gland stones, generally single (75% of cases), ranges from 0.2 to 3 centimetres. Double stones are seen in 20% of cases, triple stones are present in 5% of cases, while the presence of multiple microstones, usually confined in the gland parenchyma, is seen in less than 3% of the cases.

The etiopathogenesis of sialolithiasis is still under debate. Saliva stagnation inside the excretory ducts of the glands (or inside the gland parenchyma) is a necessary but not sufficient condition for stone formation; it appears that a concomitant local inflammation should be present. The results of ultrastructural analysis on salivary gland stones support this hypothesis: studies have demonstrated the presence of an organic central nucleus (10-20% of the total volume) formed by organic entities such as bacteria, fungi, glandular epithelial cells, inflammatory cells, cellular debris and lipids, over which concentric layers of inorganic components (calcium phosphate and carbonate) stratify, thus forming the peripheral portion (80-90% of the total volume).

Therefore, deposition of the inorganic components represents the conclusive event of salivary gland stone formation; this phase is preceded by inflammatory phenomena determined by saliva stagnation that causes local chemical and physical alterations leading to an increase of pH values and phosphate/carbonate precipitation.

Moreover, both local (anatomic) and systemic (pathologic) factors may contribute to the formation of salivary stones.

LOCAL FACTORS

As far as the submandibular gland is concerned, the formation of salivary stones seems to be correlated with the position of the gland itself that, being located below the level of its duct, is more prone to backflow and stasis of the saliva inside the duct. Moreover, the submandibular duct presents two sharp bends that, in association with its anti-gravitational course and the narrow excretion orifice, may also favour saliva stasis and a possible obstruction. Furthermore, the saliva produced by the submandibular gland is dense and viscous, and presents a high concentration of mucin and calcium ions that may influence the formation of salivary stones.

Additionally, trauma, foreign bodies, and gland cysts may interfere mechanically with the excretive function of the gland and duct, determining stasis and favouring the formation of salivary stones.

SYSTEMIC FACTORS

In addition to local factors, existing systemic diseases that influence their occurrence at a local level may favour salivary stone formation.

Hyperparathyroidism, for instance, causes an increase in calcium ions that may result in the precipitation of calcium salts and subsequent salivary stone formation.

Alterations in the activity of the sympathetic nervous system may favour the formation of salivary stones with a threefold action:

- increase of the salivary flow leading to a reduction in the reabsorption of electrolytes with subsequent increase in their concentration;
- alteration of the sphincter function and alteration of the periductal musculature;
- secretive alterations of the gland parenchyma.

A statistically significant correlation between sialolithiasis and arterial hypertension, chronic liver pathoses, renal and biliary lithiasis, and diabetes mellitus has been observed, notwithstanding that a possible etiopathogenetic correlation was not clarified.

Salivary stone formation occurs through three well-defined phases.

- The *first phase* is represented by dischilia. The presence of chronic and aspecific irritative stimuli can induce squamous metaplasia of the epithelium lining the duct with an increase in mucin secretion. This may increase saliva viscosity and concentration of mucin-associated electrolytes.

Alterations in the intraductal mechanisms of calcium ions reabsorption can cause:

- pH rise due to the interruption in the activity of natural pH buffers (calcium dependent mechanisms);
- block of the pyrophosphate pathway (calcium dependent enzymes).

- The *second phase* is represented by microlithiasis, and is characterised by a high concentration of calcium ions and the subsequent precipitation of these and other oligoelements over an organic nucleus to form the so-called spheroliths. Spheroliths, following a further deposition of inorganic components, increase in size and transform into microliths that determine duct ectasia and saliva stagnation inside the duct, leading to the formation of a periductal inflammatory infiltrate that may cause the onset of the first symptoms.
- The *third phase* is represented by *"frank" sialolithiasis*. Symptoms experienced in the second phase (pain and swelling when the gland activity is stimulated, for example, while eating) worsen, and inflammation of the gland parenchyma (sialoadenitis) may occur. In the advanced stages, particularly for long-standing, untreated lithiasis, a disruption of the gland architecture and subsequent functional involution are observed, leading to the final stage of gland scleroatrophy.

Clinical examination: analysis of signs and symptoms

Sialolithiasis is characterised by a number of specific signs and symptoms that may vary according mainly to the duration of the duct obstruction, but also to the dimension and localisation of the salivary stone.

Two types of duct obstruction can be observed: primary obstruction (mechanical obstructive block caused by the salivary stone and directly dependent on its dimension) and secondary obstruction (inflammatory oedema of the duct wall with subsequent lumen shrinkage). Symptoms deriving from the mechanical obstacle may be acute (salivary colic) and chronic (sialodochitis and/or sialadenitis).

Signs and symptoms of the salivary colic are:

- sudden increase of the gland volume in the presence of stimuli that induce an increase in salivation (meals, psychological factors, smoke, beverages, etc.);
- pain irradiated to the floor of the mouth, the tongue, and the body of the mandible for sialolithiasis of the submandibular gland; to the auriculo-temporal and/or pharyngeal region for sialolithiasis of the parotid gland;
- spontaneous remission of the symptoms within a variable time frame, with an abundant spill of thick saliva or, more rarely, the spontaneous expulsion of the salivary stone.

The salivary colic usually manifests itself only when the salivary stone is big enough to determine the occlusion of a main duct. When the salivary stone is small, or is located inside the gland parenchyma, symptoms may be less evident and characterised by intermittent swelling of the salivary gland and a sense of tension in the gland region during meals.

In some cases, sialolithiasis may be asymptomatic due to the small size of the salivary stone, or to its intraparenchymal localisation; in this event, identification of the condition may occur fortuitously in the course of examinations performed for different reasons (radiographic exams, ultrasonographies of the head and neck district, etc.).

Sialolithiasis

Symptoms	Typical signs
• Salivary colic	• Gland volume increase during meals • Possible thick secretion (corpusculated or purulent) from the duct • Pain irradiated to the floor of the mouth, the tongue, and the body of the mandible for sialolithiasis of the submandibular gland; to the auriculo-temporal and/or pharyngeal region for sialolithiasis of the parotid gland. • Possible ulceration of the duct wall, morphofunctional alterations of the gland and/or the duct.
• Sialodochitis and/or sialadenitis	• Possible pain on palpation • Hyperaemia of the duct sphincter • Possible evolution towards gland scleroatrophy and/or cutaneous fistula formation

Therefore, the absence of symptoms such as acute pain does not correspond to the absence of the condition. In fact, the onset of an asymptomatic degenerative process of the gland parenchyma with subsequent chronic functional involution (sialadenitis, gland scleroatrophy, purulent colliquation) may occur. Malignant degeneration of the gland epithelium due to chronic irritative stimuli has rarely been described.

Diagnosis

Diagnosis of sialolithiasis is based on medical history, clinical examination, and instrumental screening.

CLINICAL EXAMINATION

Intraductal sialolithiasis manifests intraorally as a hyperaemic area on the mucosa overlaying the salivary stone, particularly in case the stone is located in proximity of the duct sphincter (10.1).

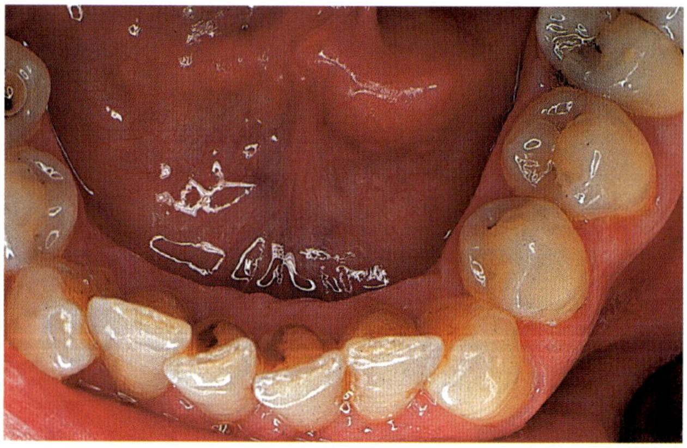

10.1 Sialolithiasis of the left submandibular duct associated with swelling and inflammation of the overlying mucosa.

Bimanual palpation of the area may provide useful information on the localisation of the stone and the patency of the duct, or its partial or total obstruction.

The saliva excreted from the duct during palpation may appear thick, corpusculated or frankly purulent, according to the degree of infection.

If the salivary stone is located superficially, spontaneous ulceration of the duct wall and intraoral fistulation may occur.

In case the salivary stone is not removed, and the chronic irritative stimulus endures, sialolithiasis can evolve into chronic sialadenitis with morphofunctional alteration of the salivary gland itself.

A further evolution may cause the transient or permanent loss of the secretive function with subsequent gland scleroatrophy, which is irreversible even if the stone is removed. In this case, the palpation of the gland will result in the individuation of a hard-elastic structure, not necessarily tender on palpation.

Instrumental examinations

Intraoral radiograph: it is the most commonly used radiographic examination to confirm the presence of intraductal salivary stones and to assess their form, dimension, and position. When the stone is located in the anterior two-thirds of the submandibular duct, or inside the sublingual gland parenchyma, the use of an occlusal radiograph is indicated (10.2). If the stone is located inside the parotid duct, a periapical radiograph positioned between the buccal mucosa and the upper posterior teeth allows identification of the stone.

Lateral cephalometric radiograph and panoramic radiograph: these exams are used to obtain information on intraglandular salivary stones of the parotid and submandibular glands. They can also offer information on the presence, location, and dimension of salivary stones located inside the posterior third of the submandibular duct, but the superimposition of the mandible may conceal the smallest stones (10.3).

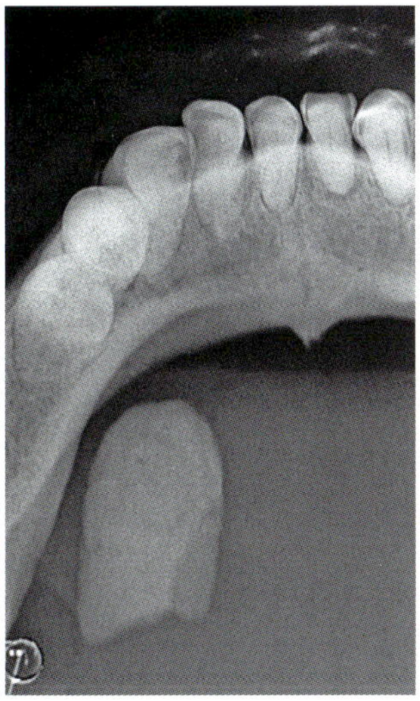

10.2 Occlusal radiograph showing the presence of a salivary stone in the left submandibular duct.

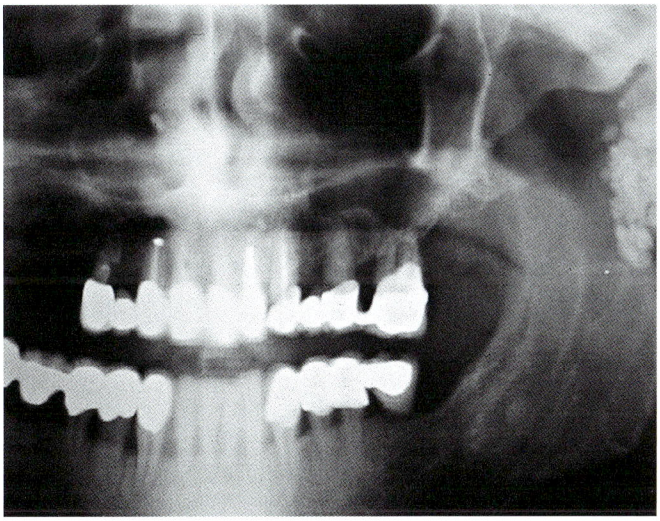

10.3 Panoramic radiograph demonstrating the presence of numerous salivary stones inside the parenchyma of the left parotid gland.

Ultrasonography: it is useful to identify radiolucent salivary stones and the echostructure of the gland parenchyma and duct. On the other hand, the interpretation of ultrasound images of the submental/submandibular and buccal/parotid regions is often difficult and, moreover, these images are not usually able to provide precise information regarding the exact location of the salivary stone (📷 10.4).

Salivary endoscopy or sialoendoscopy: introduced in the 1990s, it allows inspection of the salivary ducts with the aid of a thin (0.8 millimetres in diameter) and flexible diagnostic endoscope and, eventually, to remove small salivary stones by means of an operating endoscope (1.1-1.6 millimetres in diameter).

Sialography: currently abandoned in favour of the sialo-MRI, it provides the exact location of the salivary stone, the level of obstruction of the duct, and identifies possible intraparenchymal and extraparenchymal duct lesions (📷 10.5).

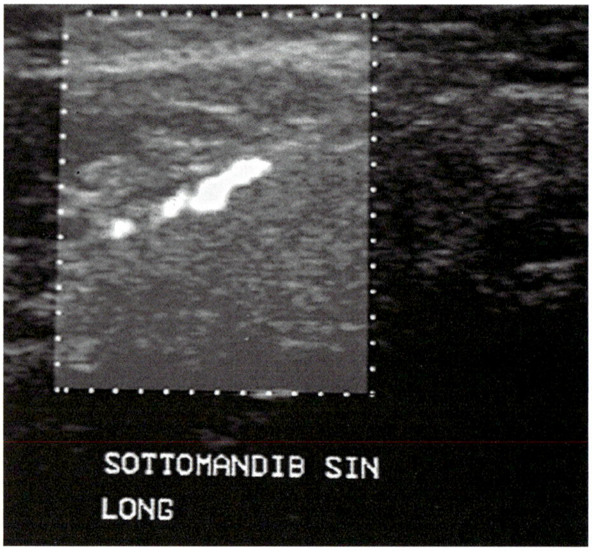

📷 **10.4** Ultrasonographic image of the floor of the mouth showing the presence of a hyperechoic structure compatible with the presence of a salivary stone.

Radiographic exams

Type	Advantages
Occlusal radiograph	Localisation of salivary stones in the anterior two-thirds of the submandibular duct
Lateral cephalometric radiograph	Identification of intraparenchymal submandibular gland stones
Panoramic radiograph	Identification of intraparenchymal stones
Ultrasonography	Evaluation of the echostructure (parenchyma and duct), and identification of radiolucent stones
Sialoendoscopy	Evaluation of the duct anatomy and removal of small salivary stones
Sialography	Precise localisation of the salivary stone, identification of intraparenchymal and extraparenchymal duct lesions
Scintigraphy	Evaluation of morphofunctional aspects of the gland
CT scan and MRI	Identification of chronic inflammatory or neoplastic lesions

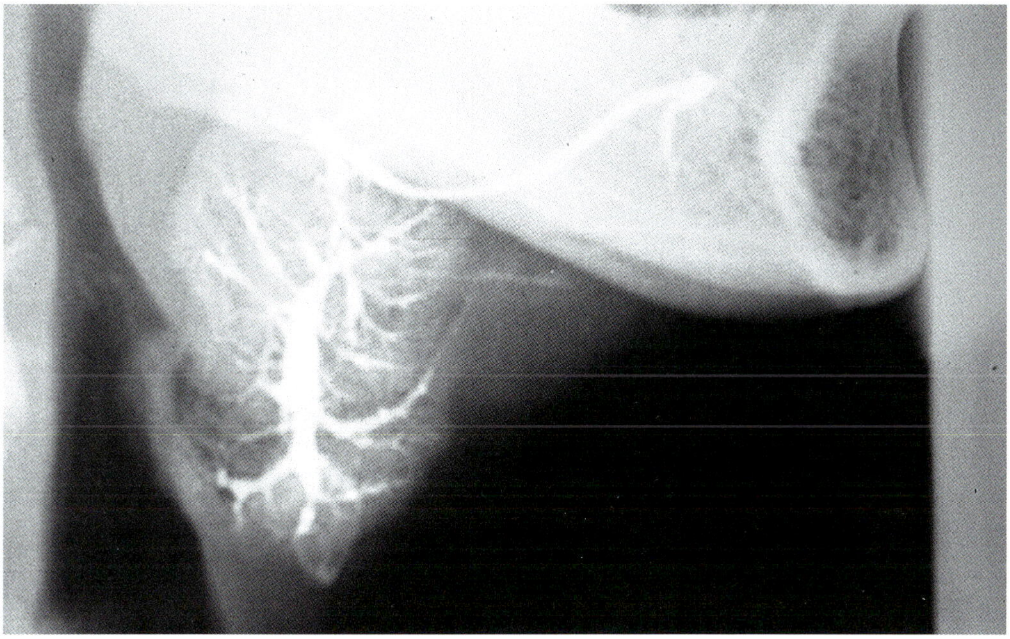

10.5 Sialography of a normal submandibular duct: the patency of the main duct and its intraparenchymal ramifications is clearly visible.

Scintigraphy: it offers useful information on the morphology and functionality of the salivary gland, but also on possible states of gland distress in case the long-lasting presence of the salivary stone may have determined functional alterations. It helps to decide if the surgical removal of the salivary gland (sialoadenectomy) is indicated.

CT and MRI: the recourse to CT scan and MRI is particularly indicated when routine radiographic exams are not sufficient for a complete evaluation of the case, and when the presence of chronic inflammatory or neoplastic lesions of the salivary gland is suspected.

Differential diagnosis

Differential diagnosis for sialolithiasis should be posed with the following:

- *sialodochitis* and *sialadenitis*: they may determine secretory alterations, both quantitative and qualitative, tenderness to palpation, and swelling in the area of the affected gland;
- *mucocele* and *ranula*: in some cases, these lesions can grow to the extent that they may determine a reduction or the interruption of saliva secretion by compression;
- *traumatic lesions*;
- *Sjögren's syndrome*: it determines xerostomy, but symptoms and structural alterations of the salivary glands are different from those occurring in cases of sialolithiasis;
- *tumours* (pleomorphic and monomorphic adenoma, papillary cystadenoma lymphomatosus or Warthin's tumour, mucoepidermoid carcinoma, adenocarcinoma, adenoid cystic carcinoma).

Whenever there is any doubt on the differential diagnosis, the recourse to specific instrumental examinations such as MRI/CT scan and/or histologic evaluation (needle aspiration, biopsy) to allow an in-depth analysis of the condition is necessary.

Treatment

The treatment of intraparenchymal sialolithiasis and its consequences on the functionality of the gland (chronic irreversible sialadenitis, gland scleroatrophy) will only be outlined; in fact, this condition generally determines the necessity to remove the salivary gland surgically (sialoadenectomy) with an extraoral approach, and it is thus performed under general anaesthesia by trained maxillofacial or ENT surgeons.

The treatment of intraductal salivary stones will be described in detail; according to the dimension of the stone, its localisation, and the possible evolution of the condition into more severe forms, the approach to the treatment of sialolithiasis may vary considerably.

MEDICAL TREATMENT

In the absence of signs of inflammation, both chronic and acute, and in the presence of small stones located in the terminal portion of the duct, the initial treatment can be based on the administration of bellafoline (which favours the relaxation of the periductal smooth musculature) and abundant oligomineral water intake.

This treatment, combined with massaging the duct upstream from the obstruction may allow the spontaneous expulsion of the stone.

SURGICAL TREATMENT

The surgical removal of salivary stones with an intraoral approach (under local anaesthesia) is indicated only when the salivary stone is located in the anterior two-thirds of the submandibular duct, or in the intraoral portion of the parotid duct, and only if no functional compromission of the gland is present.

If the salivary stone is located in the posterior third of the submandibular duct, surgical removal with an intraoral approach is possible; however, due to the difficulties in obtaining adequate retraction of the tongue, to the relative deep position of the gland, and to the presence of several important anatomic structures in the area (such as the lingual nerve, the lingual veins, and the lingual artery and its branches), the procedure should be performed only by a specifically trained maxillofacial surgeon under general anaesthesia.

SIALOADENECTOMY

The surgical removal of a salivary gland (sialoadenectomy) is necessary when morphologic and/or functional alterations of the gland are associated with the presence of one or more stones inside the gland parenchyma.

Sialoadenectomy of a major salivary gland is performed under general anaesthesia; an intraoral approach is used to reach the sublingual glands, while an extraoral approach is used to reach the submandibular and parotid glands. These surgical interventions are to be performed by trained maxillofacial or ENT surgeons in an adequate environment (hospital), and thus fall outside the duties of the oral surgeon; for this reason, they will not be described in detail in this textbook.

When sialolithiasis involves a minor salivary gland, the salivary stone is always removed together with the entire gland.

Alternatives to surgery

SALIVARY ENDOSCOPY OR SIALOENDOSCOPY

It is possible to remove small salivary stones (generally < 4 millimetres in diameter) with the aid of a flexible operating endoscope, which allows the introduction of irrigants (sterile saline) and dedicated instruments (fibre optics, microcamera, and micro-forceps).

SALIVARY LITHOTRIPSY BY EXTRACORPOREAL SHOCKWAVE APPLICATION

It is the same technique used to treat kidney stones. Under ultrasound guidance, shock waves produced by a miniaturised electromagnetic lithotripter are focused on the salivary stone with the aim of breaking it into smaller pieces to favour their spontaneous expulsion with the salivary flow, or to facilitate their removal by means of sialoendoscopy.

However, this method is rarely used due to the length of the treatment (several sessions are needed), the uncertain results, and the discomfort/pain experienced by the patient.

Surgical anatomy

The knowledge of local anatomy is imperative for the planning and execution of a correct surgical treatment of sialolithiasis, due to the presence of numerous important anatomic structures in the area of the major salivary glands, and the absence of a bony plane of reference. Therefore, the anatomic peculiarities of every area are summarised below.

PAROTID GLAND

The parotid gland is located below the subcutaneous plane in the preauricular region, superficially to the masseter muscle, and anteriorly to the sternocleidomastoid muscle and the mastoid process. The facial nerve (VII cranial nerve), with its main ramifications, passes through the gland, thus representing a plane of reference that allows identification of the superficial lobe and deep lobe of the parotid. Inside the gland, a series of small ducts merge to form the main parotid duct (Stensen duct), which emerges from the gland and runs forward along the lateral side of the masseter muscle. The duct then takes a steep turn at the anterior border of the masseter muscle and passes through the buccinator muscle, opening into the vestibule of the mouth at the parotid papilla, in the area of the first and second maxillary molars (10.6).

SUBMANDIBULAR GLAND

The submandibular gland is located between the anterior and posterior belly of the digastric muscle, and the inferior border of the mandible. The roof of its lodge is mainly composed by the mylohyoid muscle, while the lateral wall is entirely composed by the muscles of the tongue. A precise knowledge of the course of the submandibular duct (Wharton duct) is mandatory, because of its relationships with important anatomic structures that must not be damaged. The duct exits from the submandibular lodge in proximity of the posterior margin of the mylohyoid muscle and runs forward along with the lingual nerve (in the area of the second mandibular molar). Then, the lingual nerve takes a turn medially, passing under the duct, and its ramifications spread to the floor of the mouth and

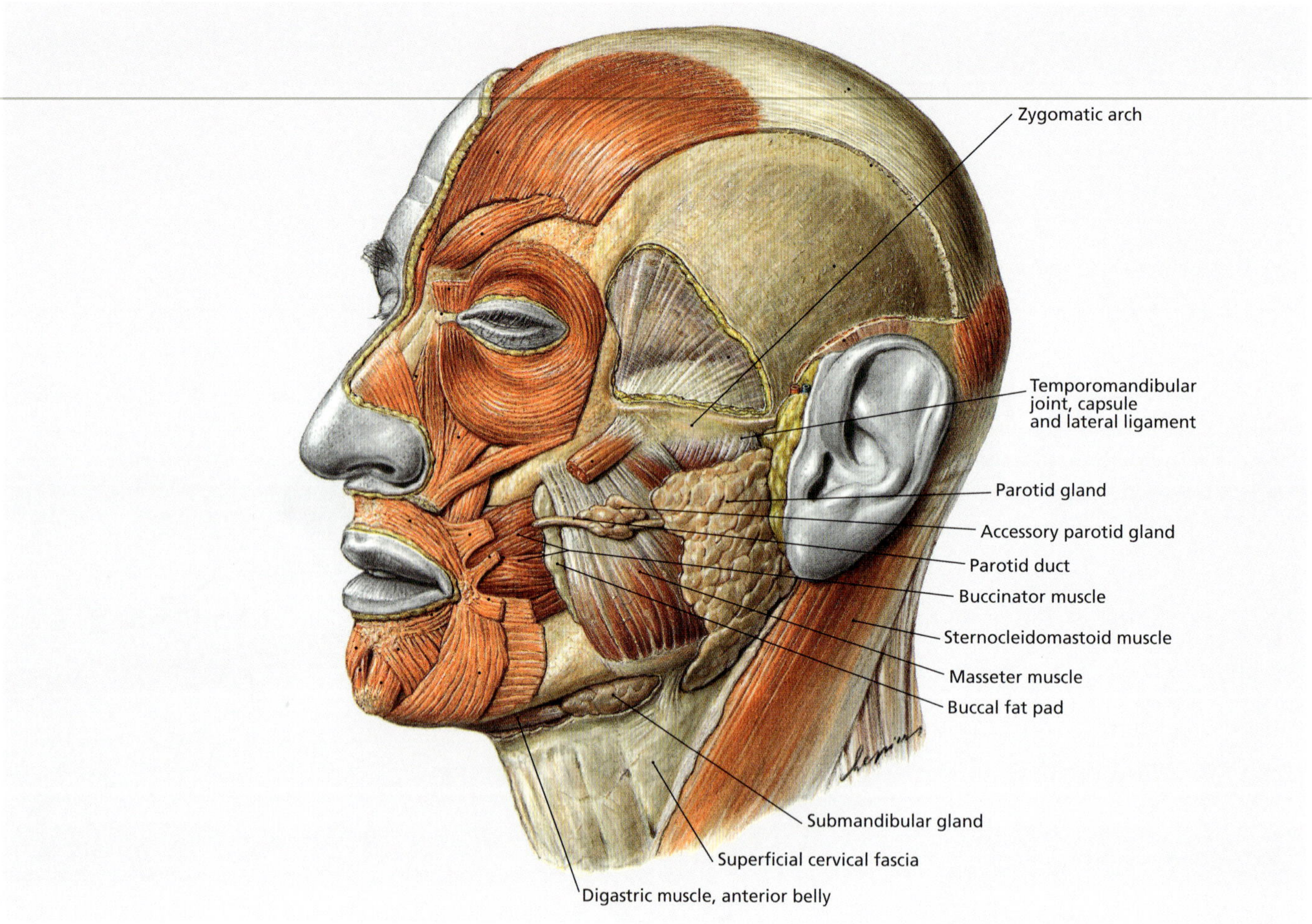

10.6 Anatomy of the parotid region and the space in which the buccal fat pad is located (modified from *Sobotta Atlante di Anatomia Umana*. Elsevier, Milano 2012).

the tongue, giving sensitive innervation to the anterior two-thirds of the ipsilateral hemitongue and floor of the mouth. Finally, the duct opens in a narrow orifice on the summit of a small papilla (sublingual caruncle) at the side of the lingual frenulum, in the anterior portion of the floor of the mouth (10.7).

SUBLINGUAL GLAND

The sublingual gland lies in the sublingual lodge, located in the anterior portion of the floor of the mouth superficially to the mylohyoid muscle. The gland presents several small ducts (ducts of Rivinus) and often a major duct (Bartholin duct) which, in some cases, merges with the submandibular duct and opens in the sublingual caruncle (10.7).

Surgical treatment

The most frequent surgical interventions for the treatment of sialolithiasis are:

- removal of a salivary stone in the anterior tract of the parotid duct;
- removal of a salivary stone in the anterior tract of the submandibular duct;
- removal of a salivary stone in the posterior tract of the submandibular duct.

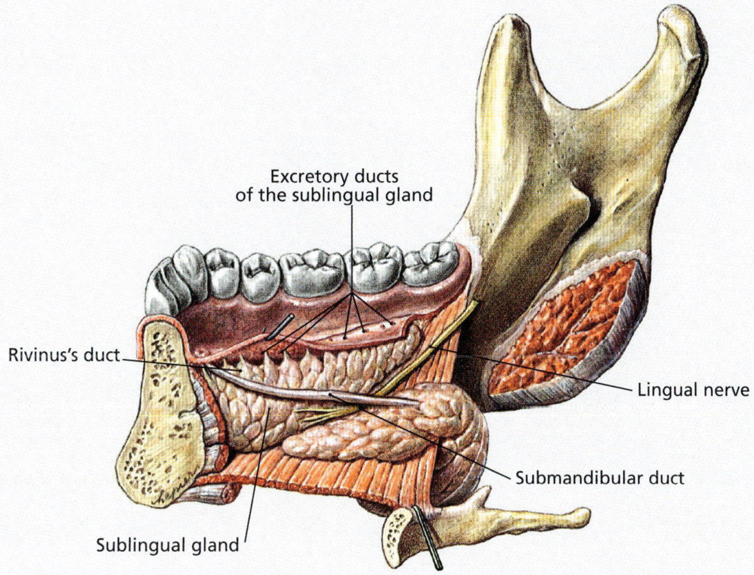

10.7 Surgical anatomy of the submandibular and sublingual glands (modified from *Sobotta Atlante di Anatomia Umana*, Elsevier, Milano 2012)

As previously mentioned, the techniques used for the complete removal of a major salivary gland or sialoadenectomy (which is necessary in cases of intraparenchymal sialolithiasis or irreversible degenerative alterations of the involved gland) are not described in this textbook, as they require an extraoral approach and should be performed under general anaesthesia by well trained maxillofacial or ENT surgeons.

Surgical armamentarium

As the removal of the salivary stone from the duct involves only the soft tissues, the surgical armamentarium is very simple:

- small retractors;
- scalpel;
- dissecting scissors;
- surgical and anatomical pliers;
- needle holder;
- non-resorbable sutures for the mucosal layer;
- resorbable sutures for the reconstruction of the duct wall;
- small-diameter surgical drain tubes.

Anaesthesia

To remove submandibular and sublingual salivary stones it is advised to perform lingual nerve block in association with a local injection of anaesthetic with vasoconstrictor (adrenalin/epinephrine), to achieve optimal visibility in the surgical field. For salivary stones located in the terminal portion of the parotid duct, local infiltration of anaesthetic is sufficient.

Basic techniques

Removal of a salivary stone located in the terminal portion of the parotid duct

This technique is generally performed under local anaesthesia obtained with periductal infiltration: an incision is made along the terminal portion of the parotid duct and the stone is retrieved with the aid of surgical probes or hooks. A surgical hook can be custom-made by bending one end of a segment of orthodontic wire; the wire is then slid along the duct wall until the bent end has passed the stone. Then, the wire is rotated until the bent end engages the stone; it is finally possible to retrieve the stone by gently pulling the wire out of the parotid duct (10.8a–g).

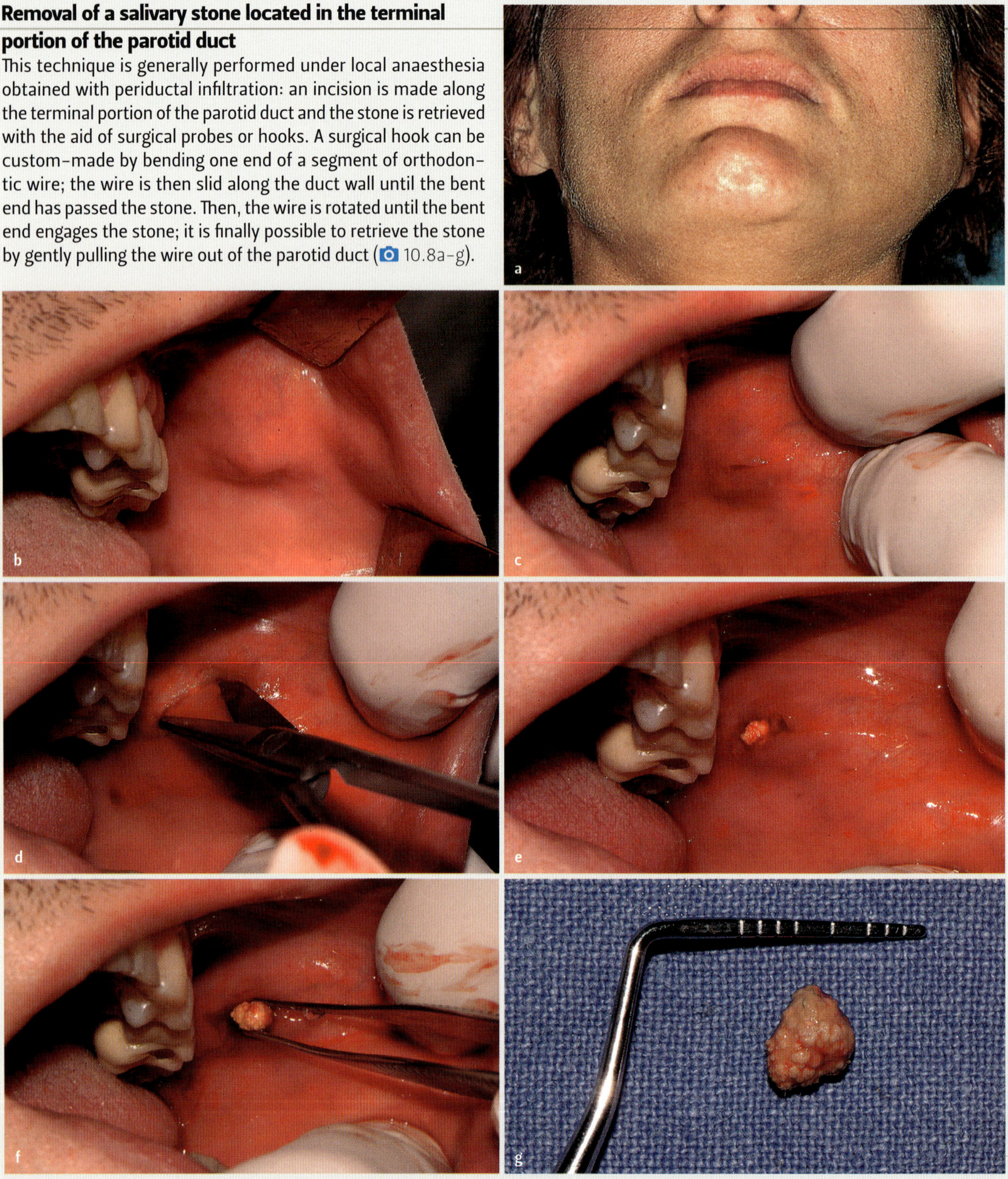

10.8 **a)** Swelling of the left parotid gland due to obstruction of the parotid duct. **b)** Swelling of the left parotid papilla. **c)** Incision of the terminal portion of the parotid duct. **d)** Blunt dissection. **e)** Identification of the salivary stone. **f)** Retrieval of the salivary stone with surgical pliers. **g)** The removed salivary stone.

Removal of a salivary stone located in the terminal portion of the submandibular duct

This technique is generally performed under local anaesthesia obtained by lingual nerve block and periductal infiltration of anaesthetic. The mucosal and submucosal layers are incised above the salivary stone and the duct is isolated from the surrounding soft tissues by blunt dissection. If the stone is not easily palpable, incannulation of the duct with a blunt probe may be of help, but care must be taken to avoid posterior dislocation of the stone. Therefore, once the duct is identified, its ligature upstream from the stone may help avoid its dislocation during the surgical manoeuvres.

After the duct is isolated, an incision is made in its wall above the salivary stone, which is then exposed and removed. The removal of the stone may be accompanied by the drainage of fluid material, either cloudy or frankly purulent, followed by clear saliva.

After evaluating the patency of the duct, a thin intraductal drainage tube can be positioned and the duct wall may be sutured with fine (6/0 or 7/0) resorbable sutures. The presence of the surgical drain avoids a possible stenosis due to scar formation, or the accidental suture of the entire duct with subsequent acute obstruction. In the event that the portion of the duct downstream from the stone appears to be stenotic due to chronic inflammatory phenomena, it is possible to modify the outlet of the duct by creating a new outlet where the surgical incision has been made (sialodochoplasty), suturing the duct wall to the mucosa of the floor of the mouth. When the salivary stone is located in close proximity to the duct ostium in the sublingual caruncle, the mucosa, submucosa and duct wall can be incised to enlarge the ostium and facilitate a simple and atraumatic removal of the stone itself (10.9a–g).

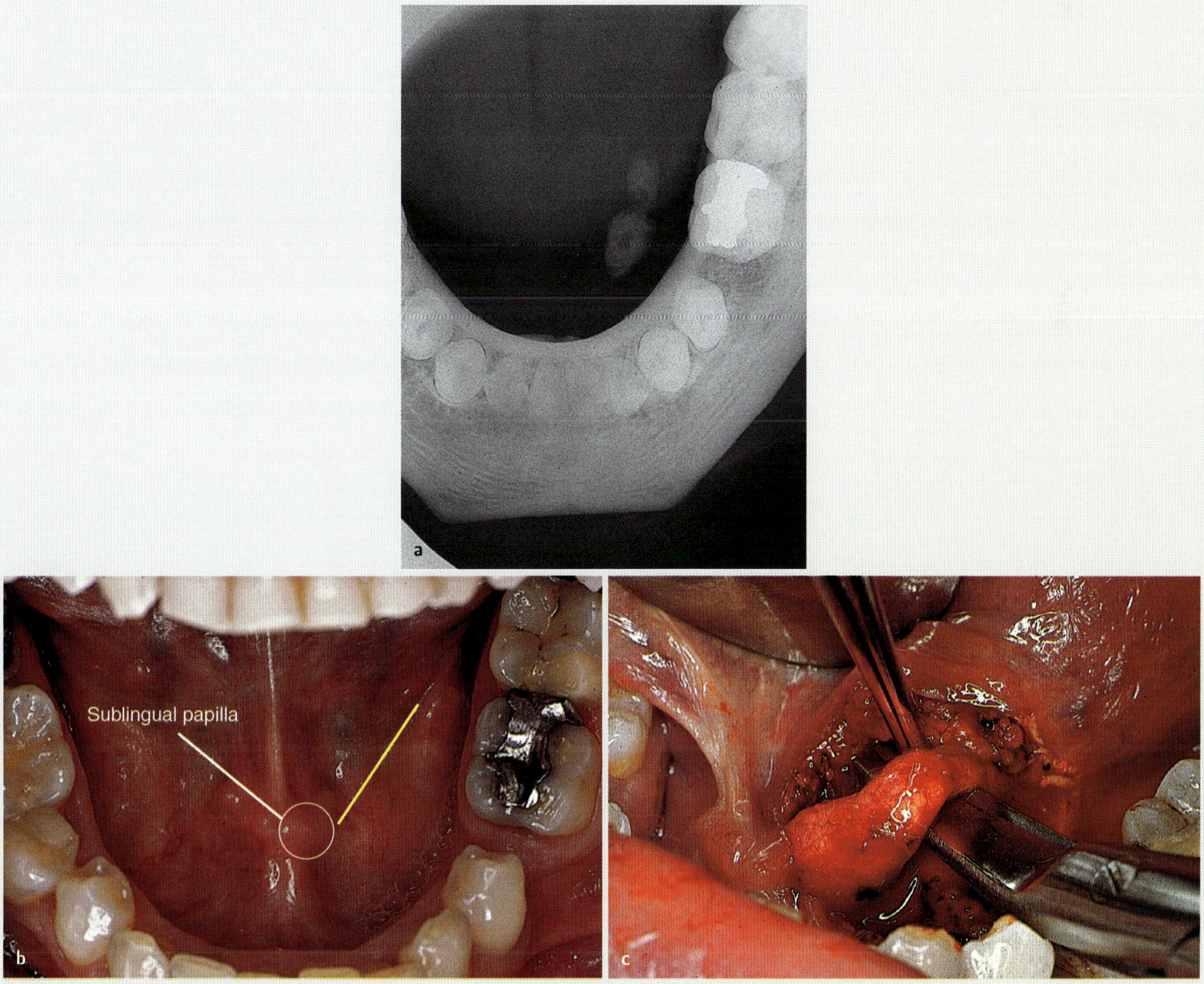

10.9 **a)** Occlusal radiograph showing two salivary stones inside the submandibular duct. **b)** Line of incision (yellow) in the floor of the mouth along the course of the submandibular duct. **c)** Isolation of the duct. (*continued*)

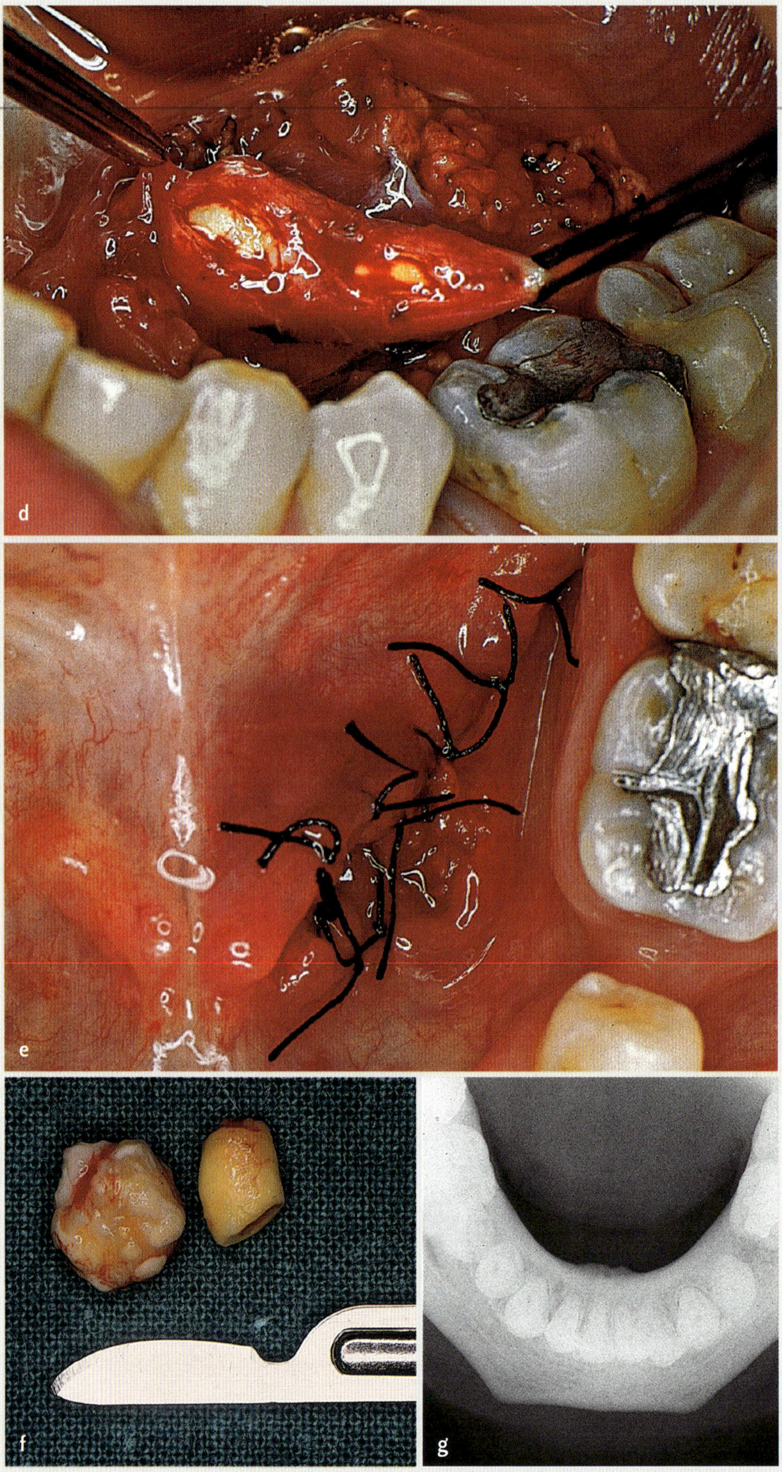

10.9 (*continued*) **d)** Incision of the duct wall to remove the salivary stones. **e)** Sialodochoplasty. **f)** The removed salivary stones. **g)** Radiographic follow-up some time after surgery.

Removal of a salivary stone located in the posterior portion of the submandibular duct

This intervention should always be conducted under general anaesthesia, and the surgeon must possess a thorough knowledge of the topographic anatomy of this area. The technique is similar to the one described for salivary stones located in the anterior portion of the submandibular duct, but special care must be taken to avoid any damage to the lingual nerve which, in this area, crosses the duct inferiorly (see Chapter 2).

Removal of the submandibular gland (sialoadenectomy)
The surgical removal of the submandibular gland (and the salivary stones inside the gland parenchyma) is performed under general anaesthesia with orotracheal or nasotracheal intubation, using an extraoral approach. The access to the submandibular lodge is obtained by means of a cutaneous incision; ideally, the incision should follow a Langer's line in the neck, 2-3 centimetres below the inferior border of the mandible to avoid any damage to the marginal branch of the facial nerve.

Once the skin, subcutaneous layer, platysma muscle and superficial cervical fascia are incised, the gland is identified and separated from the surrounding soft tissues by blunt dissection. Care must be taken during the dissection, because the gland receives its blood supply from a branch of the facial artery: ligature of this vessel must be performed before the gland can be removed. The ligature of the submandibular duct is also performed, to avoid possible migration of bacteria from the oral cavity into the neck (10.10a-f).

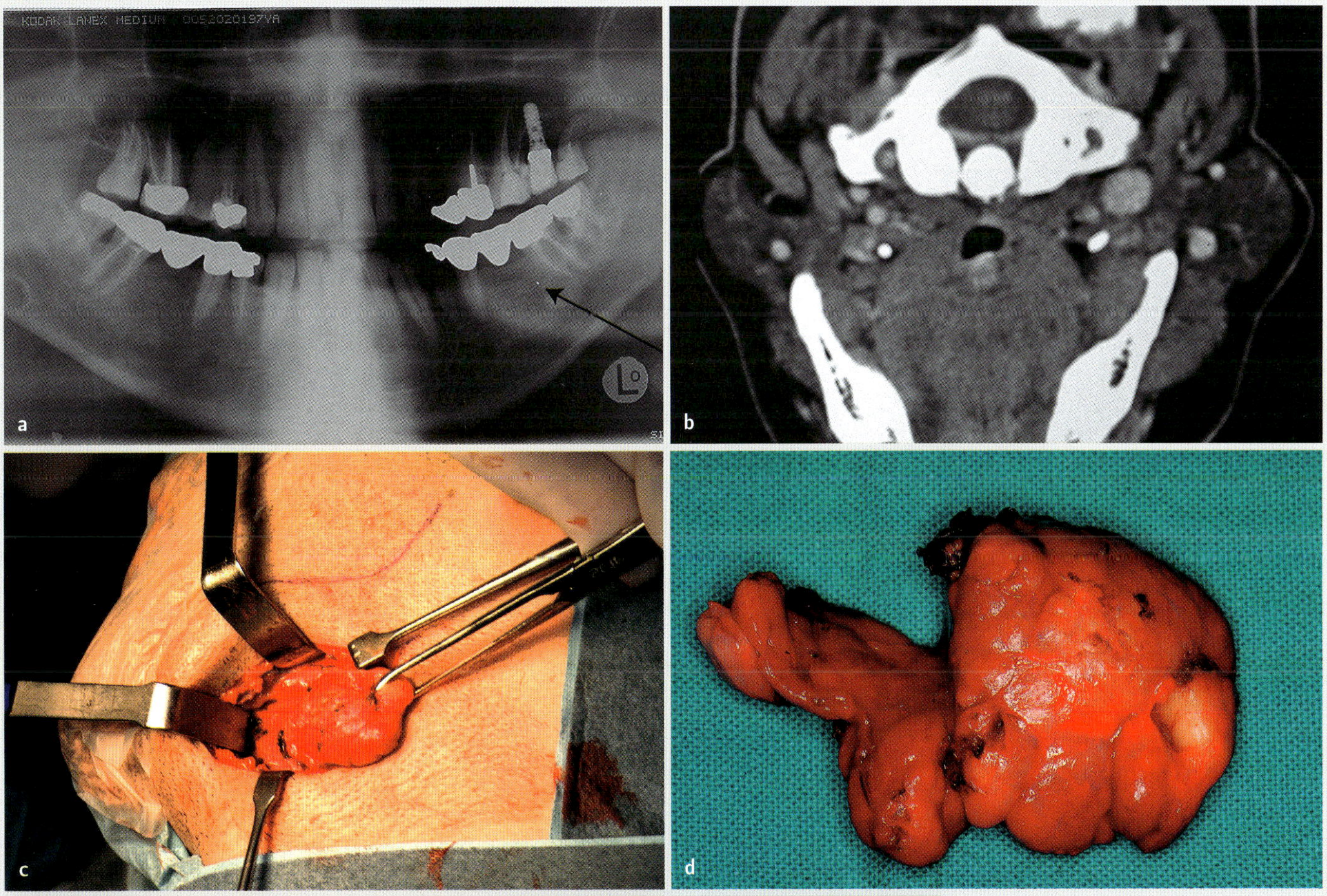

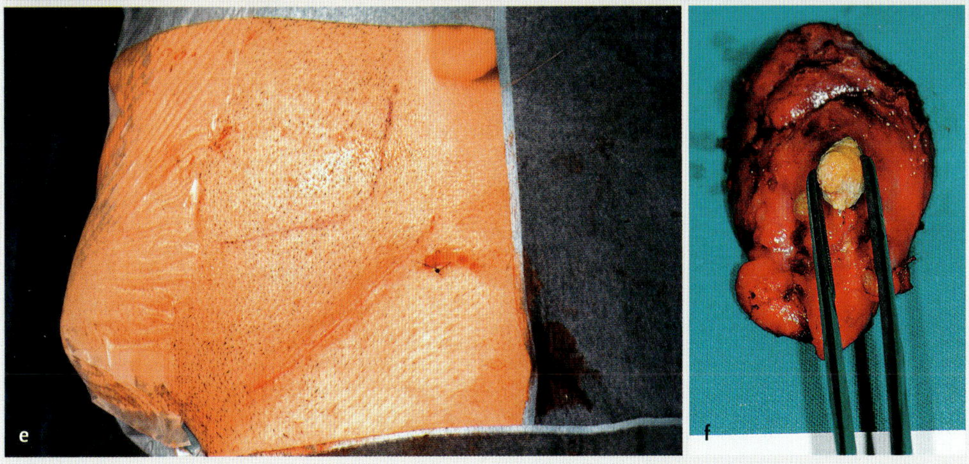

10.10 a) Panoramic radiograph showing the presence of salivary stones in the submandibular gland. The stones are barely visible due to the superimposition of the mandible. **b)** CT scan showing a salivary stone and signs of degeneration of the submandibular gland. **c)** Submandibular sialoadenectomy with an extraoral approach. **d)** The removed submandibular gland. **e)** Suture of the access incision with a surgical drain in place. **f)** The removed salivary stone.

Postoperative follow-up

After the surgical intervention, patients should be followed over time, and habits that may favour a relapse (formation of a new salivary stone) must be modified (e.g. food and water with a high content of Ca^{++} should be avoided). Radiographic controls should be performed every 6 months for the first 2 years after surgery, while an assessment of the functionality of the gland parenchyma should be performed 12 months after surgery in case the salivary stone had caused functional alterations of the gland.

Cysts and pseudocysts of the minor salivary glands

Epidemiology and etiopathogenesis

Minor salivary glands are numerous in the oral cavity; they lie in the submucosal tissues of the lips, of the buccal mucosa, of the floor of the mouth, and of the palatal mucosa. They contribute, together with the major salivary glands (submandibular, sublingual, and parotid) to the secretion of adequate quantities of saliva (10.11a–b).

These glands are never affected by sialolithiasis but, for gland rupture or obstruction of their excretory ducts, they may develop into cystic or pseudocystic lesions filled with mucous fluid produced by the gland itself. These lesions have a similar clinical presentation

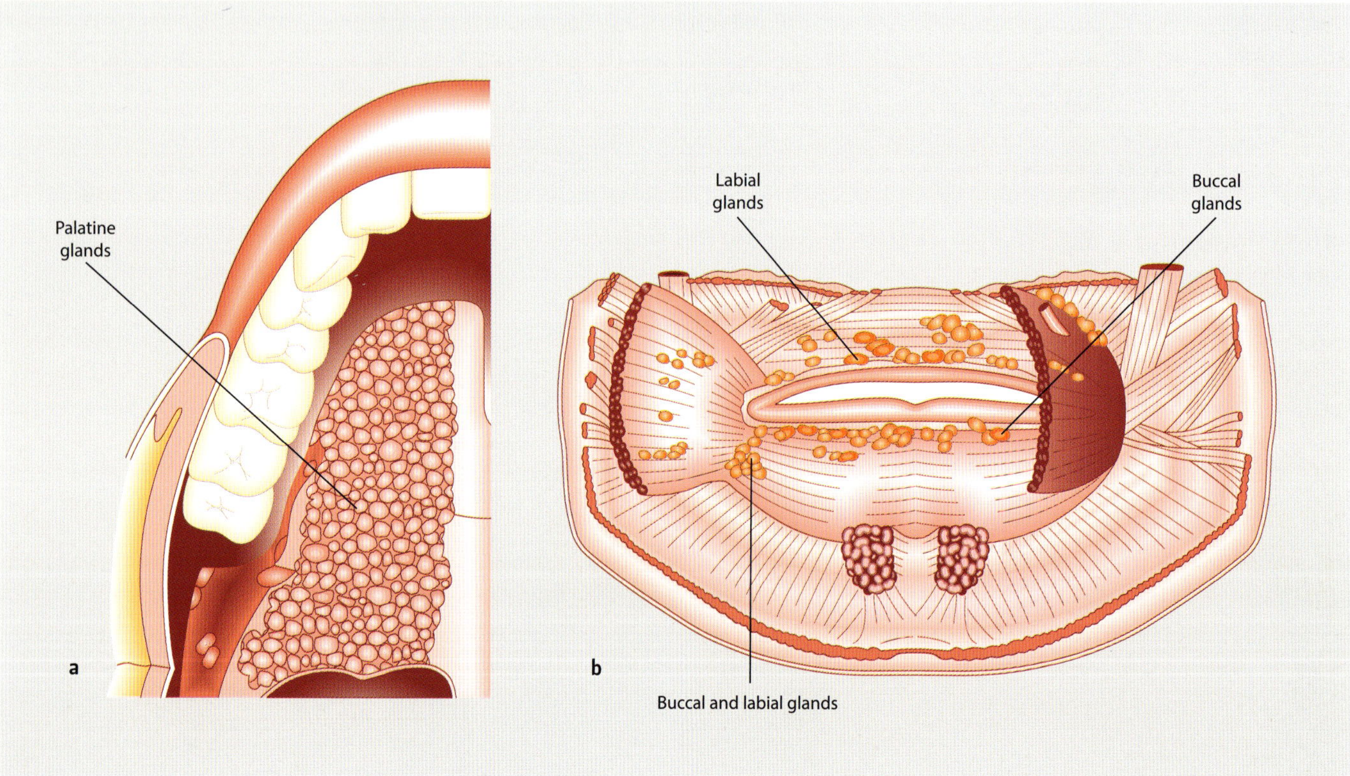

10.11 a–b) Topographic anatomy of some minor salivary glands.

and similar treatment modalities, but according to their origin and histologic appearance, they are classified as:

- mucocele or pseudocyst (also known as ranula when the lesion is located in the floor of the mouth), which have a traumatic origin;
- true retention cyst, with an obstructive etiology.

In the first case, the lesion is caused by the rupture of a salivary gland duct with subsequent extravasation of salivary fluid in the submucosal connective tissues, whereas in the second case, an obstruction causes swelling of the duct and the formation of a cavity filled with fluid and lined with epithelium ("true" retention cyst). Occasionally, a pseudocyst (which, by definition, does not have an epithelial wall) may exhibit a "pseudo-epithelium" formed by "compressed" connective cells: these cells look similar to the cuboidal epithelial cells.

Retention cysts, although similar to the extravasation cysts, tend to develop at an older age.

These lesions are more frequently observed in areas where a trauma to the oral mucosa may easily occur. In descending order of frequency, they involve: the inner mucosa of the lips, the buccal mucosa, the floor of the mouth, the tip and inferior surface of the tongue, and the palatine mucosa.

Clinical examination: analysis of signs and symptoms

The signs and symptoms of cysts and pseudocysts are very similar. These lesions typically appear as an asymptomatic round or oval swelling, with greater diameter ranging from a few millimetres to several centimetres. On palpation, they may appear fluctuant but can also be firm, and they tend to enlarge progressively. As a rule, the overlying mucosa has a normal appearance when the lesion is located deeply in the soft tissues, while it is slightly transparent with a blue tinge when the lesion is located just below the mucosal layer (10.12). A typical characteristic of these lesions is the possibility of rapid variations in their dimensions: they can quickly enlarge, but also swiftly decrease in size, thus simulating a spontaneous disappearance. Mucoceles of the lip, cheek, and palate may be observed in every sector of the involved area; ranulas, however, are located in the anterior portion of the floor of the mouth, laterally to the midline (10.13).

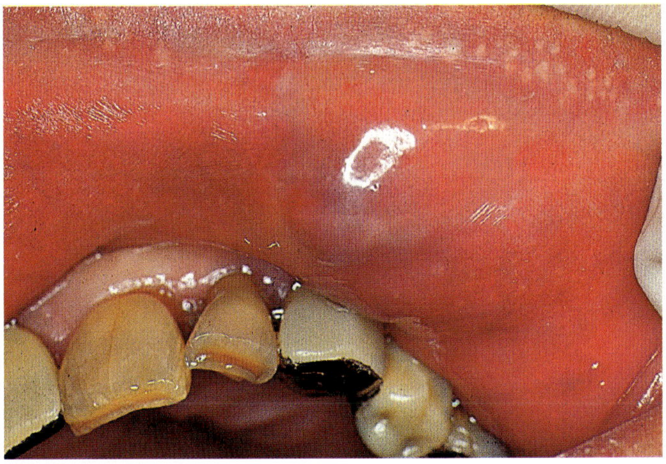

10.12 Salivary cyst of the upper lip.

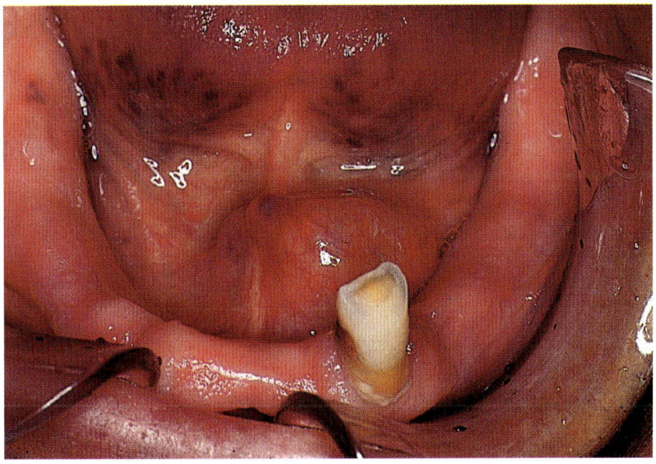

10.13 Salivary cyst of the sublingual gland (ranula).

Symptoms reported by patients may be represented by a sense of encumbrance or intraoral foreign body, or a sense of tension in the area of the lesion.

Pain is very rarely reported, except in cases of infection due to laceration of the wall of the lesion determined by trauma (e.g. accidental self-biting).

Diagnosis

Diagnosis of these lesions is usually simple, due to their well-defined clinical characteristics. Nevertheless, asking the patient about a possible trauma in the area (often represented by accidental self-biting) and looking for evidence of parafunctional habits may be of help.

It is not possible to distinguish a pseudocyst and a retention cyst based solely on their clinical appearance; histologic examination is the only way to confirm the type of lesion.

Instrumental screening is often unnecessary: only in cases of large cysts of the floor of the mouth may ultrasonography be of help in determining the limits and dimensions of the lesion.

Differential diagnosis

Although these lesions are easily diagnosed in the majority of cases, it is nonetheless important for planning the surgical treatment to distinguish them from other lesions that may present similar clinical features, particularly angiomas and papillary cystadenoma lymphomatosum (Warthin's tumour).

Angiomas, especially when large and if mistaken for salivary cysts and pseudocysts, can cause profuse bleeding during their surgical removal (10.14). If there is any doubt regarding the nature of the lesion, needle aspiration helps to verify the content; if the content is frankly haematic, further examinations should be made and the surgical approach modified accordingly.

The papillary cystadenoma lymphomatosum is a proper tumour and, before treatment is planned, incisional biopsy and histologic evaluation of the retrieved sample is necessary. If the nature of the neoplasm is confirmed, then the treatment of large lesions by trained maxillofacial surgeons should be considered (10.15).

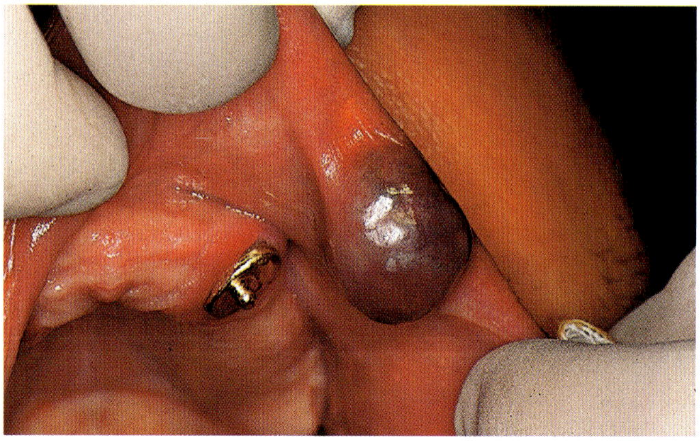

10.14 Angioma of the upper lip.

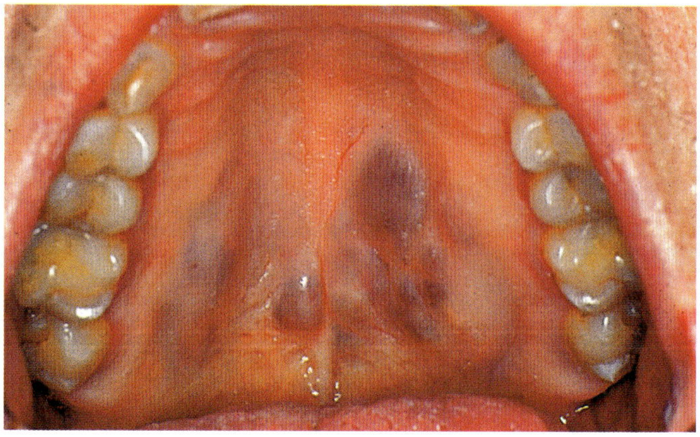

10.15 Papillary cystadenoma lymphomatosum (Warthin's tumour) of the palate.

Surgical treatment of cysts and pseudocysts

Salivary cysts and pseudocysts are always treated with a surgical approach consisting in the excision of the lesion when it is located on the lips, cheeks, and palate, while the recourse to marsupialisation may be indicated when the lesion is located on the floor of the mouth.

Excision

Surgical armamentarium

As the surgical intervention involves only the superficial soft tissues, the surgical armamentarium is very simple:

- scalpel;
- dissecting scissors;
- fine surgical and anatomical pliers;
- needle holder and sutures.

Anaesthesia

Anaesthesia is obtained by perilesional infiltration or, for large lesions, by local anaesthetic block of the corresponding nerve (mental nerve for the inferior lip, buccal nerve for the buccal mucosa, major palatine nerve and nasopalatine nerve for the hard and soft palate). Perilesional anaesthesia should be performed by infiltrating the anaesthetic at a distance from the margins of the lesion to avoid alteration of the local anatomy and subsequent loss of surgical landmarks.

Surgical anatomy

As a rule, mucoceles are superficial lesions located in the submucosal layer; therefore, surgical risks are usually limited.

For large lesions, the presence and adequate management of important anatomic structures such as nerves and arteries in the area must be taken into consideration:

- superior and inferior labial arteries and mental nerve branches in the labial region;
- palatine arteries and their ramifications in the palatal region;
- small arterial branches in the buccal region.

Details on the anatomy of these regions are reported in Chapter 2.

Basic techniques

Excision

This procedure is generally performed under local anaesthesia obtained by perilesional infiltration, which should be injected at a distance from the margins of the lesion to avoid alterations of the local anatomy and subsequent loss of surgical landmarks due to swelling and formation of small haematomas caused by the lesion of small vessels during needle penetration. In some cases, local anaesthetic block of the nerve responsible for the sensory innervation of the area may be indicated (mental nerve for the inferior lip, buccal nerve for the buccal mucosa, major palatine nerve, and nasopalatine nerve for the hard and soft palate).

Excision of the lesion is obtained by means of a delicate incision of the thin mucosal layer above the lesion, taking care not to damage the fine epithelial wall of the cyst. The incision must be conducted, for labial mucoceles, perpendicularly to the direction of the orbicularis oris muscle fibres to avoid visible scars (principle of incision along Langer's lines).

The lesion is then isolated from the surrounding soft tissues by blunt dissection; traction with surgical pliers helps to detect the correct cleavage plane. Once the lesion is excised and haemostasis is obtained, the surgical incision is sutured.

In cases of repeated trauma, separating the cyst wall from the thin overlying mucosa may be difficult, but it is possible to perform a lozenge incision comprising both the mucosa and the lesion. In the labial and buccal regions, a tension-free suture is easily achieved: the mucosa around the border of the surgical wound is separated from the submucosal plane by blunt dissection, and thus mobilised enough to allow primary closure of the surgical access. In the palatine region, the wound resulting from a lozenge excision is left to heal by secondary intention; re-epithelisation occurs in a few days without any sequelae (10.16a-h).

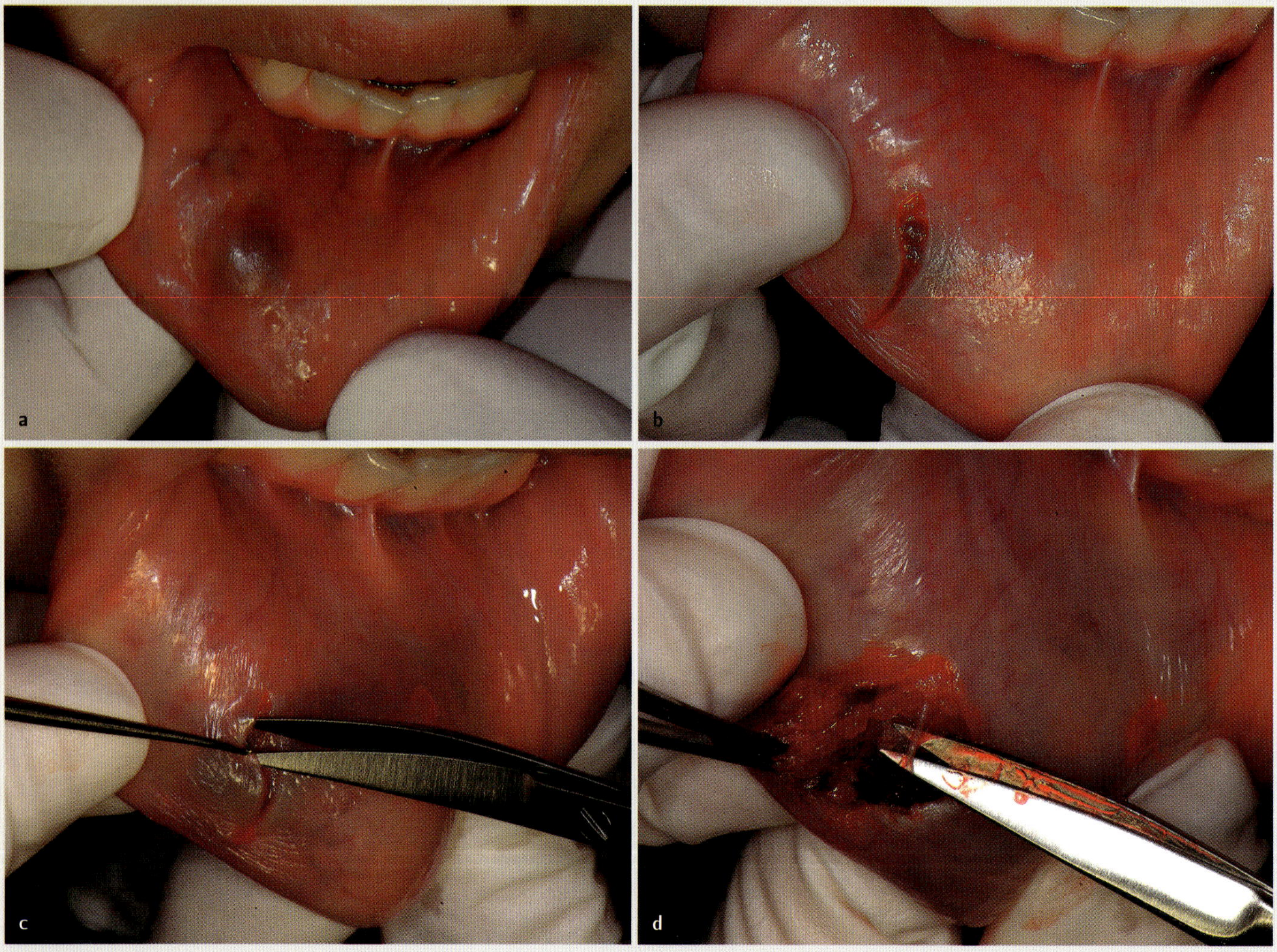

10.16 **a)** Salivary cyst of the inferior lip. **b)** Incision of the mucosa with preservation of the cyst wall. **c)** Blunt dissection. **d)** Identification and isolation of the terminal branches of the mental nerve (labial branches). (*continued*)

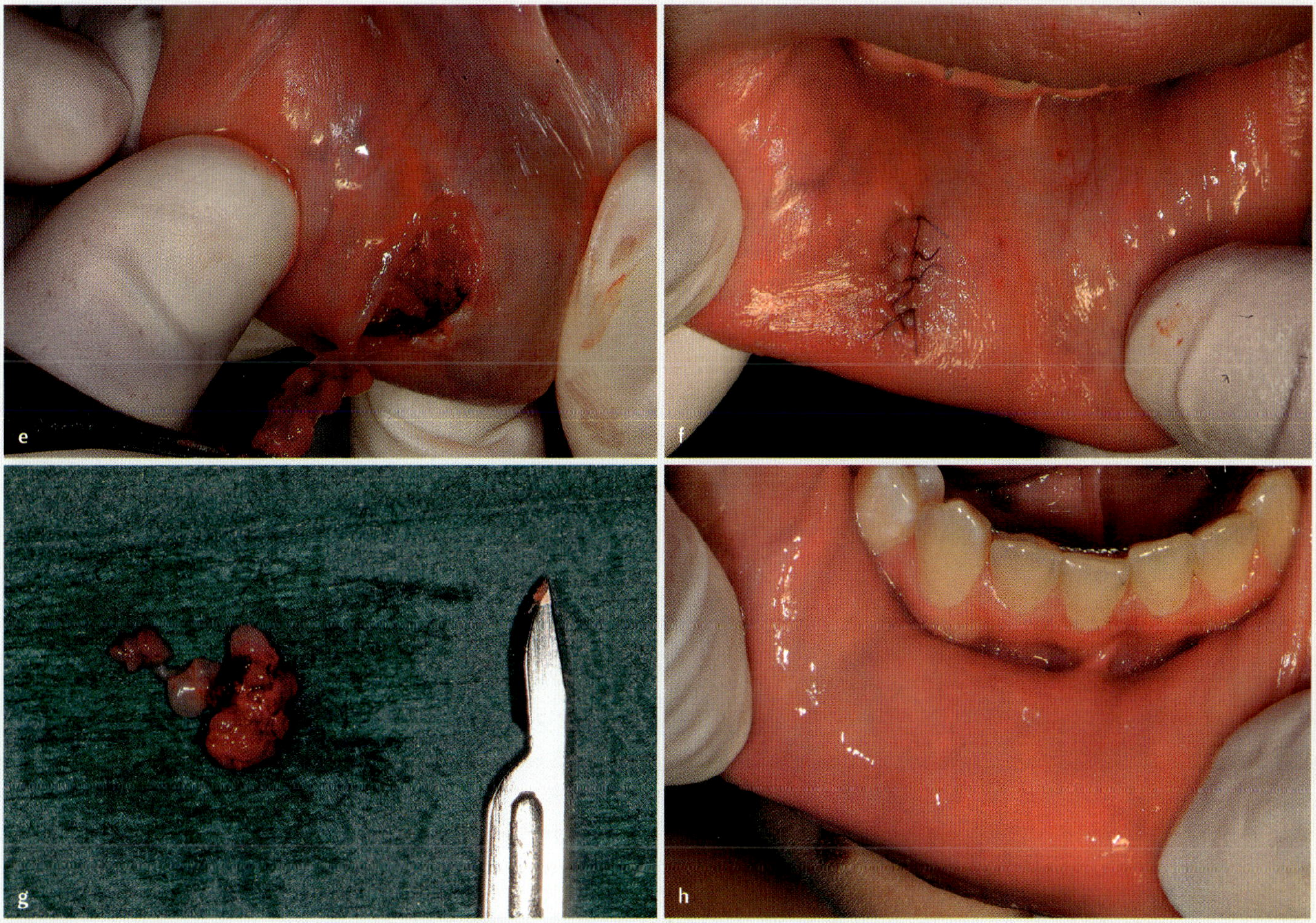

10.16 (*continued*) **e)** Excision of the minor salivary gland. **f)** Suture. **g)** The removed lesion. **h)** Clinical control some time after surgery.

Surgical treatment of sublingual ranulas

Treatment of sublingual ranulas deserves an in-depth analysis, due to the larger size of these lesions and their relationships with important surrounding anatomical structures, such as the submandibular duct, the lingual nerve, and the sublingual veins and arteries. Unlike cysts and pseudocysts of the minor salivary glands, ranulas can be treated with different surgical approaches: a) the ranula is excised; b) the ranula is excised in association with sialoadenectomy of the sublingual gland; or c) the ranula is marsupialised (with or without packing).

Excision of the ranula in association with sublingual sialoadenectomy

This is the most effective treatment of sublingual ranulas. However, the dissection may be challenging due to the difficulties in finding the correct cleavage plane, and the risk of damaging the aforementioned anatomical structures. The risk-benefit ratio is not always favourable; therefore, this technique does not represent the first choice in the treatment of a ranula. On the other hand, sublingual sialoadenectomy may be indicated for multiple relapses of the lesion after conservative treatment (simple excision, marsupialisation).

Excision of the ranula

Although feasible, in some cases it may prove difficult to perform, as the wall of the ranula can be difficult to separate from the surrounding soft tissues. The surgical technique is the same as described above for the excision of other salivary cysts (10.17a-f).

Marsupialisation

This is the most frequently applied treatment option, because it is relatively simple to perform and allows a reduction in postoperative morbidity. It entails the surgical removal of only the roof of the ranula; this allows the immediate decompression of the lesion, due to the discharge of fluid contained inside the cyst, while leaving the deepest portion of the lesion intact. The residual cavity temporarily becomes an accessory cavity of the floor of the mouth, and undergoes spontaneous healing by secondary intention. The recourse to marsupialisation eliminates the risk of damaging important anatomical structures, and maintains a favourable risk-benefit ratio. However, the main disadvantage of this technique is represented by the non-negligible incidence of relapse, which can be as high as 90%. To reduce the risk of relapse, which is caused by the caving in of the walls of the residual cavity leading to its early closure, the marsupialisation of the lesion is associated with the packing of the residual cavity. Once the roof of the ranula is removed and its fluid content is discharged, a strand of iodoform gauze is placed inside the cavity to avoid early closure of the surgical wound. The recourse to the packing significantly reduces the incidence of relapse to less than 10% (10.18a-e).

Basic techniques

Excision of a ranula associated with sublingual sialoadenectomy

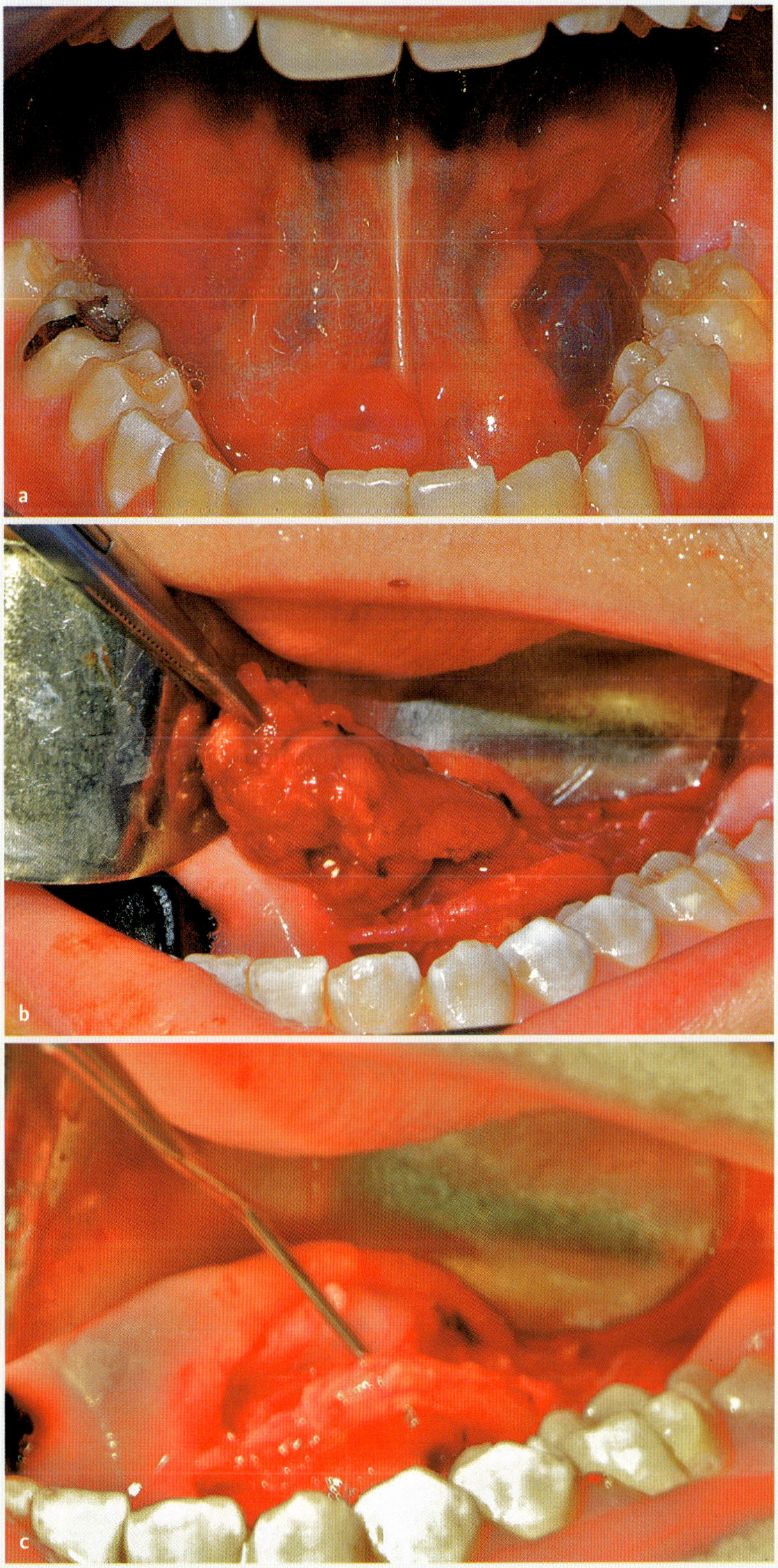

10.17 **a)** Relapsing ranula in the left side of the floor of the mouth: two marsupialisations were previously performed. **b)** Excision of the ranula in association with the removal of the sublingual gland with an intraoral approach. **c)** Preservation of the integrity of the left submandibular duct. (*continued*)

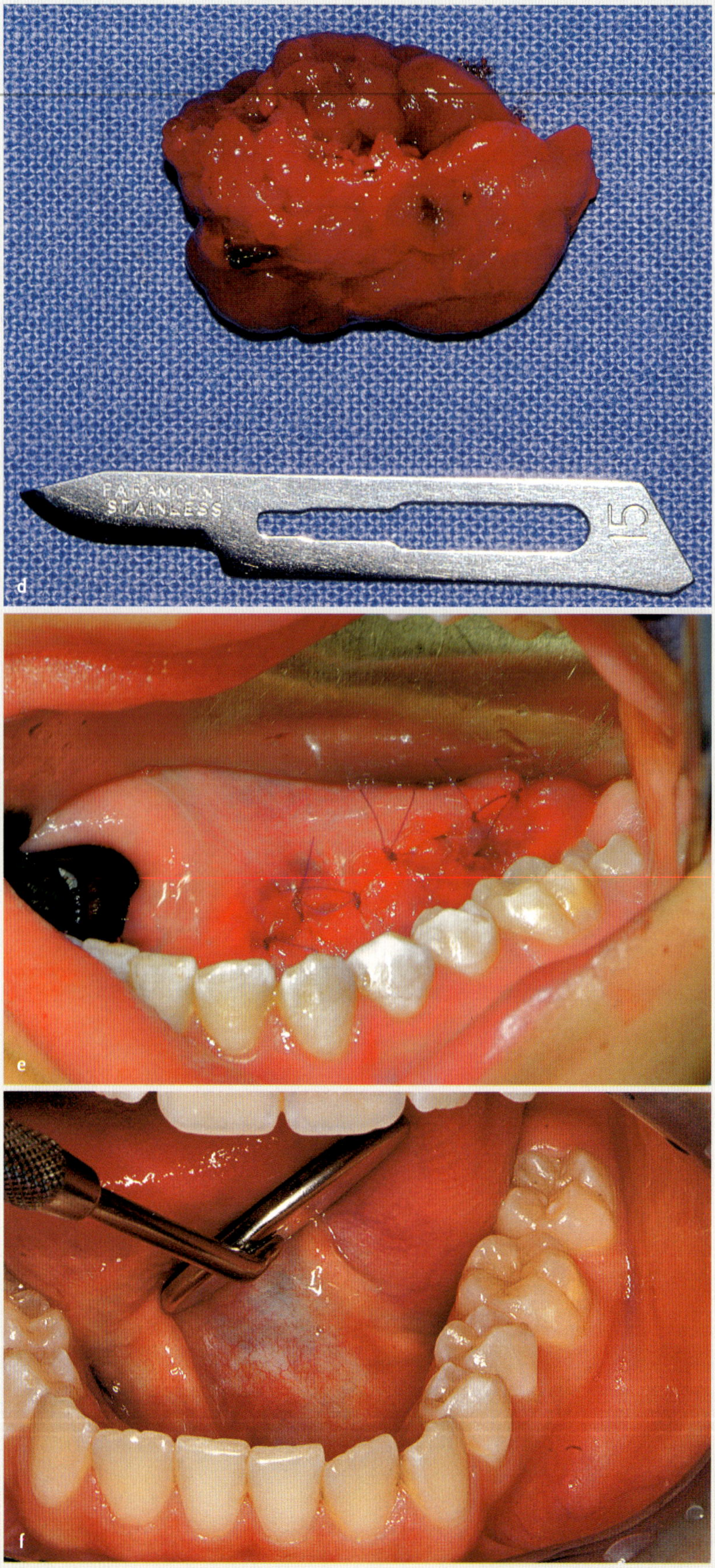

10.17 (*continued*) **d)** The removed sublingual gland. **e)** Suture. **f)** Clinical situation one year after surgery.

Marsupialisation associated with packing of the residual cavity

The roof of the lesion is generally marked with methylene blue to keep an adequate reference point for the completion of surgical incision after the collapse of the lesion, which occurs as soon as the incision induces the discharge of fluid inside the cyst. The scalpel blade or scissors should follow the line to assure that the entire roof of the lesion is removed. The margins of the ranula floor are then sutured to the oral mucosa. The length that the suture threads are cut to should facilitate subsequent ligatures to keep the iodoform gauze packing in place.

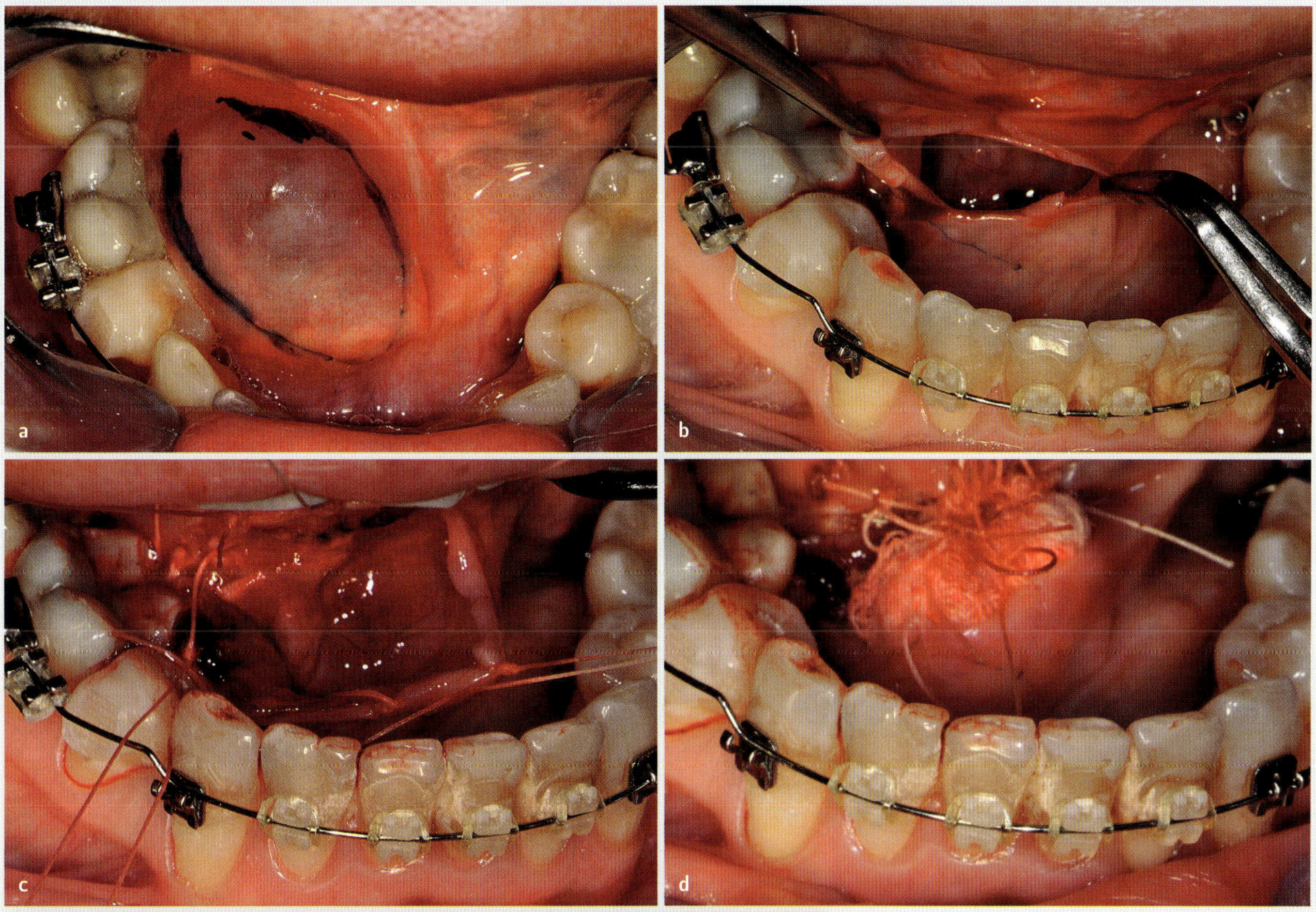

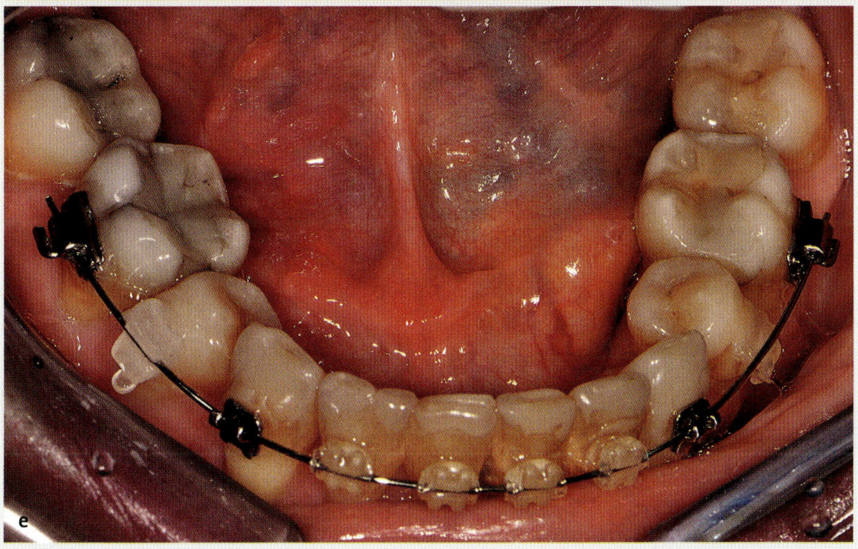

10.18 **a)** Salivary cyst of the right sublingual gland (ranula). Incision lines are marked with methylene blue. **b)** Incision of the roof of the ranula: the roof is then removed. **c)** The walls of the lesion are sutured to the mucosa of the floor of the mouth. **d)** The residual cavity is packed with iodoform gauze. **e)** Clinical situation some time after surgery demonstrating complete healing.

Surgical anatomy

Ranulas develop in the superficial planes of the floor of the mouth, an area in which important anatomical structures such as the submandibular ducts and sublingual arteries are present. Details on the anatomy of this region are reported in Chapter 2.

Surgical armamentarium

The surgical armamentarium is the same as that described for the treatment of cysts and pseudocysts of the minor salivary glands.

Anaesthesia

The most effective technique is the lingual nerve block; this approach helps prevent any alteration of the local anatomy and the subsequent loss of important anatomical landmarks.

Postoperative follow-up

Patients should be followed for at least one year after surgery, to allow early detection of possible relapses.

Generally, marsupialisation associated with packing provides reliable long-term results; only in cases of repeated relapses should marsupialisation be associated with sublingual sialoadenectomy.

Multiple relapses may lead to fibrosis of the roof of the gland and subsequent dripping from the inferior surface. If this is associated with the perforation of the mylohyoid muscle, the fluids excreted by the gland may spread in the deep tissues and form the so-called "plunging ranula". The treatment of the plunging ranula can be difficult and an extraoral approach may be necessary.

REFERENCES

Baurmash HD. Marsupialization for treatment of oral ranula: a second look at the procedure. *J Oral Maxillofac Surg* 1972; 50:1274-9.

Chiapasco M, Ferrieri G, Achilli A. Studio prospettico sull'efficacia della marsupializzazione nel trattamento delle ranule sottolinguali. *Rivista Italiana di Chirurgia Maxillo-Facciale* 1994; 3:35-9.

Chiapasco M, Tassarotti S, Tassarotti B, Abati S. La sialolitiasi della ghiandola sottomandibolare. Etiopatogenesi, considerazioni cliniche, problematiche diagnostiche. Analisi della casistica e studio ultrastrutturale. *Rivista Italiana di Chirurgia Maxillo-Facciale* 1993; 6(2):35-44.

Crysdale WS, Mendelsohn JD, Conley S. Ranulas-Mucoceles of the oral cavity: experience in 26 children. *Laryngoscope* 1988; 98:296-8.

Feinberg SE. The diagnosis and surgical management of salivary gland disorders. In: Peterson LJ, Indresano AT, Marciani RD, Roser SM. Principles of oral and maxillofacial surgery. *JB Lippincott Co.*, Philadelphia, 1992; 34:863-5.

Harrison JD, Epivatianos A, Bhatia SN. Role of microliths in the aetiology of chronic submandibular sialadenitis: a clinicopathological investigation of 154 cases. *Histopatology* 1997; 31(3):237-51.

Lustmann J, Regev E, Melamed Y. Sialolithiasis: A survey on 245 patients and a review of the literature. *Int J Oral Maxillofac Surg* 1990; 19:135-8.

Quick CA, Lowell SH. Ranula and the sublingual salivary glands. Arch Otolaryngol 1977; 103:397-400.

Thomas BL, Brown JE, McGurk M. Salivary gland disease. *Front Oral Biol* 2010; 14:129-46.

Wallace E, Tauzin M, Hagan J, Schaitkin B, Walvekar RR. Management of giant sialoliths: review of the literature and preliminary experience with interventional sialendoscopy. *The Laryngoscope* 2010 Oct; 120:1974-8.

Zui YT. The study of sialolithiasis and the microstructure of salivary calculus: clinical analysis of 55 cases. *Chin J Stom* 1993; 28(5):295-6.

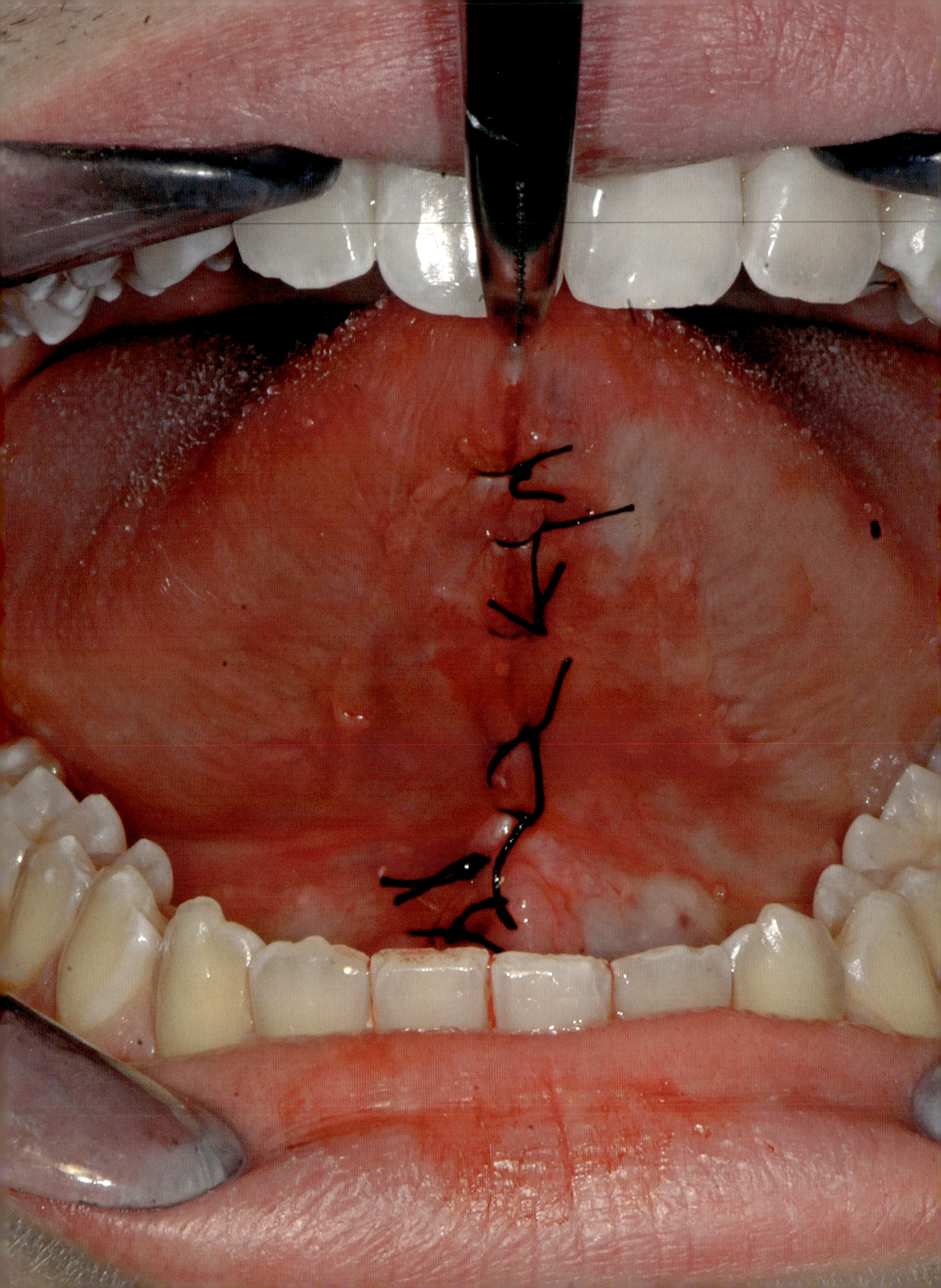

Surgery of the oral frenula and minor preprosthetic surgery

M. Chiapasco ▪ M. Zaniboni

Introduction

In the field of oral surgery, an important role is played by procedures aimed at solving problems that might interfere with a correct orthodontic, periodontal or prosthetic treatment plan. These procedures are performed to improve the hard and/or soft tissues in cases in which their morphology represents an obstacle to the oral rehabilitation of the patient, or when it can jeopardise the results.

In this chapter, a detailed description is presented about the surgical procedures aimed at correcting:

- frenula that may be responsible, due to their position or dimension, for organic or functional problems (diastema, periodontal tissues recessions, tongue hypomobility), or incompatible with an adequate prosthetic rehabilitation;
- alterations of the hard (alveolar ridge and basal bone) and soft tissues (keratinised mucosa and alveolar mucosa) of the jaws that may interfere with an adequate removable prosthetic rehabilitation (pre-implant and peri-implant surgical procedures of the hard and soft tissues are discussed in the next chapter).

Frenula

Frenula are thin bands of soft tissue: they are located on the buccal side of the jaws (particularly on the midline) and on the floor of the mouth and tongue, and are formed by oral mucosa, connective tissue, and muscle fibres. The three frenula that are more frequently a target for surgical treatment are the *superior labial frenulum*, the *inferior labial frenulum*, and the *lingual frenulum*. The removal of one or more of these frenula may be a part of an orthodontic, periodontal, or prosthetic treatment plan, or it may be indicated to correct a functional problem.

Superior labial frenulum

The superior labial frenulum extends from the internal surface of the upper lip to the interincisive area, on the midline. A great interindividual variability exists as far as the level at which the insertion of the frenulum is located; in the majority of cases, it is located on the buccal side of the alveolar ridge near the muco-gingival junction, a few millimetres apically to the interincisive papilla. However, in some cases the insertion of the frenulum may be more coronal, to the point where it can reach the interincisive papilla. If a midline diastema is present, the insertion may even extend on the palatal side of the alveolar ridge.

Correlated issues

Orthodontic issues: presence of an interincisive (midline) diastema. The cause of the interincisive diastema may be the presence of a hypertrophic frenulum. However, it is worth noting that the transient presence of the midline diastema may be considered normal during the transition between primary and permanent dentition, particularly before the eruption of the permanent canines. Once other possible causes have excluded (e.g. presence of a supernumerary tooth, presence of a cyst), it is imperative that the traction manoeuvre be performed on the frenulum to assess the possible mobility and ischaemia of the palatine interincisive papilla. If those signs are present, an active role of the frenulum in the formation and maintenance of the diastema is possible and, in this case, its removal is indicated.

The choice regarding the surgical removal of the frenulum should be carefully evaluated in cooperation with the orthodontist, because frenulectomy represents only the initial (preparatory) phase for the closure of the diastema, which is obtained with orthodontic appliances.

Functional issues: obstacle to lip movements. In rare cases, when the frenulum is very short and inextensible, due to the presence of fibrous connective tissue or thick muscle fibres, it can hinder lip mobility.

Prosthetic issues: obstacle to the making of an upper removable prosthesis. Alveolar bone resorption in partially and totally edentulous patients causes a relative position of the frenulum in an area that is critical for the stability of a partial or complete removable prosthesis. In these cases the insertion of the frenulum may actually be found near the top (or, eventually, on top) of the residual alveolar crest; therefore, lip movements will cause dislocation of the prosthesis.

Periodontal issues: the traction caused by the frenulum on the periodontal tissues may represent, in some cases, a predisposing factor to the development of gingival recessions on the central incisors.

Surgical techniques

Several surgical techniques are available for the removal of labial frenula (both superior and inferior). However, the following measures are valid for all of them:

- before performing a frenulectomy, it is important to limit the infiltration of local anaesthetic, because an excess of liquid modifies the local anatomy of the soft tissues and renders a precise visualisation of the frenulum very difficult, thus complicating the following surgical manoeuvres;
- in the course of surgery, the lip should be tractioned and rotated outwards, to correctly highlight the anatomy of the frenulum;
- it is advisable to control intraoperative bleeding by compressing the surgical wound with sterile saline soaked gauzes, as this manoeuvre, compared to surgical suction, can significantly reduce bleeding.

Basic techniques

Simple excision of the frenulum

The simplest technique for the excision of the labial frenulum is represented by a lozenge-shaped incision involving the mucosal layer, the connective tissue, and the muscle fibres; the extent of the excision towards the alveolar ridge is dictated by the dimension of the frenulum. If a midline diastema is present, and the frenulum develops towards the palate, the incision will run past the centre of the alveolar ridge up to the palatal interincisive papilla: care should be taken to avoid any damage to the nasopalatine neurovascular bundle. Next, the frenulum is removed with a scalpel or fine-pointed scissors, taking care to remove all tissue layers except from the periosteum.

Once excision is completed, a lozenge-shaped wound remains, with an area of exposed periosteum at the bottom. Since the margins of the wound are separated by a distance, simply suturing them may leave a residual exposed area that could cause both an augmented postoperative morbidity and a slower healing of the wound by secondary intention. For this reason, it is indicated to perform a blunt dissection along the margins of the wound to separate the mucosa from the deeper tissue layers allowing a tension-free closure; a water-tight suture guarantees healing of the surgical wound by primary intention. The first stitch must be placed in the deepest point of the fornix, below the nasal spine, and must involve both of the wound margins and the underlying periosteum; this reduces the risk of postoperative haematoma formation, and allows a more favourable anatomy to be obtained. Closure of the surgical wound is then completed with a simple interrupted suture.

Another technique, among those proposed for the excision of labial frenula, involves clamping the margins of the frenulum with haemostatic forceps at the labial and alveolar insertions. The portion of soft tissues comprised between the two forceps is then easily excised. Completion of the surgical procedure is performed with the same modalities described for the previous technique (11.1a–h).

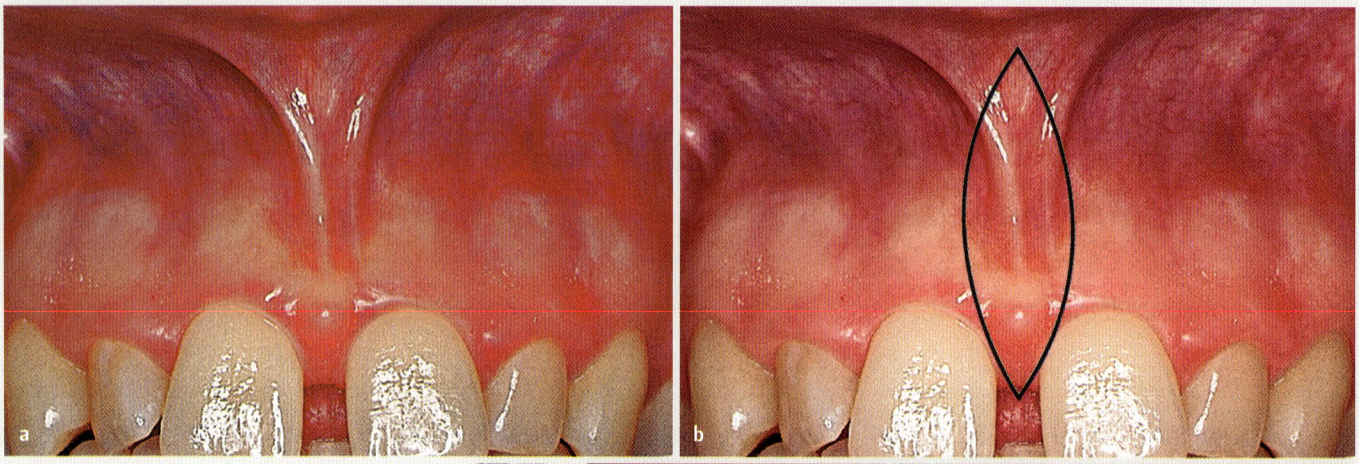

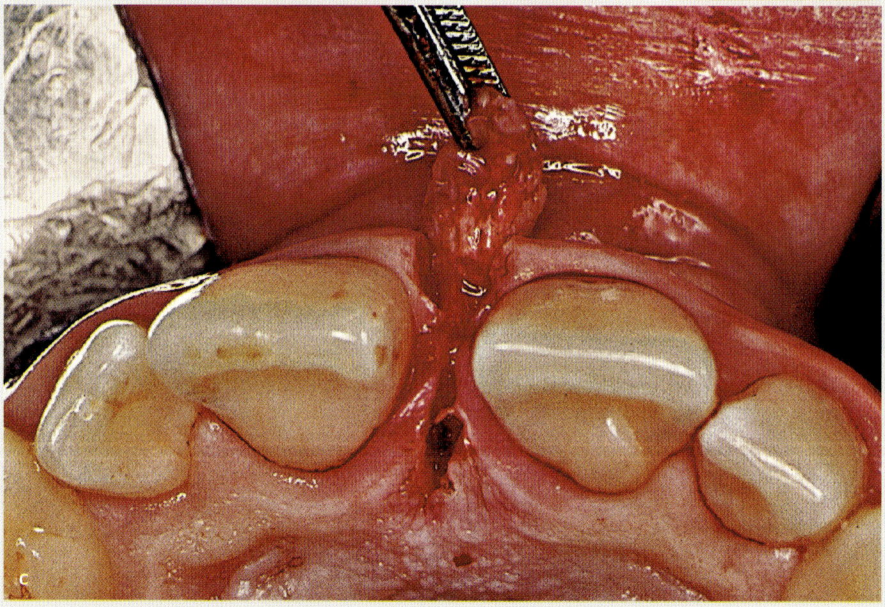

11.1 **a)** Superior labial frenulectomy: preoperative situation. **b)** The surgical incision is outlined: due to the presence of a midline diastema, the excision involves also the palatal papilla. **c)** The incision starts from the palatal papilla. (*continued*)

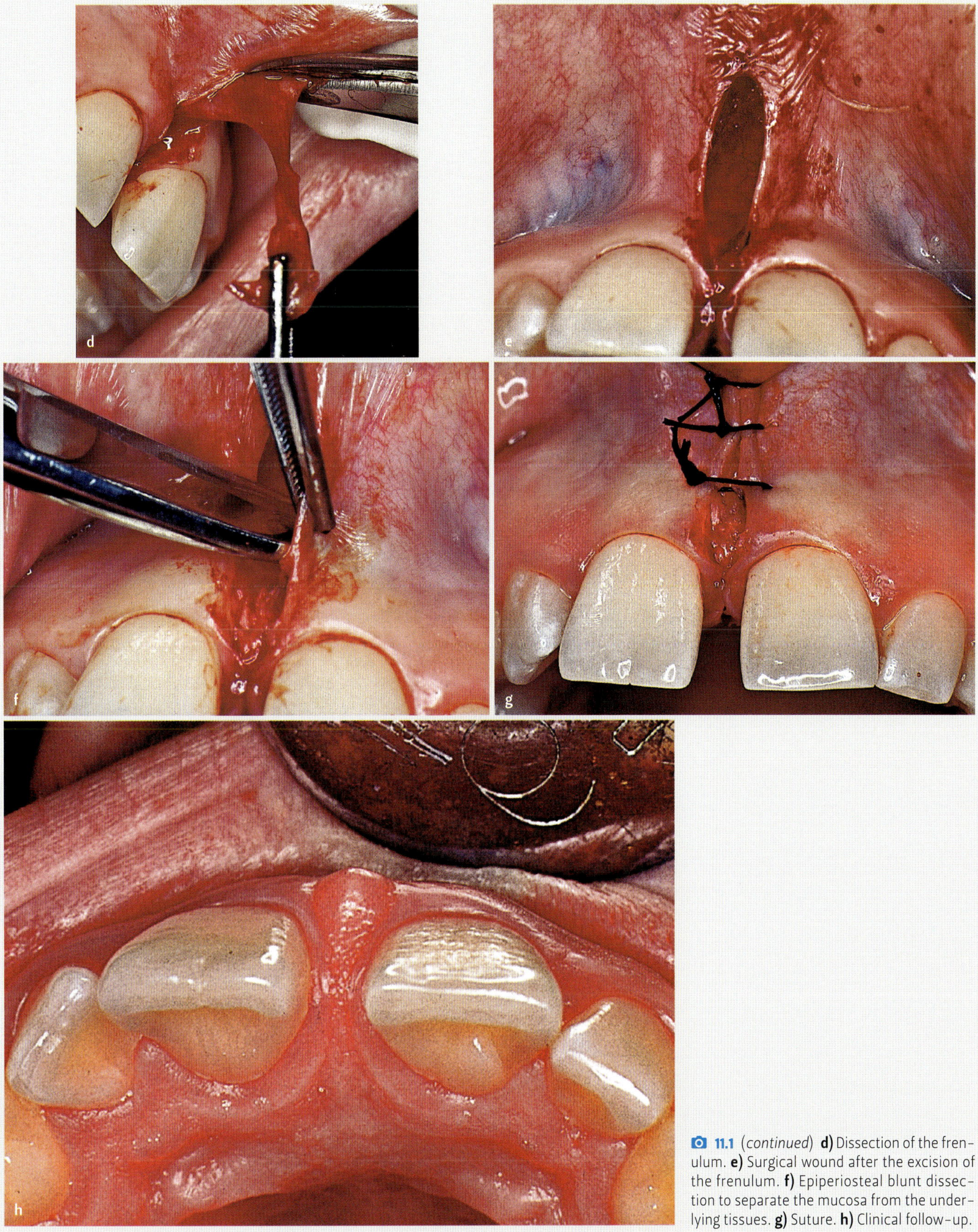

11.1 (*continued*) **d)** Dissection of the frenulum. **e)** Surgical wound after the excision of the frenulum. **f)** Epiperiosteal blunt dissection to separate the mucosa from the underlying tissues. **g)** Suture. **h)** Clinical follow-up.

Frenulectomy in association with Z-plasty

The recourse to this technique reduces the risk of formation of a contracting scar along the main axis of the removed frenulum (according to one of the basic principles of plastic surgery) and provides a deeper repositioning of the bottom of the fornix. Once the frenulum is excised, two parallel oblique incisions (at a 60° angle with respect to the midline) are made pointing in opposite directions, starting from the superior and inferior apex of the surgical wound. The mucosal layer of the two triangular flaps resulting from these incisions is then separated from the underlying tissues, allowing the flaps to be mobilised and transposed to obtain the primary closure of the wound (11.2a–g).

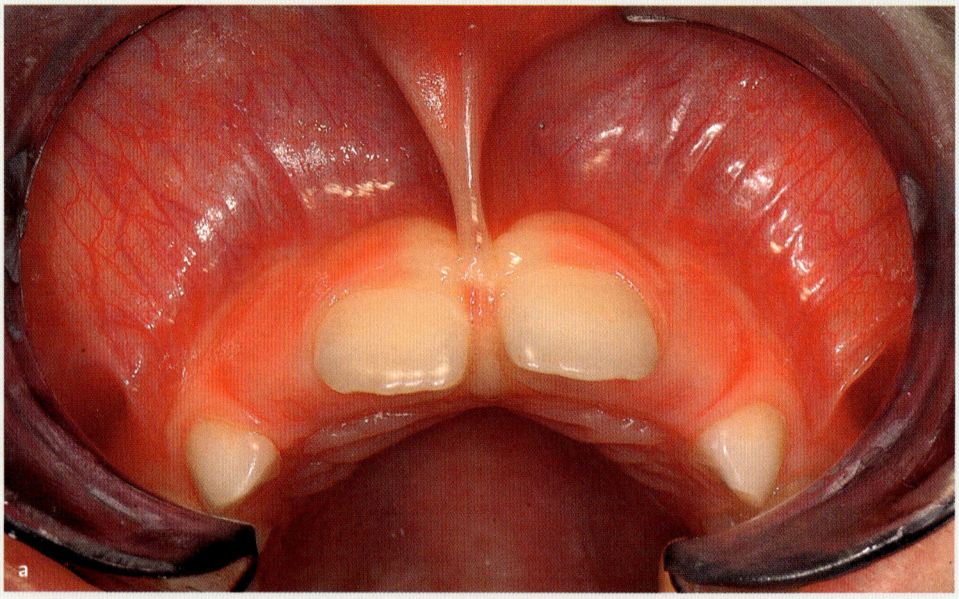

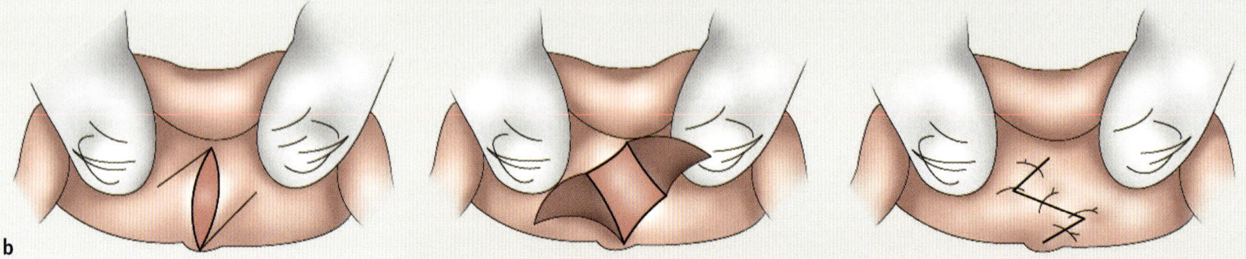

b

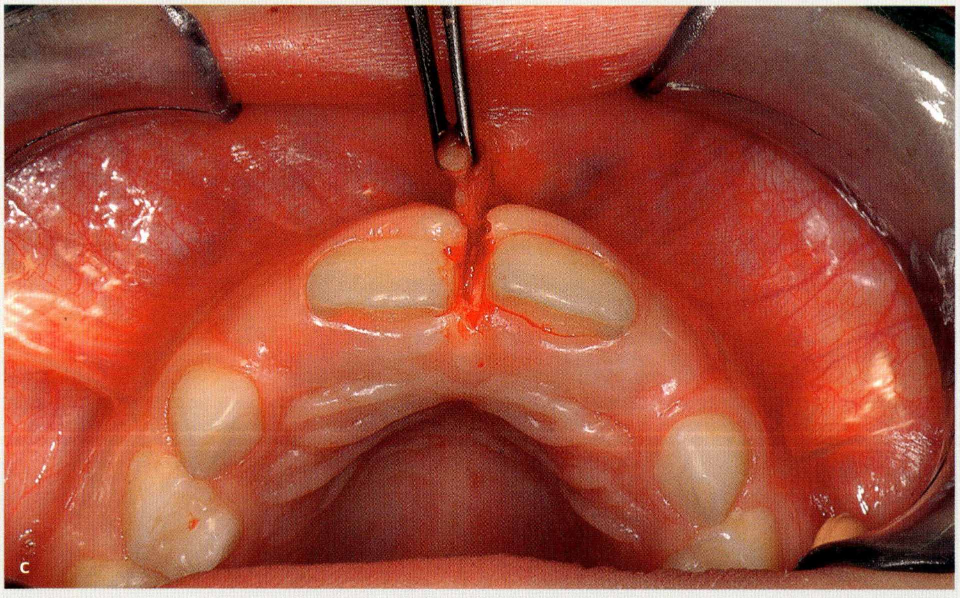

11.2 **a)** Wide superior labial frenulum. **b)** Incision outline: Z-plasty. **c)** Incision and mobilisation of the frenulum. (*continued*)

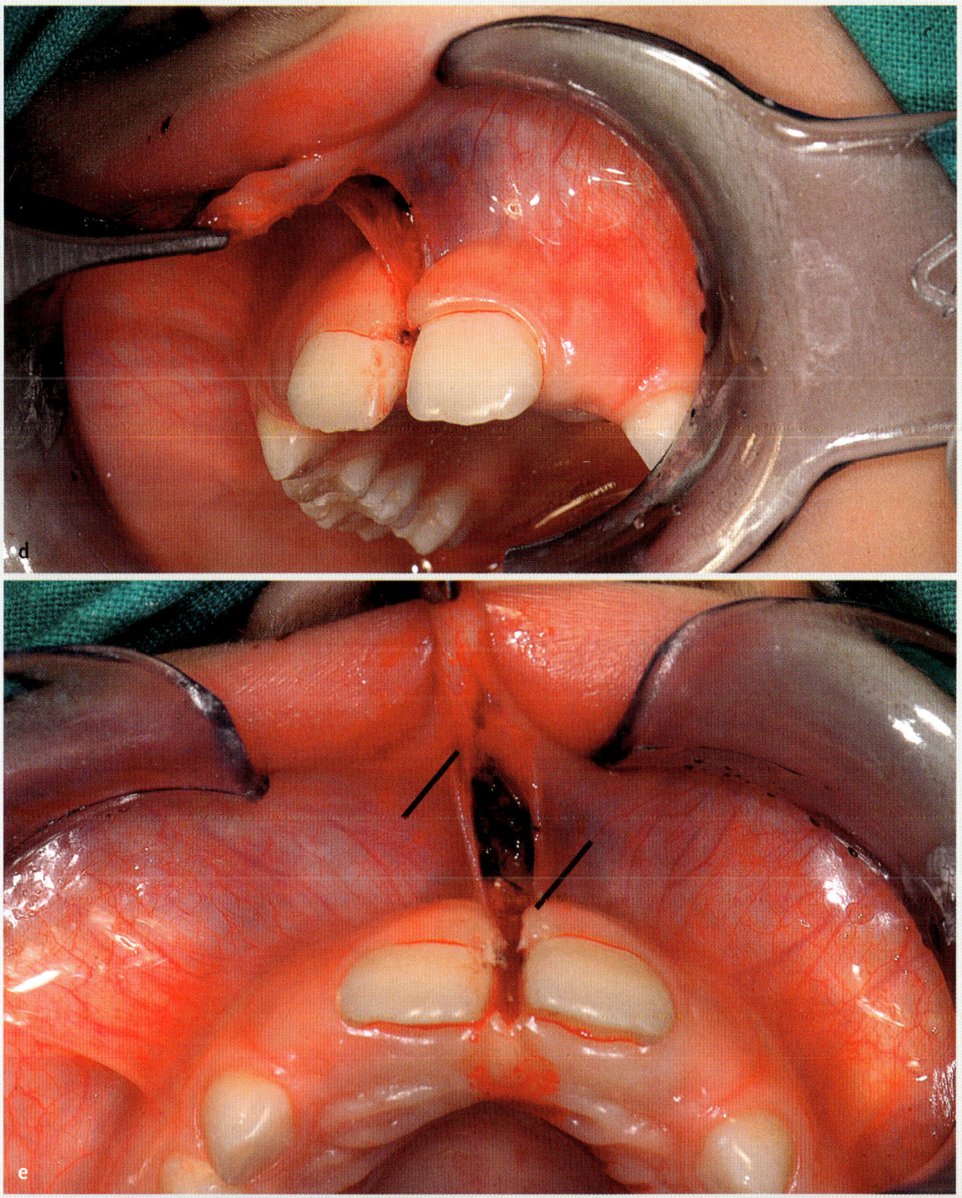

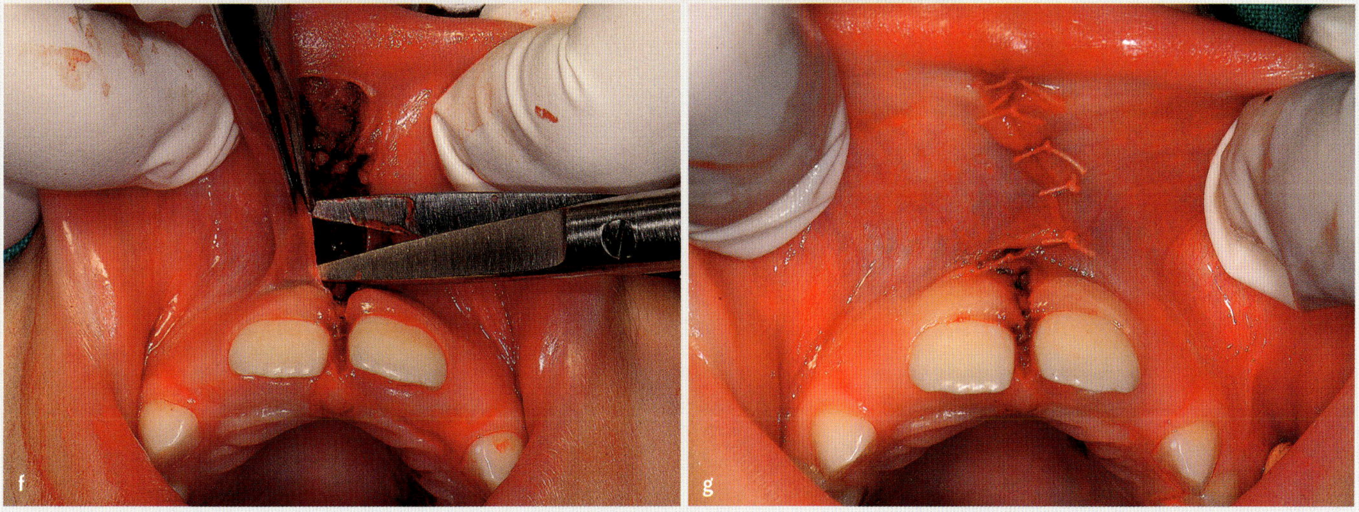

11.2 (*continued*) **d)** Dissection of the frenulum. **e)** Surgical wound after the excision of the frenulum: the incisions for the Z-plasty are outlined. **f)** Epiperiosteal blunt dissection for the separation of the mucosal layer from the underlying tissues. **g)** Suture after Z-plasty.

Frenulectomy in association with V-plasty

This surgical technique is indicated in the presence of a hypertrophic frenulum with a large insertion on the labial side. It allows the vestibular fornix to be deepened in a more predictable way, compared to the aforementioned techniques. However, healing occurs by secondary intention, involving greater discomfort for the patient. The procedure begins with two partial-thickness incisions following the margins of the base of the frenulum, forming an upright "V". If the frenulum extends towards the palate, the two incisions become parallel in the area of the midline diastema, and are joined on the palatal side with a short perpendicular incision. Blunt dissection of the epiperiosteal soft tissues is performed by means of specifically designed scissors. After the frenulum is excised, a triangular surface of bone covered by periosteum is obtained; the mucosa of the lip, which represents the upper side of the triangle, is fixed to the periosteum at the deepest point of the vestibular fornix (a few millimetres under the nasal spine) with a resorbable suture. The surgical wound is then left to heal by secondary intention (11.3a–g).

Frenulum excision with CO2 laser

As far as the advantages are concerned, the use of the laser requires less anaesthetic infiltration and reduces intraoperative bleeding. Healing occurs by secondary intention, and is generally associated with mild discomfort.

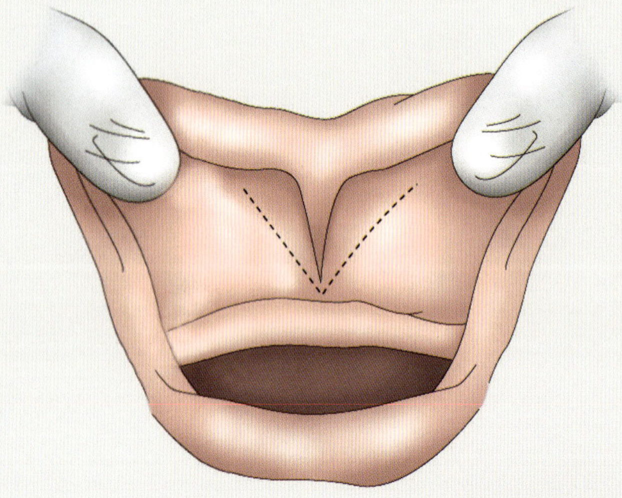

a

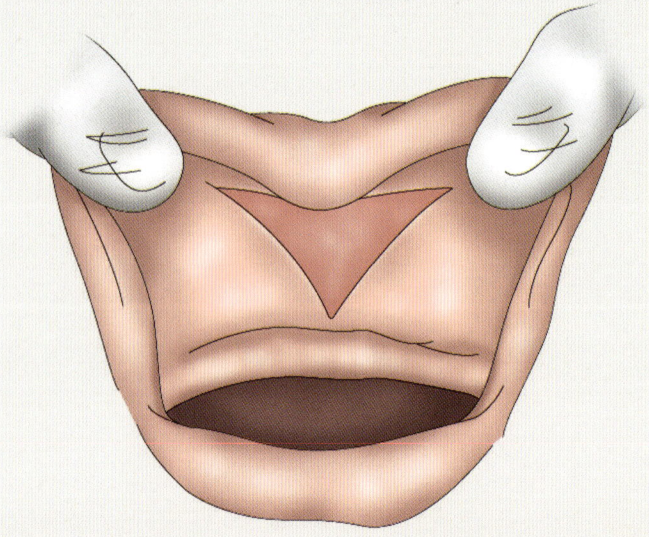

b

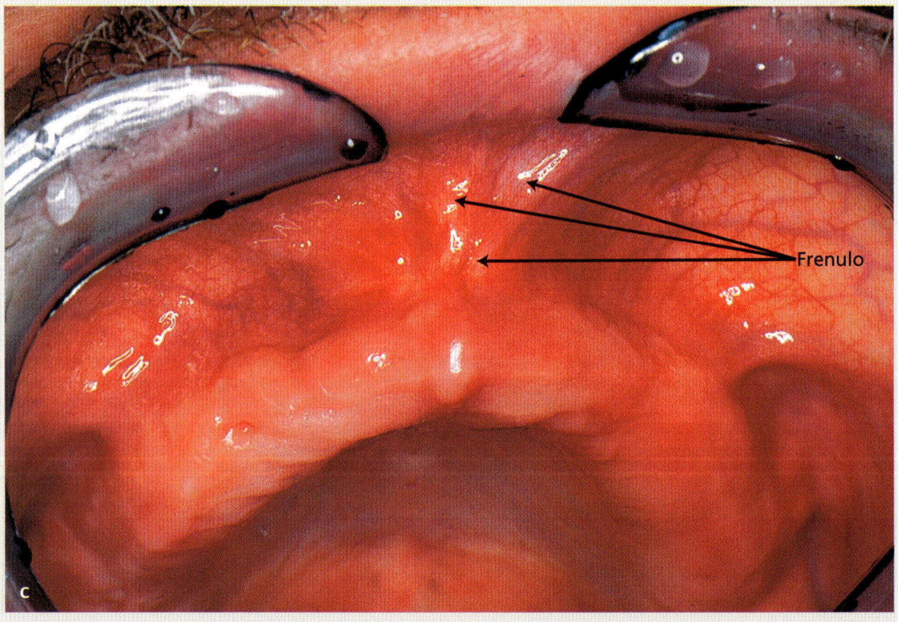

c

11.3 **a)** The V-plasty incision is outlined. **b)** Result after V-plasty. **c)** Superior labial frenulum with ample insertion that causes dislocation of the removable prosthesis. (*continued*)

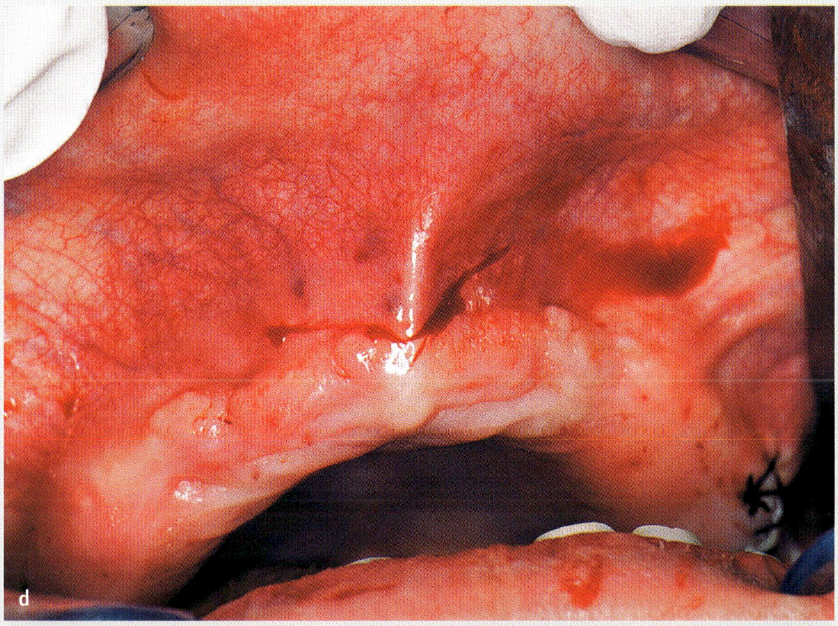

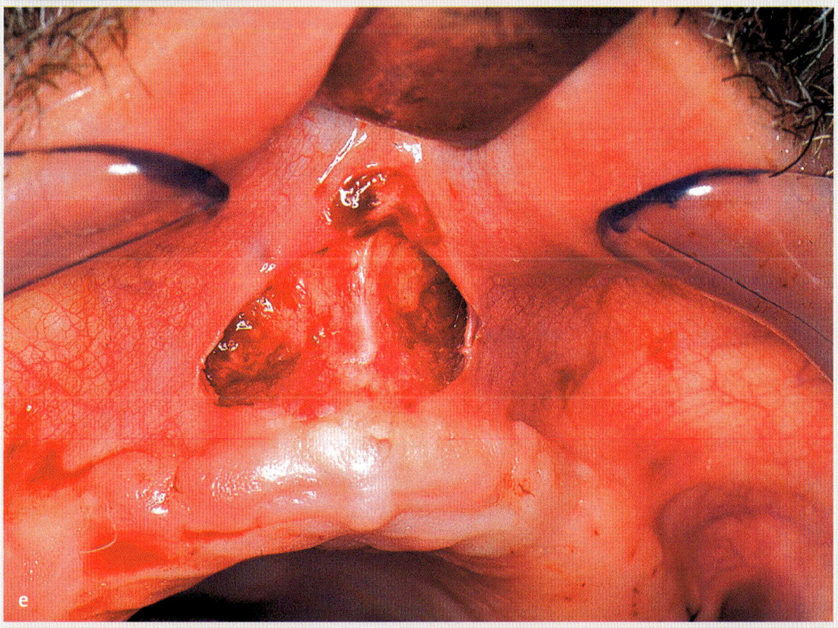

11.3 (*continued*) **d)** V-shaped incision. **e)** Epiperiosteal dissection. **f)** The mucosa is fixed apically with resorbable sutures. **g)** Clinical follow-up.

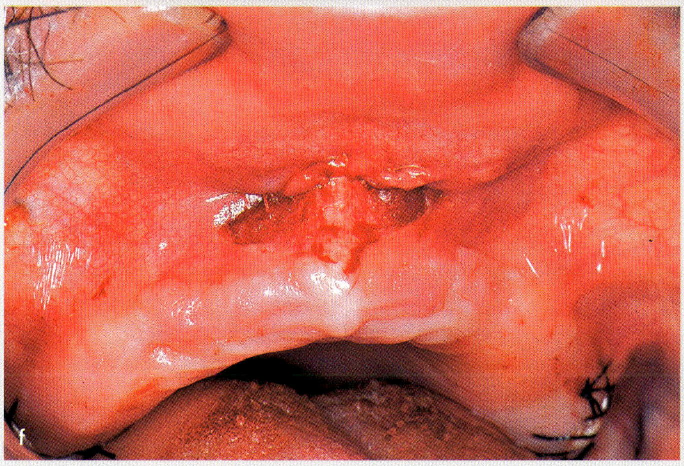

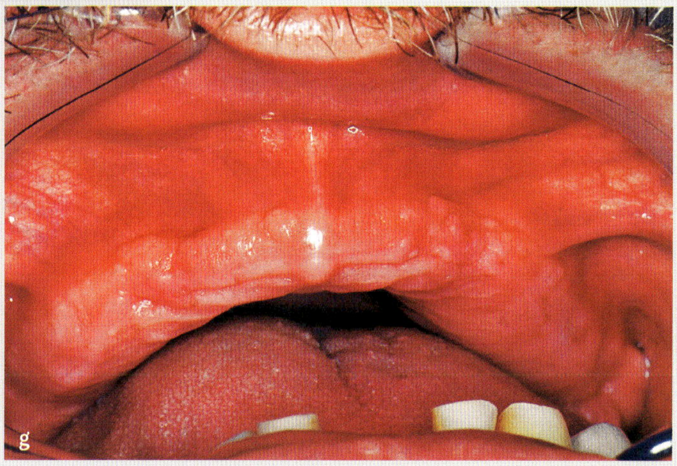

Inferior labial frenulum

The inferior labial frenulum extends from the oral surface of the lip to the inferior alveolar ridge, at the midline, having its insertion on the interincisive papilla or apically to it. Surgical correction of the inferior labial frenulum is rarely indicated, because clinical problems associated with its presence are infrequent.

Correlated issues

Periodontal issues: they represent the main indication for the inferior labial frenulectomy. The presence of a pulling frenulum, associated with a thin or absent band of keratinised mucosa, represents a predisposing factor to the development of gingival recessions on the central incisors. Once the recession is present, the frenulum represents an aggravating factor.

Surgical techniques

FRENULECTOMY ASSOCIATED WITH VESTIBULOPLASTY

In the surgical treatment of the inferior labial frenulum, it is often indicated to associate vestibuloplasty to frenulum excision, because it makes it possible to augment the width of the keratinised mucosa. The surgical technique is identical to the one previously described for the excision of the superior labial frenulum, leading to the creation of a surface covered by periosteum that is left to heal by secondary intention.

FRENULECTOMY ASSOCIATED WITH FREE GINGIVAL GRAFT

When keratinised mucosa is absent, it is recommended to associate a free gingival graft to the excision of the frenulum. A detailed description of this technique is reported in Chapter 13 of this book and in periodontology textbooks.

Lingual frenulum

The lingual frenulum extends from the floor of the mouth to the midline of the undersurface of the tongue; anteriorly, the insertion of the frenulum is located on the lingual surface of the mandibular alveolar crest and, in some cases can reach the interincisive papilla. Inside the frenulum, superficial fibres of the genioglossus muscle may be present.

Correlated issues

Ankyloglossia caused by the presence of a short, thick or tight frenulum: diagnosis is mainly based on the impossibility for the patient to reach the palate with the tip of the tongue while keeping their mouth open, and to protrude the tongue more than 1-2 centimetres beyond the inferior incisors. The presence of ankyloglossia may cause phonation impairment, atypical swallowing, orthopaedic-orthodontic alterations, and a predisposition to develop caries.

Phonation impairment: the pronunciation of dental-lingual-labial consonants (d, l, n, r, s, t, z) may be altered. In these cases, the surgical removal of the frenulum represents only the first phase of the treatment; when healing of the surgical wound is achieved, the patient can undergo speech therapy sessions.

Frenula-related issues

Type	Issues
Superior labial frenulum	Midline diastema Impaired lip movements Dislocation of removable prosthesis
Inferior labial frenulum	Gingival recession
Lingual frenulum	Gingival recession Ankyloglossia (impaired phonation, atypical swallowing, and orthodontic alterations) Dislocation of removable prosthesis Periodontal issues

Atypical swallowing and orthopaedic-orthodontic issues: tongue ankylosis favours the onset and persistence of atypical swallowing and associated orthodontic alterations. The position of the tongue on the floor of the mouth can cause excessive pressure on the inferior incisors and reduce the normal stimulation exerted for the growth of the maxilla. Consequently, cross-bite of the lateral-posterior dentition and open bite in the anterior region may develop.

Predisposition to develop caries of the inferior molars: the issue is caused by the reduced self-cleansing of the teeth surfaces due to the hypomobility of the tongue.

Prosthetic issues: the lingual frenulum, like the labial frenula, may represent an obstacle to the fabrication and use of a complete denture prosthesis, especially when its anterior insertion on the alveolar ridge is coronal or reaches the top of the crest. In fact, in these cases the movements of the tongue put the frenulum under tension causing dislocation of the prosthesis.

Periodontal issues: the insertion of the frenulum in proximity to the lingual surface of the central incisors may promote the onset of periodontal issues such as gingival recession, as previously described for the labial frenula.

Surgical techniques

The surgical procedures for the excision of the lingual frenulum involve the floor of the mouth and the undersurface of the tongue. In these areas, notable anatomic structures are present (e.g. submandibular ducts, submandibular vessels, terminal branches of the lingual nerves, ascending branches of the sublingual arteries) and the utmost care must be taken to prevent any damage to them. A detailed description of the anatomy of the region is reported in Chapter 2.

Basic techniques

Lingual frenulectomy

Anaesthesia in the area is obtained by simple submucosal infiltration of local anaesthetic, while anaesthesia of the body of the tongue, if necessary, is obtained by lingual nerve block. A suture going through the tongue apex allows elevation and extrusion of the tongue, facilitating the surgical manoeuvres. The frenulum can be isolated with the aid of haemostatic forceps: one is placed along the insertion of the frenulum on the tongue, while another is placed along the insertion of the frenulum on the floor of the mouth. However, it is imperative that involvement of the outlets of the submandibular ducts be avoided, the latter of which are located at the base of the lingual frenulum, in the isolation manoeuvres. Once the haemostatic forceps are in place, the frenulum can be excised with a scalpel or sharp scissors; the forceps are then removed to reveal a lozenge-shaped wound. Bleeding from the small vessels can be easily managed by means of bipolar coagulation, taking care not to use the bipolar pliers in proximity to the submandibular ducts or nerve branches, to prevent direct and indirect damage to these anatomical structures. Cleavage of the mucosa from the underlying muscles is then performed to obtain a tension-free suture of the wound and to prevent restrictions in muscle contraction. Once adequate mobility of the tongue is obtained, the mucosa is sutured. The use of resorbable sutures is preferable, because suture removal in this area may be difficult and can cause discomfort, particularly in paediatric patients (11.4a–f).

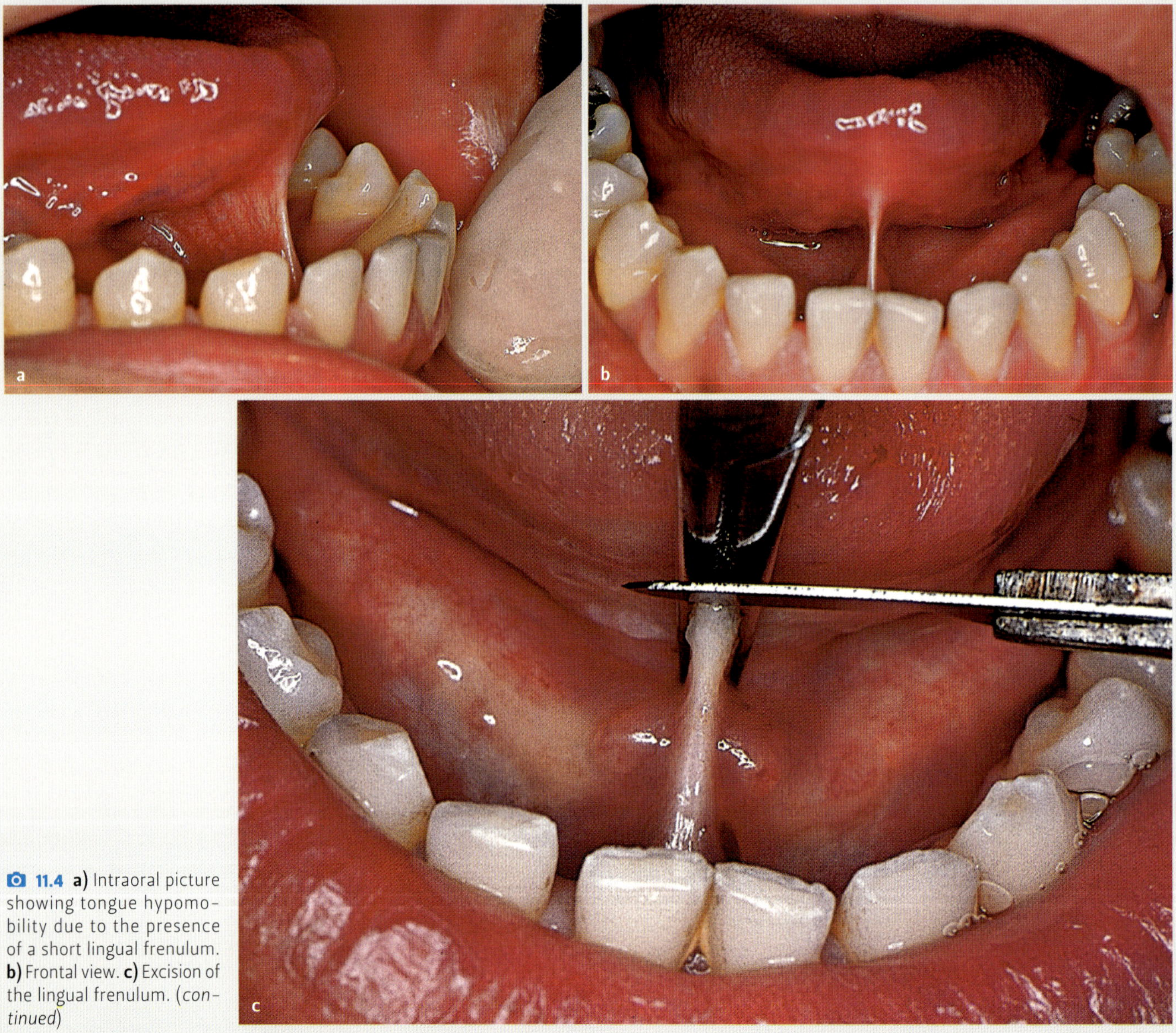

11.4 **a)** Intraoral picture showing tongue hypomobility due to the presence of a short lingual frenulum. **b)** Frontal view. **c)** Excision of the lingual frenulum. (*continued*)

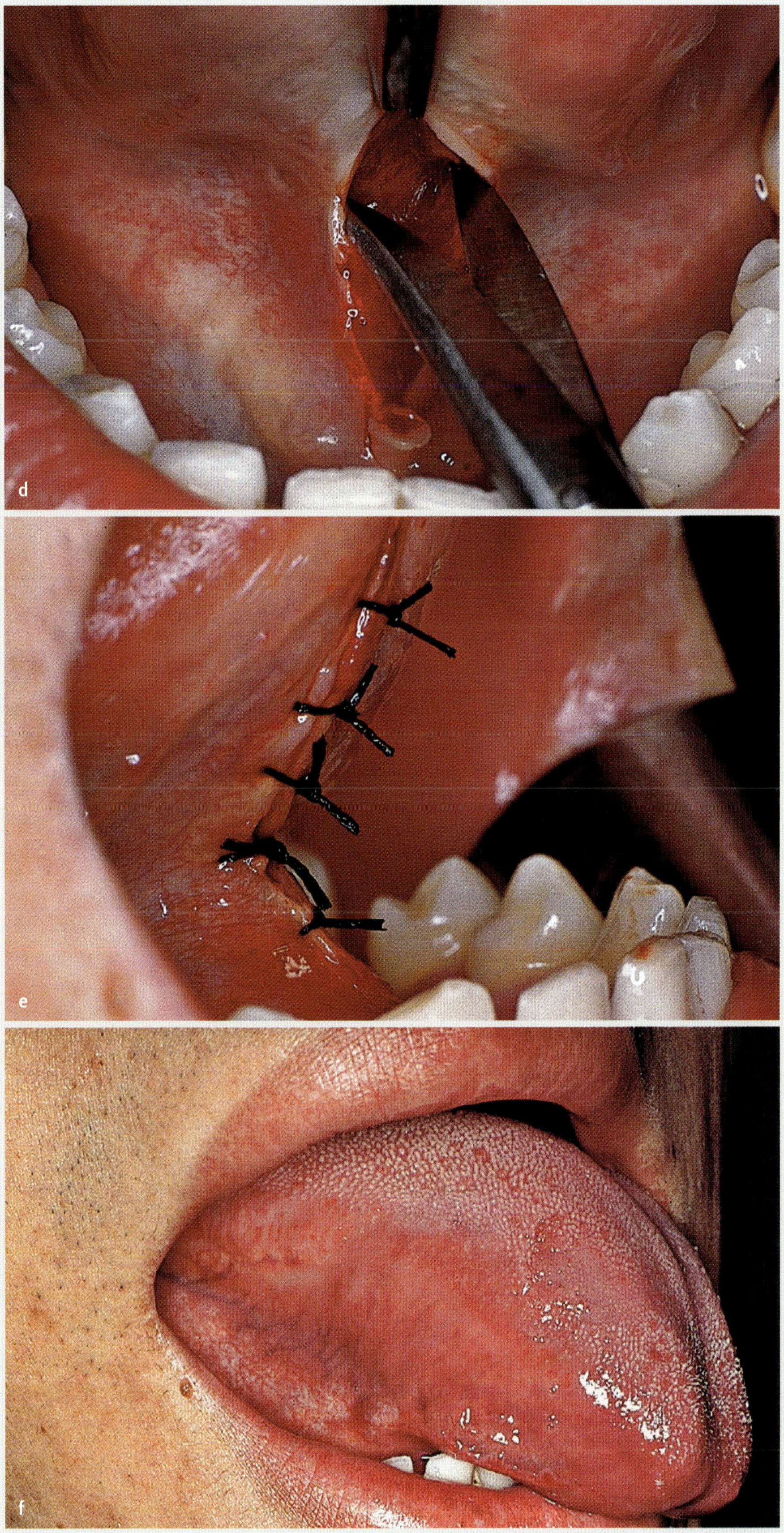

11.4 (*continued*) **d)** Blunt dissection is performed to separate the mucosal layer from the genioglossus muscle insertions. **e)** Suture. **f)** Clinical follow-up: normal tongue mobility is evident.

Minor preprosthetic surgery

Minor preprosthetic surgical procedures are aimed at creating or restoring, in partially or totally edentulous patients, a local anatomy of the hard and soft tissues, which can offer adequate support to removable prostheses. Preprosthetic surgical procedures aimed at correcting bone defects prior to implant rehabilitation are described in detail in Chapter 12.

Clinical conditions that may interfere with an adequate prosthetic rehabilitation of edentulous areas can be classified as follows:

- unfavourable morphology and/or presence of alterations of the hard tissues (alveolar ridge and basal bone);
- unfavourable morphology and/or presence of alterations of the soft tissues (gingiva and alveolar mucosa).

However, it is worth remembering that alterations of the local morphology often involve both the hard and soft tissues.

The majority of these alterations are a direct consequence of the modifications that the jaws undergo after the loss of teeth, or the result of endodontic and/or periodontal disease, while in some cases they can be caused by lesions that interfere with the prosthetic rehabilitation (e.g. exostoses and tori, exophytic lesions of the soft tissues, tumours, trauma or tumour resection sequelae, etc.). In the first place, modifications of the hard and soft tissues due to teeth loss and endodontic and periodontal disease are analysed; these, generally, result in atrophy.

Classification of atrophies of the edentulous jaws

Edentulism, both partial and total, results in a progressive resorption of the alveolar ridges and the overlying keratinised mucosa. This process is due to the loss of the supporting function that the alveolar bone and the keratinised gingiva accomplish according to the functional matrix principle, an organ that for any reason loses its function undergoes progressive atrophy. It has been demonstrated that these processes, notwithstanding the interindividual variability, follow predictable models and are thus easily classifiable.

Among the different classifications proposed over the years, one that is widely known and used due to its simplicity and the possibility of being applied to both the mandible and the maxilla is the Cawood and Howell classification published in 1988.

These authors have made the following observations:

- the morphology of *basal bone* does not change significantly after tooth loss, if no external incongruous or irritative stimuli are applied (e.g. inadequate removable prostheses);
- the *alveolar ridges* undergo atrophy according to constant, area-specific patterns.

In the maxilla, resorption of the alveolar ridge typically follows a horizontal trend, both in the anterior and the posterior areas. In the interforaminal area of the mandible, horizontal bone resorption is more pronounced on the buccal side, while in the posterior areas vertical bone resorption is more significant. Cawood and Howell identified six classes for mandibular atrophy, and five classes for maxillary atrophy, associated with different morphologies according to the area in which they occur (anterior or posterior maxilla, anterior or posterior mandible) (📷 11.5, 11.6). Different areas of the same jaw can present different classes of atrophy at the same time.

The use of incongruous removable prostheses, causing chronic irritative stimuli, can accelerate and/or modify the bone resorption process.

Endocrine and metabolic factors, as well as eating habits, may also play an important role in the process of atrophy. The progressive reduction in the mineral content of bone after the 5th decade, particularly in postmenopausal women, a diet with low contents of calcium and D vitamin, caffeine and tobacco abuse accentuate the normal resorption rate. In addition, the soft tissues undergo considerable alterations because of alveolar ridge resorption:

- insertions of the muscles of the floor of the mouth and of the perioral muscles become more superficial with respect to the centre of the residual alveolar crest, and the depth of the buccal vestibules is reduced (for severe bone atrophy, the vestibule can completely disappear);
- the band of keratinised mucosa undergoes progressive reduction (11.7, 11.8).

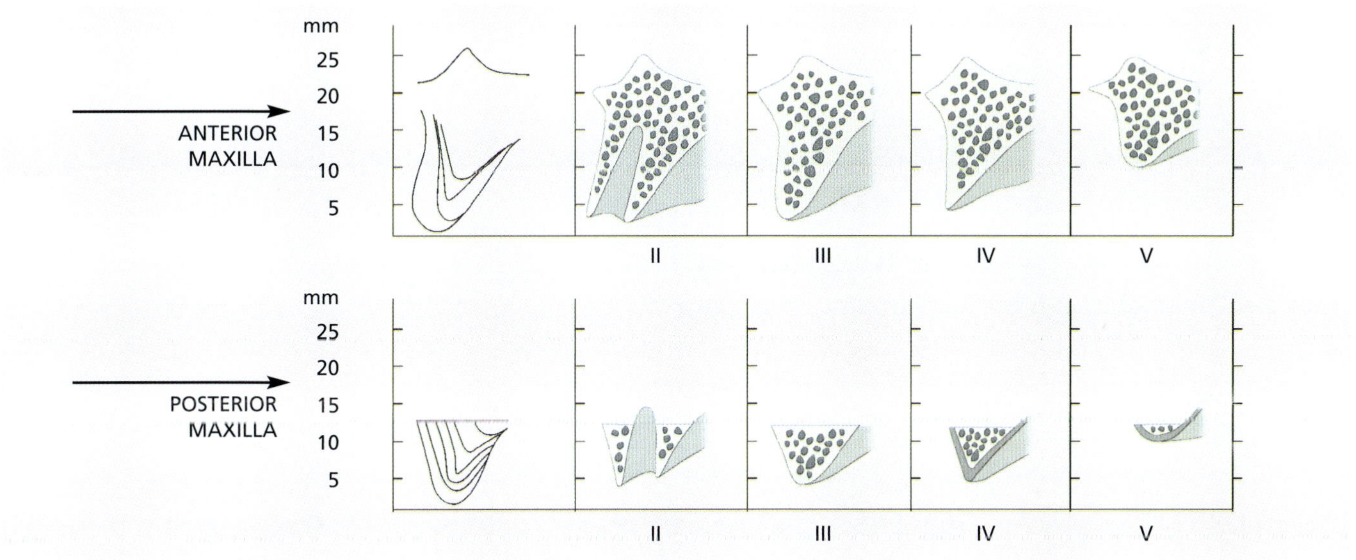

11.5 Cawood and Howell classification of the atrophic edentulous maxilla.

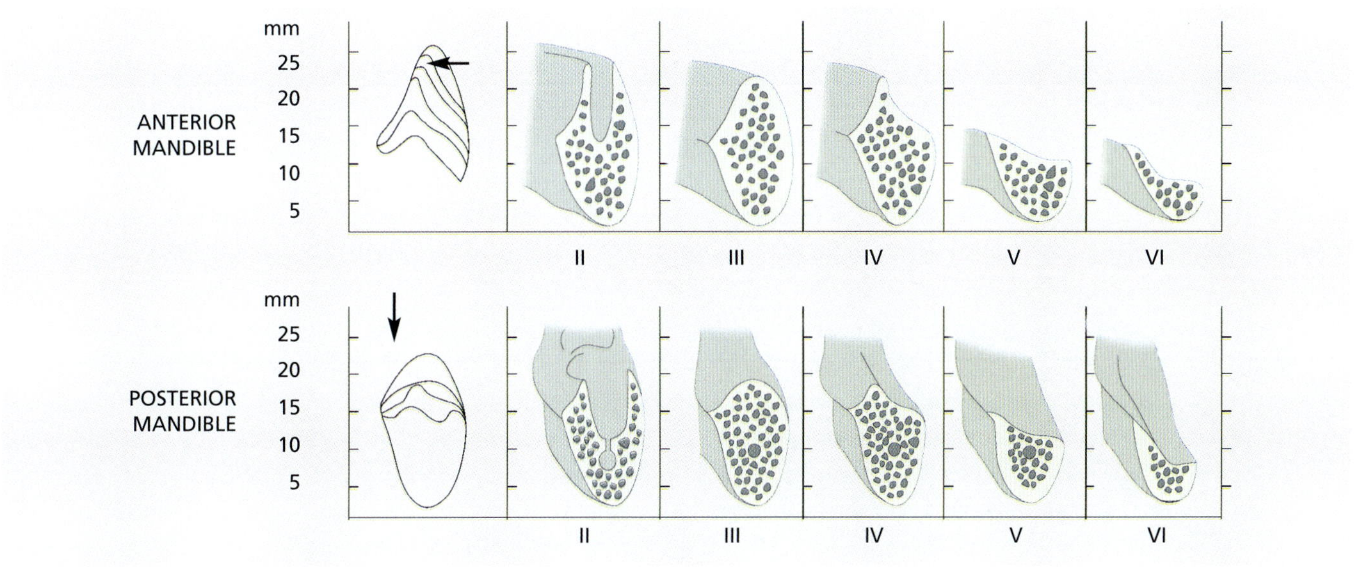

11.6 Cawood and Howell classification of the atrophic edentulous mandible.

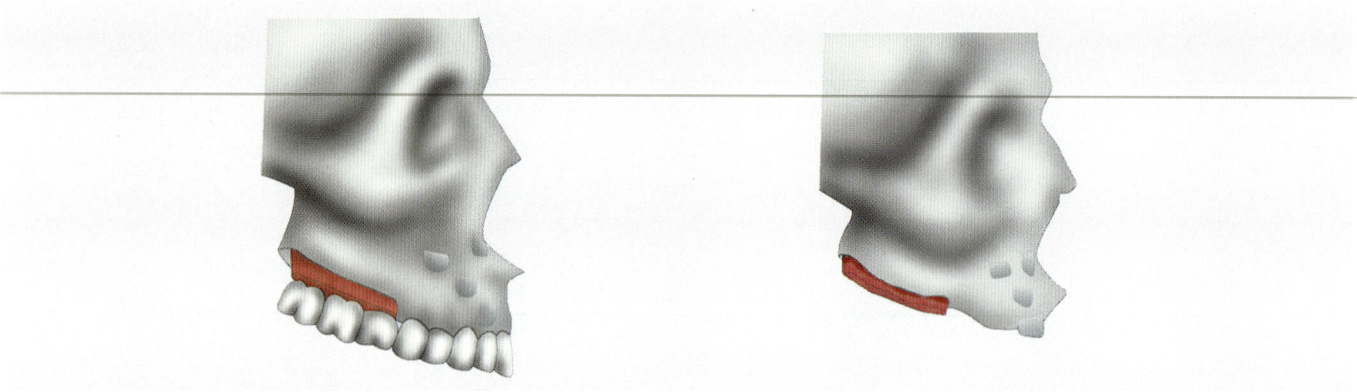

11.7 Relative superficialisation of muscle insertions following bone atrophy (maxilla).

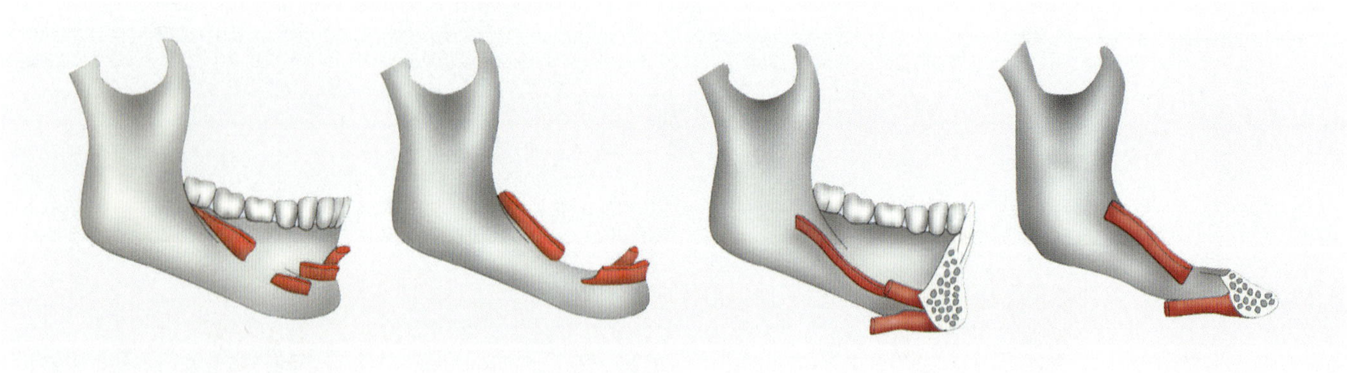

11.8 Relative superficialisation of muscle insertions following bone atrophy (mandible).

In cases where bone resorption occurs rapidly, or the removable prostheses used by the patient are incongruous, a clinical situation of relative excess of soft tissues can occur, leading to the formation of mobile soft tissue crests know as *flabby ridges*.

The modifications of the oral tissues have a significant impact on *face morphology*. It is well-known that perioral and mimic muscles imbricate at the labial commissure creating the so-called modiolus. Tooth loss and resorption of the alveolar ridges cause a change of direction and loss of tone of these muscles, causing the modiolus to collapse backwards and downwards (11.9, 11.10). The association between bone atrophy and facial tissue collapse leads to the increase and accentuation of perioral wrinkles, and to the reduction or disappearance of the vermilion border of the lip, resulting in an "old" appearance of the face.

Classification of the atrophic alveolar ridges

- **Class I** Dentate patient
- **Class II** Immediate post-extractive alveolar ridge
- **Class III** Late post-extractive alveolar ridge with reossification of the alveoli and rounded profile of the crest, which retains adequate height and width.
- **Class IV** The alveolar crest retains adequate height but insufficient width (knife-edge ridge)
- **Class V** Flat alveolar ridge, insufficient height and width
- **Class VI** Depressed alveolar ridge, with atrophy of the basal bone (only in the mandible)

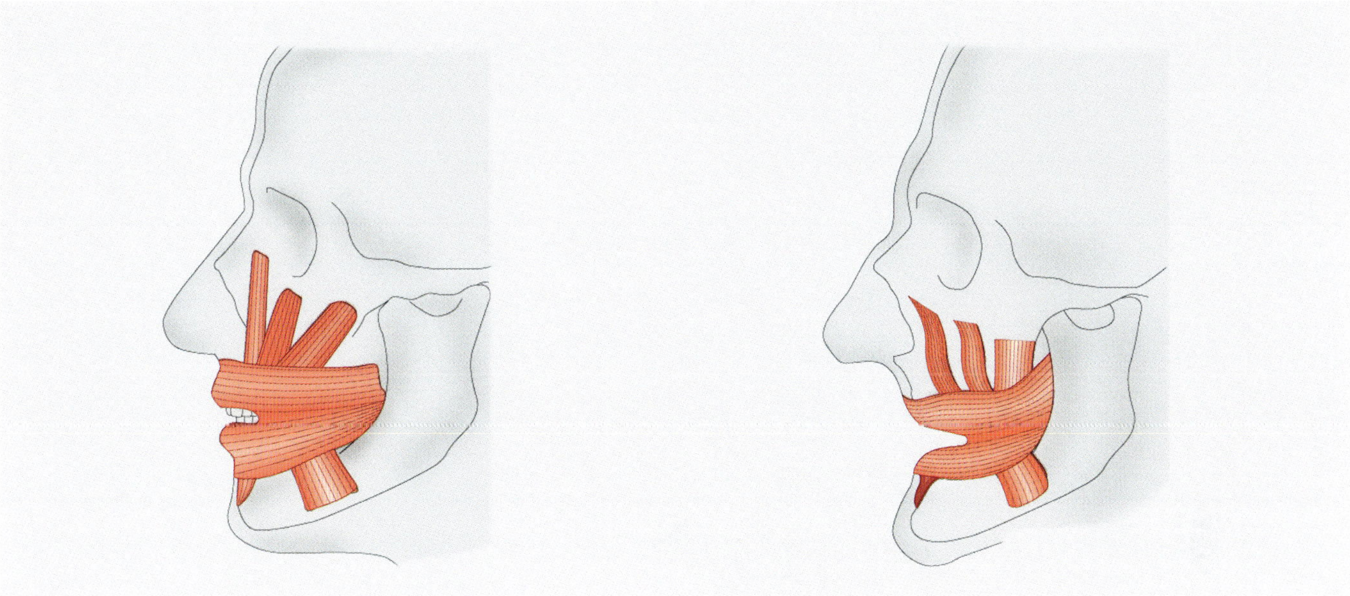

11.9 Alteration of the facial morphology (extraoral view).

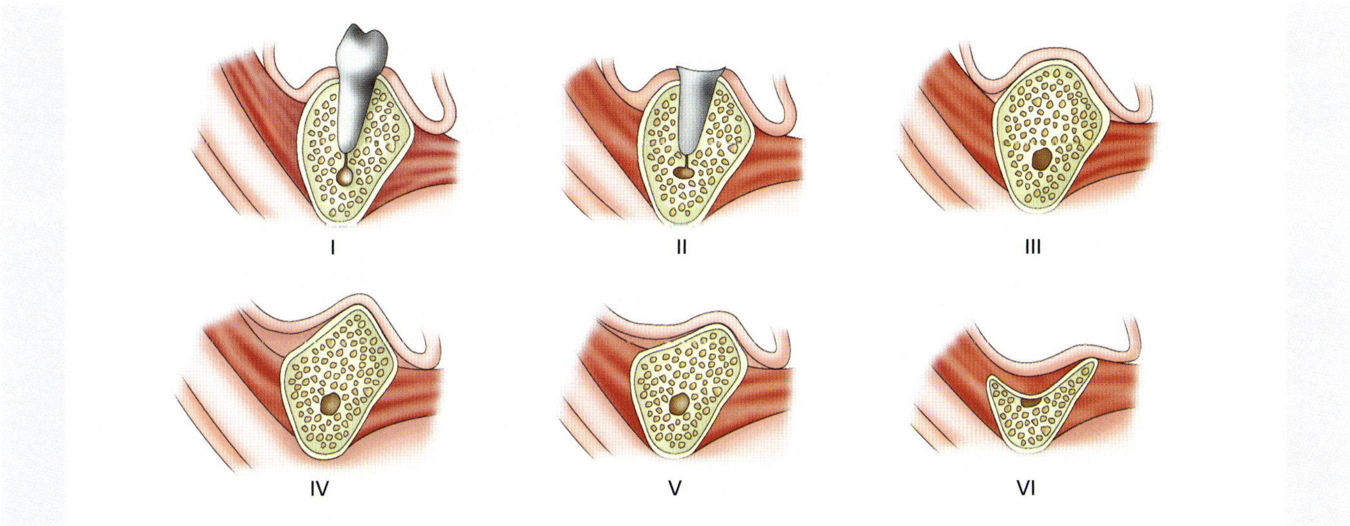

11.10 Musculoskeletal alterations according to Cawood and Howell classification.

Clinical examination: analysis of signs and symptoms

The treatment plan for the correction of hard and soft tissue defects of the jaws for preprosthetic purposes must not only take into account the altered local morphology, but should also include an accurate evaluation of the benefits achievable with surgery. Functional and aesthetic expectations of the patient must be adequately considered, and compared to the results that the planned treatment may achieve. Preoperative planning includes an accurate anamnesis aimed at highlighting possible local or systemic contraindications to the surgical treatment and a thorough intra and extraoral evaluation.

Extraoral examination allows assessment of possible dysmorphisms caused by edentulism and bone atrophy to the facial and perioral muscles, and the sagittal, vertical and transverse intermaxillary relationships.

Intraoral examination is performed with the methods of traditional semiology, particularly inspection and palpation. Palpation should involve the entire area of the alveolar crest to discover possible irregularities of the hard and soft tissues that may interfere with the planned prosthetic rehabilitation, such as bone undercuts and flabby ridges.

Instrumental screening

The panoramic radiograph allows the morphology of both mandible and maxilla to be evaluated, particularly the vertical bone modifications, while it is not suitable for the evaluation of horizontal bone defects or sagittal discrepancies.

The lateral cephalometric radiograph may be useful for evaluating, on both the vertical and anterior-posterior planes, possible alterations of the anatomy of the jaws and of their relationships, as well as modifications of the facial profile; on the other hand, superimposition of the left and right sides of the maxilla and mandible represents the main limit of this examination.

Computed tomography, particularly when a tridimensional reconstruction is performed with the aid of medical image processing software, is certainly able to provide the most information regarding both the hard and soft tissues (11.11).

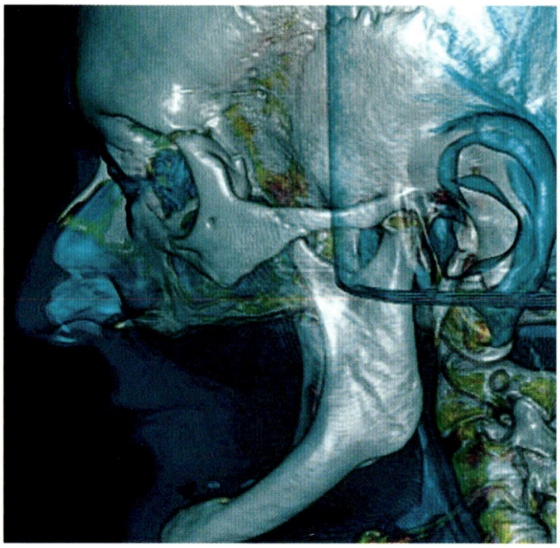

11.11 Tridimensional reconstruction and rendering of the face: specific filters allow both hard and soft tissues to be highlighted.

Radiographic examinations

Type	Advantages	Disadvantages
Panoramic radiograph	Good overall view of the jawbones	Impossible to evaluate sagittal and transverse defects
Lateral cephalometric radiograph	Good evaluation of anatomic alterations, of the intermaxillary relationships, and of the facial profile, both in the vertical and anteroposterior aspects.	Superimposition of the two profiles
Computed tomography	Complete tridimensional information	Higher radiation dose Higher economic costs

Clinical presentations

Different clinical presentations requiring surgical treatment can be observed, that are a consequence of:

- atrophy of the soft tissues;
- atrophy of the hard tissues;
- post-traumatic iatrogenic bone defects (e.g. tooth extraction with fracture and/or removal of portions of alveolar bone);
- neoplasms of the hard tissues, such as maxillary and mandibular exostoses (tori);
- neoplasms of the soft tissues;
- presence of dislocating frenula.

Soft tissue atrophy sequelae

Flabby ridges: when resorption of the alveolar ridge occurs more rapidly than atrophy of the overlying soft tissues, a relative excess of soft tissues is observed. As these crests of mucosa have no bone support, they are mobile with respect to the alveolar crest; therefore, they represent an unstable base for any removable prosthesis, and surgical correction is often necessary. As far as the maxilla is concerned, frequently involved areas include the molar region and the anterior buccal vestibule, while for the mandible the interforaminal region is often interested (11.12).

Fibrous hyperplasia: it represents a hypertrophic-hyperplastic response of the mucosa and submucosa to a chronic irritative stimulus caused by the friction exerted by unstable and/or incongruous removable prostheses.

Hyperplastic formations appear as mobile flanges of folded soft tissue that can reach considerable dimensions, and interfere with the stability of removable prostheses (11.13).

In the presence of ulcerated lesions, it is indicated to retrieve a bioptic sample and perform histologic examination of the collected specimen, to exclude the possibility of malignant degeneration in the form of squamous cell carcinoma.

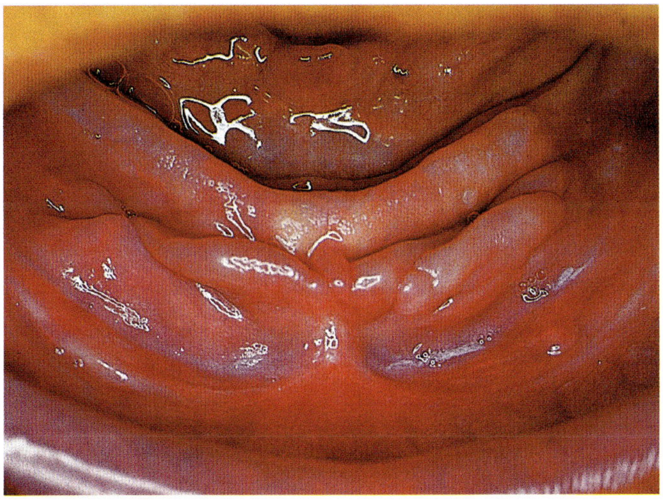

11.12 Mandibular flabby ridge in a totally edentulous patient.

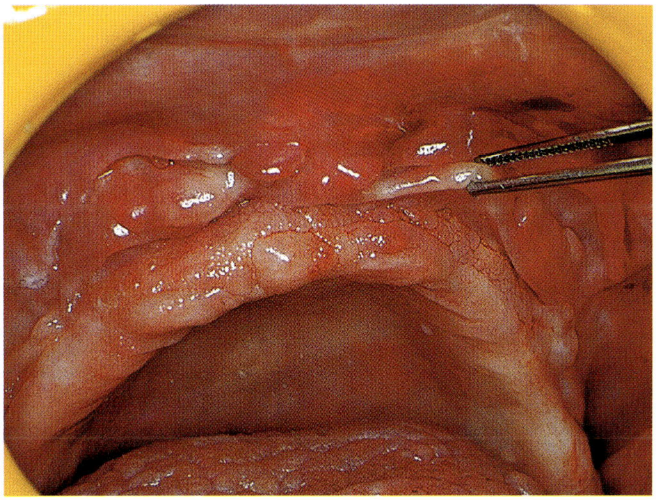

11.13 Fibrous hyperplasia of the maxillary alveolar mucosa.

Tuber maxillae hyperplasia: in some patients, hyperplasia-hypertrophy of the palatal connective tissue in the molar and retromolar area may be observed. The hyperplastic tissue has the same colour of the normal palatal mucosa, a hard-elastic consistency, and can exhibit a considerable development towards the midline in the palate, and distally towards the tonsil pillar.

In the bilateral forms, an almost complete obliteration of the palatal vault may occur (11.14). These lesions may render the prosthetic rehabilitation difficult or impossible.

Hard tissue atrophy sequelae

Irregular morphology of the alveolar ridges: the presence of irregularities of the alveolar ridges, such as acute angles or knife-edge profile (Cawood and Howell class IV atrophy), may cause painful decubiti and ulcerations of the overlying soft tissues in patients wearing removable prostheses (11.15, 11.16a-b).

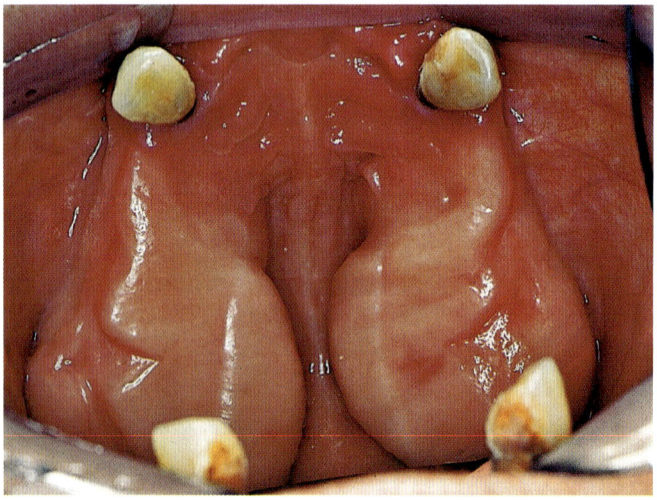

11.14 Tuber maxillae hyperplasia.

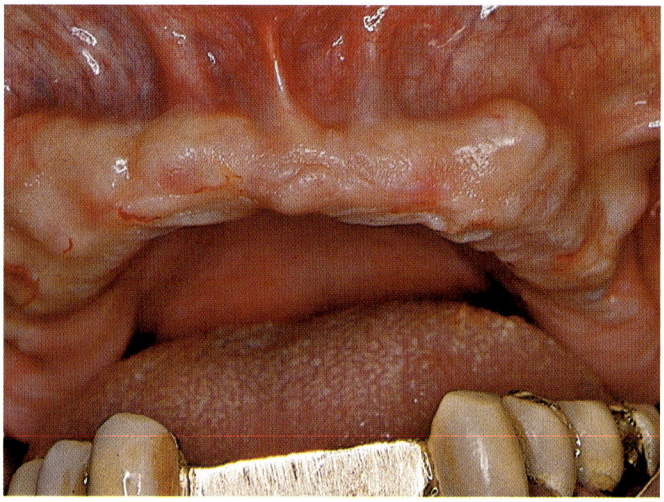

11.15 Irregular maxillary alveolar ridge: exostoses and undercuts are incompatible with a removable prosthetic rehabilitation.

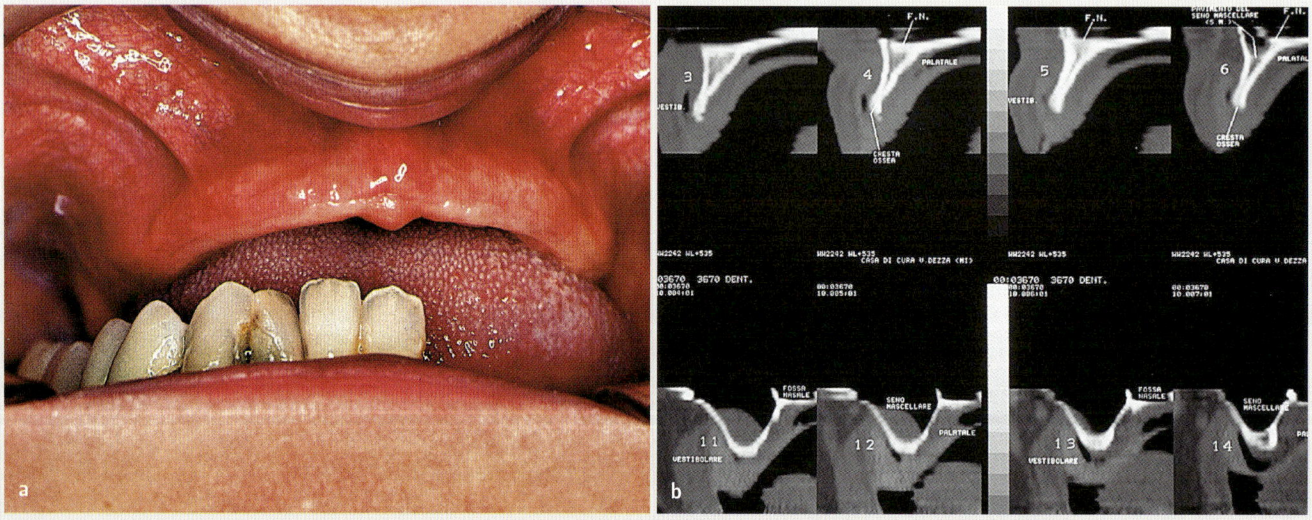

11.16 Knife-edge alveolar ridge (Cawood and Howell class IV): **a)** clinical appearance; **b)** radiographic appearance.

Severe tridimensional bone resorption (Cawood and Howell class V-VI defects): extensive bone atrophy may cause the partial or total disappearance of the alveolar ridges and both the vestibular and lingual fornix, with a subsequent reduction of the mechanical retention offered to removable prostheses. This problem is particularly evident with complete mandibular edentulism, because the movements of the mandible and tongue during phonation, chewing, swallowing, etc. emphasise the instability of the prosthesis. In the maxilla, severe bone atrophy causes flattening of the palatal vault and reduction of the retrotuberal undercut, jeopardising the retention of the removable prostheses (11.17a-b).

Post-traumatic and post-extractive defects

Dentoalveolar trauma, as well as inappropriate manoeuvres during tooth extraction, may be associated with loss of alveolar bone and/or healing of malpositioned bone fragments, and may result in morphologic alterations of the alveolar ridges, either in the form of bone defects or in the form of exostoses, with subsequent functional and/or aesthetic sequelae, particularly in the anterior regions of the jaws (11.18).

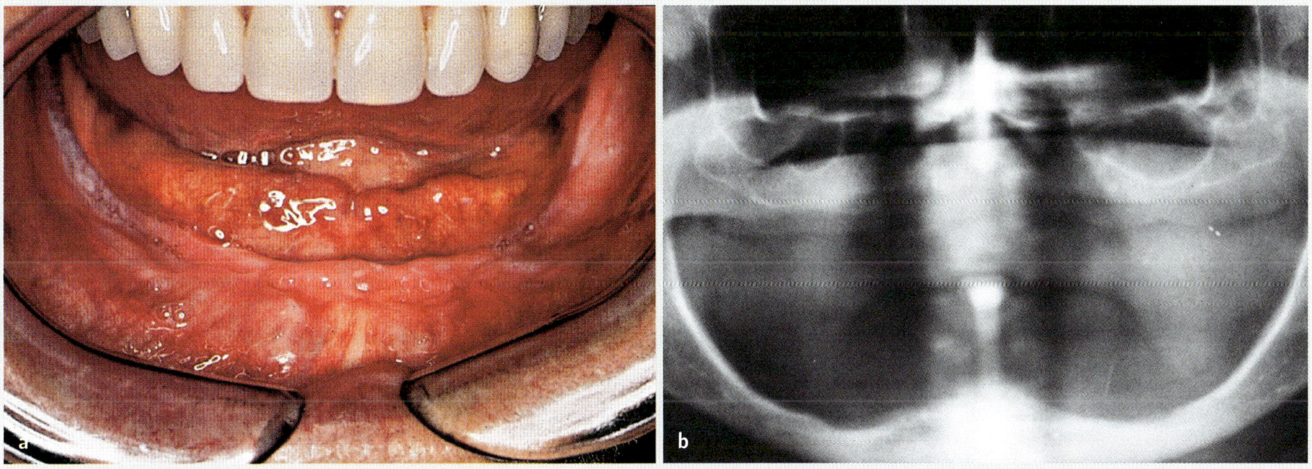

11.17 a) Severe vertical resorption: the buccal fornix and lingual sulcus have disappeared. **b)** Panoramic radiograph shows significant bone resorption.

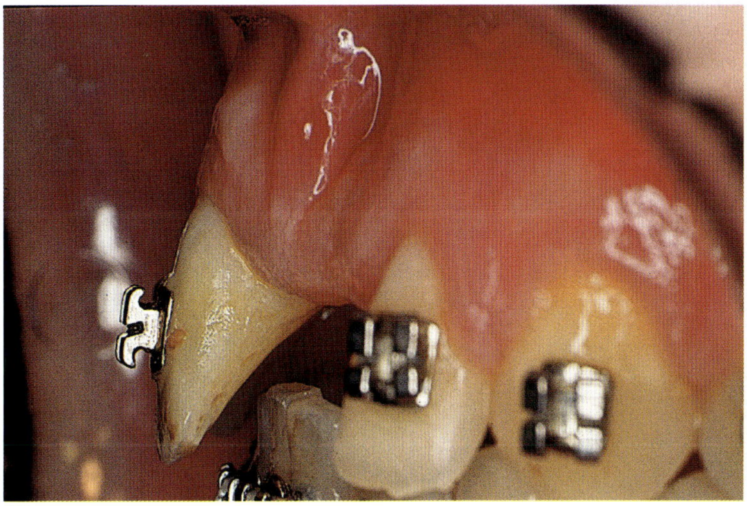

11.18 Traumatic extraction sequelae: compromised aesthetics.

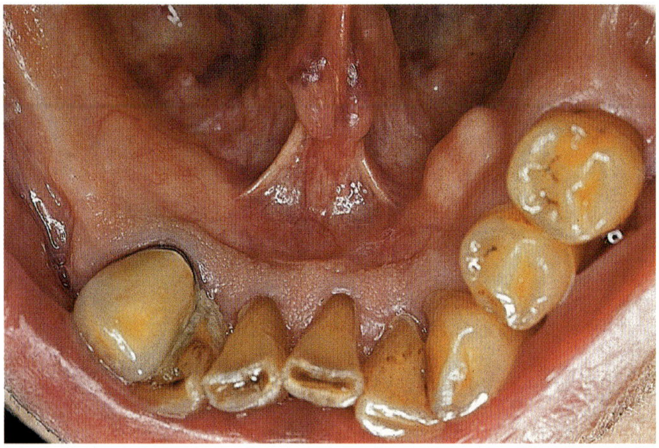

11.19 Exostosis (torus) on the lingual side of the mandible.

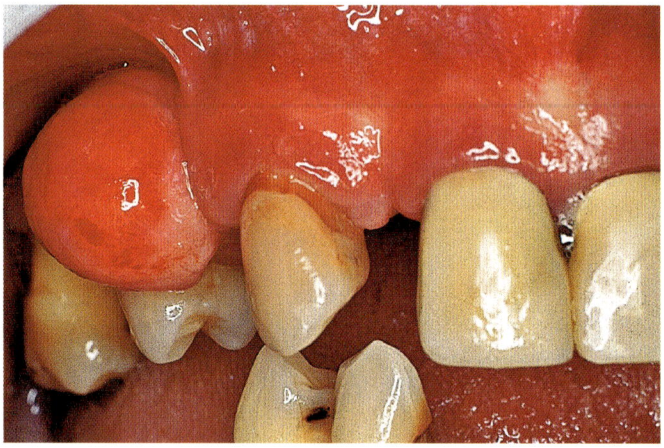

11.20 The presence of a giant cell epulis prevents the fabrication of a removable prosthesis.

Neoplasms of the hard tissues

Apart from proper benign tumours such as osteomas (see Chapter 9), one of the most frequent neoplasms of the jaws is the *torus* (plur. *tori*). The tori are exostoses, and their growth is typically self-limiting; nonetheless, they may interfere with maxillary and mandibular removable prostheses. They show a gender predilection for females (incidence is double that found in males), and the most frequent localisations are the palate (along the midline) and the lingual side of the mandible, laterally to the midline. From a histologic point of view, the tori are formed by mature bone with a significant development of the cortical layer; clinically, they appear as a hard swelling covered by a normal mucosa (11.19). Only if incongruous mechanical stimuli exerted by removable prostheses are present, the overlying mucosa may manifest signs of inflammation and can present ulcerations.

Neoplasms of the soft tissues

Apart from flabby ridges and fibrous hyperplasia, benign lesions such as fibropapillomas, epulides, angiomas etc. may render the use of removable prostheses difficult or impossible (11.20) (a detailed description of these lesions is reported in Chapter 9).

Frenula

Apart from the labial and lingual frenula described in the first section of this chapter, other frenula can be present on the buccal side of the maxilla and mandible; due to their dimensions and/or proximity to the alveolar ridge, they may contribute to the dislocation of removable prostheses. The surgical protocol for their excision is the same as previously described for the treatment of labial and lingual frenula.

Treatment

The most common surgical procedures that can be performed under local anaesthesia will be described in detail, while complex procedures requiring general anaesthesia will be briefly summarised. It is worth noting that these procedures, albeit following the general principles illustrated in Chapter 3, require additional precautions due to the local condition of the involved tissues and their vascularisation. Minor preprosthetic surgery, in fact, is frequently performed on older patients, whose tissues are generally more fragile, less vascularised, and take longer to heal.

In particular:

- in *young patients*, the maxilla and mandible receive both an endosteal vascularisation provided by alveolar arterial branches, and a periosteal vascularisation provided by perforating vessels;
- in *older patients*, periosteal vascularisation is maintained while *a significant reduction of the endosteal blood supply* is observed (11.21a-b).

Surgical techniques

SOFT TISSUES

Surgical procedures for the correction of the soft tissues include:

- flabby ridges excision;
- fibrous hyperplasia excision;
- vestibuloplasty;
- reduction of the maxillary tuberosity;
- frenula excision (described in the first section of this Chapter).

Surgical armamentarium

Basic surgical armamentarium should include thin retractors and dissecting scissors, to provide better control during soft tissues excision.

Locoregional anaesthesia

It follows the same principles as those described in Chapter 3.

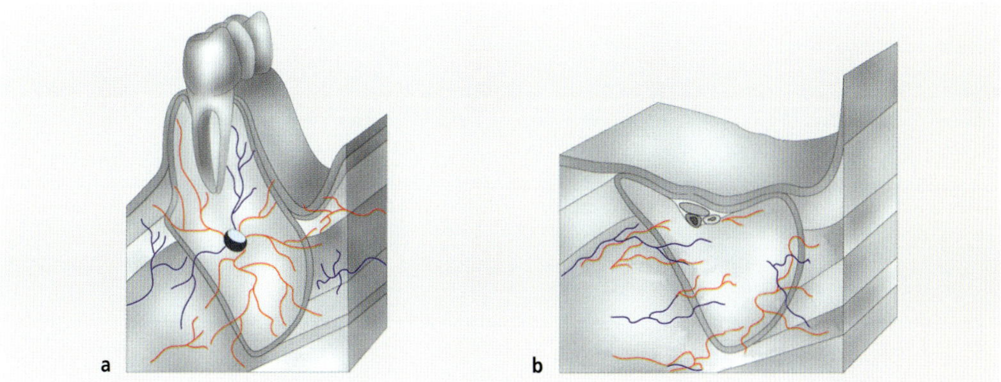

11.21 Vascularisation of the jaws: **a)** young patient; **b)** older patient.

HARD TISSUES

Surgical procedures for the correction of the soft tissues include:

- horizontal reduction alveoloplasty;
- intraseptal alveoloplasty;
- vertical reduction alveoloplasty;
- exostoses (tori) removal;
- correction of post-extractive and post-traumatic defects.

It is worth noting that, due to the widespread diffusion of implant therapy in the last decades, minor prosthetic surgery procedures are rarely indicated today.

Basic techniques – Soft tissues

Flabby ridges excision

This surgical procedure allows removal of a portion of the soft tissues that is not supported by bone; however, it should be considered that this implies the loss of residual keratinised gingiva, thus exposing to the prosthetic load the thin alveolar mucosa. Particularly for Cawood and Howell class IV alveolar ridges, this choice may expose the area to a high risk of decubitus ulcers. In these cases, when complex reconstructive surgery (autologous bone grafting) is not an option, vestibuloplasty or subperiosteal positioning of alloplastic materials (such as hydroxylapatite) without soft tissue reduction may be preferable. On the other hand, indications to this latter surgical procedure have significantly decreased over the years, both due to the evolution and diffusion of endosseous implants, and to the instability of the alloplastic material that migrates under prosthetic load, thus nullifying the initial result. Moreover, the presence of the alloplastic granules may further increase the risk of decubitus ulcers and perforation of the overlying soft tissues with graft exposure and infection.

Two full-thickness incisions are made lingually and buccally to isolate the flabby tissue, which is then gently separated from the underlying bone with the aid of a periosteal elevator. The margins of the surgical wound are then sutured to allow healing by primary intention. When concomitant vestibuloplasty is indicated, a partial-thickness incision and elevation of the buccal side of the flap is performed, and the buccal margin of the surgical wound is moved apically to be sutured to the periosteum. Healing occurs by secondary intention; if it is necessary, a free keratinised mucosa graft can be sutured to the exposed periosteum (11-22a-f).

It is worth remembering that, with severe atrophy, notable anatomical structures may be relatively superficial (particularly if reference points such as the centre of the alveolar ridge are considered). Therefore, errors in the evaluation of the local anatomy and/or in the surgical manoeuvres may cause a high risk of intraoperative complications.

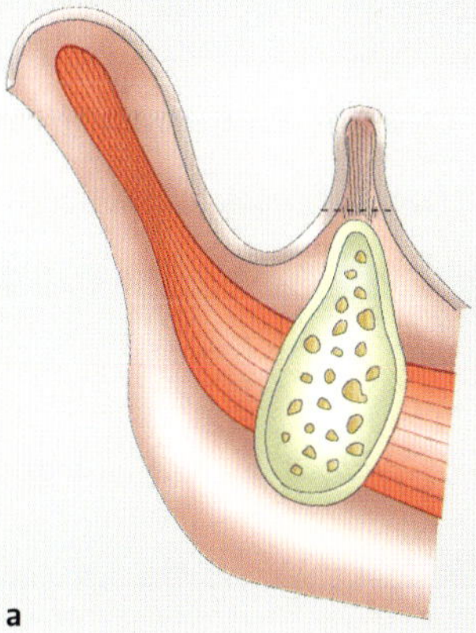

a

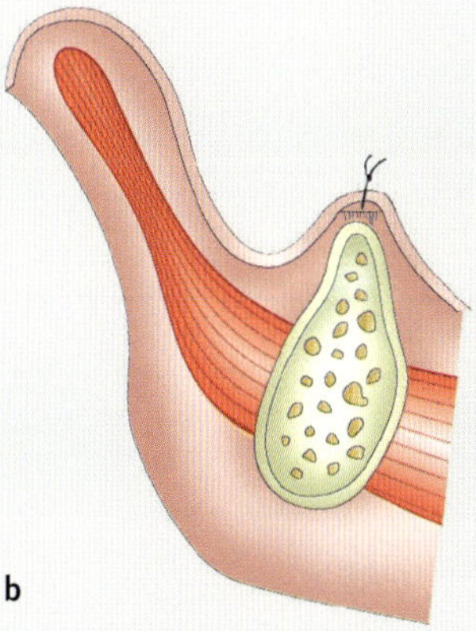

b

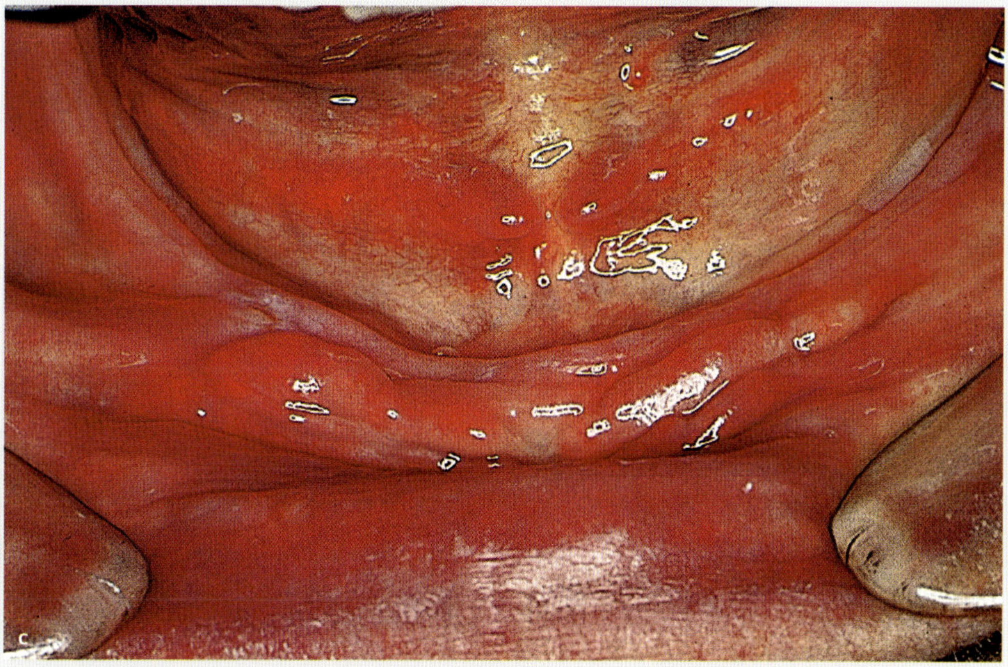

c

11.22 a) Flabby ridges removal: incision. **b)** Excision. **c)** Initial clinical situation: presence of a flabby ridge on the alveolar crest. (*continued*)

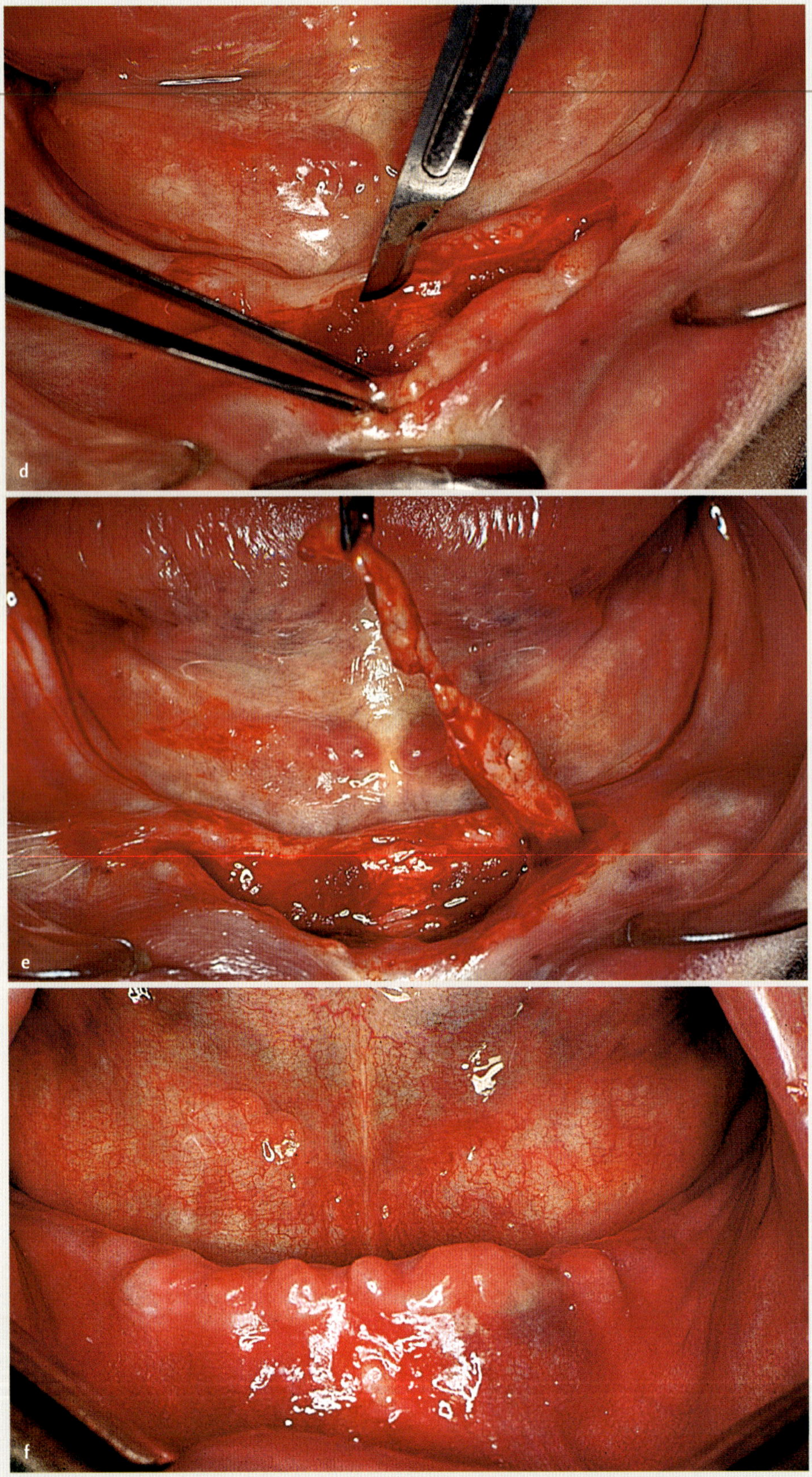

11.22 (*continued*) **d)** Lozenge-shaped incision. **e)** Excision of the unsupported soft tissue crest. **f)** Clinical follow-up (vestibuloplasty was performed in conjunction with flabby ridge excision).

Fibrous hyperplasia excision

An epiperiosteal incision is made to isolate the hyperplastic tissues from the surrounding mucosa. After excision is completed with the aid of a scalpel or dissecting scissors, the surgical wound may be left to heal by secondary intention. If the depth of the fornix is reduced, vestibuloplasty can be performed in conjunction with the excision of the hyperplastic tissues; in this case, the superficial muscle fibres are sectioned and then sutured apically to the periosteal layer. If the extent of the resulting surgical wound is limited, healing by secondary intention can be achieved. However, the risk of prompt reduction of the fornix depth is significant; therefore, it is indicated to suture a free keratinised mucosa graft on the exposed periosteal layer (11-23a-f).

In the majority of cases, the diagnosis of these conditions can be based solely on clinical data; however, if inflammation and/or ulceration of the soft tissues are present, it is recommended to perform an incisional biopsy prior to the excision of the hyperplastic tissues. Histologic examination of the tissue sample is essential to excluding the neoplastic nature of the lesion (e.g. squamous cell carcinoma).

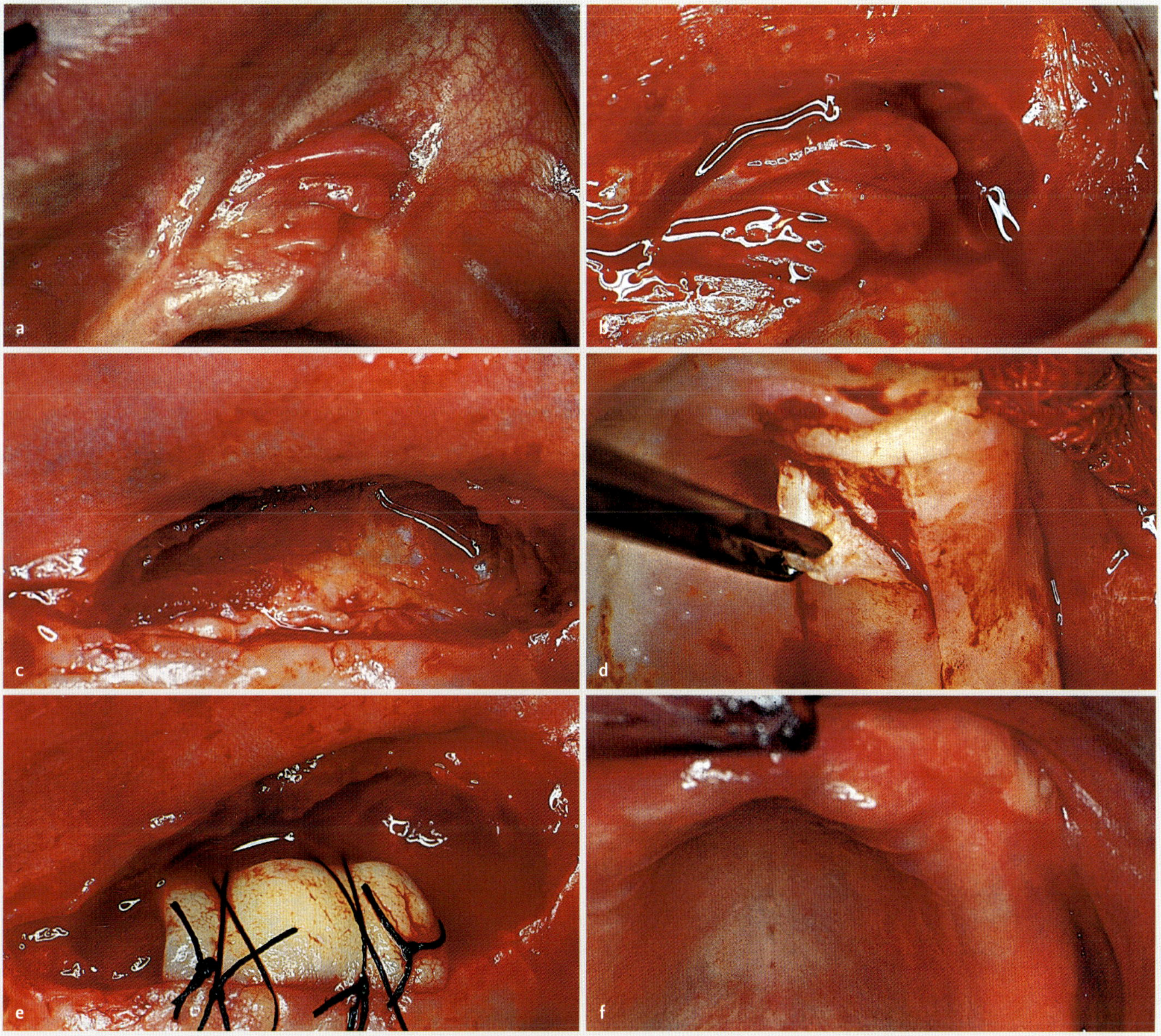

11.23 **a)** Initial clinical situation. **b)** Epiperiosteal incision isolating the hyperplastic tissues. **c)** Surgical wound after the excision of the hyperplastic tissues, and the epiperiosteal dissection of muscle insertions. **d)** Harvesting of a free keratinised mucosa graft from the palate. **e)** Fixation of the graft. **f)** Clinical follow-up: appearance of the treated area 6 months after surgery.

Vestibuloplasty

Vestibuloplasty is indicated when the alveolar ridge is atrophied to the point where a significant reduction of the fornix depth is present, and muscle insertions are thus relatively superficial; satisfactory results can be achieved only if adequate residual height of the alveolar ridge is preserved. The surgical procedure begins with an epiperiosteal incision of the soft tissues: partial-thickness elevation of the surgical flap allows the interruption of the insertions of the most coronal muscle fibres and their apical repositioning. The area in which the periosteum is exposed can be left to heal by secondary intention. However, the risk of reduction of the fornix depth due to coronal migration of the muscle insertions is significant; therefore, it is indicated to suture a palatal keratinised mucosa graft on the exposed periosteal layer to prevent the possibility of relapse. Free skin grafts, once widely used in these cases, now have limited indications due to the quality of the tissue, which is not suitable for the oral environment. While no relevant anatomic structures are present on the buccal side of the maxilla, with severe mandibular resorption it is imperative that the relative position of the mental foramina be considered, the latter of which may be found near the top of the residual alveolar crest or, in cases of extreme resorption, in the centre of the ridge. Consequently, vestibuloplasty in the premolar area may not be always feasible, as it would inevitably lead to nerve damage and subsequent permanent anaesthesia of the lip and chin regions. In the other areas of the mandible, vestibuloplasty can be performed following the general principles previously described (11.24a–f).

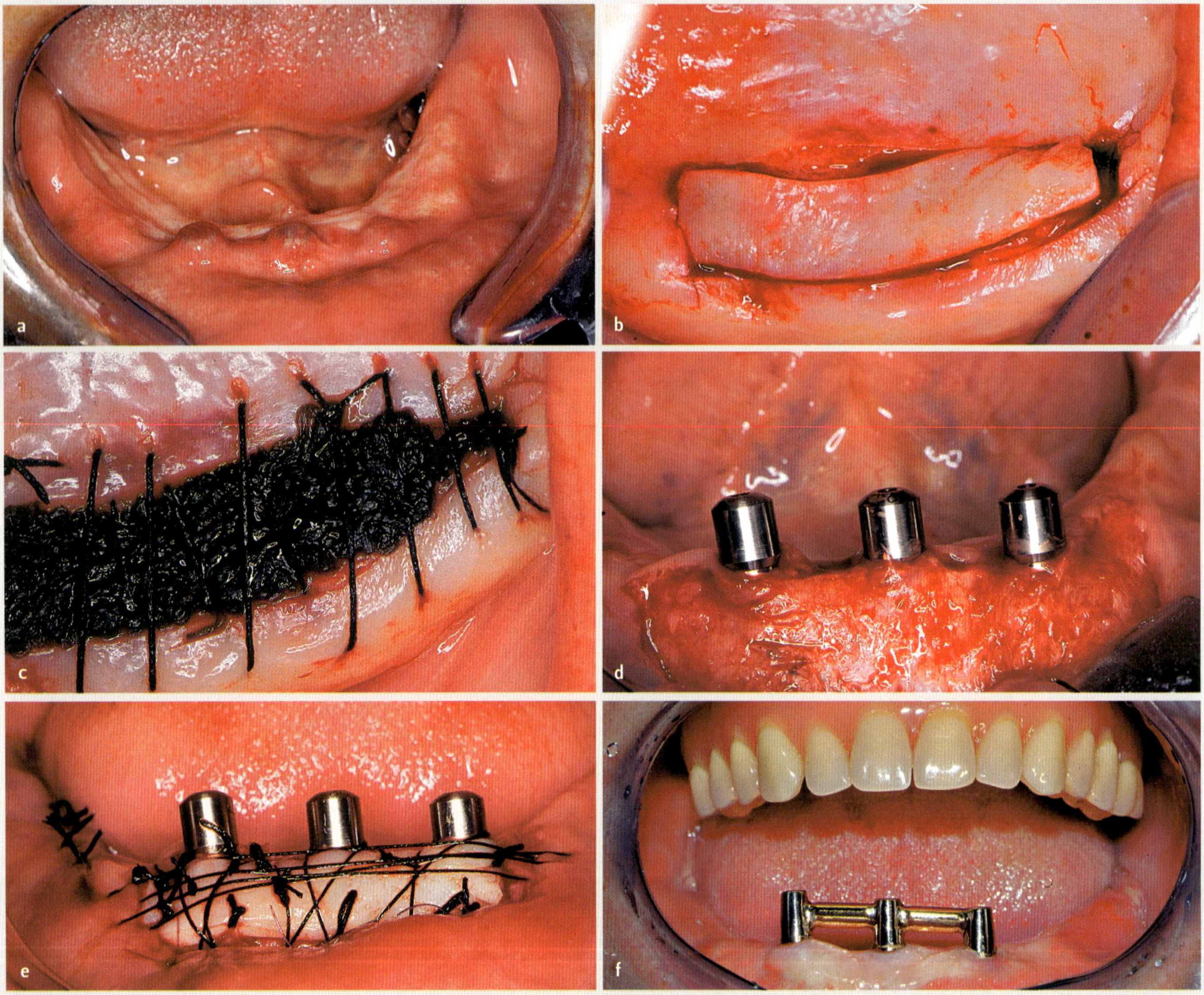

11.24 **a)** Peri-implant keratinised mucosa graft. Initial clinical situation: total absence of keratinised mucosa is evident around three submerged implants. **b)** Keratinised mucosa is harvested from the palate. **c)** Protection of the donor site by means of resorbable haemostatic material stabilised with a continuous suture. **d)** A split-thickness flap is raised and a recipient bed is created (healing abutments are connected to the implants). **e)** The keratinised mucosa graft is fixed to the recipient bed by means of non-resorbable sutures. **f)** Clinical follow-up.

An alternative, albeit rarely used today, technique for mandibular vestibuloplasty is the Edlan procedure. In the interforaminal region, a split-thickness flap is raised on the labial mucosa: the flap is separated from the underlying muscles and sutured apically after an epiperiosteal recipient bed is prepared in the mental region, and the exposed labial surface is left to heal by secondary intention. Theoretically, this technique could be used also for the maxilla (11.25a–b). Whenever an apical repositioning of the lingual sulcus is necessary, it is crucial to remember that, due to the presence of notable anatomic structures in the area (particularly, branches of the sublingual and mylohyoid artery), the procedure should not be performed under local anaesthesia, and generally falls outside the duties of the oral surgeon. The technique, proposed by Trauner in 1952, entails a partial-thickness incision and elevation of the soft tissues on the lingual side of the mandible, and the lingual reflection of the flap. Once exposed, the most superficial insertions of the genioglossus and mylohyoid muscles are sectioned by means of a diathermic knife to reduce bleeding; the mucosa of the floor of the mouth and muscle insertions are then kept in an apical position with the aid of transcutaneous osteosynthesis wires fixed in place with surgical buttons. The periosteum covering the most coronal portion of the lingual side of the mandible is left exposed, and the area undergoes healing by secondary intention. It is worth remembering that this technique, used in the past for total edentulism with extreme mandibular atrophy, is rarely indicated today, due to the widespread use of endosseous implants.

Reduction of maxillary tuberosity

The excision of hyperplastic tissue alone is not sufficient to correct the alteration of the local anatomy, because the soft tissues are excessively thick. Therefore, submucosal connective tissue is removed from both sides of the surgical wound with the aid of a scalpel: this makes it possible to reduce the thickness while preserving the integrity of the mucosa. Branches of the major palatine artery may be involved in this manoeuvre, but the resulting bleeding may be controlled by means of bipolar coagulation. Once the planned reduction is obtained, the mucosa is sutured to obtain healing by primary intention. However, it is imperative that excessive reduction be avoided, as this may result in an unfavourable alteration of the tuber anatomy with subsequent prosthesis instability (11.26a–g).

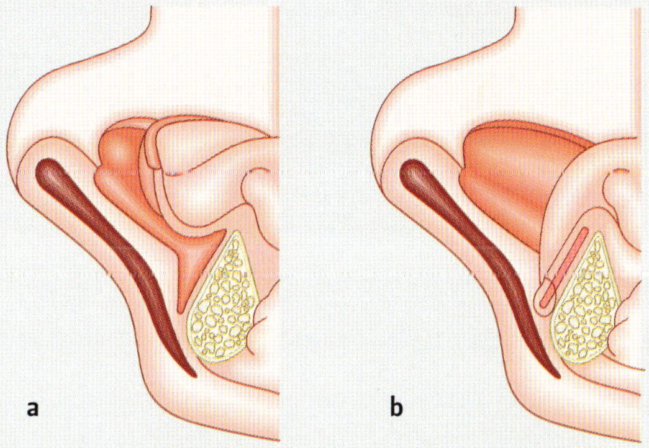

11.25 a) Vestibuloplasty according to Edlan: elevation of a labial mucosal flap and epiperiosteal dissection of the mental muscle. **b)** The flap is sutured apically, on the bottom of the newly created fornix.

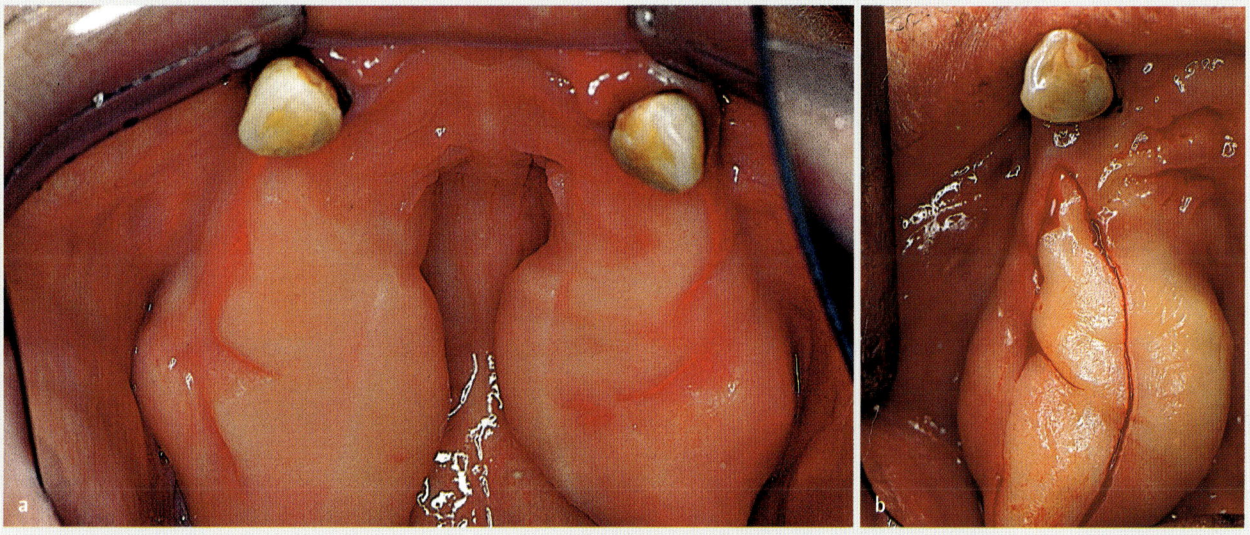

11.26 a) Reduction of tuber maxillae hyperplasia. Initial clinical situation: extensive bilateral hyperplasia of the maxillary tuberosities. **b)** Lozenge-shaped incision of the mucosa. (*continued*)

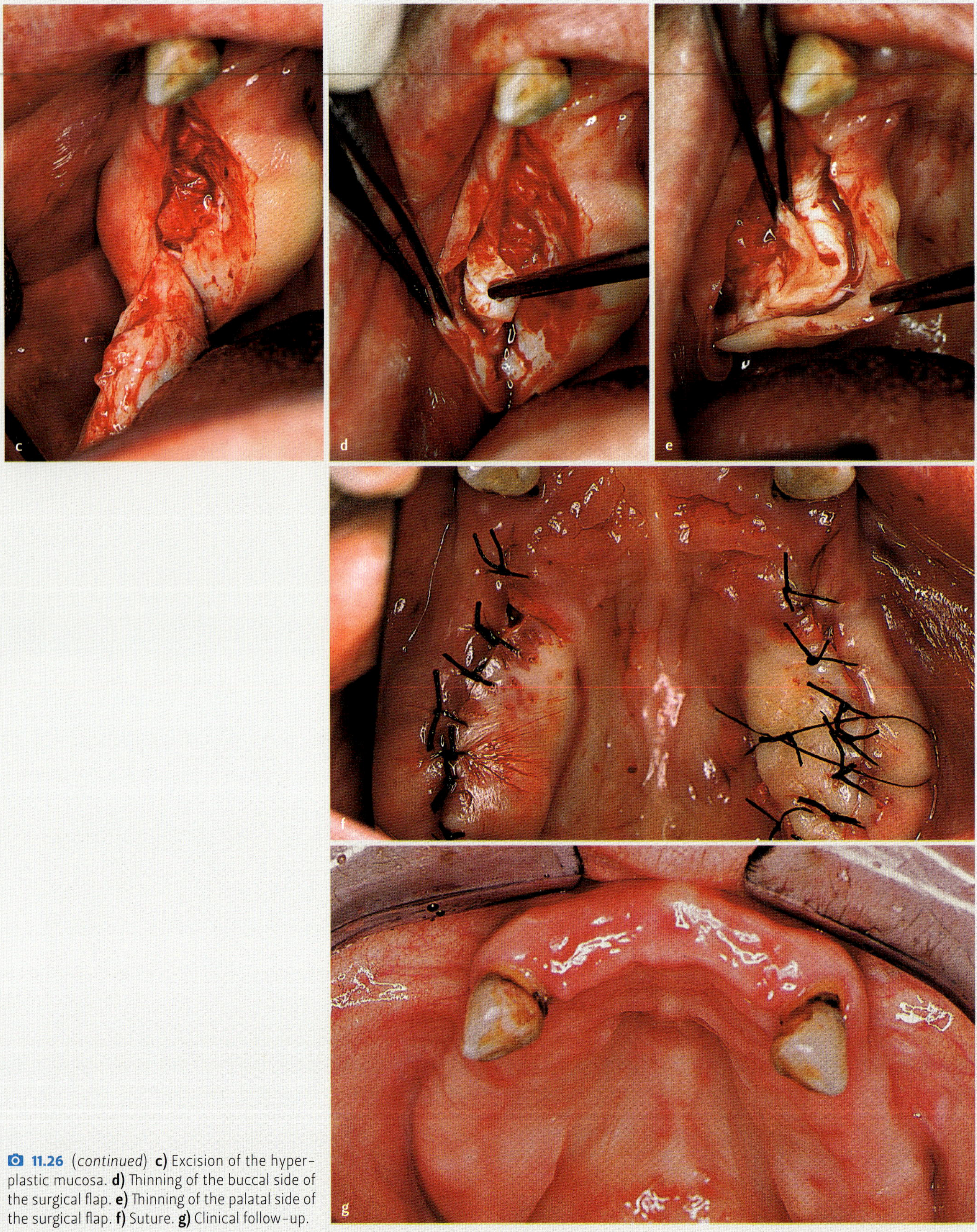

11.26 (*continued*) **c)** Excision of the hyperplastic mucosa. **d)** Thinning of the buccal side of the surgical flap. **e)** Thinning of the palatal side of the surgical flap. **f)** Suture. **g)** Clinical follow-up.

Basic techniques – Hard tissues

Alveoloplasty (horizontal reduction)

Whenever the buccal cortical plate of the alveolar ridges presents irregularities, such as protuberances causing undercuts that render the use of removable prostheses impossible, alveoloplasty for horizontal bone reduction is indicated. A full-thickness incision and elevation of the surgical flap is performed to allow adequate exposure of the underlying alveolar crest. Correction of the bone protuberances may be performed with bone burs mounted on a straight handpiece, with specifically designed piezoelectric instruments, or with bone rongeurs and files. After profuse irrigation of the surgical field with sterile saline, the soft tissues are repositioned on the alveolar ridge to evaluate a possible excess that, if necessary, should be removed with great care to limit the loss of keratinised mucosa as much as possible. A thorough palpation of the alveolar crest is a useful means to assess the suitability of the new bone morphology (11.27a–e).

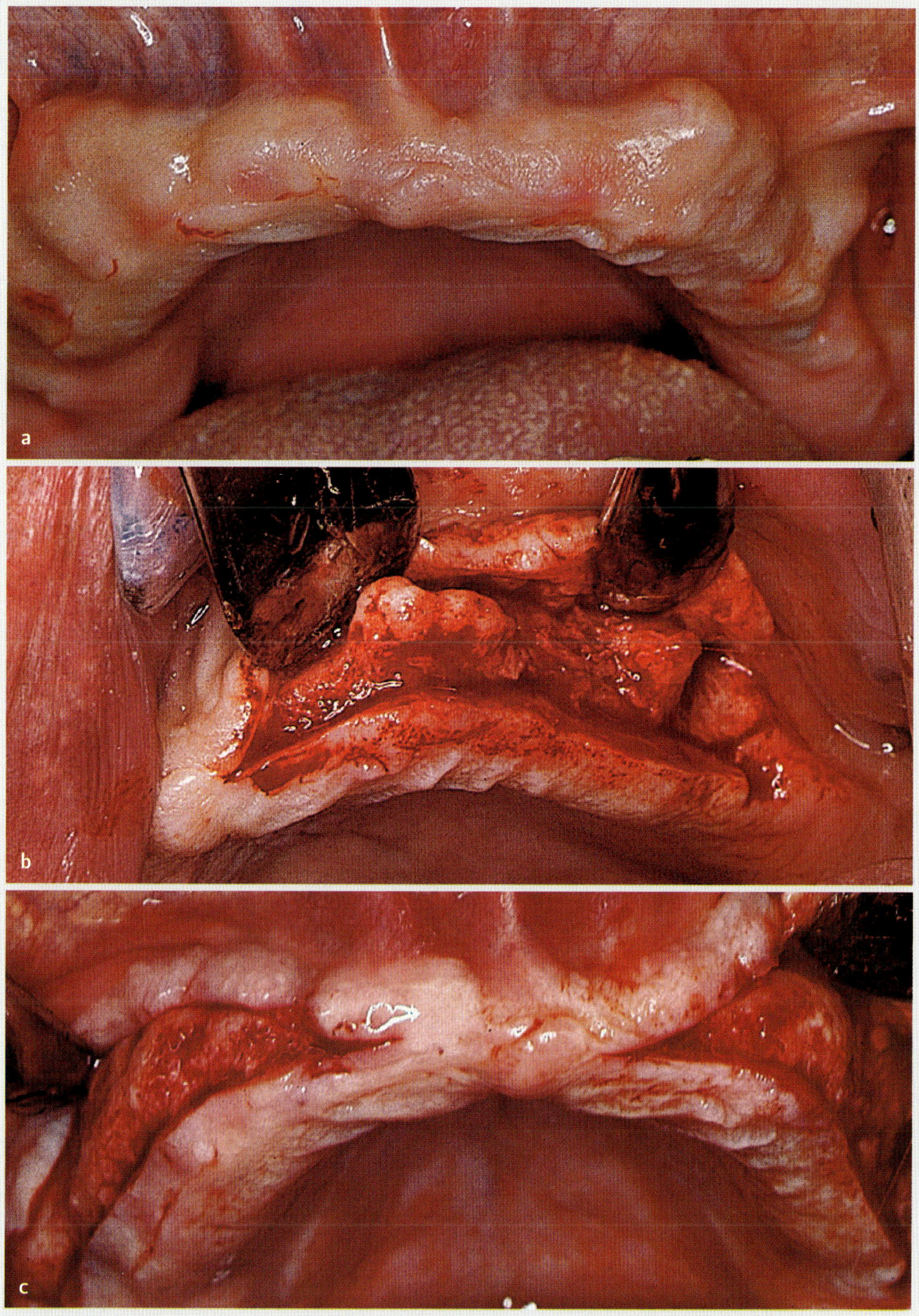

11.27 **a)** Buccal alveoloplasty. Exostoses and undercuts are incompatible with a removable prosthetic rehabilitation. **b)** Crestal incision and exposure of the buccal cortical plate. **c)** Clinical appearance of the alveolar crest after the elimination of the exostoses with a bone bur. (*continued*)

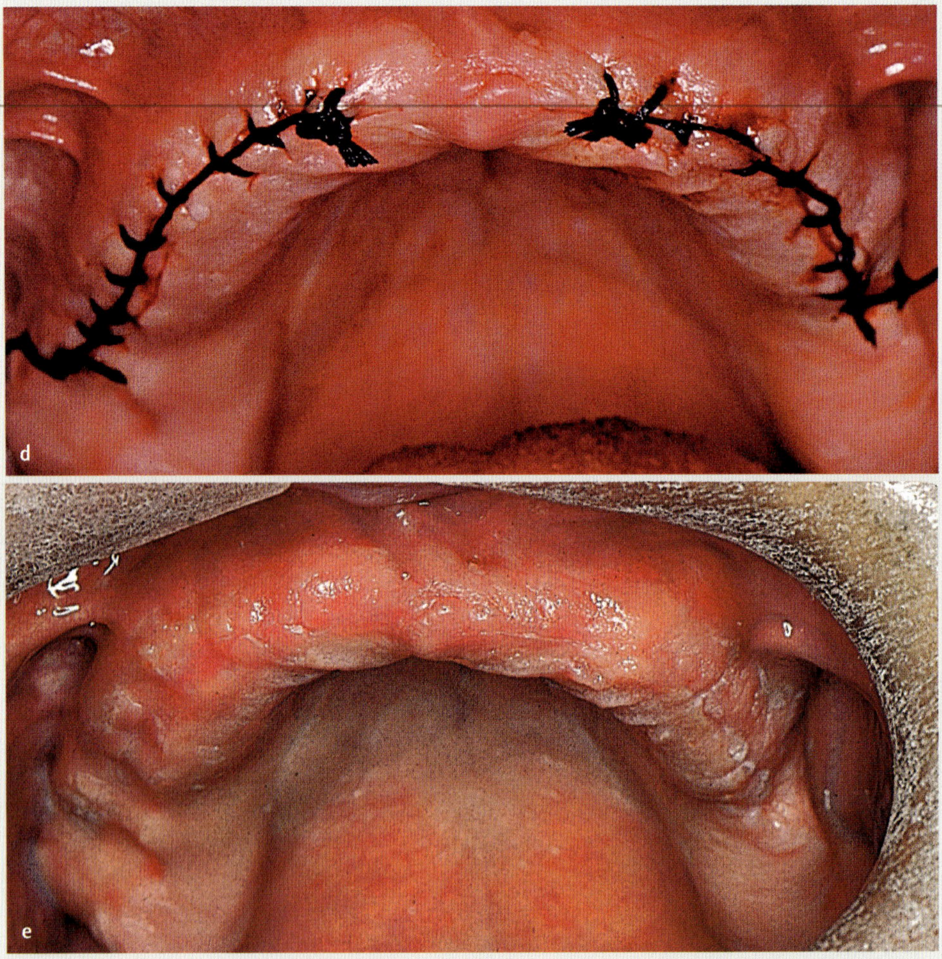

11.27 *(continued)* **d)** Suture. **e)** Clinical follow-up.

Intraseptal alveoloplasty

In the past, when tooth extractions were performed in patients presenting significant undercuts of the alveolar ridges, intraseptal alveoloplasty was performed to obtain a reduction of the width of the crests. However, in the last decades, widespread use of endosseous implants has significantly reduced its indications, due to the resulting reduction of the available bone volume. Therefore, it may only be indicated if a removable prosthetic rehabilitation is planned.

After tooth extractions are completed, a full-thickness incision of the soft tissues is performed; elevation of the surgical flap should be limited to the coronal portion of the alveolar ridge. Interalveolar septa are eliminated with a bone rongeur, while possible irregularities are corrected with rotary or piezoelectric instruments, or with bone files. A "greenstick fracture" of the buccal cortical plate is produced by manual compression of the alveolar ridge; wound margins are then sutured to allow healing by primary intention (11.28a–d).

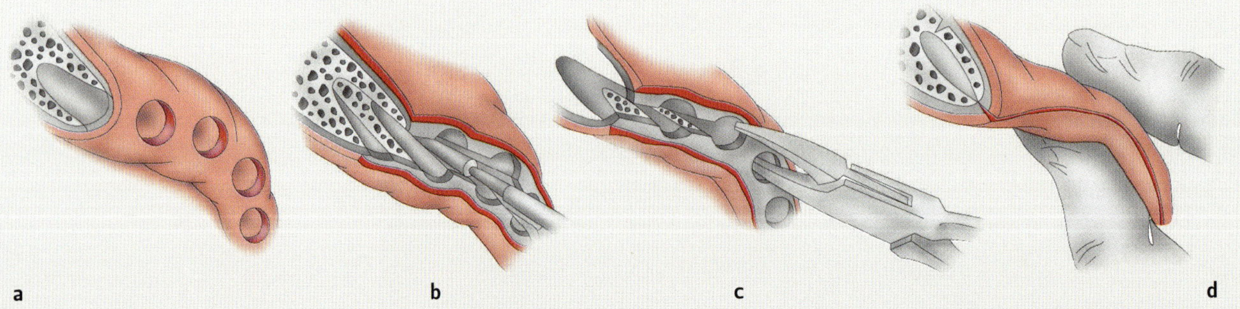

11.28 **a)** Intraseptal alvoloplasty: tooth extractions. **b–c)** Removal of the interdental septa with a bone bur or bone rongeur. **d)** Manual compression of the alveolar ridge.

Alveoloplasty (vertical reduction)

This technique is indicated when the height of the alveolar ridge is preserved but horizontal bone resorption has caused a knife-edge profile (Cawood and Howell class IV), which can cause decubitus ulcers on the mucosa in patients wearing removable prostheses. However, care must be taken in the vertical reduction of the alveolar crest to avoid excessive bone removal, which may result in a significant reduction of the fornix depth. Vertical remodelling can be performed in conjunction with tooth extraction, when the irregular morphology of the edentulous ridge may interfere with the following prosthetic rehabilitation. Unlike other minor preprosthetic surgery procedures, which saw a drastic reduction of their indications with the advent of endosseous implants, the recourse to alveoloplasty for vertical reduction still retains a specific indication, particularly when implant placement in the interforaminal area of the mandible is planned for the rehabilitation of complete mandibular edentulism. In fact, notwithstanding the atrophy of the edentulous ridge, the residual bone volume available in this area is generally sufficient to harbour implants of adequate dimensions; moreover, alveoloplasty eliminates the need for complex reconstructive procedures, thus reducing the economical and biological costs of the treatment. On the other hand, the recourse to this procedure for the vertical correction of the alveolar ridge in the posterior areas of the maxilla and mandible is not indicated, due to the risk of an excessive reduction of the distance between the superior margin of the alveolar crest and important anatomic structures such as the inferior alveolar nerve, the maxillary sinus, and the nasal cavity.

A full-thickness incision of the soft tissues along the centre of the alveolar ridge is performed, and the surgical flap is cleaved from the underlying bone with the aid of a periosteal elevator. The exposed alveolar crest is modelled with rotary instruments (a large bone bur mounted on a straight handpiece); excision of soft tissues in excess must be evaluated with great care, to avoid unnecessary loss of keratinised mucosa. Palpation of the alveolar crest allows the suitability of the new bone morphology to be assessed before suturing the surgical wound (11.29a–d).

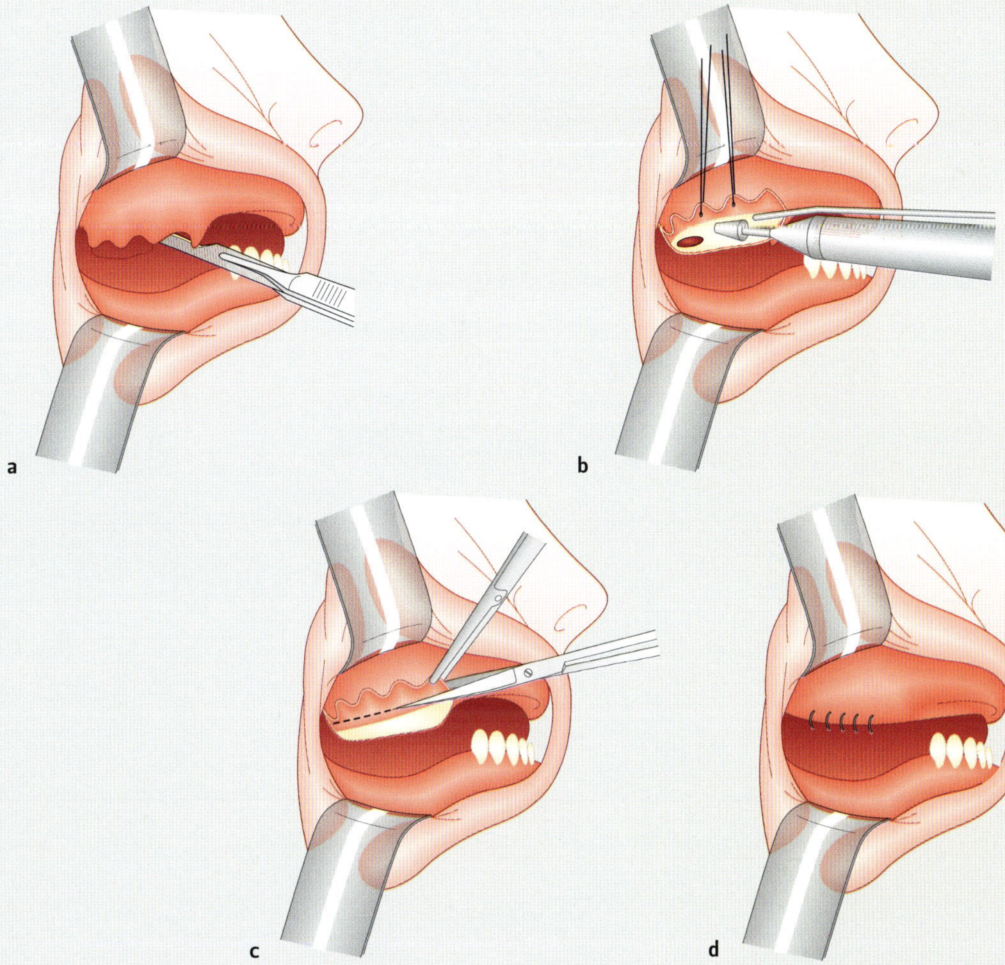

11.29 **a)** Alveoloplasty (vertical reduction). Knife-edge alveolar ridge (Cawood and Howell class IV). **b)** Vertical reduction is performed with a pear-shaped bone bur mounted on a straight handpiece. **c)** If it is necessary, soft tissues are trimmed. **d)** Suture.

Exostoses (tori) removal

Techniques for the removal of the palatal and mandibular tori are described, as they present peculiar aspects. For a different localisation of the torus, the same procedure is followed.

Palatine torus removal

After block anaesthesia of the major palatine and nasopalatine nerves, a full-thickness incision along the palatal midline is made, extending 1 centimetre beyond the torus both anteriorly and posteriorly. Two releasing incisions, forming a 120° angle, are made at both ends of the primary incision, to allow better retraction and complete exposure of the torus. Flap elevation must be conducted with great care, due to the thinness of the soft tissues overlying the lesion, and the possible presence of depressions or undercuts; full-thickness elevation prevents damage of the palatine neurovascular bundle. Once the exposure of the torus is obtained, the torus is removed with bone burs mounted on a straight handpiece, or piezoelectric instruments. Palpation makes it possible to highlight residual irregularities that must be eliminated prior to flap repositioning; a possible relative excess of soft tissues should be corrected before suturing the surgical wound (11.30a–h). A compressive dressing of iodoform gauze can be sutured to the palatal mucosa to reduce the risk of postoperative haematoma and the dressing is generally kept in place for 2–3 days.

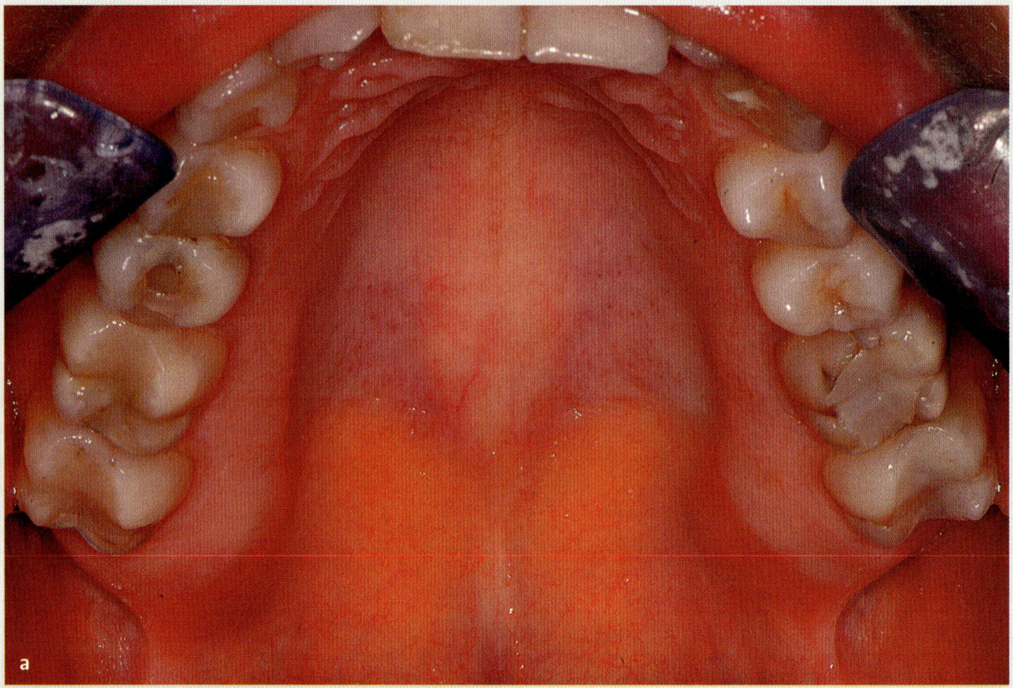

11.30 a) Initial clinical situation. **b)** CT scan: coronal image showing the presence of the exostosis on the palatal midline. **c)** Surgical incision along the palatal midline: v-shaped releasing incisions are made at both ends. (*continued*)

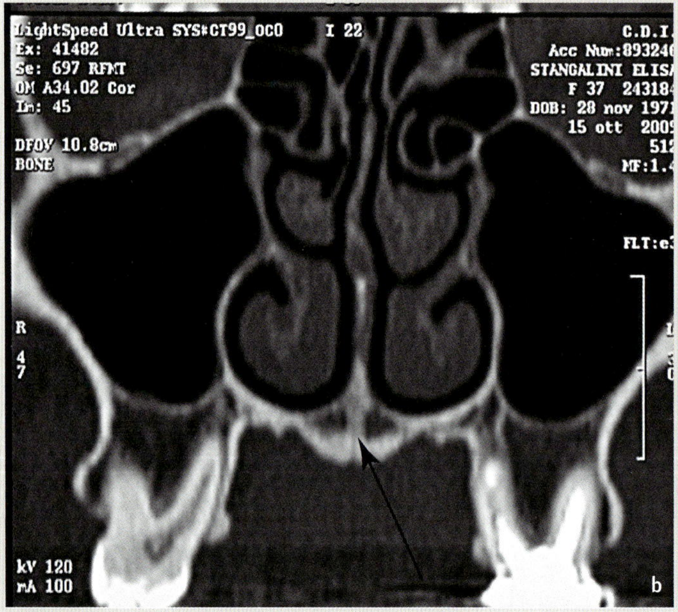

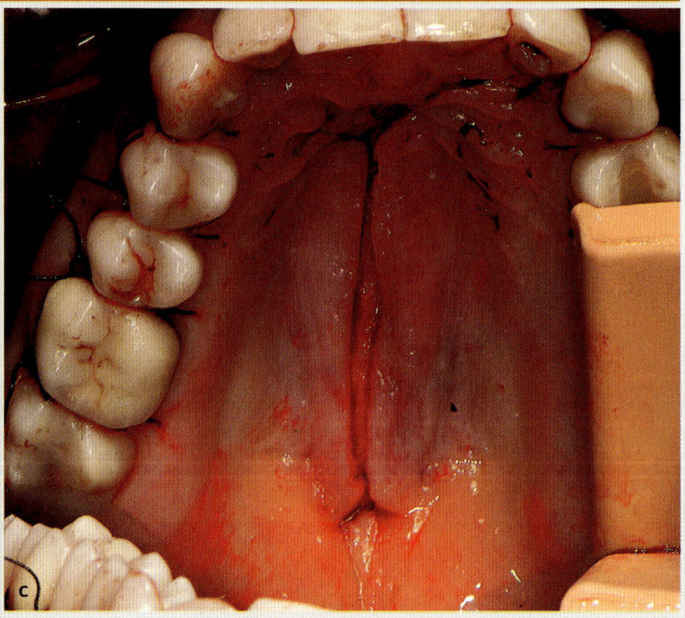

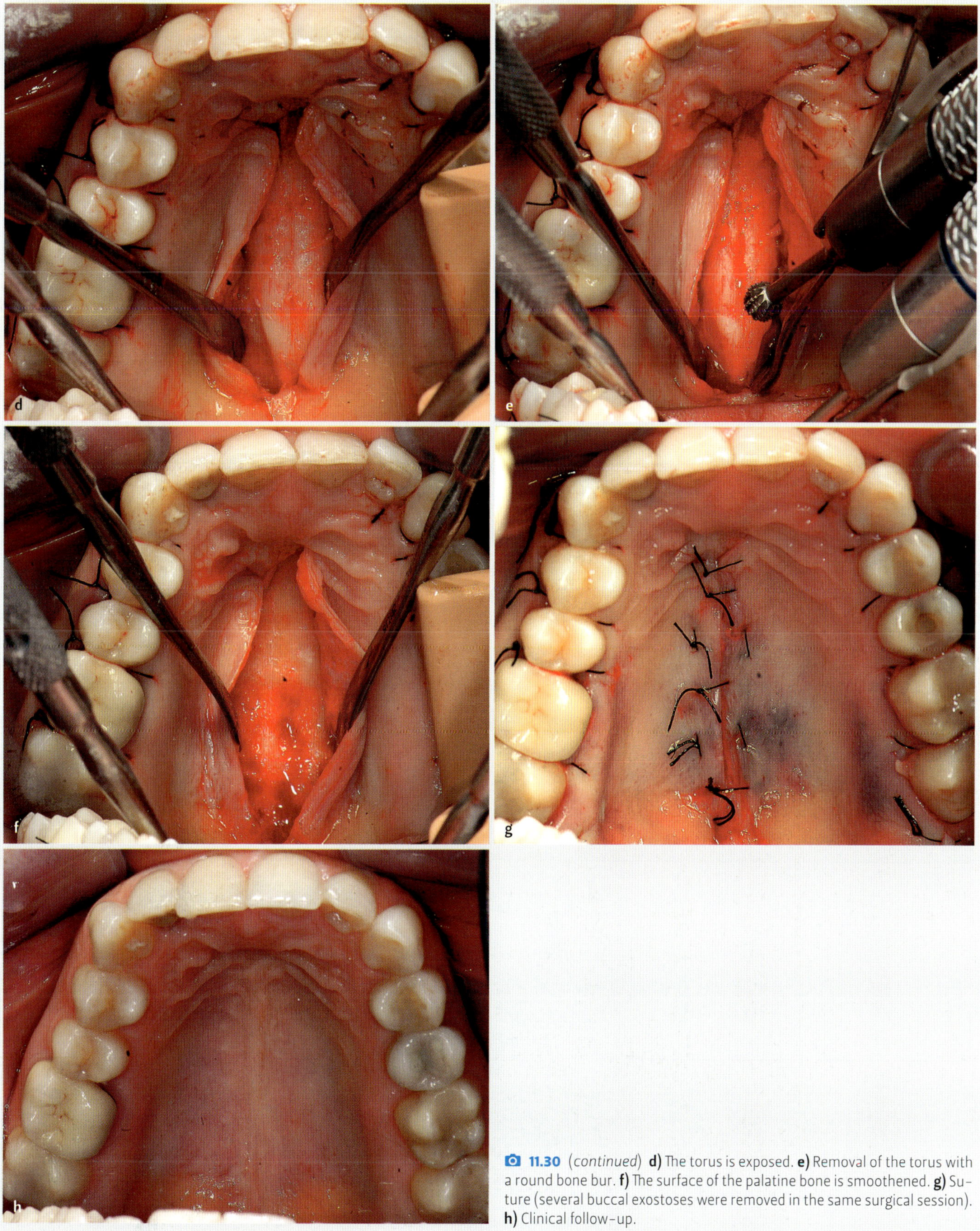

11.30 (*continued*) **d)** The torus is exposed. **e)** Removal of the torus with a round bone bur. **f)** The surface of the palatine bone is smoothened. **g)** Suture (several buccal exostoses were removed in the same surgical session). **h)** Clinical follow-up.

Mandibular torus (lingual side)

According to the apical-coronal position of the torus, a sulcular or submarginal full-thickness incision is chosen for dentate patients, while a crestal incision is the choice for edentulous patients. Full-thickness elevation of the soft tissues facilitates exposure of the exostosis. Tissue retractors or malleable spatulas are used to retract and protect the surgical flap, to avoid potentially dangerous damage to relevant anatomic structures of the floor of the mouth (see Chapter 2), while the torus is separated from the lingual cortical plate with a fissure bur, or consumed with a round or pear-shaped bone trimming bur. Once a smooth surface is obtained, the surgical wound is sutured (11.31a–f).

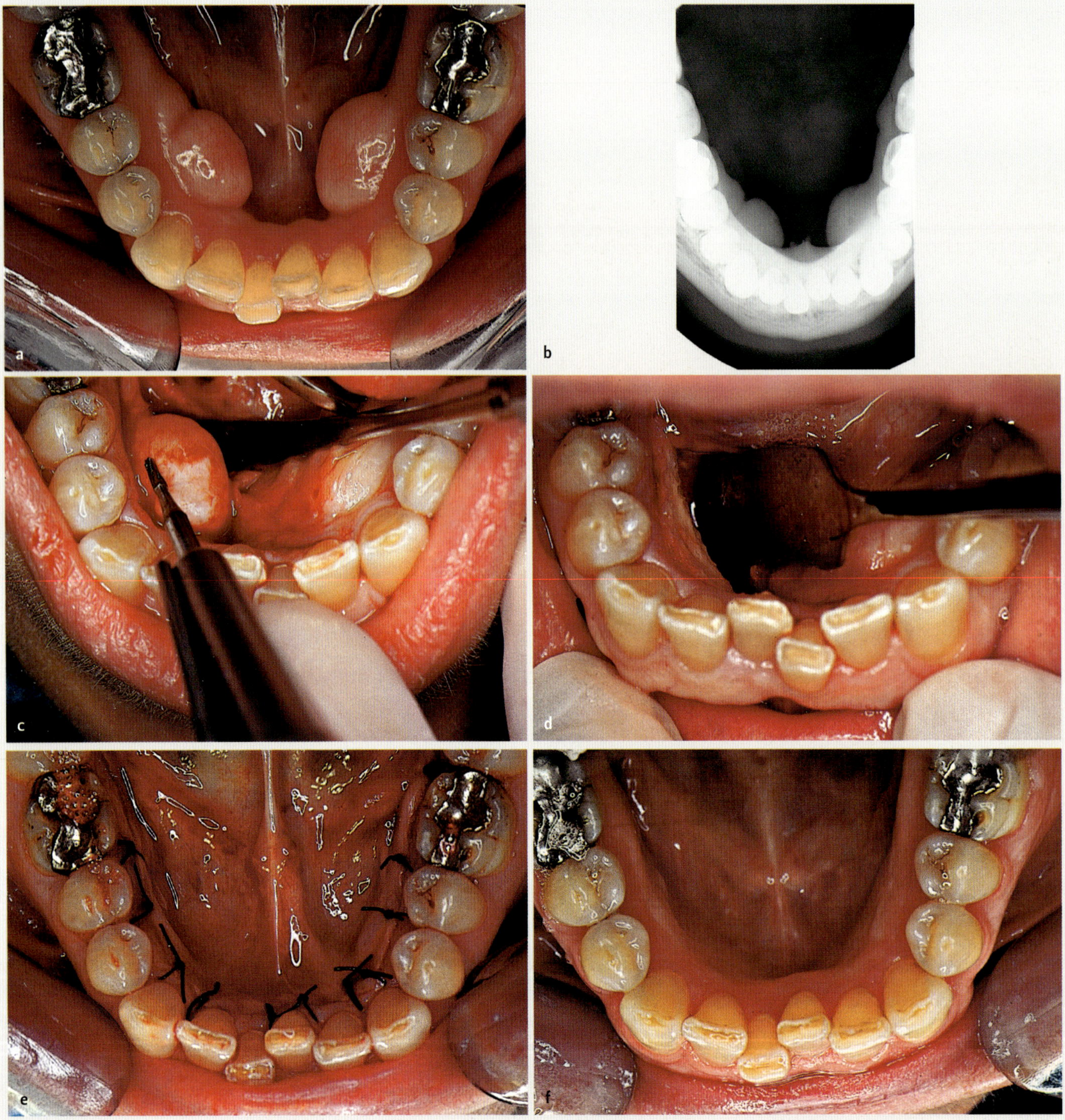

11.31 **a)** Initial clinical situation. **b)** Preoperative occlusal radiograph. **c)** The torus is exposed, and is then separated from the lingual cortical plate of the mandible with a fissure bur mounted on a straight handpiece. **d)** Surgical field after the removal of the torus. **e)** Suture. **f)** Clinical follow-up.

Correction of post-extractive defects

As previously mentioned, only the treatment of limited defects will be described in this chapter; large bone defects are treated under general anaesthesia in a protected environment (hospital), and thus a detailed description of these procedures is beyond the scope of this manual. Pre-implant hard and soft tissue reconstructions are treated in detail in Chapter 13.

The most common techniques used to treat small defects are as follows:

- correction by means of soft tissue grafts;
- correction by means of autologous bone grafts;
- correction by means of alloplastic grafts.

Correction by means of soft tissue grafts

The basic technique consists in the preparation of local rotation flaps to correct the defect: if the rotation flap alone does not allow adequate correction, connective tissue grafts harvested from the palate or tuber maxillae can be used as a base layer to thicken the soft tissues. A clinical case is presented together with the description of the technique; this latter may be subjected to modifications according to specific clinical indications (11.32a–f).

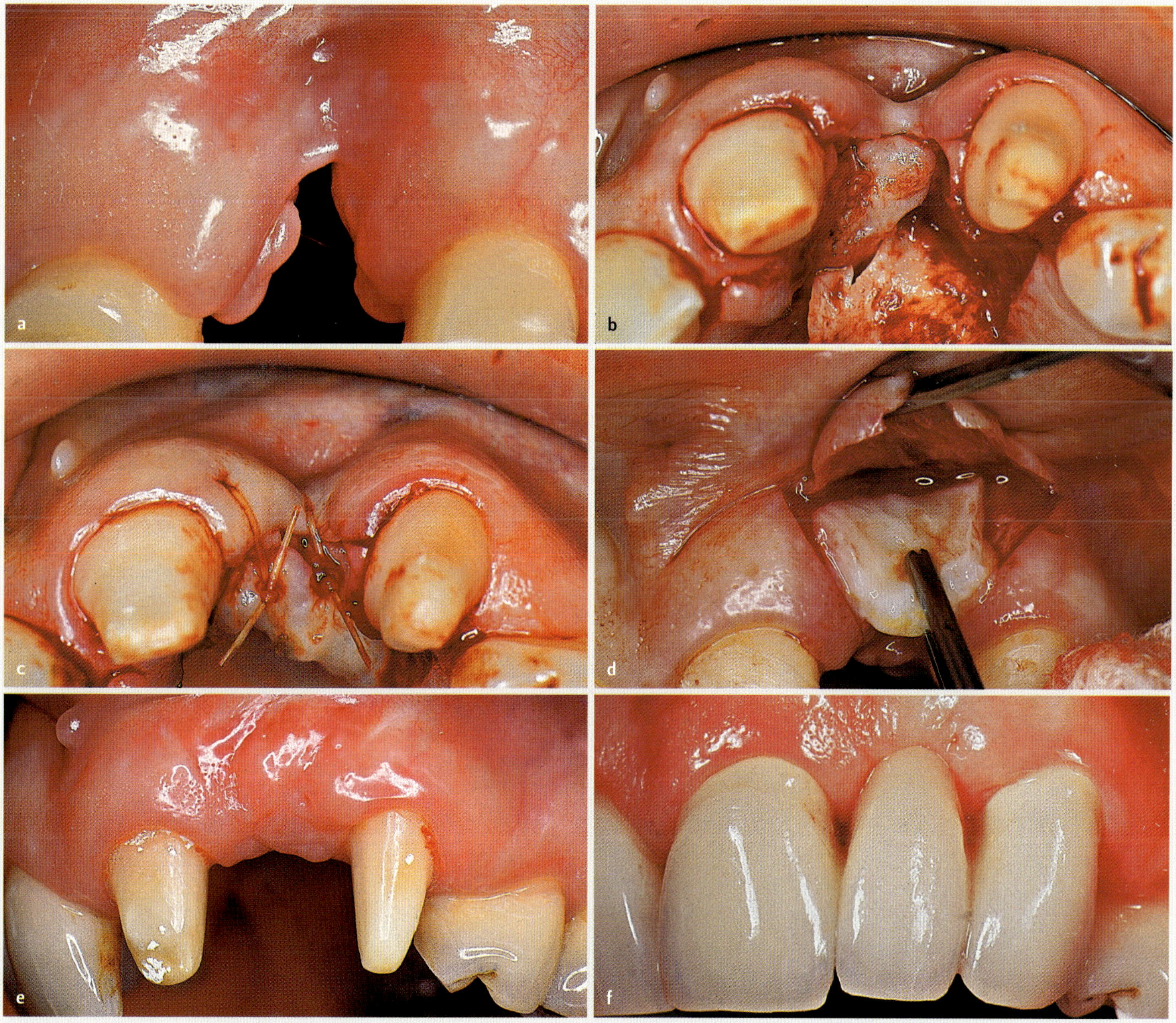

11.32 **a)** Correction of a defect by means of soft tissue plasty: the full-thickness alveolar defect resulted from the surgical excision of a desmoplastic fibroma, determining aesthetic impairment. **b)** Two surgical flaps are raised on the palatal side: one is disepithelialised and placed under the other to close the defect on the palate. **c)** Suture. **d)** One month later, a split-thickness flap is raised on the buccal side: a connective tissue graft is harvested from the palate and fixed under the flap to obtain adequate thickening of the soft tissue and the complete correction of the defect. **e)** Soft tissue maturation. **f)** Final result after fixed prosthetic rehabilitation.

Correction by means of autologous grafts

Autologous bone grafts harvested from intraoral (mandibular ramus, chin) or extraoral (iliac crest, calvaria) donor sites represent, at present, the most versatile and reliable technique for the reconstruction of bone defects of the jaws prior to implant placement.

Between the 1950s and 1970s, before the advent of titanium endosseous implants, autologous onlay grafts were used to correct defects of the alveolar ridges with the aim to recreate a retentive morphology that was necessary to guarantee the stability of removable prostheses. Unfortunately, notwithstanding good initial results, the resorption rate of the reconstructed bone volume was significant (70% to 100% within 3 years). For this reason, autologous bone grafts are described in Chapter 13 among the techniques used to treat bone defects prior to implant placement.

Correction by means of alloplastic grafts

These surgical procedures were originally proposed for the correction of horizontal (Cawood and Howell class IV) and tridimensional (class V–VI) defects of the alveolar ridges. A subperiosteal tunnel was created on the alveolar crest and the alloplastic bone substitute (such as hydroxylapatite), either in the form of granules or blocks, was positioned inside, to create adequate volume and morphology for the stabilisation of removable prostheses. This technique was proposed to overcome the problems caused by the resorption of autologous bone grafts under prosthetic loading (removable prostheses) and to reduce postoperative morbidity associated with autologous bone harvesting. Moreover, porous alloplastic materials were believed to have an intrinsic osteoconductive potential, and due to this characteristic, they were to be colonised and then substituted by newly formed autologous bone.

However, in recent decades the indications to the use of these methods have seen a significant reduction, due to the following:

- relevant risk of exposure and subsequent infection of the alloplastic graft (particularly when used in the form of blocks), both in the postoperative period and after prosthetic loading, requiring removal of the grafting material;
- compaction and/or migration of the alloplastic material (particularly when used in the form of granules) with partial or total impairment of the initial result, and with the risk of unfavourable alterations of the local ridge morphology.

Moreover, the use of alloplastic materials may render the prosthetic rehabilitation of the patient more difficult, in case the removable prosthesis is to be substituted by a fixed, implant-supported prosthesis at a later stage. In fact, although biocompatible, these materials are not resorbed (or are slowly resorbed), and are colonised by newly formed autogenous bone not only with great difficulty, but also only at the periphery of the grafted mass, thus resulting in incomplete osteointegration of the grafting material. However, this technique may still be useful for the correction of small defects.

A small, vertical incision is made in proximity to the mesial end of the deficient area, and a periosteal elevator is used to create a subperiosteal tunnel. Care must be taken when using blind techniques, to avoid perforations of the soft tissues and any damage to relevant anatomic structures, such as the mental nerve. Once the planned space is obtained, the alloplastic material is placed inside the subperiosteal tunnel and the access incision is sutured. The patient must not be allowed to wear removable prostheses for one month, to allow consolidation of the grafting material and avoid early migration due to prosthetic loading (11.33a–f).

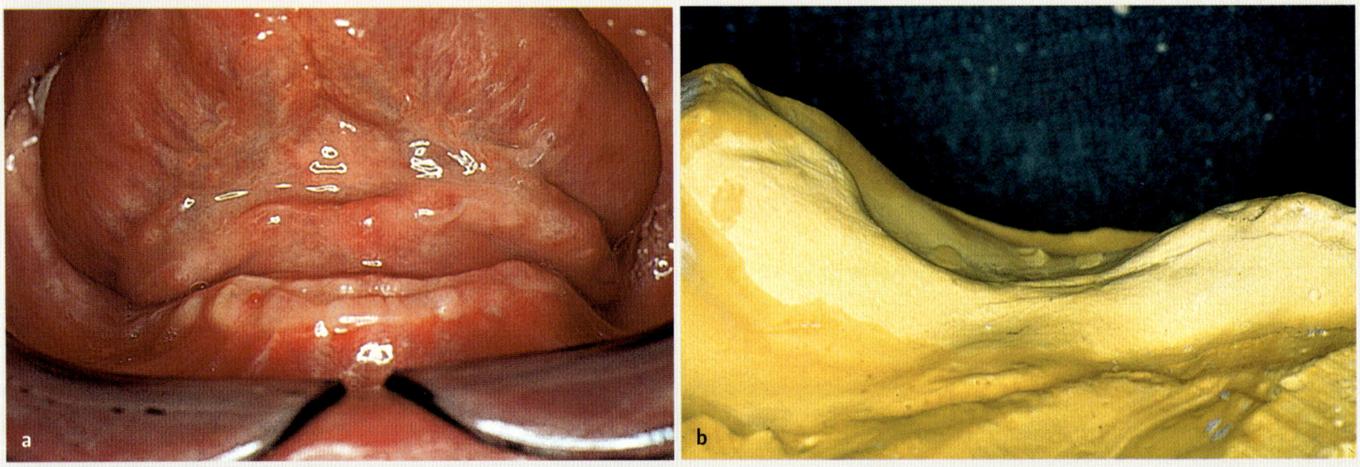

11.33 **a)** Reconstruction of the vertical defect with alloplastic materials (hydroxylapatite). Initial clinical situation: a large depression is visible in the lower left hemimandible. **b)** Plaster cast showing the extent of the vertical defect. (*continued*)

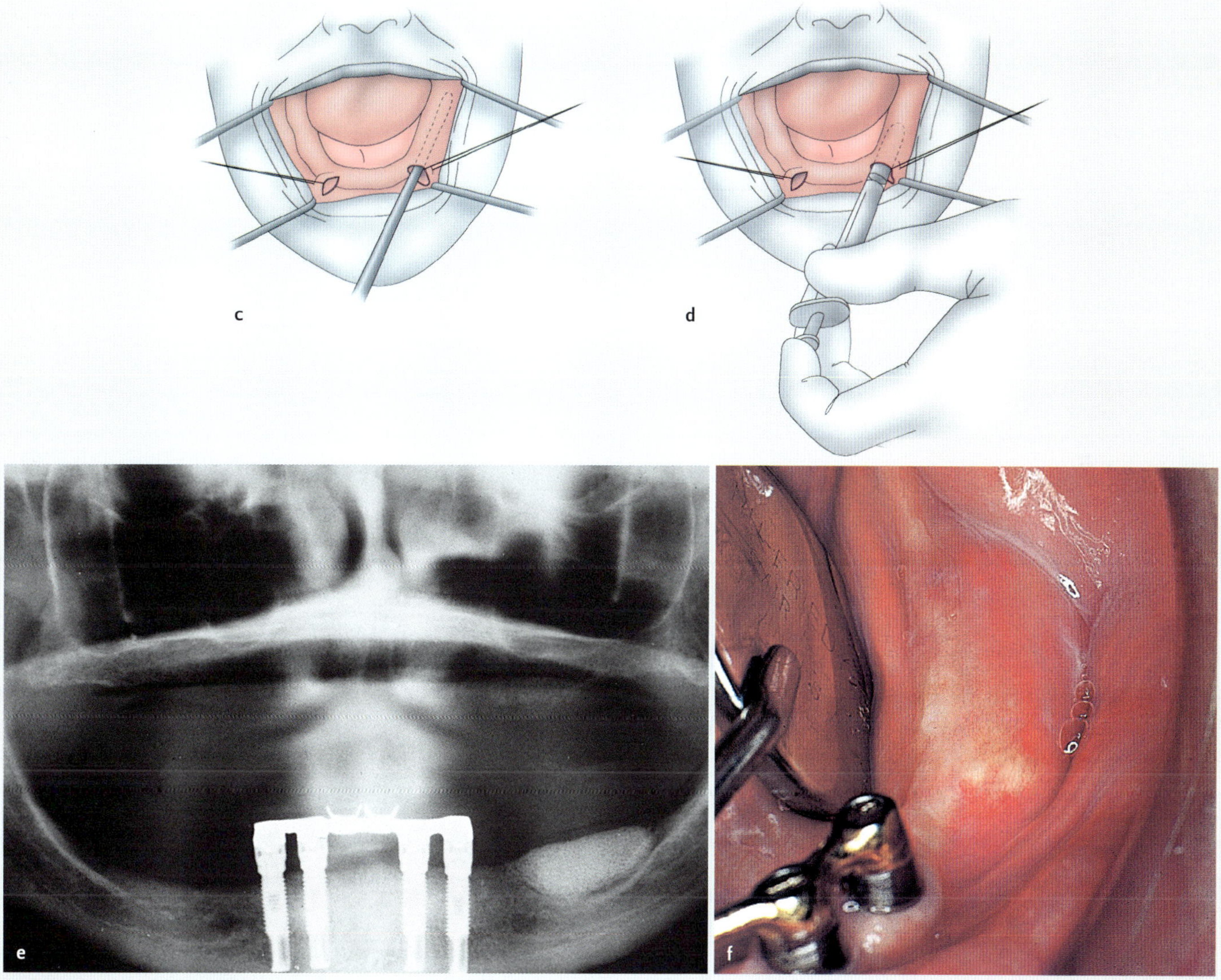

11.33 (*continued*) **c–d)** The blind subperiosteal tunnel technique. **e)** Radiographic follow-up after the completion of an implant-supported prosthetic rehabilitation. **f)** Clinical follow-up demonstrating adequate correction of the defect.

REFERENCES

Andreasen JO, Storgard Jensen S, Kofod T, Schwartz O, Hillerup S. Oper or closed repositioning of mandibular fractures: is there a difference in healing outcome? A systematic review. *Dent Traumatol* 2008 Feb; 24(1):17-21.

Brusati R. Attuali indirizzi in chirurgia preprotesica maggiore. *Dental Cadmos* 1985; 4:9.

Brusati R, Capozzi L, Curioni C. Chirurgia odontostomatologica e maxillo-facciale. Vol. 1 e 2, Piccin, Padova 1986.

Brusati R, Chiapasco M, Ronchi P. Riabilitazione dei mascellari atrofici mediante: trapianti ossei, osteotomie, impianti. *Dental Cadmos* 1997; 13:11-45.

Brusati R, Chiapasco M. Elementi di chirurgia oro-maxillo-facciale. Masson, Milano 1999.

Cawood JI, Howell RA. A classification of the edentulous jaws. *Int J Oral Maxillofac Surg* 1988; 17:232-6.

Chiapasco M, Romeo E, Vogel G. Three-dimensional reconstruction of a knife-edge edentulous maxilla by sinus elevation, only grafts, and sagittal osteotomy of the anterior maxilla: preliminary surgical and prosthetic results. *J Oral Maxillofac Impl* 1998; 13:394-9.

Chiapasco M, Romeo E. Riabilitazione implantoprotesica nei casi complessi. Utet, Torino 2003.

Cohenca N, Simon JH, Roges R, Morag Y, Malfaz JM. Clinical indications for digital imaging in dento-alveolar trauma. Part 1:traumatic injueries. *Dent Traumatol* 2007 Apr; 23(2):95-104.

Coulthard P, Esposito M, Worthington HW, Jokstad A. Interventions for replacing missing teeth: preprosthetic surgery versus dental implants. Cochrane Database of Systematic Reviews 2002; (4):CD003604.

Hillerup S, Eriksen E, Solow B. Reduction of mandibular residual redge after vestibuloplasty. *Int J Oral Maxillofac Surg* 1989; 18:271-6.

Kahnberg KE, Nyström E, Bartholdsson L. Combined use of bone grafts and Brånemark fixtures in the treatment of severely resorbed maxillae. *Int J Oral Maxillofac Impl* 1989; 4:297-304.

Mehta N, Butala P, Bernstein MP. The imaging of maxillofacial trauma and its pertinence to surgical intervention. *Radiol Clin North Am.* 2012 Jan; 50(1):43-57.

Peterson LJ, Ellis III E, Hupp JR, Tucker MR. Contemporary oral and maxillofacial surgery. 2nd ed. Mosby, St Louis 1993.

Peterson LJ, Indresano AT, Marciani RD, Roser SM. Principles of oral and maxillofacial surgery. JB Lippincott Company, Philadelphia 1992.

Seah YH. Torus palatinus and torus mandibularis: a review of the literature. *Aust Dent J* 1995; 40(5):318-21.

Starshak TJ. Corrective soft tissue surgery. Preprothesic Oral and Maxillofacial Surgery. Mosby, St. Louis 1980.

Terry BC, Hillebrand DG. Minor preprosthetic surgical procedures. *Dent Clin North Am* 1994 Apr; 38(2):193-216.

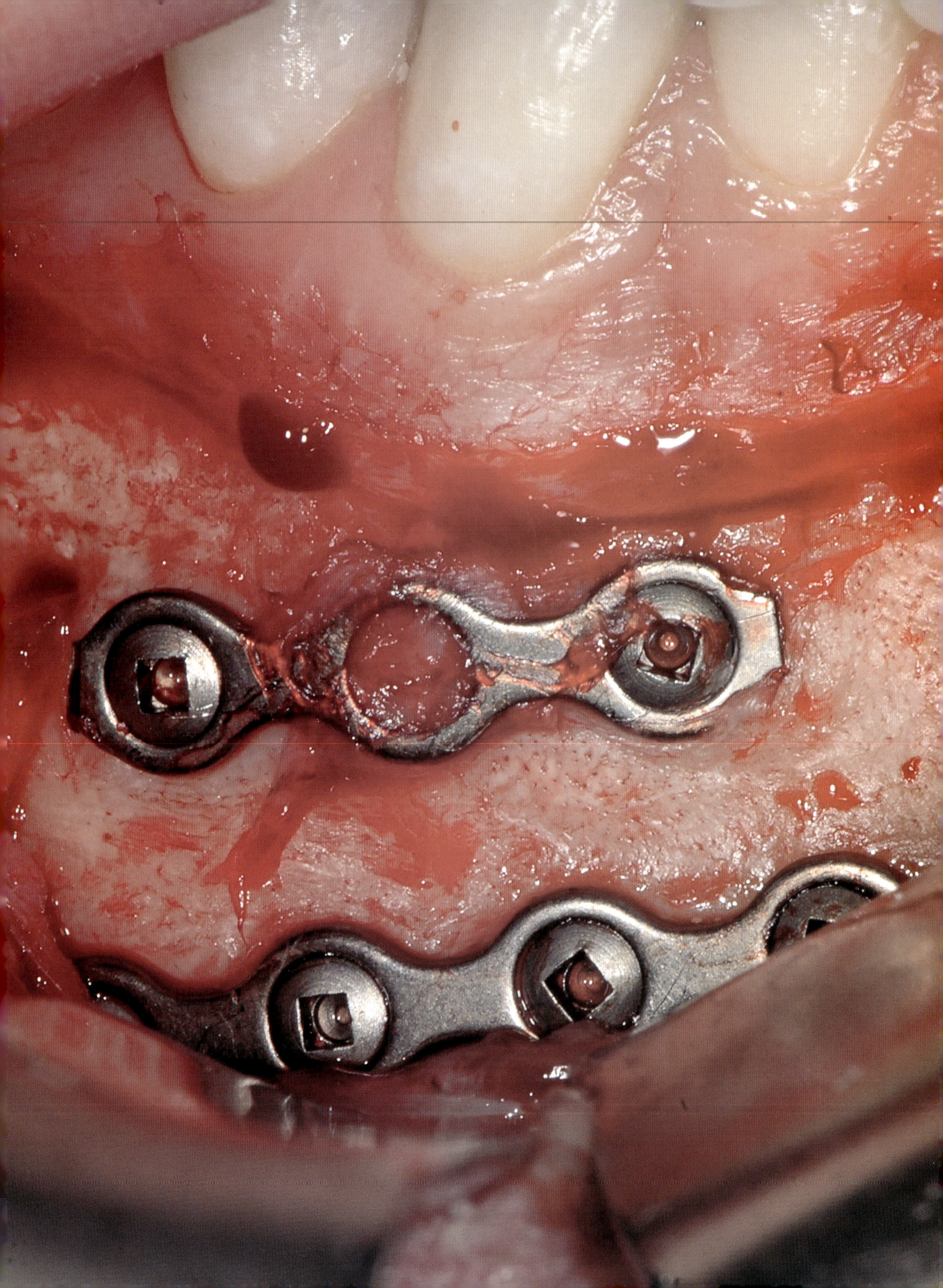

Dentoalveolar trauma

M. Chiapasco ▪ M. Zaniboni ▪ A. Coggiola

Introduction

Facial trauma is a relatively common occurrence, and the dentist is frequently the first specialist involved in the management of the consequences. A comprehensive description of complex facial trauma and the respective treatment modalities are not within the scope of this manual: a detailed description of these subjects can be found in maxillofacial surgery textbooks (see Peterson et al. 2004). Likewise, an in-depth description of dental trauma causing crown fractures that can be treated with restorative and endodontic techniques can be found in restorative dentistry and endodontics textbooks. In this chapter the diagnosis and treatment of traumatic avulsion of teeth and dentoalveolar fractures are presented, and rationale guidelines for the management of the patient from the first examination to clinical and radiographic follow-up.

Trauma classification

Because of facial trauma, the following conditions may result:

LESIONS OF THE HARD TISSUES AND PULP OF THE TOOTH

- *Crown crack*: incomplete enamel fracture without loss of tooth substance.
- *Enamel fracture*: partial or complete, without pulp exposure.
- *Enamel and dentin fracture*: loss of tooth substance without pulp involvement.
- *Enamel, dentin and pulp fracture*: loss of tooth substance with pulp involvement.
- *Crown-root fracture without pulp exposure*: enamel, dentin and cementum are involved, but the pulp is not exposed.
- *Crown-root fracture with pulp exposure*: enamel, dentin, cementum and pulp are involved.
- *Root fracture*: cementum, dentin and pulp are involved (12.1).

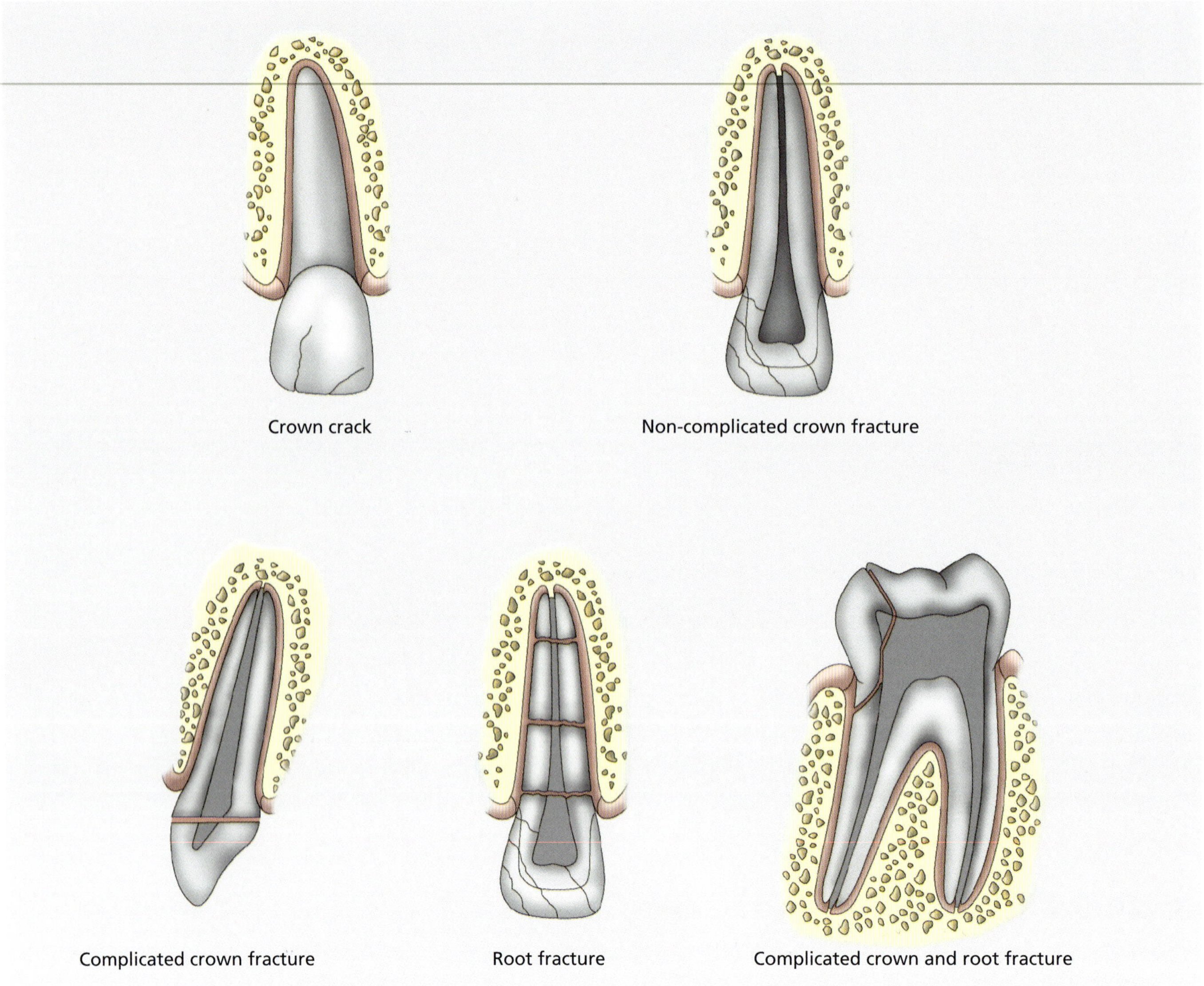

12.1 Complicated and non-complicated crown and root fractures.

LESIONS OF THE PERIODONTAL TISSUES

- *Concussion*: lesion of the tooth supporting structures without abnormal mobility or dislocation, and sharp pain upon compression.
- *Subluxation*: lesion of the tooth supporting structures with abnormal mobility, but without dislocation.
- *Extrusive luxation*: partial dislocation of the tooth outside its alveolus.
- *Lateral luxation*: dislocation of the tooth in a non-axial direction; the presence of a comminuted lesion of the alveolus is frequent.
- *Intrusive luxation*: dislocation of the tooth in the alveolar bone; the association with a comminuted fracture of the alveolus is frequent.
- *Complete avulsion* (12.2).

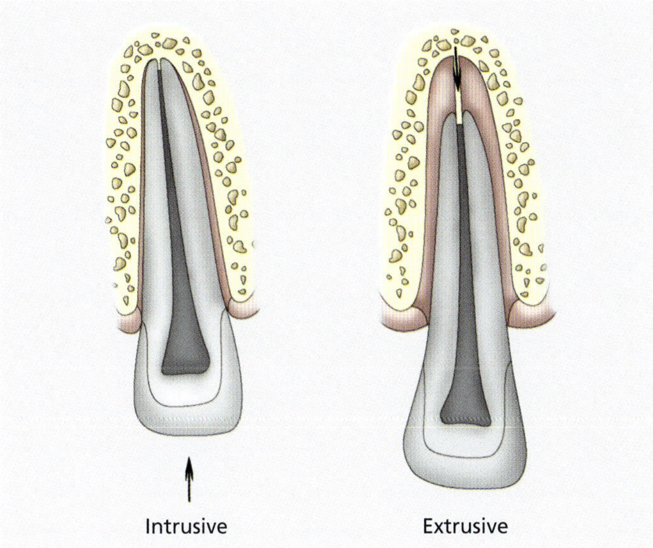

12.2 Traumatic luxation of the tooth.

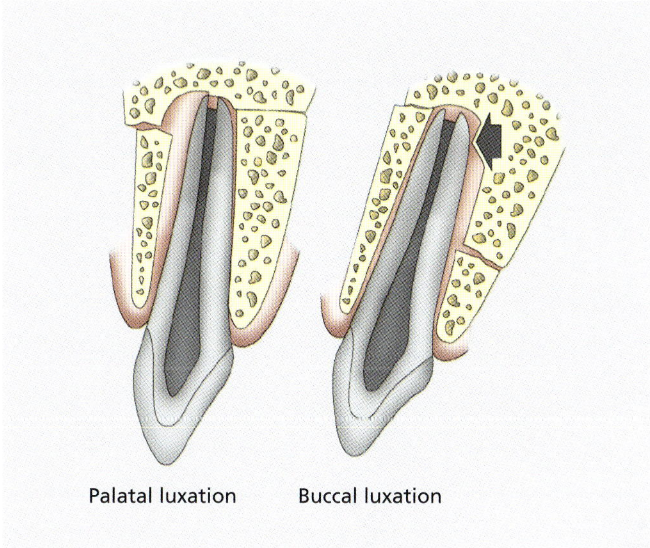

12.3 Fracture of the alveolar process.

LESIONS OF THE GINGIVA AND ORAL MUCOSA

Facial trauma may cause *abrasion*, *contusion* and *laceration* of the gingiva and oral mucosa.

BONE FRACTURES

- *Fracture of the alveolus wall or comminuted fracture of the alveolar crest* subsequent to tooth luxation (12.3).
- *Fracture of the mandible or maxilla*: involves both the alveolar ridge and the basal bone of the upper or the lower jaw.

According to the extent and the type of trauma, fracture paths may show a great variability. However, it is possible to classify jaw fractures by considering the paths that fracture lines follow in the majority of cases.

A classification of *maxillary fractures* was proposed by Le Fort in 1901, when the author identified the paths of least resistance along which fractures most frequently develop.

- *Le Fort I* fractures: the fracture line extends horizontally above the alveolar ridges, from the piriform aperture to the zygomatic pillar and pterygopalatine suture, running above the teeth apexes, along the anterolateral wall of the maxillary sinus. Complete detachment of the maxilla from the cranial base occurs, with loss of the occlusion, mobility of the maxilla and, eventually, the presence of an open and/or cross-bite (12.4).
- *Le Fort II* fractures: the fracture line extends cranially, determining the detachment of the frontonasal suture, before running caudally along the medial wall of the orbital cavity to rejoin the same line of the Le Fort I fracture. Mobility of the maxilla and nose can be observed (12.4).
- *Le Fort III* fracture: this is the more complex maxillary fracture, also known as craniofacial dissociation. The fracture line begins from the frontonasal suture following the same path of the Le Fort II fracture, but at the infraorbital foramen, it runs along the orbital floor, and then cranially along the lateral wall of the orbital cavity, interrupting the frontozygomatic suture. It then descends along the infratemporal fossa to reach the pterygoid process (12.4).

Type of fracture

Greenstick fracture	The fracture involves only the external cortical plates, while the cancellous bone remains intact. Spontaneous healing may occur.
Simple (non-dislocated) fracture	Complete fracture of the involved bone: the two segments remain in their original position, and the fracture appears radiographically as a radiolucent line.
Dislocated fracture	Complete fracture of the involved bone with dislocation of the fractured segments.
Comminuted fracture	Disintegration of the involved bone in several fragments.
Closed fracture	Integrity of the soft tissues surrounding the fractured bone is maintained.
Compound fracture	The soft tissues surrounding the fracture are lacerated and the fracture fragments are exposed

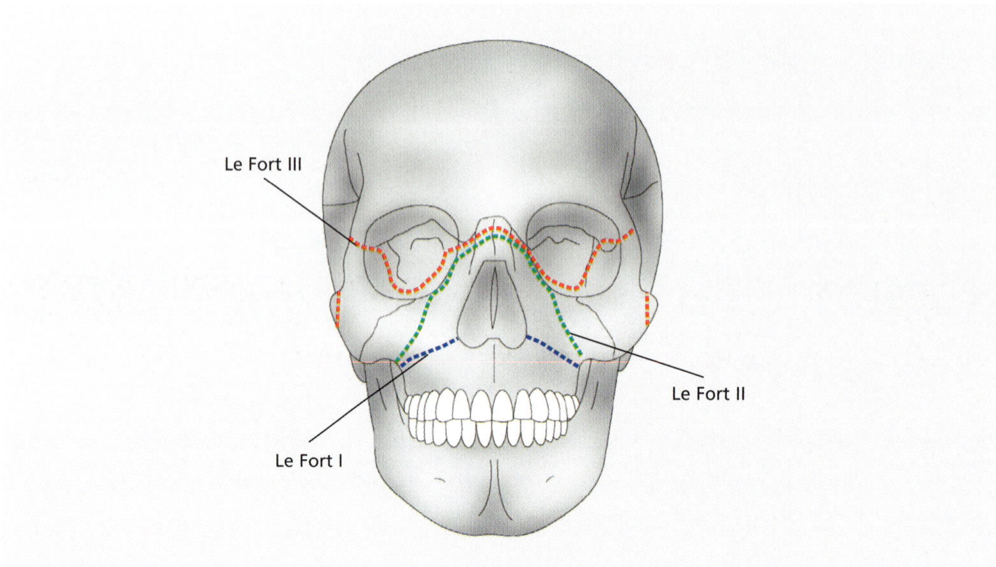

12.4 The most common fracture paths in the upper maxilla/midface, as classified by Le Fort.

Mandibular fractures also occur more frequently along distinct paths of least resistance, represented by the mandibular angle, the neck of the condyle, and the mandibular body in the area of the premolars (12.5, 12.6).

- *Panfacial fracture*: it involves the lower, middle, and upper face. Management of these lesions is complex because fractures are frequently comminute, and bone fragments may be dislocated in the soft tissues and inside the paranasal sinuses. Panfacial fractures also cause significant alterations of the facial features (12.7). Important neurosurgical implications arise whenever the skull is involved.

Dentoalveolar trauma is rare in the first year of life; a significant increase in their incidence is seen in pre-school children, due to accidental falls, while peak incidence is seen among teenagers and adults, typically due to sporting activities, road traffic accidents, work accidents, domestic accidents, and social conflict (scuffles).

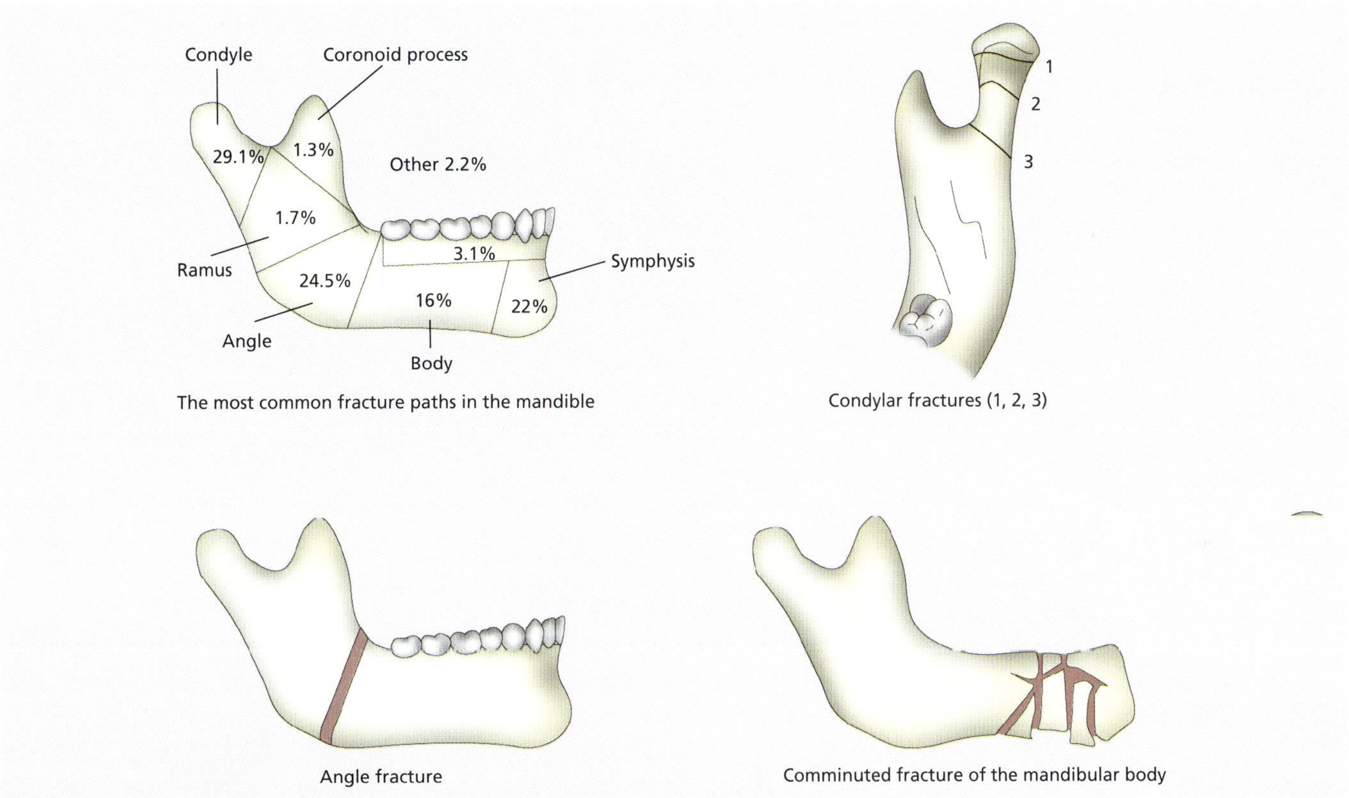

12.5 Mandibular fractures.

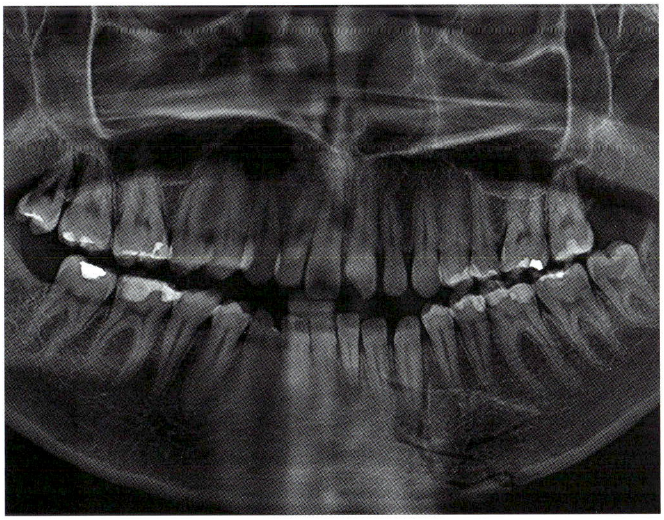

12.6 Complete mandibular body fracture: the fracture lines can be observed in the area between 3.3 and 3.5.

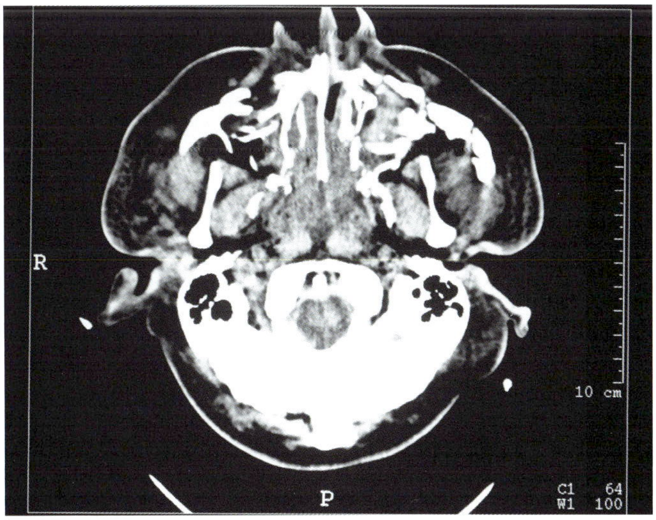

12.7 Panfacial fracture: disintegration of the maxillofacial complex led to the presence of tens of comminuted bone fragments.

As previously mentioned, a comprehensive description of complex facial trauma and the respective treatment modalities, including dental trauma causing crown fractures that can be treated with restorative and endodontic techniques, is not within the scope of this manual. On the other hand, clinical scenarios and guidelines for the management of dentoalveolar trauma are described in the following sections, to serve as a reference for the oral surgeon in the treatment of the trauma patient.

Clinical examination: analysis of signs and symptoms

The patient's medical history should be accurately gathered and analysed, particularly with regard to the following:

- *timing*: if the treatment is immediate the prognosis is good, while delayed treatments are burdened with a worsened prognosis; therefore, it is very important to know exactly when the trauma occurred;
- *place*: it is important to know where the trauma occurred, to evaluate possible chemical or bacterial contamination of the wounds;
- *how the trauma occurred*;
- *possible treatments performed elsewhere*;
- *history of (possible) previous dentoalveolar trauma.*

Once the patient's medical history is recorded, clinical examination must be performed.

CLINICAL EXAMINATION: EXTRAORAL SOFT TISSUES

Lacerations, abrasions, and contusions can be observed in facial trauma and dentoalveolar fractures. Prior to clinical examination, irrigation of the wounds with sterile saline allows removal of blood clots or debris (tooth fragments and/or foreign bodies such as glass, metal, or concrete fragments) that may cause infection, and grant adequate visualisation of the area. Extraoral lesions may present as incised or, more frequently, contused and lacerated wounds. Dimension and localisation of all wounds must be assessed, and the possible involvement of notable anatomic structures (parotid duct, facial nerve, mental nerve, etc.) must be thoroughly evaluated. Palpation of the soft tissues allows verification of the presence of dislocated tooth fragments or foreign bodies.

CLINICAL EXAMINATION: INTRAORAL SOFT TISSUES

In facial trauma, lesions of the intraoral soft tissues are frequent and the same principles described for extraoral wounds apply. Irrigation with sterile saline and removal of debris, blood clots and/or foreign bodies to allow a precise clinical evaluation, the elimination of infectious material, and the identification of tooth fragments or exposed portions of alveolar bone.

PALPATION OF THE ALVEOLAR CREST AND BASAL BONE

Dentoalveolar fractures may be easily identified with palpation, although the recourse to this manoeuvre is frequently limited by the pain experienced by the patient. Bleeding from the buccal fornix or from the floor of the mouth may suggest the presence of a fracture of the alveolar crest.

EXAMINATION OF THE CROWNS

Examination of the visible portion of the teeth (crowns) makes it possible to assess the possible presence of crown or crown-root fractures and to classify them correctly, to choose the most appropriate treatment modality.

TEETH MOBILITY

All teeth should be examined to assess mobility, even in the absence of proper luxation. Mobility of several adjacent teeth may suggest the presence of a dentoalveolar fracture.

TEETH LUXATION

Teeth extrusion and intrusion, together with lateral luxation, are the most frequent consequences of direct dental trauma. Occlusion tests can be helpful to recognise subluxations which may not be evident during tooth examination.

TEETH PERCUSSION

Percussion tests allow verification of possible damage to the periodontal ligament; in such a case, tooth percussion elicits sharp pain.

PULP VITALITY TESTS

The significance of vitality tests performed immediately after the occurrence of the trauma is low; in fact, the trauma may induce a phase of "stupor" in the pulp, leading to false positive results.

Instead, a certain time after the trauma, the absence of reactions to thermal and/or electric stimuli suggests the loss of vitality of the pulp due to the trauma, influencing the treatment of the involved tooth (endodontic therapy).

SYMPTOMS

Typically, symptoms reported by the patient *include pain and possible teeth mobility, or mobility of the alveolar ridge* in the area involved in the trauma. Sensory disturbances may be present with concomitant involvement of superficial branches of the trigeminal nerve (e.g. the mental nerve). Furthermore, extrusive luxation of teeth may cause premature contacts and loss of the established occlusion. The patient may also exhibit and/or report the loss of the established occlusion with displaced fractures, involving the alveolar crest alone or the alveolar crest and the basal bone.

SIGNS

Signs vary according to the type and extent of the occurred trauma.

- *Concussion*: typically, no peculiar signs can be observed upon inspection, but the patient experiences sharp pain upon palpation and percussion.
- *Subluxation*: no peculiar signs can be observed upon inspection, but palpation allows the involved teeth to be assessed and elicits pain.
- *Luxation*: according to the type of trauma (intrusive, extrusive, lateral), displacement of the involved teeth in the direction of the trauma, in conjunction with the loss of the established occlusion, can be observed upon inspection. Tooth luxation is typically associated with fractures of the alveolar crest; in this event, palpation makes it possible to recognise morphologic alterations in the area of the fracture.
- *Avulsion*: accurate inspection of the alveolus and of the avulsed tooth (if retrieved), in association with radiographic examinations, make it possible to diagnose the possible

presence of residual root fragments. Moreover, lesions of the soft tissues such as contusions, abrasions, and lacerations can be present.

- *Fracture of the alveolar crest*: typically, fractures of the alveolar crest occur in the anterior region of the jaws. In edentulous patients, due to bone atrophy, fracture of the alveolar ridge is less frequent; in cases of severe trauma, complete fracture of the basal bone may occur. Migration of one or more teeth in association with dislocation of the alveolar ridge can be observed upon inspection; a non-displaced fracture may be appreciated upon palpation of the alveolar crest, while displaced or compound fractures can be recognised upon inspection. Contusions, abrasions, and lacerations of the soft tissues may be present. Palpation makes it possible to evaluate the extent of the fracture, the mobility of the fractured dentoalveolar segment, and the possibility of reduction. All of this information should be gathered, if possible, immediately after the trauma and before swelling of the overlying soft tissues occurs, as this latter may impede a correct clinical evaluation (12.8a–c, 12.9a–f).

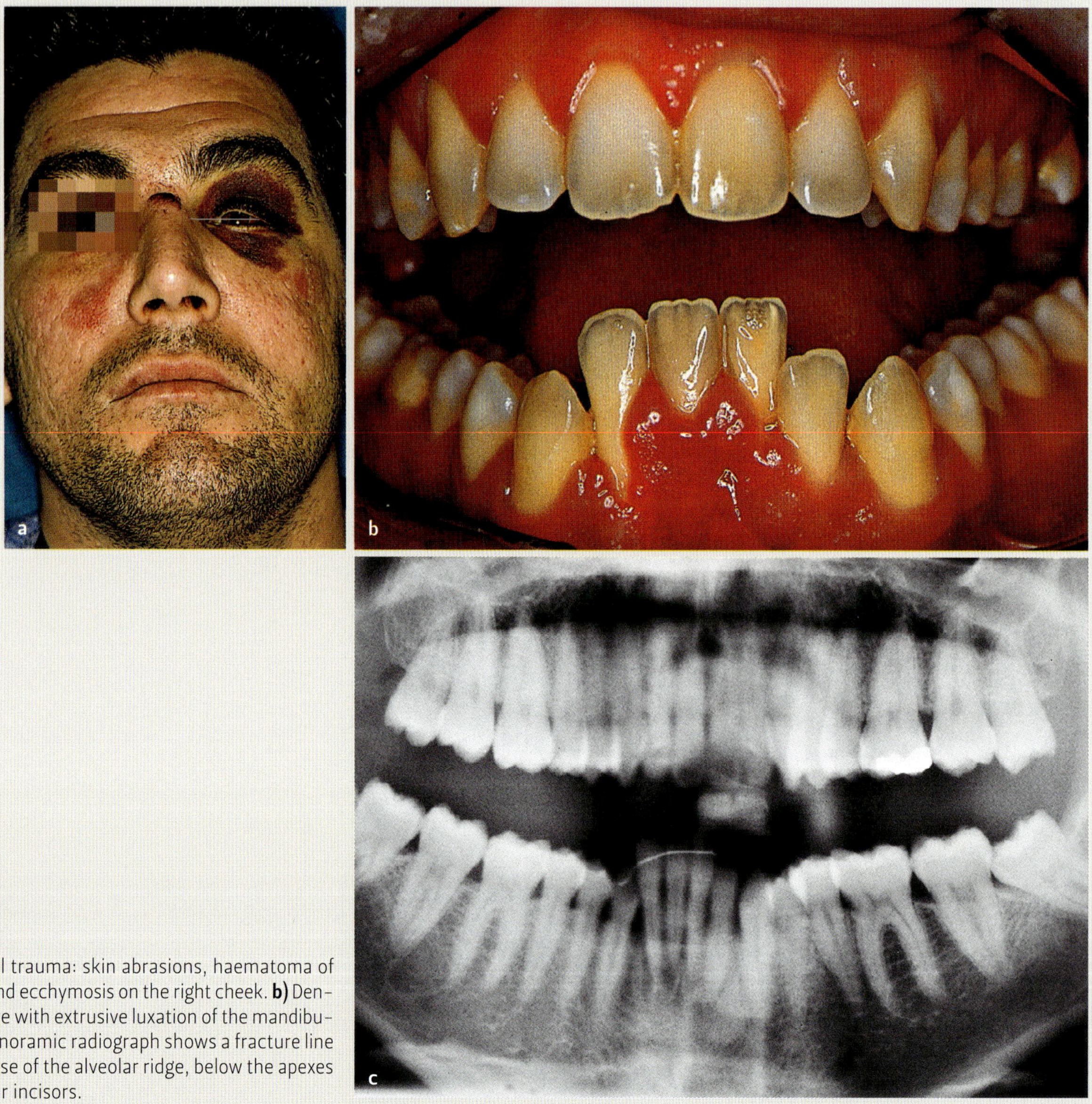

12.8 **a)** Facial trauma: skin abrasions, haematoma of the left eyelids, and ecchymosis on the right cheek. **b)** Dentoalveolar fracture with extrusive luxation of the mandibular incisors. **c)** Panoramic radiograph shows a fracture line running at the base of the alveolar ridge, below the apexes of the mandibular incisors.

It is worth remembering that while the treatment of complex facial fractures falls beyond the duties of the oral surgeon, the diagnosis of these lesions and the prompt referral of the patient to a maxillofacial unit should be adequately managed. Therefore, clinical examination should not be limited to the evaluation of the teeth and periodontal tissues, but should also include inspection and palpation of the jaws and facial bones. For example, a dentoalveolar fracture in the anterior mandible can be associated with a complete mandibular fracture in the premolar region and/or a condylar fracture, and with typical signs such as loss of the established occlusion, trismus, lateral deviation of the mandible towards the side of the fractured condyle.

Dentoalveolar trauma: signs and symptoms

Trauma	Signs	Symptoms
Concussion	No peculiarities	Relevant pain
Subluxation	No peculiarities	Tooth mobility and pain
Luxation	Tooth dislocation	Local pain
Complete avulsion	Loss of the normal occlusion Empty alveolus Gingival lesions	
Dentoalveolar fracture	Tooth and alveolar process dislocation Soft tissues oedema	Local pain

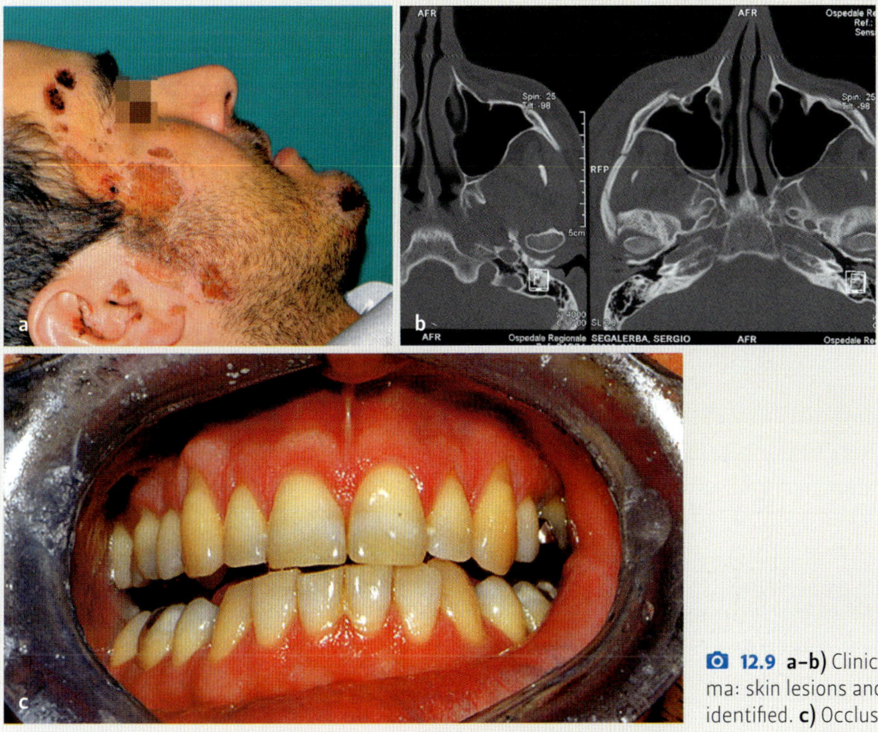

12.9 a–b) Clinical and radiographic examination after facial trauma: skin lesions and fractures of the zygoma and zygomatic arch are identified. **c)** Occlusion is checked. (*continued*)

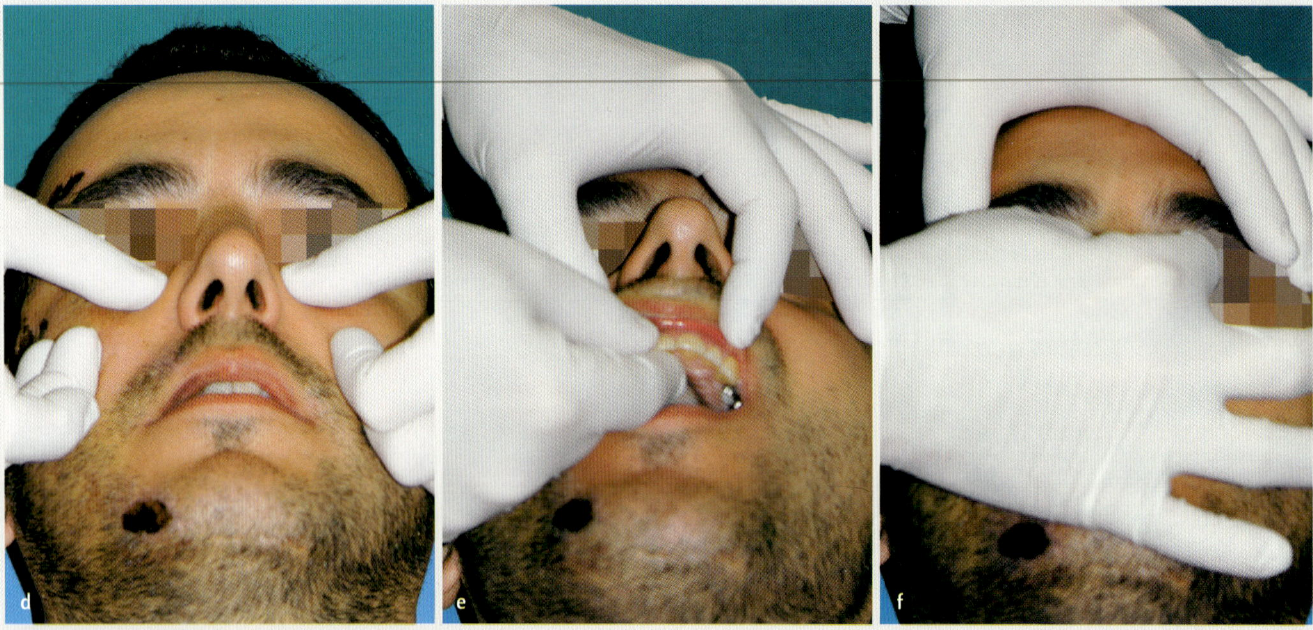

12.9 (*continued*) **d)** The inferior orbital rims are palpated to evaluate possible dislocations. **e–f)** Possible dental, maxillary, and nasal mobility is evaluated. Eyeballs are also checked to exclude the possible incarceration of the inferior rectus muscle in the fracture line, for fractures involving the inferior orbital rim and/or the orbital floor.

Radiographic examinations

	Advantages	Disadvantages
Periapical radiograph	+ Accurate evaluation of tooth and alveolar process fractures	+ Small visible area
Panoramic radiograph	+ Visualisation of the maxillomandibular complex + Complete visualisation of fracture paths	+ Superimposition of anatomic structures
CT scan	+ Tridimensional visualisation of the maxillofacial complex	+ Higher radiation dose

Instrumental screening

Radiographic examinations are fundamental for a correct diagnosis of dentoalveolar trauma. The combined use of different radiographic techniques provides a more precise evaluation of the clinical situation. Information on the local anatomy of the involved area, as well as evidence of pre-existing conditions, can be obtained together with information on the consequences of the trauma, such as:

- presence of root fractures;
- degree of extrusion or intrusion of the involved teeth;
- presence of fractures of the alveolar crest;
- presence of complete fractures of the basal bone;
- presence of (radiopaque) foreign bodies in the soft tissues.

Periapical radiographs allow evaluation of damage to the teeth and alveolar crest. Possible fractures appear as radiolucent lines.

As regards larger lesions, *the panoramic radiograph* can offer a complete visualisation of the maxillomandibular complex; therefore, the localisation and paths of maxillary and mandibular fractures can be assessed (12.6).

If bidimensional radiographs are not sufficient to clearly visualise all the necessary details of the involved areas (particularly the maxilla, where the superimposition of many anatomic structures may render evaluation of the image difficult), the recourse to *computed tomography* is indicated. In cases of severe trauma, when complex maxillary and mandibular fractures are present, computed tomography represents the gold standard for a comprehensive evaluation of the clinical situation and for the adequate planning of the following treatment. In this event, a CT scan of the entire maxillofacial region and skull should be requested.

Treatment

Dentoalveolar trauma must always be considered an emergency condition; as such, immediate treatment should be performed to alleviate pain, facilitate the reduction of dislocated teeth and/or alveolar ridges, and improve the prognosis. Clinical evaluation can become difficult when swelling of the soft tissues sets in (24-48 hours after the trauma). In this event, a waiting period of 7-10 days makes it possible to achieve complete oedema remission and allows clinical examination to be accurately performed. Waiting periods longer that 15 days are contraindicated, because during the third week after trauma maturation of the callus occurs: if bone segments/fragments are dislocated or malpositioned they can heal in an incorrect position and reduction of the luxated teeth may be impossible.

General principles

PRINCIPLES OF FRACTURE HEALING

Bone fracture healing is a complex process that follows specific regenerative patterns. Following the initial trauma, bone may undergo either direct (primary) healing by proliferation of the Haversian canals across the line of fracture or indirect (secondary) healing by callus formation. Indirect healing is the most common occurrence, since primary healing requires anatomical reduction and rigid stabilisation of the fracture, which are generally obtained by open reduction and internal fixation. However, the evolution and duration of the healing process are determined by the type and severity of the fracture, by the conditions of the overlying soft tissues, by the type of treatment chosen or available, and by individual factors (e.g. age, history of radiotherapy, etc.). In children, the metabolic rate is higher and, thus, fractures heal faster than in older patients. If bone has been exposed to radiotherapy (particularly for doses exceeding 45 Gy), the regenerative potential may be greatly reduced.

Primary healing

Primary bone healing requires an anatomical reduction and rigidly stable conditions, commonly obtained by open reduction and internal fixation. When such conditions are achieved, Haversian canals can proliferate directly across the line of fracture; if minimal space is present along the line of fracture, however, blood vessels proliferate to carry osteoblasts that produce newly formed lamellar bone until stability of the fractured fragments is obtained. In the second healing phase, new osteons are formed to fill the interstices completely.

Secondary healing

Secondary healing is characterised by the formation of fibrous bone (callus) in the line of fracture, and by the formation of periosteum on the cortical plate of the fractured fragments.

In the healing process, the following phases can be identified:

- in the first phase (1st-6th day), haematoma formation in the line of fracture occurs, determining a connective tissue response in the form of active hyperaemia;
- in the second phase (6th-12th day) the blood clot is infiltrated by granulation tissue migrating from the open medullary canals and from the periosteum;
- the third phase is characterised by the formation of osteoid tissue that gradually transforms; in fact, fibroblasts and chondroblasts produce an extracellular organic matrix of fibrous tissue and cartilage wherein woven bone is deposited by osteoblasts, leading to the formation of the callus. The formation of the periosteal callus is more evident than that of the endosteal callus;
- from the 4th week after the trauma, fibrous bone gradually transforms into lamellar bone, characterised by the typical arrangement of the lamellae along the pressure or traction vectors (remodelling).

The general principles for the treatment of bone fractures may be summarised as follows:

- the traumatised area is carefully cleaned;
- the fracture is reduced;
- rigid fixation of the bone fragments is performed.

CLEANING

The traumatised area must be cleaned to remove foreign bodies (dirt, grass, glass fragments, etc.) and to decontaminate open wounds to reduce the risk of infection. Cleaning is performed with the aid of sterile pliers and irrigation with sterile saline.

REDUCTION

The reduction manoeuvre consists in the repositioning of the tooth/teeth, of the dislocated dentoalveolar fragment, or of the fractured bone fragments into their correct position. It is performed manually and, when conditions are favourable, can be performed without the need for a surgical access.

As regards tooth luxation with acceptable preservation of the anatomical integrity of the alveolus, a purposefully activated orthodontic wire can be used in association with dedicated brackets fixed on the patient's teeth to reposition the luxated tooth gradually, until a precise realignment is obtained.

Whenever complex lesions that require a direct visualisation of the traumatised area are present, particularly for displaced or comminuted fractures, open reduction of the fracture is indicated.

However, closed reduction should always represent the first choice in the treatment of a fracture, as it is the less invasive approach, makes it possible to maintain the blood supply in the traumatised area unaltered, and avoids exposure of the fractured bone to the external environment, thus reducing the risk of infection.

RIGID FIXATION

Rigid fixation makes it possible to lock the luxated teeth and/or the fractured dentoalveolar segment in their original position, to restore occlusion and permit healing and consolidation of the fracture.

It is obtained with the use synthesis materials such as interdental metallic ligatures, orthodontic brackets and wires, arch bars, titanium plates and screws; the type of fixation depends on the type and extent of the trauma, and on the degree of stabilisation needed. For open reduction of bone fractures, titanium plates and screws are the first choice for osteosynthesis.

To obtain optimal healing, it is necessary that the fractured segments be prevented from moving during the entire healing period, to avoid transformation of the granulation tissue formed inside the fracture interface into connective tissue, with subsequent formation of a pseudarthrosis.

Generally, the fractured segments are kept immobilised for 4-6 weeks to allow adequate healing. During this period, it is indicated to protect the traumatised area also by "physiologic trauma", such as occlusion/chewing.

Surgical armamentarium for closed reduction (12.10a-b)

- Materials for bracket fixation.
- Orthodontic wires.
- Arch bars.
- Steel wires for interdental ligatures.

Surgical armamentarium for open reduction

- Materials for closed reduction.
- Standard armamentarium for bone surgery.
- Titanium plates and screws.

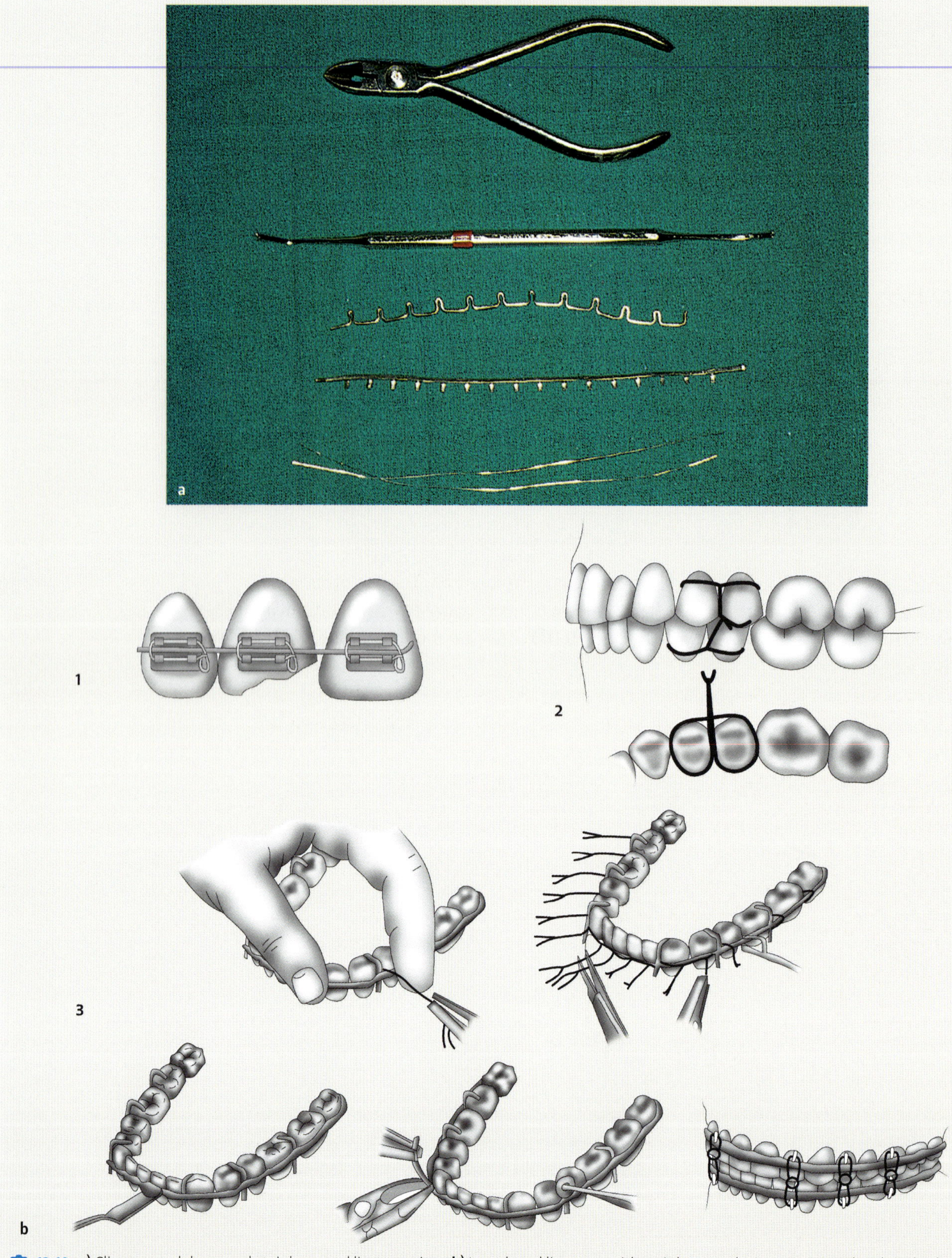

12.10 **a)** Clippers, arch bars, and stainless steel ligature wires. **b)** Interdental ligatures with stainless steel wires associated with orthodontic brackets or arch bars.

Surgical protocols

Surgical procedures to treat the different types of traumatic injuries will be summarised according to the type of lesion.

CONCUSSION

As no modifications of the teeth position are present, it is sufficient to wait for spontaneous healing, while preventing any mechanical stress to be exerted on the traumatised area. Tooth vitality must be monitored over time.

SUBLUXATION

While the teeth are not dislocated, marked tooth mobility is appreciable. The treatment consists in the rigid fixation of the subluxated teeth for 3-4 weeks, to allow the damaged periodontal ligament and possible microfractures of the alveolar bone to heal spontaneously. Rigid fixation can be easily achieved when non-traumatised teeth are present mesially and distally to the subluxated tooth: brackets are fixed to the teeth and connected with an orthodontic wire or arch bar. Tooth vitality must be monitored over time.

LUXATION

As regards teeth luxation, the correct position of each tooth must be first restored, and closed reduction of the possible fracture of the alveolar bone must be performed with manual manoeuvres. Rigid fixation is then achieved with the same technique described for subluxated teeth.

With luxation or subluxation, possible lesions to the soft tissues should be treated at the same time. Bite guards engaging the non-traumatised dentition should be fabricated to free the traumatised teeth from occlusion and mastication.

Two step-by-step clinical cases illustrating the described procedure are presented (12.11a-d, 12.12a-d).

COMPLETE AVULSION

Typically, traumatic avulsion is observed in the anterior areas of the maxilla and mandible, and it is quite frequent in young patients. Simple avulsion without fractures of the alveolar ridge is more frequent in preschool and school-aged children, due to the incomplete formation of the roots, and to the flexibility of the alveolar bone, which allows it to tolerate significant stress without fracturing.

Generally, the traumatic avulsion of deciduous teeth is not treated; the tooth is not reimplanted, and the eruption of the permanent tooth is monitored.

For complete avulsion of a permanent tooth, on the other hand, the treatment of choice is represented by tooth *reimplantation*. The success of this treatment depends on the following criteria:

- how the tooth was preserved prior to reimplantation;
- how long the tooth was preserved out of the oral cavity;
- degree of contamination of the tooth;
- degree of root formation.

Clinical case 1 – Extrusive luxation of 1.2-1.1-2.1

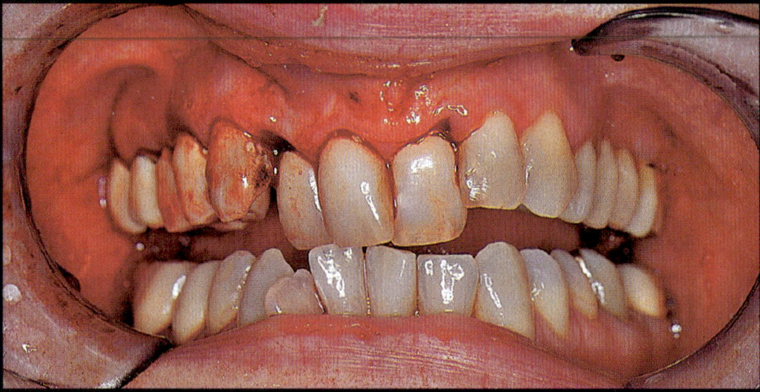

12.11.a Extrusive luxation of 1.2-1.1-2.1: palatal inclination of the luxated teeth and marked alteration of the normal occlusion due to premature contacts are evident.

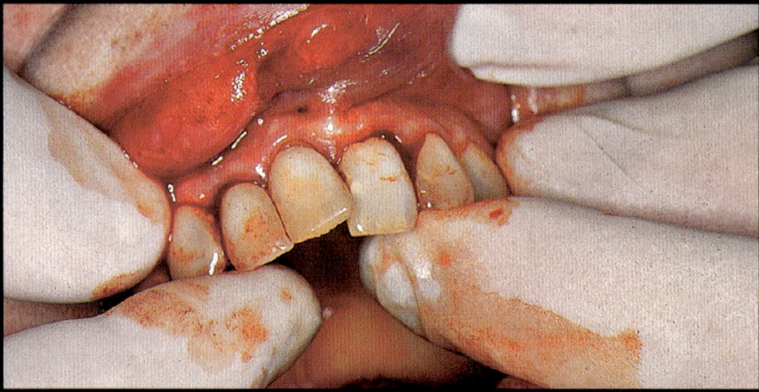

12.11b Closed reduction.

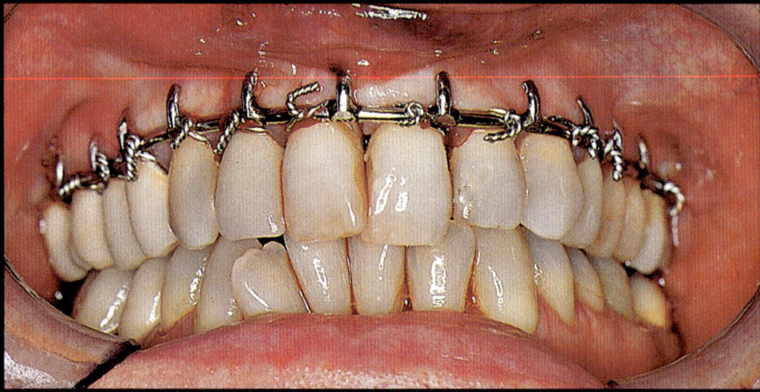

12.11c Rigid fixation with an arch bar and ligature wires.

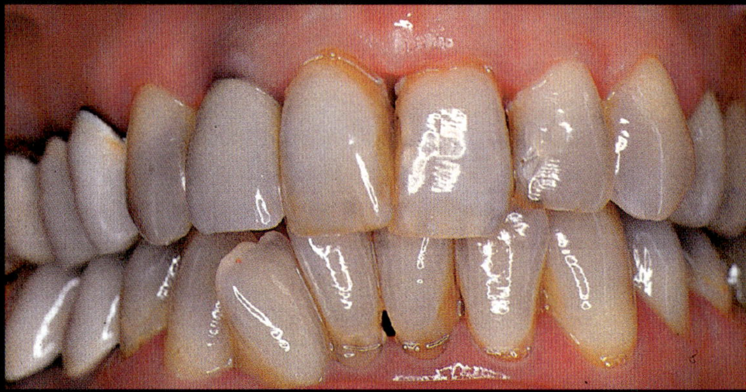

12.11d Follow-up time after the removal of the arch bar.

Clinical case 2 – Intrusive luxation of the maxillary incisors

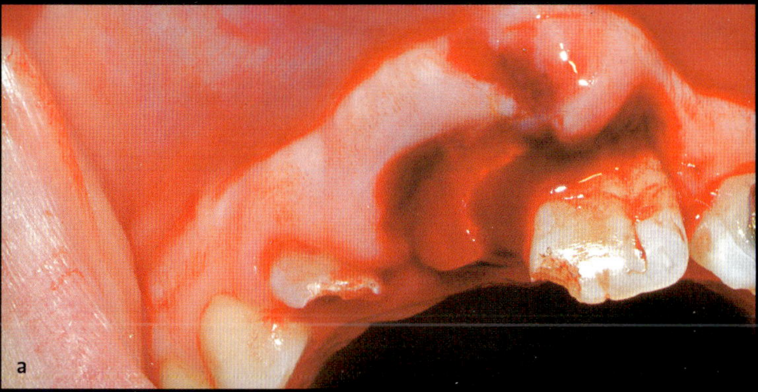

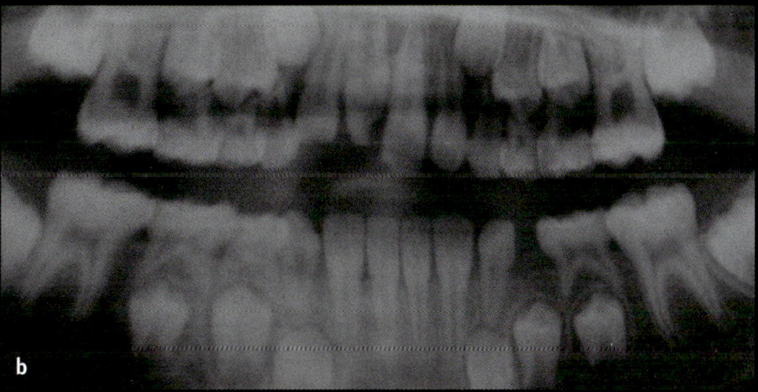

12.12a–b Facial trauma in a child has caused the intrusive luxation of the maxillary incisors and crown fractures.

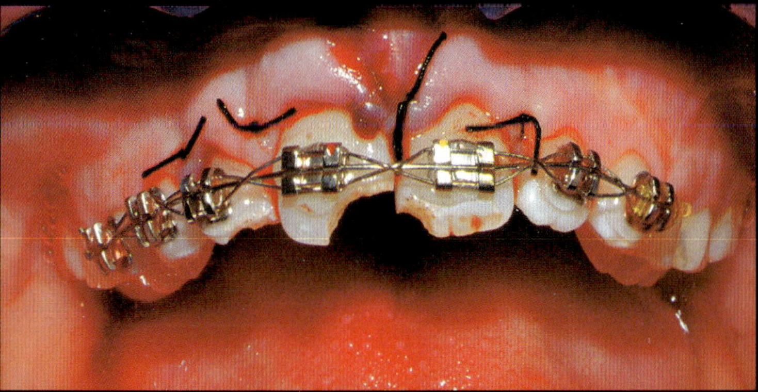

12.12c Closed reduction allowed the repositioning of the dentoalveolar segment; rigid fixation is obtained by means of orthodontic brackets and wires.

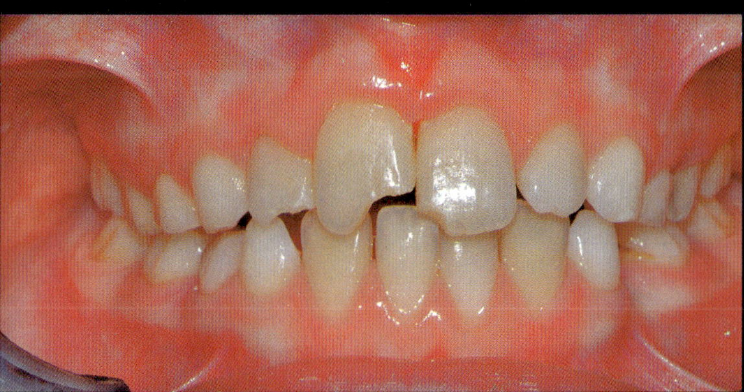

12.12d Complete healing of the dentoalveolar fracture: restorative techniques will allow the treatment of crown fractures.

Preservation of the tooth prior to reimplantation: the tooth can be effectively preserved by submerging it in sterile saline, blood, milk, or saliva. It is important to avoid non-isotonic solutions, which could cause further damage to the pulp.

Preservation time: chances of complete healing are inversely proportional to the length of time the tooth is preserved out of the oral cavity.

Degree of contamination of the tooth: the avulsed tooth must be carefully cleaned with sterile saline to remove the majority of contaminants on its surface. Root planing, recommended in the past, is currently advised against, as it results in the complete elimination of residual fibres of the periodontal ligament and part of the root cement fundamental to obtaining the complete reattachment of the periodontal ligament.

Degree of root formation: teeth with partially formed roots can be immediately reimplanted, as the open apex facilitates revascularisation and reinnervation of the tooth, with subsequent periodontal ligament reattachment. Contrarily, endodontic treatment must be performed after reimplantation of teeth with completely formed roots, with the exception of teeth with an apex diameter wider than 1 millimetre; in these cases, a waiting period of 4-6 weeks after reimplantation makes it possible to monitor the possible recovery of the pulp vitality.

MANAGEMENT OF TEETH INVOLVED IN THE LINE OF FRACTURE

The tooth involved in the line of fracture can be maintained in situ only if no severe periodontal, endodontic or carious lesions are present, and if it does not significantly interfere with fracture reduction.

This is particularly important for trauma involving the anterior areas of the maxilla and mandible, which are particularly exposed to dentoalveolar fractures and the related functional and aesthetic implications.

Implant rehabilitation after tooth loss due to trauma

IMMEDIATE REPLACEMENT OF THE AVULSED TOOTH

In some cases an avulsed tooth, if immediately retrieved and adequately preserved, may be reimplanted (see previous section). On the contrary, with vertical root fractures, or multiple root fractures, the long-term prognosis is significantly worse; the pulp may lose its vitality and root resorption may develop years after the trauma and the reimplantation. Another possible consequence is represented by variations in the position of the reimplanted tooth, with possible aesthetic sequelae. Whenever it is impossible to retrieve the avulsed tooth, or reimplantation is not possible, prosthetic rehabilitation of the edentulous area is necessary.

Traditional removable prostheses may cause functional and psychological problems, particularly in young patients, as well as accelerate bone resorption in the traumatised area. Bone resorption, in these cases, is compensated with artificial gingiva to avoid the use of long and disharmonic teeth.

Tooth-supported fixed prosthetic restorations eliminate the functional and psychological disadvantages of removable prostheses, but imply the preparation of neighbouring teeth.

Endosseous implants represent a safe and reliable alternative for the correction of edentulism caused by trauma sequelae, and permit the prosthetic rehabilitation of the edentulous area while maintaining the integrity of the neighbouring teeth.

Basic techniques

Traumatic avulsion

Once the tooth is cleansed with sterile saline, the alveolus is inspected to evaluate its shape and the integrity of its walls, and to identify possible bone fragments or foreign bodies that may contaminate the area or impede a successful reimplantation of the tooth. Irrigation with sterile saline is performed to cleanse the alveolus before the avulsed tooth is repositioned and rigidly fixed to the adjacent teeth by means of brackets and an orthodontic wire or an arch bar, after endodontic treatment has been completed. Unlike bone fractures, which necessitate several weeks of rigid fixation to allow the formation of the callus, rigid fixation of the reimplanted tooth can be limited to 1-2 weeks; in fact, early functionalisation of the periodontal ligament prevents root ankylosis (12.13a-d).

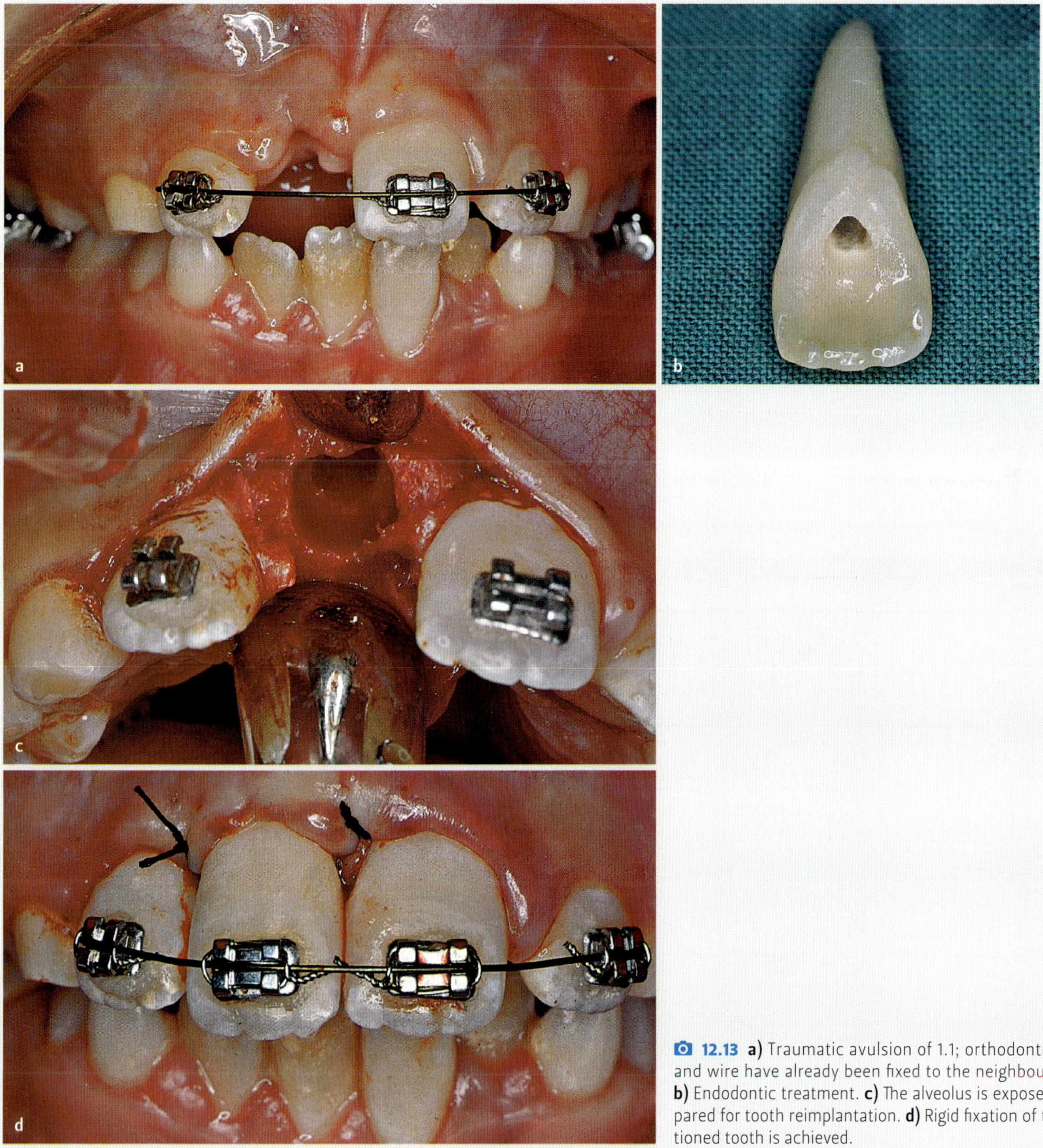

12.13 a) Traumatic avulsion of 1.1; orthodontic brackets and wire have already been fixed to the neighbouring teeth. **b)** Endodontic treatment. **c)** The alveolus is exposed and prepared for tooth reimplantation. **d)** Rigid fixation of the repositioned tooth is achieved.

Lesions of the intraoral soft tissues

Contusions and abrasions do not need specific treatments, except thorough cleansing and disinfection.

Lacerations of the gingiva and oral mucosa must be cleaned to assess the condition of the tissues. Necrotic or severely lacerated portions, when present, should be removed with a conservative approach. Vital flaps should be sutured in their correct anatomical position, limiting the number of stitches to avoid further ischaemia of the soft tissues.

Fracture of the alveolar ridge

Typically, fractures of the alveolar ridge occur when teeth are present. In edentulous patients, the alveolar ridge is usually atrophic and, in these cases, fractures of the basal bone are more frequent (a detailed description of these fractures and their treatment can be found in maxillofacial surgery textbooks). Fractures of the alveolar ridge can be treated with closed reduction or open reduction.

Closed reduction

This is the treatment of choice for dentoalveolar fractures, even if dislocated, whenever the integrity of the overlying soft tissues is preserved.

After thorough cleansing of the traumatised area is completed, manual reduction of the fracture is performed with delicate and gradual movements. This manoeuvre is relatively simple in the presence of a single fractured segment, whereas with a comminuted fracture the presence of several bone fragments can represent an obstacle to correct repositioning.

Once the fracture is reduced, adequate restoration of the patient's occlusion must be verified, and the possible presence of premature contacts must be determined.

The fractured dentoalveolar segment is finally locked into its original position by rigid fixation with brackets and orthodontic wires or arch bars and interdental ligatures.

Open reduction

When excessive dislocation or comminution of the fractured fragments and laceration and contamination of the soft tissues are present, it is indicated to perform an open reduction of the dentoalveolar fracture.

Generally, surgical access is designed to exploit the lacerations of the soft tissues to avoid further devascularisation that would be caused by new incisions performed on intact soft tissues.

After thorough cleansing of the traumatised area, the fracture is reduced and the patient's occlusion is restored. For comminuted fractures, the use of osteosynthesis means, such as titanium micro or miniplates and screws, may be indicated to obtain a rigid fixation of the fractured segments. The soft tissues are then sutured in their correct anatomical position. The same postoperative recommendations described for the closed reduction apply (12.14a–e).

> It is not always possible to obtain an exact repositioning of all the dislocated fragments in a single surgical session; in these cases, small corrections can be performed in the first days after surgery with the aid of orthodontic appliances.
> For contamination of intraoral and/or extraoral wounds, administration of an antibiotic therapy and tetanus prophylaxis are advised.

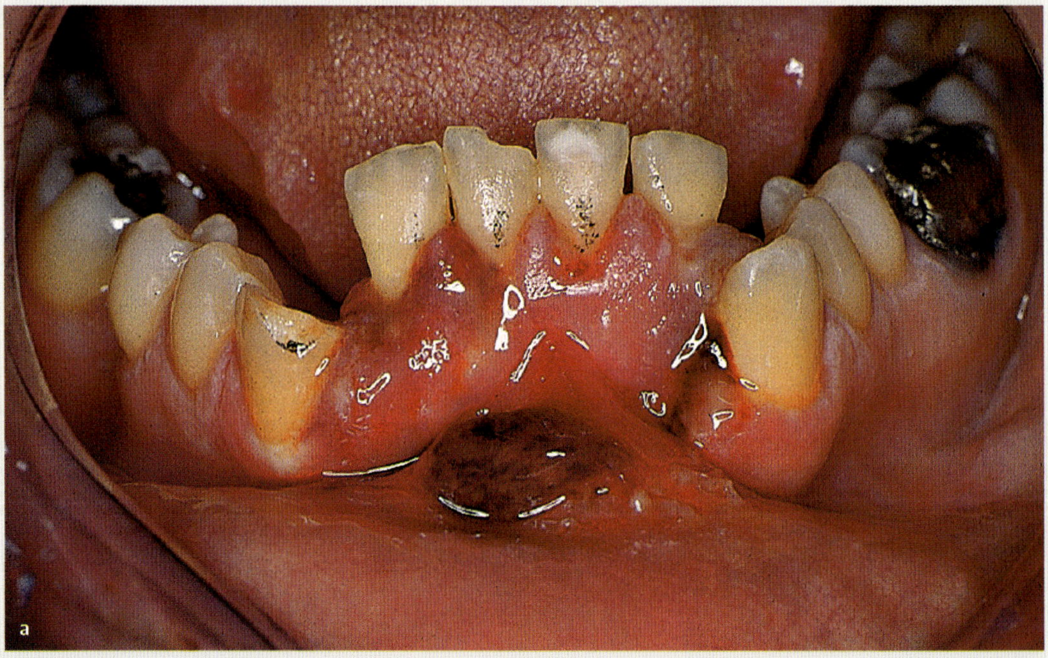

12.14 a) Dentoalveolar fracture in the area of the mandibular incisors, with significant dislocation of the fractured segment, and loss of the normal occlusion. (*continued*)

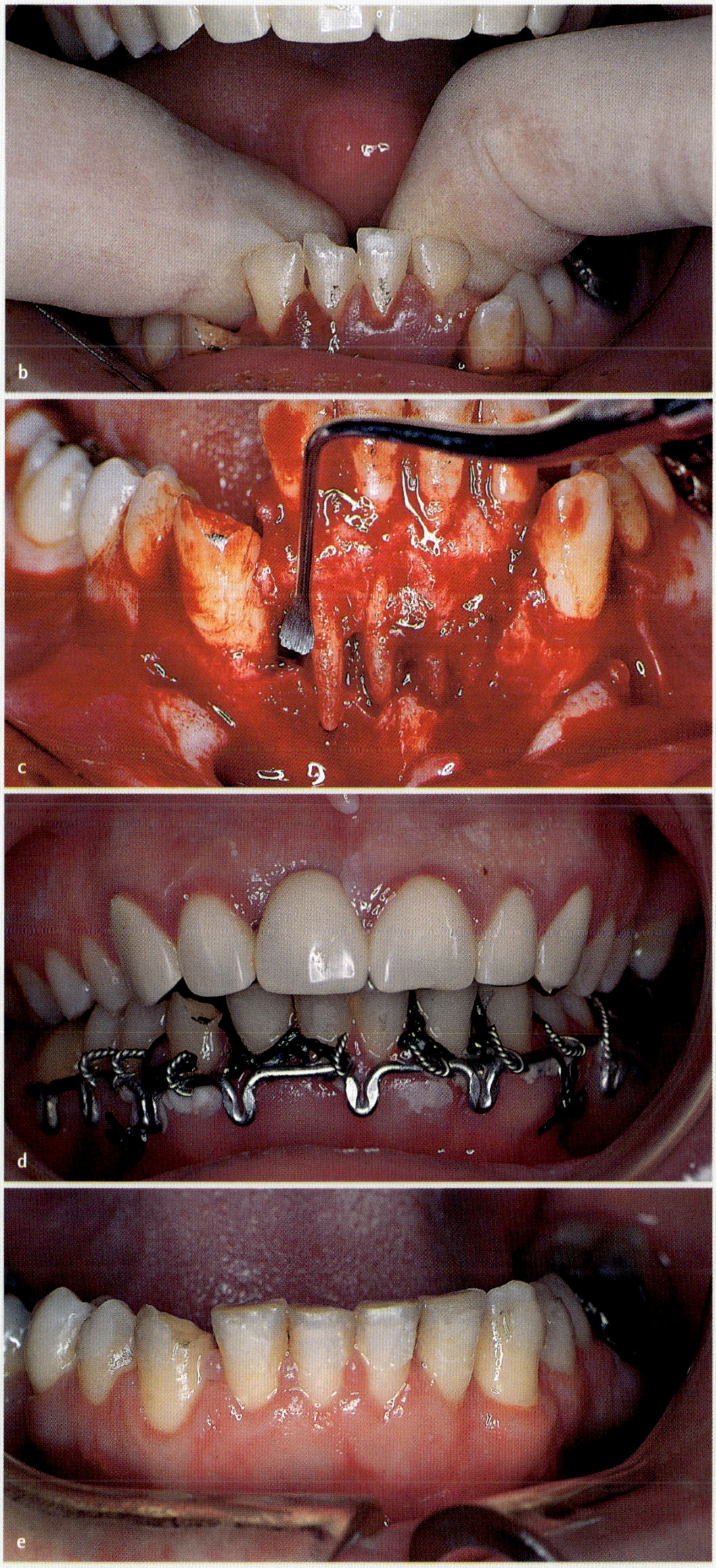

12.14 (*continued*) **b)** Closed reduction does not allow adequate repositioning of the fracture segment. **c)** A surgical flap is elevated to expose the traumatised area: devascularised bone fragments preventing the correct repositioning of the fractured segment are eliminated with the aid of a bone curette. **d)** Fracture reduction, rigid fixation, and suture: the normal occlusion is restored. **e)** Follow-up time after surgery.

Fracture of the basal bone

For complete fracture of the basal bone, the treatment follows the same principles outlined for dentoalveolar fractures (reduction and rigid fixation). As for dentoalveolar fractures, in favourable cases (e.g. non-displaced fractures) it is possible to perform a closed reduction followed by intermaxillary fixation, particularly with mandibular fractures. However, since intermaxillary fixation should be maintained for a minimum of 4 weeks (with relevant discomfort for the patient), open reduction and rigid fixation with titanium plates and screws is currently indicated. Open reduction is particularly indicated in the case of displaced fractures and fractures in the anterior maxilla, where intermaxillary fixation is contraindicated due to the risk of displacement of the reduced fractured segments with involuntary movements of the mandible. A detailed description of the surgical procedures is reported in textbooks of maxillofacial traumatology; a step-by-step clinical case is presented to illustrate the reduction and rigid fixation techniques (12.15a–j).

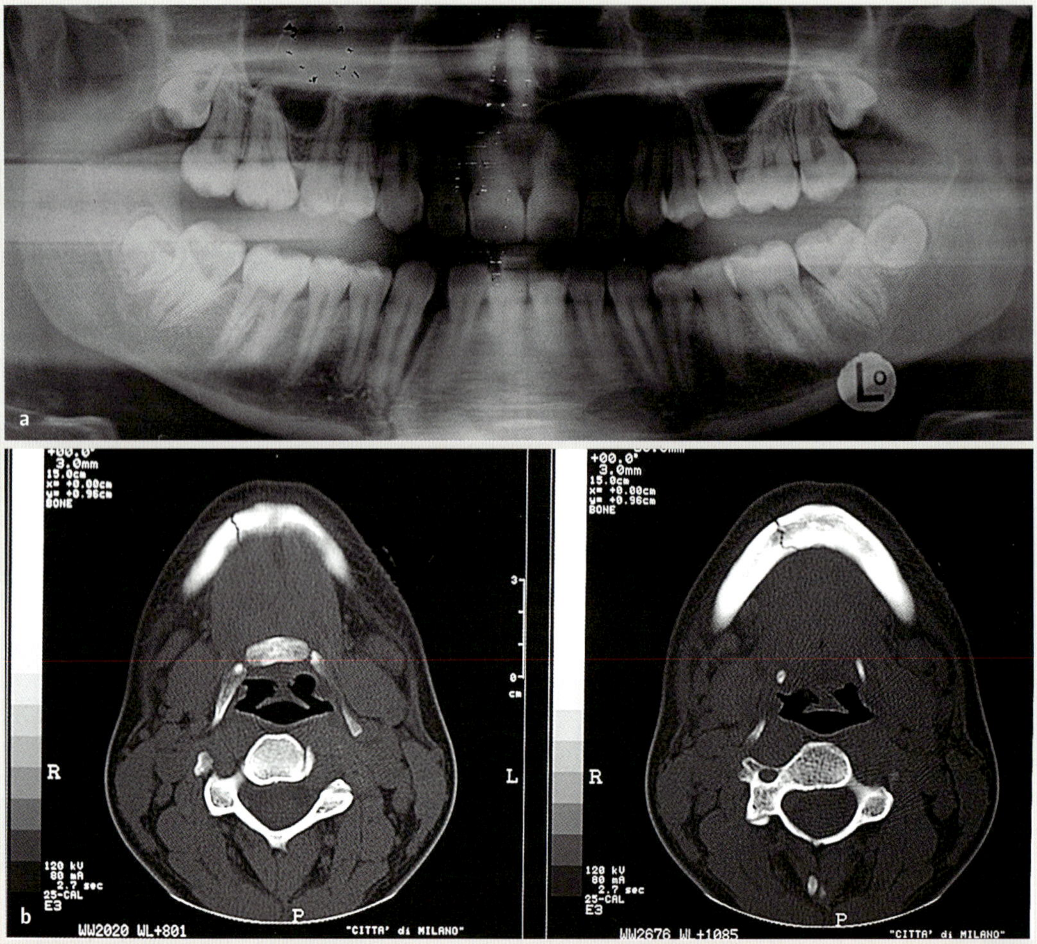

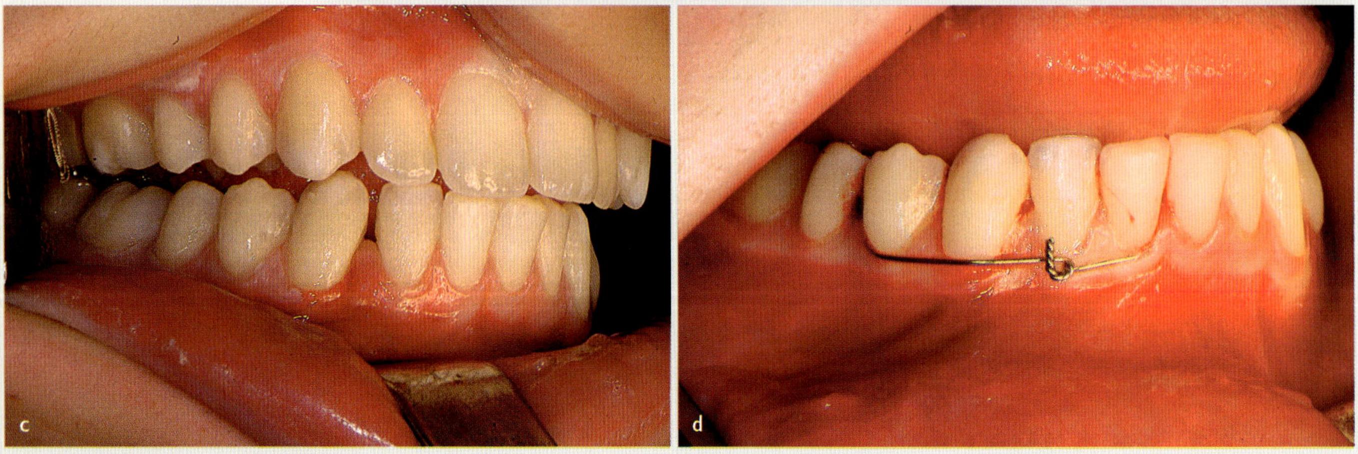

12.15 **a)** Panoramic radiograph showing a mandibular fracture in the area between 4.3 and 4.2. **b)** CT-scan demonstrates the complete fracture of the mandibular body. **c)** Preoperative clinical situation with loss of the normal occlusion. **d)** An interdental ligature is used to stabilise the dentoalveolar fracture. (*continued*)

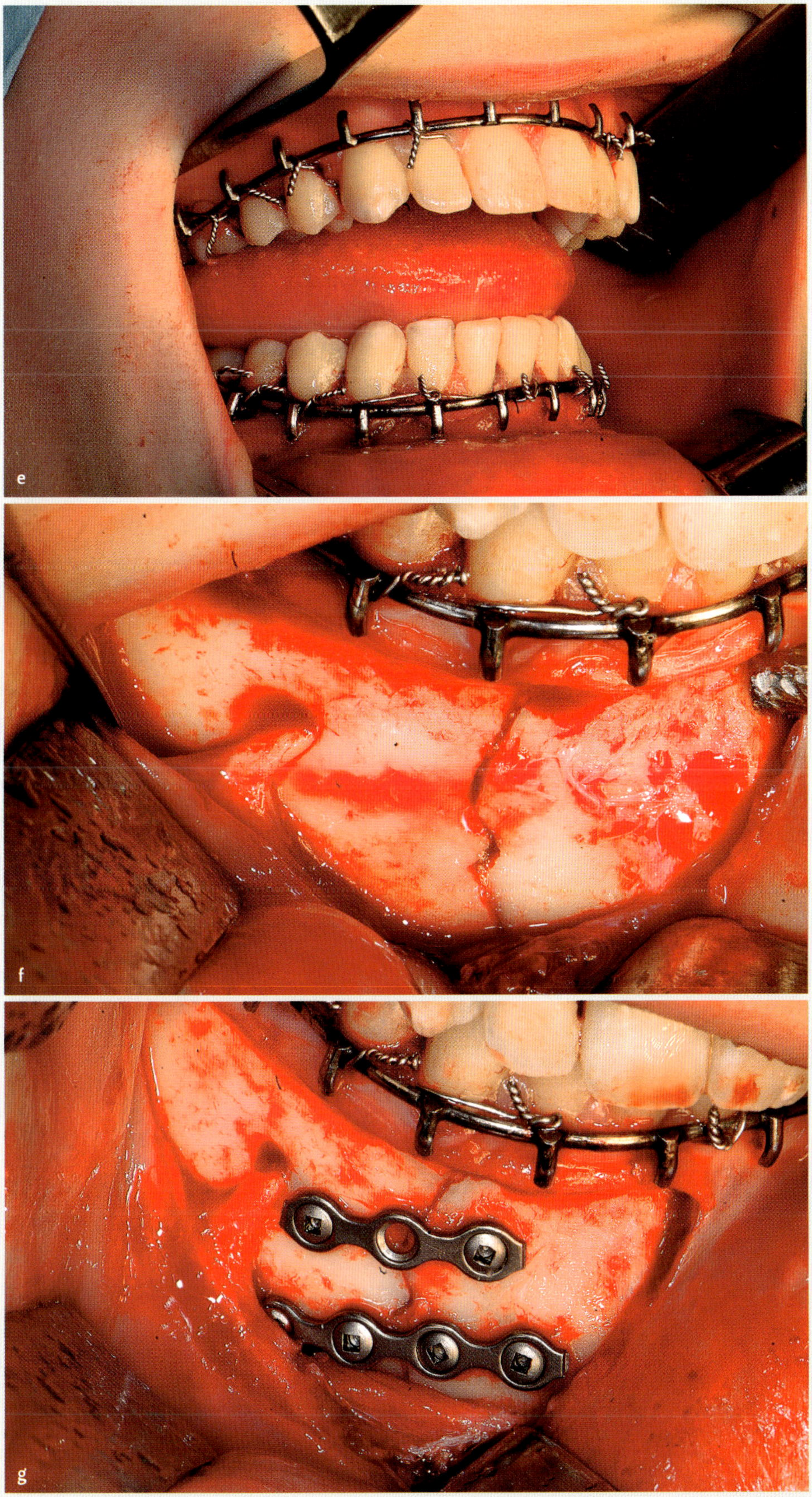

12.15 (*continued*) **e)** Two arch bars are fixed to the dental arches by means of ligatures. **f)** Intraoperative view of the fracture, and identification of the mental foramen and nerve. **g)** Rigid fixation of the fracture with two titanium miniplates and osteosynthesis screws. (*continued*)

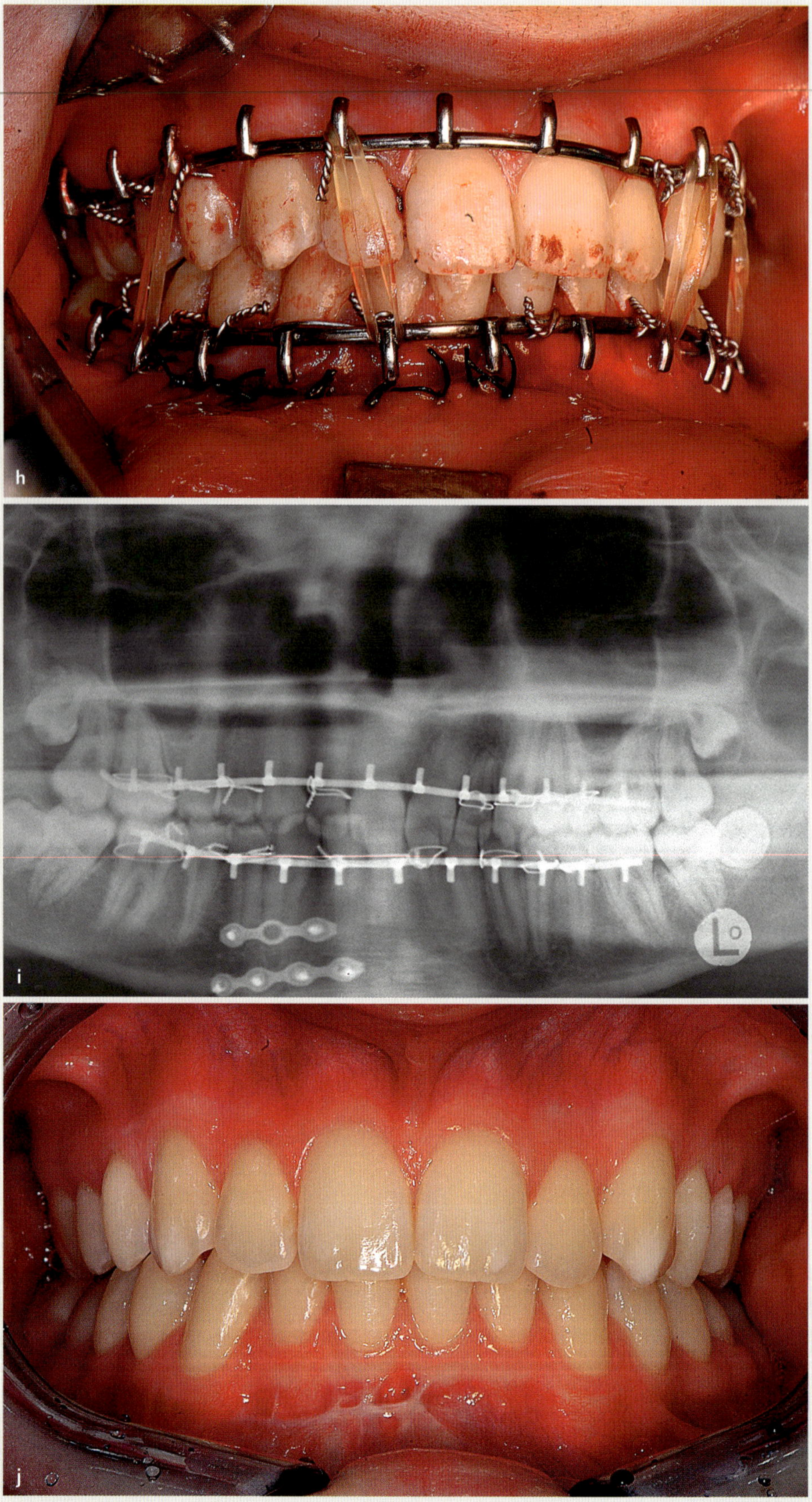

12.15 (*continued*) **h)** Intermaxillary fixation is obtained by means of orthodontic elastic bands. Normal occlusion is restored. **i)** Postoperative panoramic radiograph. **j)** Follow-up time after surgery: the correct occlusion is maintained.

The early replacement of a fractured tooth with an immediate post-extractive implant is possible when local conditions, such as the anatomy of the alveolus, the integrity of the buccal bone plate, and the gingival biotype are favourable. A step-by-step clinical case is presented to illustrate the replacement of a fractured maxillary central incisor with a post-extractive implant (12.16a-i).

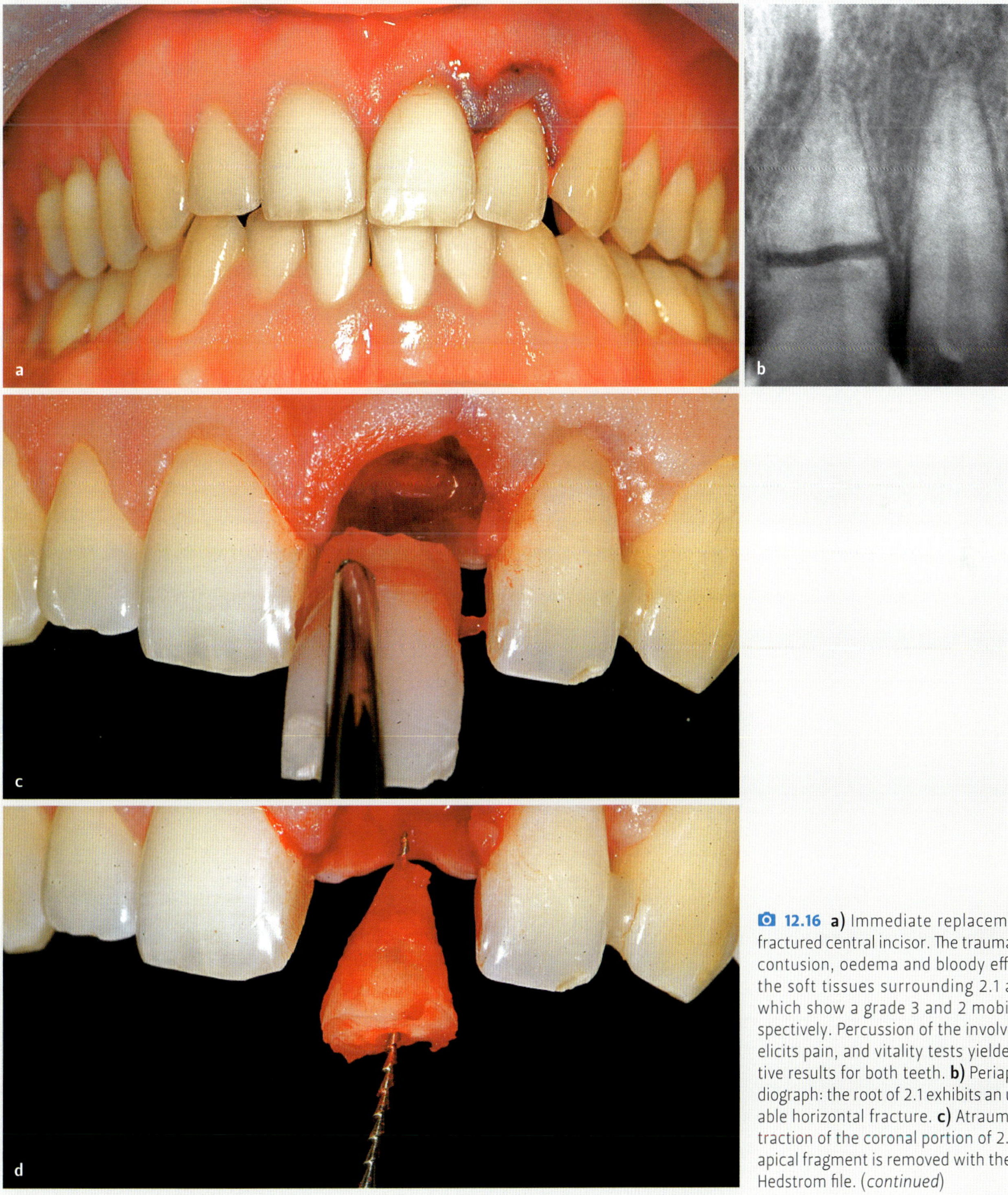

12.16 **a)** Immediate replacement of a fractured central incisor. The trauma caused contusion, oedema and bloody effusion in the soft tissues surrounding 2.1 and 2.2, which show a grade 3 and 2 mobility, respectively. Percussion of the involved teeth elicits pain, and vitality tests yielded negative results for both teeth. **b)** Periapical radiograph: the root of 2.1 exhibits an untreatable horizontal fracture. **c)** Atraumatic extraction of the coronal portion of 2.1. **d)** The apical fragment is removed with the aid of a Hedstrom file. (*continued*)

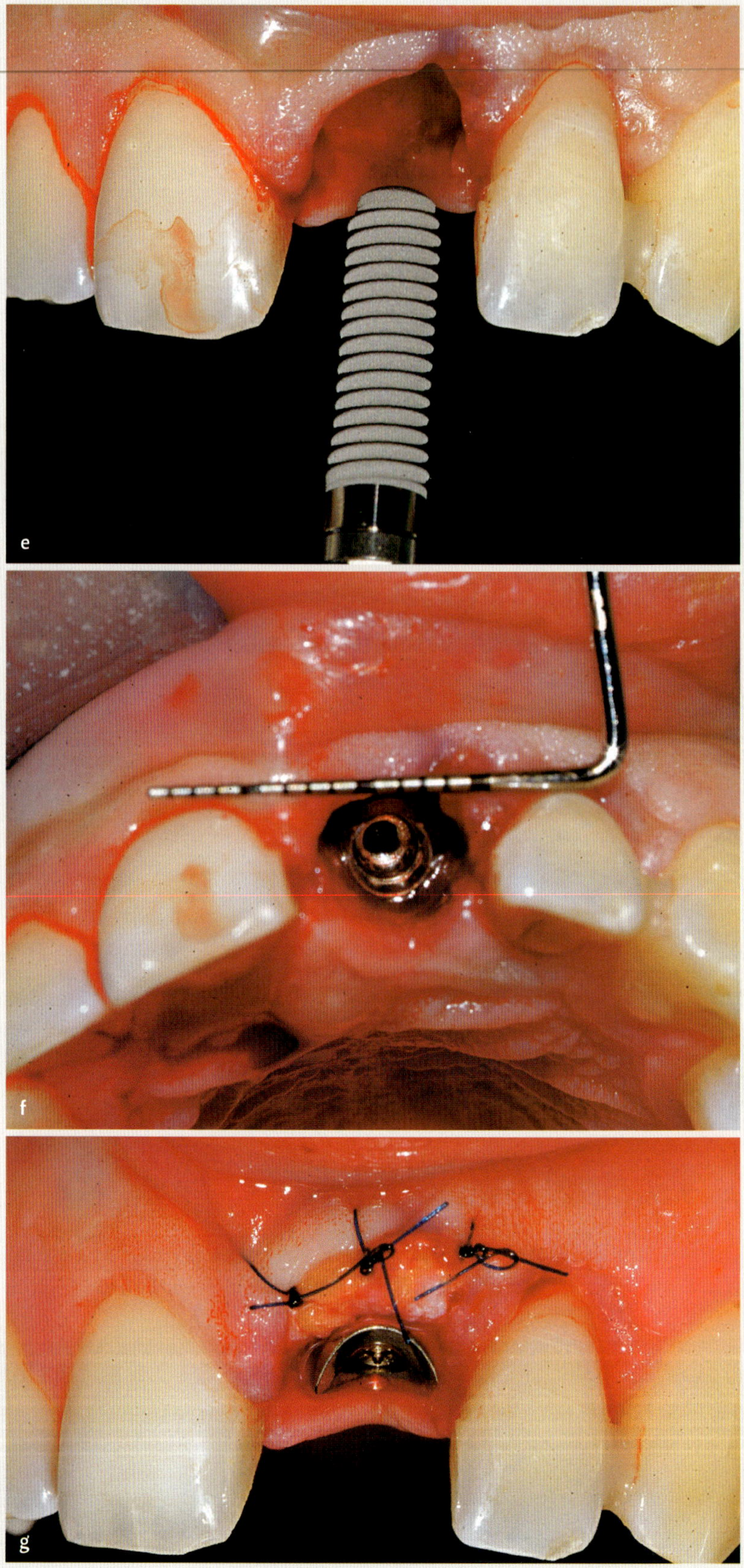

12.16 (*continued*) **e)** Immediately after tooth extraction, the implant site is prepared and an endosseous implant is placed (Straumann TE). **f)** Exact positioning of the implant is obtained by following the guidelines for prosthetically guided implant placement. **g)** A connective tissue graft makes it possible to augment the thickness of the peri-implant soft tissues and enhance the final aesthetics (implant surgery: Dr. Paolo Casentini). (*continued*)

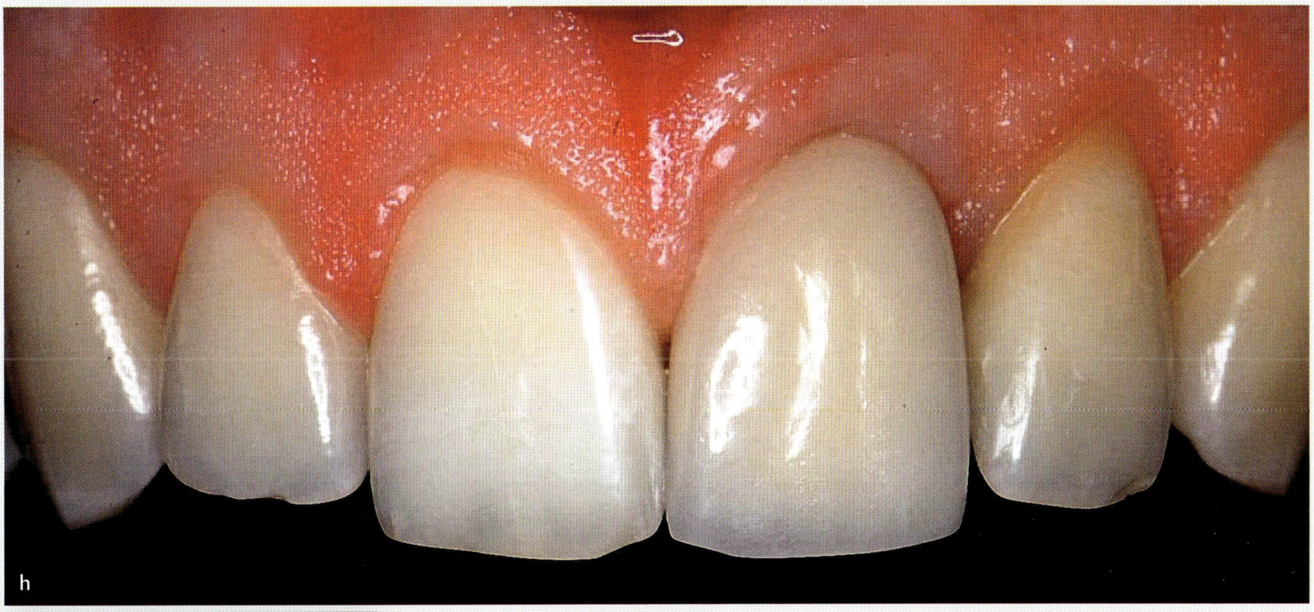

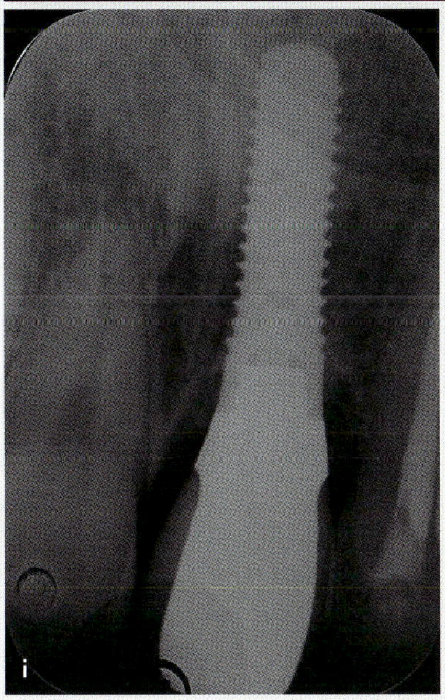

12.16 (*continued*) **h)** The implant-supported prosthetic rehabilitation shows a good integration with the patient's natural dentition (prosthetic rehabilitation: Dr. Dario Mezzanzanico). **i)** Radiographic follow-up after prosthetic loading.

If the traumatic avulsion of teeth has also caused the loss of both alveolar and basal bone, traditional fixed and removable prostheses may prove inadequate to rehabilitate the edentulous area satisfactorily, due to anatomic alterations of the hard and soft tissues caused by bone loss and atrophy. Moreover, bone defects may render placement of the implants in a correct position difficult or impossible. The recourse to regenerative/reconstructive procedures using autologous bone as a grafting material has led to significant improvements in the management of these clinical situations. In fact, these procedures make it possible to recreate adequate bone volume and morphology in the deficient areas, thus rendering implant-supported rehabilitations not only reliable from a functional viewpoint, but also aesthetically satisfying. Details on the planning of this type of rehabilitation and the surgical techniques involved are presented in Chapter 13 (Chiapasco and Romeo, 2003).

Follow-up

A liquid or semi-liquid diet is recommended for 4 weeks after fracture reduction, to avoid any mechanical stress in the area of the fracture.

Adequate oral hygiene is essential to avoiding postoperative infections; the use of chlorhexidine mouthwashes in association with tooth brushing is indicated.

Four weeks after surgery, rigid fixation means (brackets, arch bars) are removed, occlusion is verified, and the normal masticatory function is gradually resumed. In cases of dental trauma (luxation, avulsion), rigid fixation is removed after 1-2 weeks to avoid tooth ankylosis.

Internal osteosynthesis devices (plates and screws) can be left in place, or they can be removed 6 months after surgery.

Every tooth that experiences trauma may lose its vitality; therefore, these teeth must be monitored over time to diagnose a possible pulpar necrosis and promptly proceed with endodontic therapy, to avoid colour alterations and periapical infections.
In cases of avulsion, ten years after trauma pulp survival in teeth with immature apexes ranges from 30% to 40%, while pulp survival in teeth with completely formed roots is 0%.
Reimplanted teeth exhibit a good mid-term (7 years) survival rate in the oral cavity. However, roots are exposed to internal and external resorption that may lead to their exfoliation.

REFERENCES

ANDREASEN JO. Etiology and pathogenesis of traumatic dental injuries. *Scand J Dent Res* 1970; 78:339.

ANDREASEN JO, ANDREASEN FM, BAKLAND LK, FLORES MT. Traumatic dental injuries: A manual. 2nd ed. Blackwell Munksgaard, Copenhagen 1999.

BRUSATI R, CHIAPASCO M. Elementi di chirurgia oro-maxillo-facciale. Masson, Milano 1999.

CABRINI GABRIELLI MA, REAL GABRIELLI MF, MARCANTONIO E, HOCHULI-VIEIRA E. Fixation of mandibular fractures with 2.0 mm miniplates: review of 191 cases. *J Oral Maxillofac Surg* 2003 Apr; 61(4):430-6.

CHIAPASCO M, ROMEO E. Riabilitazione implanto-protesica nei casi complessi. Utet, Torino 2003.

COULTHARD P, ESPOSITO M, WORTHINGTON HV, JOKSTAD A. Interventions for replacing missing teeth: preprosthetic surgery versus dental implants. *Cochrane Database Syst Rev* 2002; (4):CD003604.

PETERSEN JK. Management of acute dento-alveolar trauma - from the viewpoint of an oral surgeon. *Aust Endodon J* 2000 Aug; 26(2):72-7.

PETERSON LJ, ELLIS III E, HUPP JR, TUCKER MR. Contemporary oral and maxillofacial surgery. 2nd ed. Mosby, St. Louis 1993, pp. 112-6.

SCHWARTZ-ARAD D, LEVIN L, ASHKENAZI M. Treatment options of untreatable traumatized anterior maxillary teeth for future use of dental implantation. *Implant Dent* 2004 Jun; 13(2):120-8.

THOR A, ANDERSSON L. Interdental wiring in jaw fractures: effects on teeth and surrounding tissues after a one-year follow-up. *Br J Oral Maxillofac Surg* 2001 Oct; 39(5):398-401.

TULI T, HACHL O, RASSE M, KLOSS F, GASSNER R. Dentoalveolar trauma. Analysis of 4763 patients with 6237 injuries in 10 years (articolo in tedesco). *Mund Kiefer Gesichtschir* 2005 Sep; 9(5):324-9.

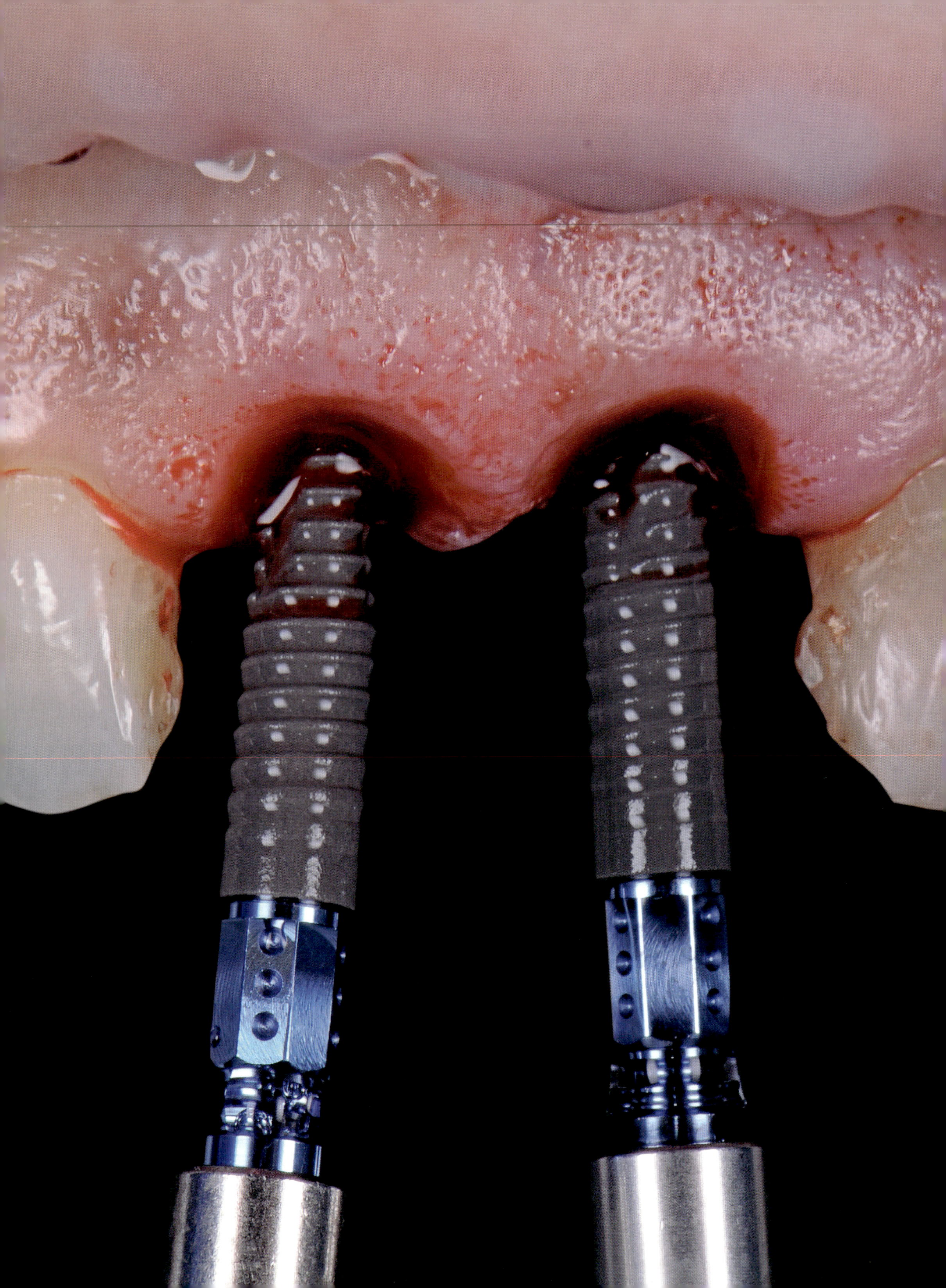

Implant surgery

M. Chiapasco, P. Casentini, M. Zaniboni

Basic implant surgery

Introduction

Over the last decades, a vast number of studies published in international scientific literature have demonstrated that oral implantology is a safe and reliable method to rehabilitate partially and totally edentulous ridges with fixed or removable prostheses supported by endosseous, osseointegrated implants.

The advent of endosseous implants has made it possible to have fixed pillars supporting prosthetic rehabilitations without involving the natural dentition (e.g. tooth preparation), or when bone resorption associated with total edentulism prevents adequate stability of removable prostheses. As implants allow the satisfactory treatment of conditions for which there was once no adequate option, and can significantly improve the functional and aesthetic outcome of others, they now represent an indispensable instrument in modern treatment plans.

Implant surgery is thus a relevant part of the oral surgeon's routine and, therefore, a description of the most common surgical techniques and their indications is presented in this chapter.

Historical overview

The last 40 years have seen a great development in oral implantology: the use of osseointegrated implants, traditionally limited to the treatment of total edentulism, has been extended to the treatment of partial edentulism and single tooth replacement. The primary objective, which was originally the creation of a bone anchorage for prostheses to restore the masticatory function, has been gradually joined by the search for a proper *restitutio ad integrum* that implies a growing consideration for aesthetics in implant-supported prosthetic rehabilitations.

A deeper knowledge has been acquired regarding the process of osseointegration, the more convenient implant morphology and surface, the timing of prosthetic loading, and the clinical, surgical, and prosthetic aspects of implantology in general.

Implant success criteria according to Albrektsson, Zarb, and Worthington (1986)

- An individual, unattached implant is immobile when tested clinically
- A radiograph does not demonstrate any evidence of peri-implant radiolucency
- Vertical bone loss is less than 0.2 mm annually following the implant's first year of service
- Individual implant performance is characterised by an absence of persistent and/or irreversible signs and symptoms such as pain, infections, neuropathies, paraesthesia, or violation of the mandibular canal
- In the context of the above, a success rate of 85% at the end of a five-year observation period and 80% at the end of a ten-year period is the minimum criterion for success

Modern oral implantology, intended for the use of endosseous titanium implants to support prosthetic rehabilitations, and the study of the osseointegration process were initiated in the 1960s by Swedish researcher Per Ingvar Brånemark and his colleagues. Brånemark was the first researcher to describe the biologic principle of osseointegration, defined as "direct contact between titanium implant and living bone without soft tissue interposition". He identified the following fundamental requisites to obtain osseointegration:

- the use of biocompatible materials, such as titanium, that do not cause rejection;
- the use of an atraumatic surgical technique to reduce the surgical and thermal trauma on the bone while allowing maximum precision in the creation of the implant site, to ensure an adequate contact area between the implant and the surrounding bone;
- a submerged healing phase to reduce the risk of infection and to avoid early loading of the implants.

Histologic confirmation of the osseointegration process of titanium implants came from the studies conducted by Swiss researcher André Schroeder and his team.

Utilising new techniques for the section and fixation of non-decalcified bone, they demonstrated the direct contact between the implant surface and the surrounding bone, which Schroeder defined as "functional ankylosis".

Years later, a group of researchers working in the Brånemark group tried to define specific criteria to evaluate implant success rates over time. Those criteria were originally proposed by Albretsson, Zarb and Worthington in 1986, and then adopted by Smith and Zarb in 1989. These criteria are still considered acceptable, even if over the following years several other methods to assess implant success rates have been proposed by different authors.

In a clinical study, the *implant success rate* corresponds to the percentage of implants satisfying those criteria.

The *implant survival rate*, on the other hand, corresponds to the percentage of implants that are still in function at a given moment, while not satisfying one or more of the success criteria.

Implant survival and success rates represent valuable information only when they are considered in relation to time: a follow-up period of at least 5 years after the start of prosthetic loading would be necessary to draw meaningful conclusions.

Biology of osseointegration

The endosseous placement of an implant, like a fracture or a trauma, activates a healing process aimed at restoring the original anatomy of the bone by means of biological repair and remodelling mechanisms that, in this specific case, do not modify bone quantity but renew its structure.

The healing process following the endosseous placement of a titanium screw-type implant has been investigated in several experimental studies; histological techniques have been used to analyse sections performed at the bone-to-implant interface at different moments in time after implant placement.

Main phases

The main phases of the healing process can be summarised as follows:

1. haematoma formation around the implant;
2. migration of mesenchymal and inflammatory cells in the area;
3. releasing and activation of mediators from the tissue subjected to the surgical trauma and from the blood;
4. differentiation of the mesenchymal cells into osteoblasts, and concurrent revascularisation and formation of granulation tissue;
5. macrophagic action of the osteoclasts on the granulation tissue;
6. woven bone formation;
7. lamellar bone formation;
8. bone remodelling.

The interval between the 2nd and 4th week after implant placement represents the most critical moment of the entire osseointegration process. In this phase, the remodelling process is prevalent in the cortical bone, while in the cancellous bone the mineralisation of newly formed bone is still insufficient. Therefore, micromovements of the implant (particularly those exceeding 100 microns) should be prevented, as they may interfere with osseointegration and cause a process of fibrous integration.

This event represents an early failure, and the involved implant must be removed. However, in selected cases where adequate primary implant stability is obtained and micromovements under 50 microns can be kept, it is possible to proceed to the immediate loading of implants. According to this protocol, the prosthesis is connected to the implants immediately after their placement is completed.

Although from a clinical point of view endosseous implants may appear to be integrated a few weeks after placement, it has been verified that the entire process of bone remodelling around implants may take up to 12 months.

Bone-implant interface and different implant surfaces

Several experimental and clinical studies have demonstrated that implants with a rough surface perform better with respect to the speed of the osseointegration process, the percentage of bone-to-implant contact, and the resistance to torsion tests when compared to implants with a machined surface. The evolution of surface treatments has caused a substantial reduction in the healing and loading time of implants (13.1).

The current surfaces, some of which are defined as chemically active due to special treatments that cause a higher hydrophilicity and, thus, an augmented capacity of attracting biofluids such as blood, have reduced the length of the osseointegration process from the initial 6-month figure (necessary for machined surfaces) to 3-4 weeks.

One or two-piece implants, one or two surgical phases

There are two main types of endosseous implants currently in use: two-piece implants and one-piece or transmucosal implants. Notwithstanding the differences between the two, as far as the interface between the implant and the peri-implant tissues (for a comprehensive review of the literature on this subject, see Esposito et al., 2009) is concerned, numerous clinical studies have demonstrated the reliability of both architectures from a clinical-prognostic point of view. However, specific indications for submerged and transmucosal types of implants exist, and will be listed below.

TWO-PIECE (OR "BONE LEVEL") IMPLANTS

This system consists of an endosseous component and a transmucosal component: the junction between the two is generally located level with the alveolar crest, where a micro-gap is present (13.2a).

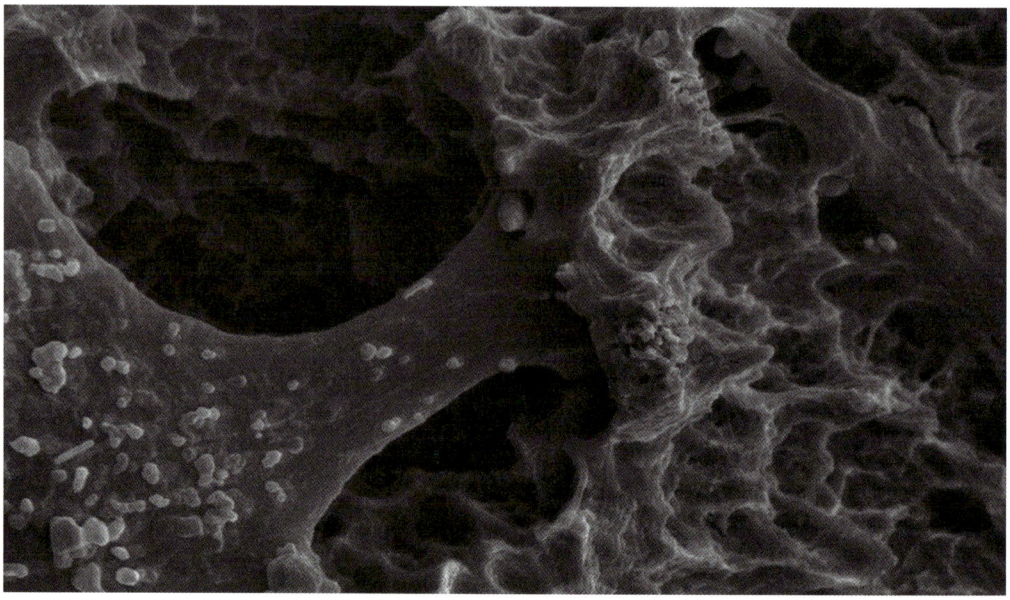

13.1 Scanning electron microscope image of a sand-blasted, acid-etched titanium surface.

The surgical protocol used for two-piece implants consists of a first phase in which the endosseous implant is placed and the overlying soft tissues are sutured to allow for a submerged healing during the osseointegration process.

According to Brånemark, submerged healing should have allowed a reduction in the risk of infection and early loading of the implant, and prevented the apical migration of the mucosa during the healing phase.

After an adequate healing period (6 months for implants placed in the maxilla and 4 months for implants placed in the mandible), the second surgical phase is performed: the implant is uncovered and is connected with the transmucosal component, which has a smooth, polished surface. It must be underlined, however, that the development of new implant surfaces and implant macro and micromorphology in the last two decades (rough surfaces instead of the original, machined surface of Branemark implants) has reduced these waiting times relevantly.

Some authors have demonstrated the presence of anaerobic bacteria inside two-piece implants and the presence of inflammatory infiltrate in the area of the micro-gap between the endosseous and transmucosal components. These factors determine the typical vertical bone remodelling up to the first implant thread, which can be observed around this type of implant.

This problem has been significantly reduced with the introduction of a new type of connection between the two components, designed according to the "platform switching" concept. The implant has an internal connection slot and the abutment is narrower and engages inside the implant; while the connection is still located level with the alveolar crest it is shifted inwards, distancing it from the bone surrounding the implant shoulder. Sophisticated internal connections and the inward shifting of the connection made it possible to eliminate the vertical bone remodelling frequently observed in the first generation of two-piece implants (13.2b).

Specific indications

- *Implants placed in conjunction with regenerative procedures*: in this case, a submerged healing protocol facilitates safer healing and integration of the regenerated bone.
- *Implants placed in the aesthetic zone*: the deeper location of the connection between the implant and the abutment allows greater flexibility in the design of the prosthetic structures.

ONE-PIECE (OR "TRANSMUCOSAL" OR "SOFT TISSUE LEVEL") IMPLANTS

In this case, the endosseous and transmucosal components form a single unit, thus eliminating any micro-gap between the two. One-piece implants are traditionally placed in a single surgical phase and are allowed a non-submerged healing; therefore, osseointegration and the formation of an interface between the soft tissues and the transmucosal portion of the implant occur at the same time (13.2c).

It is worth noting that the endosseous portion of these implants has a rough surface, while the transmucosal portion has a smooth surface.

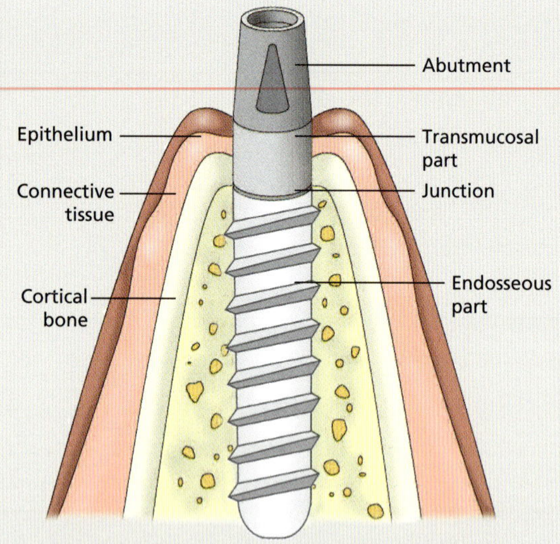

a

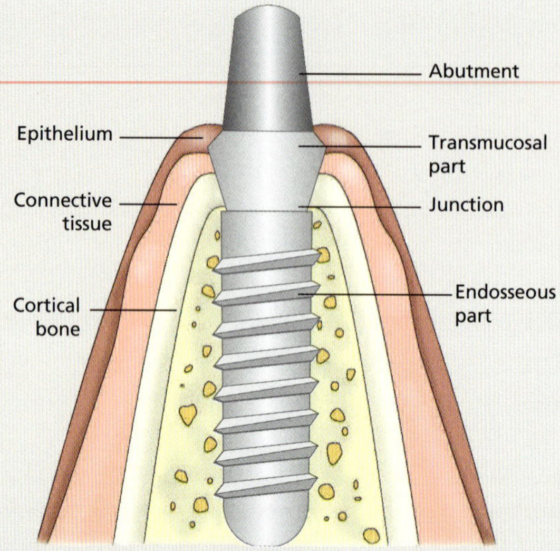

b

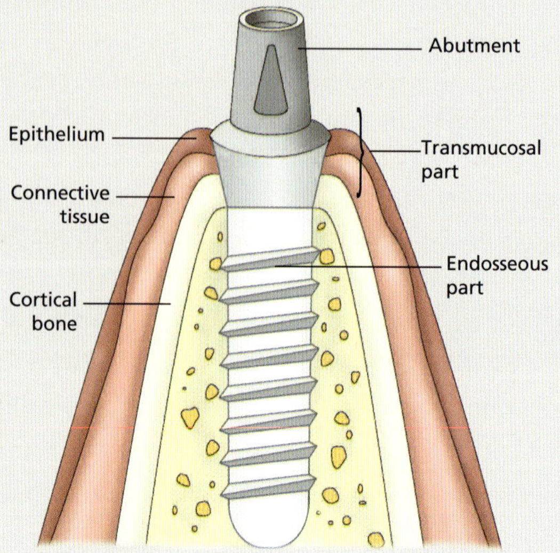

c

13.2 a) Schematic representation of the structure of a two-piece implant: the micro-gap between implant and mesostructure is level with the alveolar crest. **b)** Schematic representation of the connection between implant and mesostructure according to the platform-switching concept. **c)** Schematic representation of the structure of a one-piece implant: the endosseous and transmucosal parts form a single unit and the prosthetic connection is supragingival or level with the soft tissues border.

Specific indications

- *Implants placed in the lateral-posterior areas of the maxilla and mandible in cases where adequate bone volume is present*: in these cases it is not necessary to resort to the submerged healing protocol, and the one-piece implant allows simultaneous osseointegration and formation of the soft tissue seal around the transmucosal portion of the implant.
- *Patients with a history of periodontal disease*: patients who suffer from periodontal disease may be rehabilitated with implants only when infection is eliminated. In these cases, the absence of a connection between the endosseous and transmucosal portion of the implant seems preferable for avoiding the possible presence of any micro-gap between the two.

Long-term results of implant-supported prosthetic rehabilitations

The reliability of an implant protocol can be assessed by evaluating the clinical outcome, in terms of success rate, over time. However, well-defined success criteria must be established beforehand. The comparison between different implant systems is often difficult because clinical studies published in the literature are planned with different modalities and inclusion criteria, and there may be significant differences as far as the parameters evaluated and success criteria are concerned. Moreover, it is difficult to exclude the possibility that commercial pressures in the field of implantology may in some ways influence the results of clinical trials published in the literature, which should consequently be interpreted with caution at all times. A useful tool to help clinicians in the evaluation of scientific data is represented by systematic reviews of the literature, particularly those published by international journals or non-profit organisations such as the *Cochrane Collaboration*. The authors of these reviews select for evaluation only those papers that meet precise scientific criteria, and underline any weak points of every clinical study.

Acts and final reports of *consensus conferences*, where world-renowned specialists define the latest advances in implantology and related subjects, may offer clinicians useful information on guidelines to follow in their clinical activity, and guarantee the expression of a multiplicity of opinions. The introduction of a new implant system should be preceded by an adequate validation through:

- documentation demonstrating osseointegration on an animal model;
- one or more multicentric, longitudinal studies on a significant patient sample producing data on success rate, survival rate, and failure rate, according to well-defined criteria, as well as precise information on complications and drop-out patients. Finally, data on peri-implant bone resorption values measured around every implant at precise moments in time should be reported, evaluated, and thoroughly discussed.

Many implant systems are currently available; however, scientific data for a large number of these is frequently insufficient to recommend their clinical use. The growing commercial competition among different companies pushes them to make claims about clinical performance that are not supported by sufficient evidence due to the lack of clinical trials. The clinician must never forget that the implant is a biomedical device whose choice and use should always be determined by ethical criteria in the pursuit of the patient's best interest. Therefore, commercial considerations should never play any role whatsoever in the care process.

Local and systemic contraindications to implant treatment

A thorough analysis of relative and absolute contraindications to implant treatment is beyond the scope of this manual: detailed information on this subject can be found in specialty textbooks. However, as a rule, implant therapy shares the same contraindications described in Chapter 1 for all other oral surgery procedures.

Contraindications to implant therapy

Absolute contraindications

- Untreated cardiovascular disease (recent myocardial infarction, unstable angina, severe cardiac insufficiency, severe valvulopathy)
- Immune deficiencies (AIDS, organ transplantation, chemotherapy)
- Severe coagulation disorders
- Severe liver disease
- Renal insufficiency
- Presence of tumours and on-going biphosphonate therapy for the treatment of bone metastases
- Osteomalacia, osteogenesis imperfecta, Paget disease
- Neurological disorders (Parkinson's disease, Alzheimer's disease, cognitive disabilities, Down's syndrome)
- Severe psychological disorders that prevent adequate compliance or cooperation in the course of the treatment and do not guarantee adequate maintenance of the implant-supported rehabilitation over time
- Alcohol and drug abuse
- History of osteoradionecrosis of the jaws following radiotherapy

Relative contraindications

- Compensated heart diseases (history of myocardial infarction, stable angina)
- History of endocarditis or valvulopathy (antibiotic prophylaxis is mandatory)
- Chronic respiratory insufficiency
- Compensated liver diseases
- Compensated renal diseases
- Diabetes mellitus
- Osteoporosis (when no biphosphonate therapy is administered)
- Anticoagulant therapy
- Arterial hypertension
- History of radiotherapy in the head and neck district (particularly for doses exceeding 48 gy)
- Anxiety and stress
- Heavy smoking habit (< 20 cigarettes/day): smoking has a negative influence on the short-term and long-term prognosis of oral implants
- Periodontal disease (implant rehabilitation is possible only after periodontal disease is treated)
- Acute or chronic inflammatory conditions involving the residual dentition
- Diseases of the oral mucosa (lichen planus, pemphigus, erythema multiforme, herpetic stomatitis)

Prosthetic-driven implant placement: treatment plan

First and foremost, to adequately plan the placement of an endosseous implant, the height and width of the edentulous alveolar ridge should be precisely measured: as a general rule, the width should exceed the diameter of the implant by at least 3-4 mm, so that a layer of 1.5-2 mm is present both on the buccal and on the lingual/palatal side once the implant is in place. The height should be no less than 7-8 mm. However, if important anatomic structures are present in the area, such as the mandibular nerve, the floor of the nasal cavities, or the floor of the maxillary sinus, an additional 2 mm should be considered as a safety distance to avoid damaging those structures.

Nonetheless, to obtain good functional and aesthetic integration between the implant-supported restorations and the residual natural dentition, the position and inclination of the implant should never be planned according to the anatomy of the alveolar ridge, but rather according to the ideal position and dimension of the final prosthetic restoration.

In fact, the concept of prosthetic-driven implant placement was based on the premise that planning implant placement according to prosthetic considerations was the best way to obtain adequate support and functional/aesthetic integration of the prosthetic restoration. Therefore, when the anatomy of the edentulous ridge does not allow the placement of an implant in the ideal position, bone regeneration/reconstruction techniques (such as onlay grafts, guided bone regeneration, sinus floor elevation and grafting, etc.) should be used to recreate an adequate bone volume and morphology (for a detailed analysis on this subject, see Chiapasco and Romeo, 2003).

From a practical point of view, the correct diagnostic path to plan a prosthetic-driven implant placement includes the following steps.

Mounting the casts on an articulator and creating a diagnostic wax-up of the missing teeth: this procedure makes it possible to evaluate the prosthetic feasibility of the implant rehabilitation. The diagnostic wax-up should reproduce the ideal morphology of the missing teeth and surrounding soft tissues, and it should be possible to remove it from the cast. Fundamental information can thus be gathered regarding possible asymmetries, intermaxillary discrepancies, and vertical and/or horizontal defects (13.3a-b). Moreover, the diagnostic wax-up can be placed directly on the edentulous ridge to obtain a preview of the final result (13.3c).

Creating a diagnostic/radiographic stent: on the basis of the diagnostic wax-up, a diagnostic/radiographic stent can be created to obtain further information on the anatomy of the alveolar ridge at the planned implant sites. Generally, a mixture of resin and barium sulphate in precise proportions is used to reproduce the missing teeth, while clear resin or thermoplastic polypropylene sheets can be used to create a retainer that fits on the residual dentition or on the mucosa in cases of totally edentulous jaws (13.3d).

Specific radiographic exams: the use of a diagnostic/radiographic stent while a CT scan is performed makes it possible to obtain a thorough tridimensional analysis at the planned implant sites (13.4a).

Surgical planning: information obtained by the CT scan performed as described enables the clinician to choose implants of appropriate length and diameter, and to plan the correct position and inclination of each implant. Ideally, the implant should be surrounded by 1.5-2 mm of bone, both on the buccal and on the lingual/palatal side. When this prerequisite is not met, the tridimensional analysis made possible by CT scan images taken with the radiographic stent in place gives a precise assessment of the bone defect and ensures the most appropriate grafting technique is selected to recreate adequate bone volume and morphology.

The choice of appropriate implant length and diameter can be made either with the aid of dedicated transparent templates placed over the printed CT scan or with dedicated software. In the latter case, digital files from the CT scan are imported and implants of different types and dimension can be chosen from a library and superimposed on the images in the planned positions (13.4b).

Use of the diagnostic/radiographic template during surgery: the same radiographic/diagnostic stent used in the diagnostic phase can also be used during implant placement, to allow precise positioning of the implants according to the prosthetic plan (13.5a-d). The implementation of this protocol is particularly important when the implant rehabilitation involves the aesthetic zone (13.6).

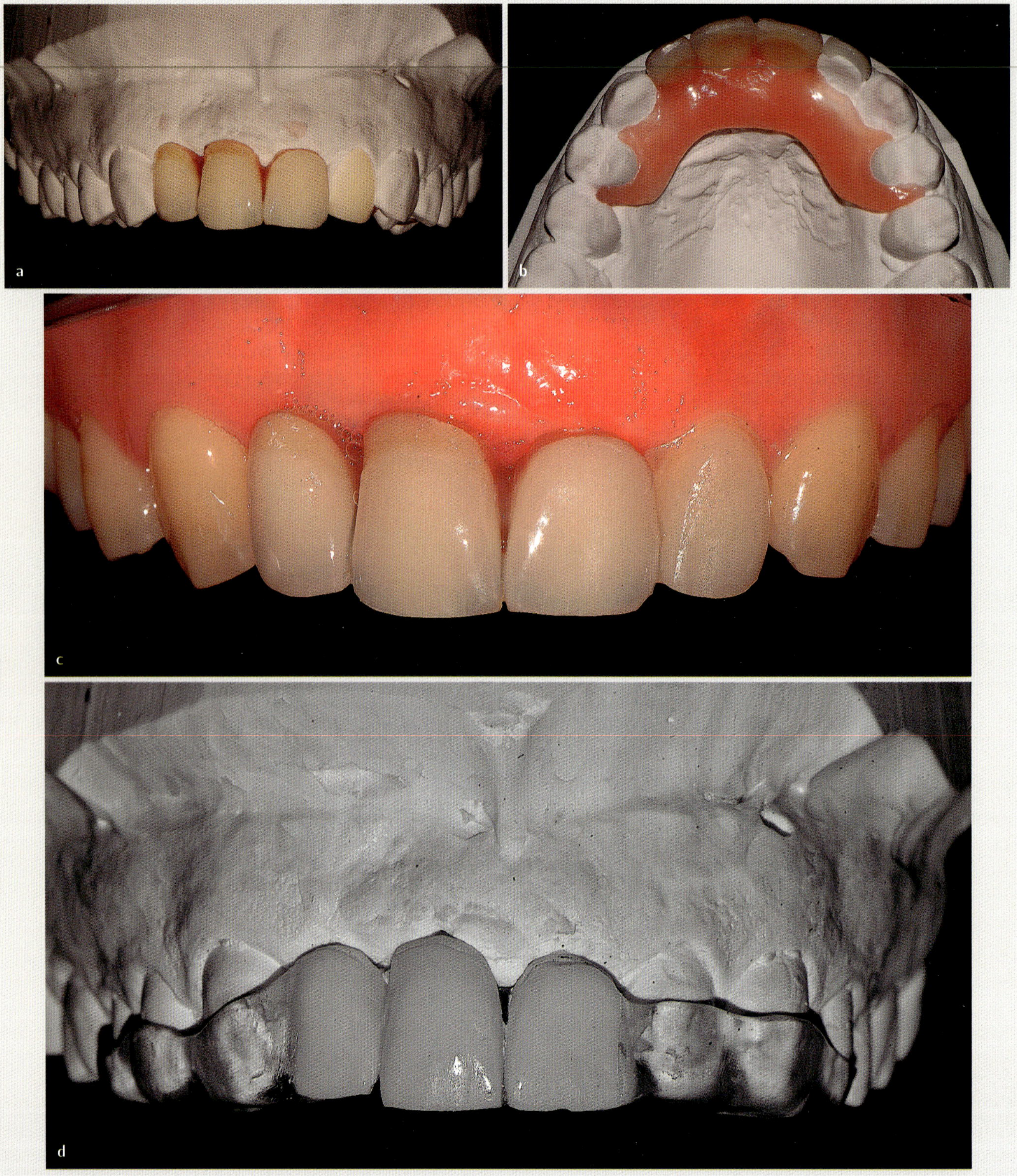

13.3 **a–b)** After the casts are mounted on the articulator, a diagnostic wax-up of the edentulous area is prepared. **c)** The diagnostic wax-up, placed in the patient's mouth, makes it possible to obtain a preview of the final result, and to verify the presence of adequate intermaxillary relationships. **d)** The diagnostic wax-up is finally transformed into a radiographic/surgical stent: the structure of the stent is made of clear resin while the missing teeth are made with a mixture of resin and barium sulphate, so that the teeth to be replaced appear as radiopaque in the CT scan. A hole is drilled in the centre of every artificial tooth to serve as a reference point for the ideal positioning of the centre of each implant, and for the ideal implant axis.

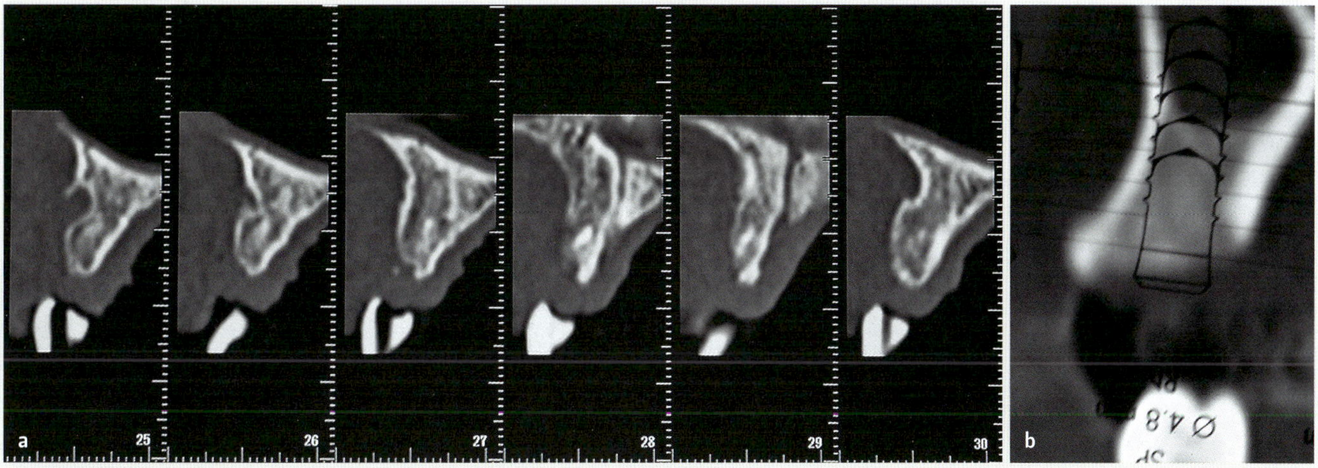

13.4 **a)** The CT scan taken with the radiographic stent in place makes it possible to verify the presence of sufficient bone volume to place the implants according to the ideal axis, which is represented by the hole drilled at the centre of the teeth on the radiographic stent. **b)** The CT scan makes it possible to choose the length and diameter of each implant: the outlines of the implants (1:1 aspect ratio) are printed on specific transparent guides that can be superimposed on the CT images.

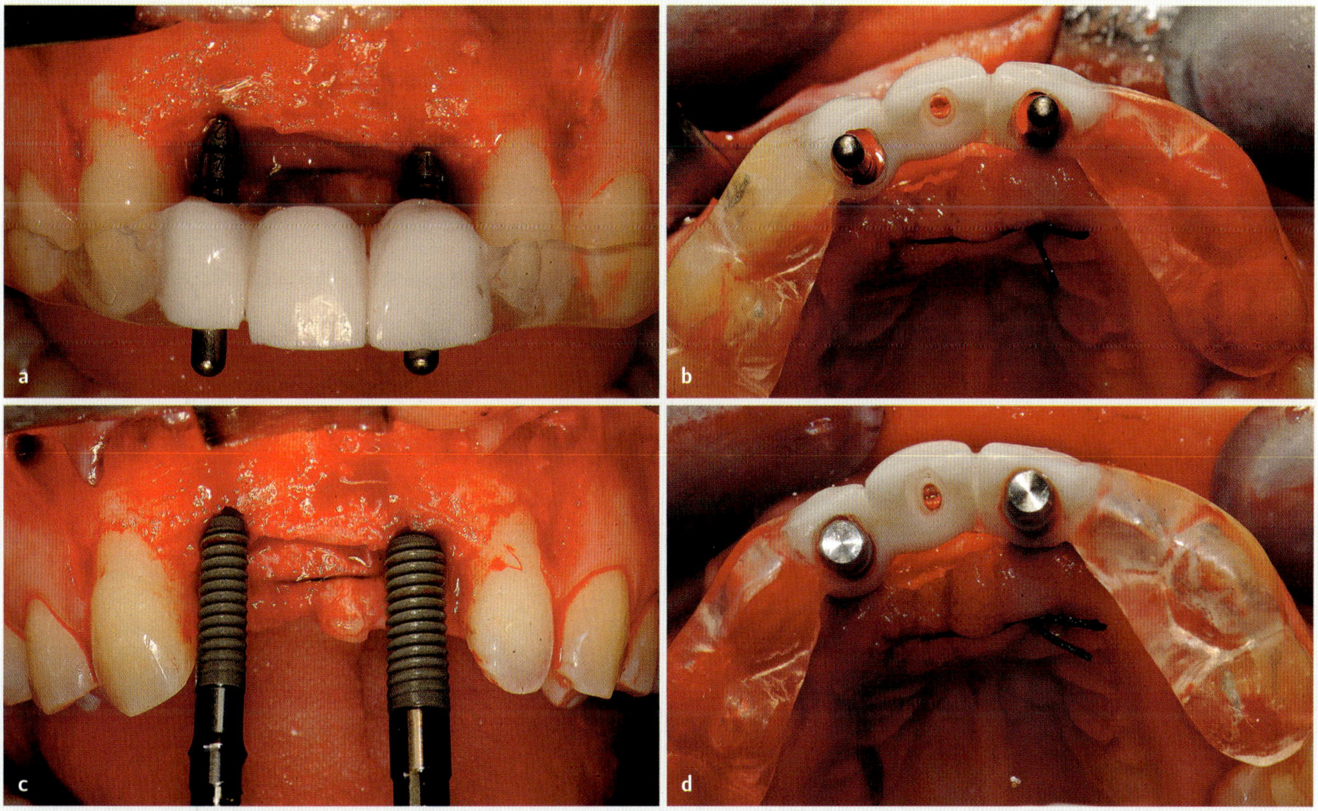

13.5 **a–b)** The radiographic stent can be used as a surgical stent to serve as a guide during implant placement: the diameter of the holes corresponding to the ideal centre and axis of the implant is enlarged, if needed, to allow the passage of the drills and guide pins. **c–d)** If the preparation of the implant sites is correct according to the indications of the surgical guide, the implant mounting devices should be centred with the holes in the stent.

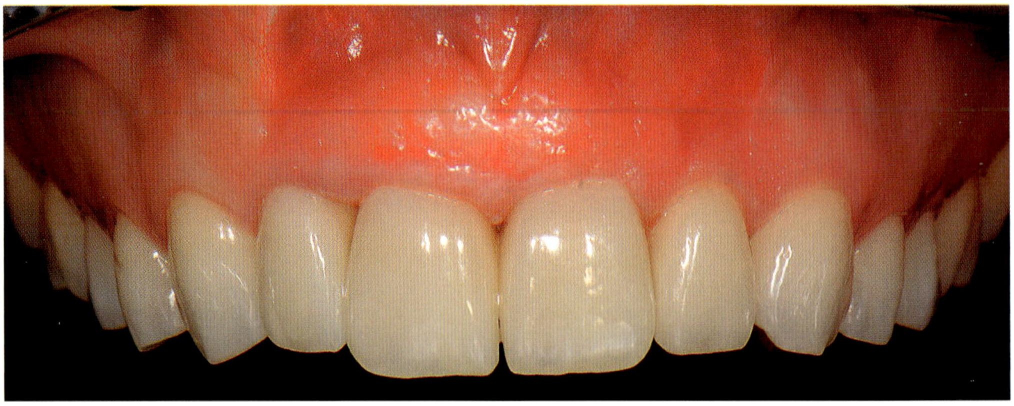

13.6 The final prosthetic restoration (clinical case presented in 13.3a-d, 13.4a, 13.5a-d) includes a cemented bridge (1.2-1.1-2.1) and a porcelain veneer (2.2)

The surgical stent should not be bulky, and it should be easy to put in place and remove; it should firmly engage the neighbouring teeth, and it should not interfere with the retraction of the surgical flaps. As regards totally edentulous patients, the surgical stent should extend to the most distal areas of the jaws (tuber maxillae, retromolar trigone) that are not involved in surgical flaps, to help a precise positioning of the stent and improve its stability.

Note: for implant rehabilitation of small edentulous areas (e.g. single tooth replacement), when the morphology of the alveolar ridge is favourable and the aesthetic zone is not involved, the diagnostic path can be simplified excluding the wax-up, diagnostic/radiographic stent, and CT scan. In these cases, inspection and palpation in association with periapical or panoramic radiographs is sufficient to obtain adequate information to guide the choice of the appropriate implant diameter and length, but it is worth remembering that the position of the implant should be planned according to prosthetic/restorative criteria.

Choice of the implant diameter: according to modern concepts of prosthetically-driven implantology, the choice of implant diameter should be based on the dimensions of the missing tooth. Generally speaking, to replace the inferior incisors and upper lateral incisors, narrow diameter implants (3-3.5 mm) are recommended, while to replace canines, premolars, and, in particular molars, wider diameter implants (3.5-6 mm) are preferred (13.7). However, this must be considered just a general rule, as the choice of the diameter is also related to local anatomy, space available between neighbouring teeth, dimensions of adjacent natural dentition, and patient biotype.

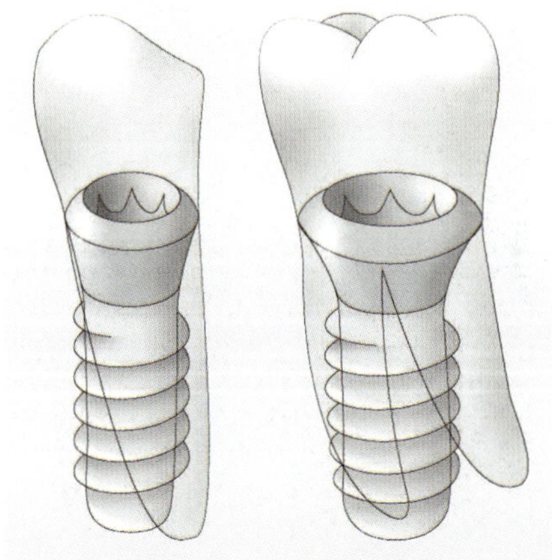

13.7 The majority of modern implant systems provide implants of different diameter to allow clinicians to choose according to the dimension of the tooth to be replaced.

Treatment plan: the use of narrow/short implants

The evolution of implant surfaces, particularly as regards the increase in the bone-to-implant contact surface obtained with rough surfaces, has allowed a reduction in the minimum implant dimensions. While 30 years ago a bicortical anchorage was deemed necessary and long implants were used to achieve that specific goal, today short implants (< 7 mm) can be used with specific indications in selected cases (Annibali et al., 2012).

The reduced length of the implant can be compensated by choosing a wider diameter (5-6 mm). However, in this case a correct tridimensional positioning of the implant and adequate intermaxillary relationships should allow axial loading and an optimal crown-to-implant ratio (13.8a-i).

Indications to the use of narrow-diameter implants have also expanded, due to improvements in the design and structure (titanium-zirconium alloys) of the implants, the latter of which have caused an increase in their mechanical resistance.

Treatment planning with the aid of specifically designed software: computer-guided surgery

A relevant evolution in the field of implantology has been represented, in recent years, by the possibility of analysing CT scans with softwares that are specifically created for the planning of implant treatments. The initial phases of the planning remain unchanged, while the CT scan is performed with a radiographic stent reproducing the ideal position/

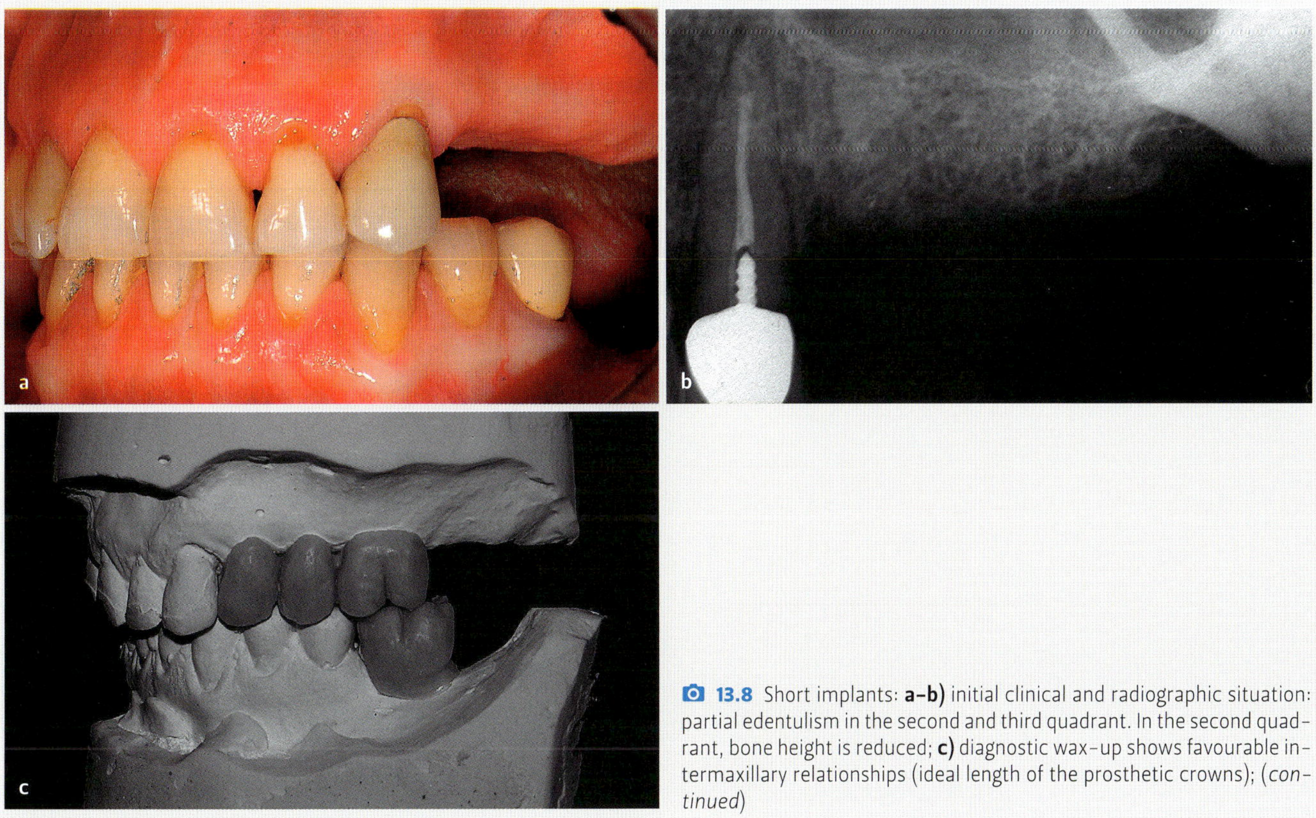

13.8 Short implants: **a–b)** initial clinical and radiographic situation: partial edentulism in the second and third quadrant. In the second quadrant, bone height is reduced; **c)** diagnostic wax-up shows favourable intermaxillary relationships (ideal length of the prosthetic crowns); (*continued*)

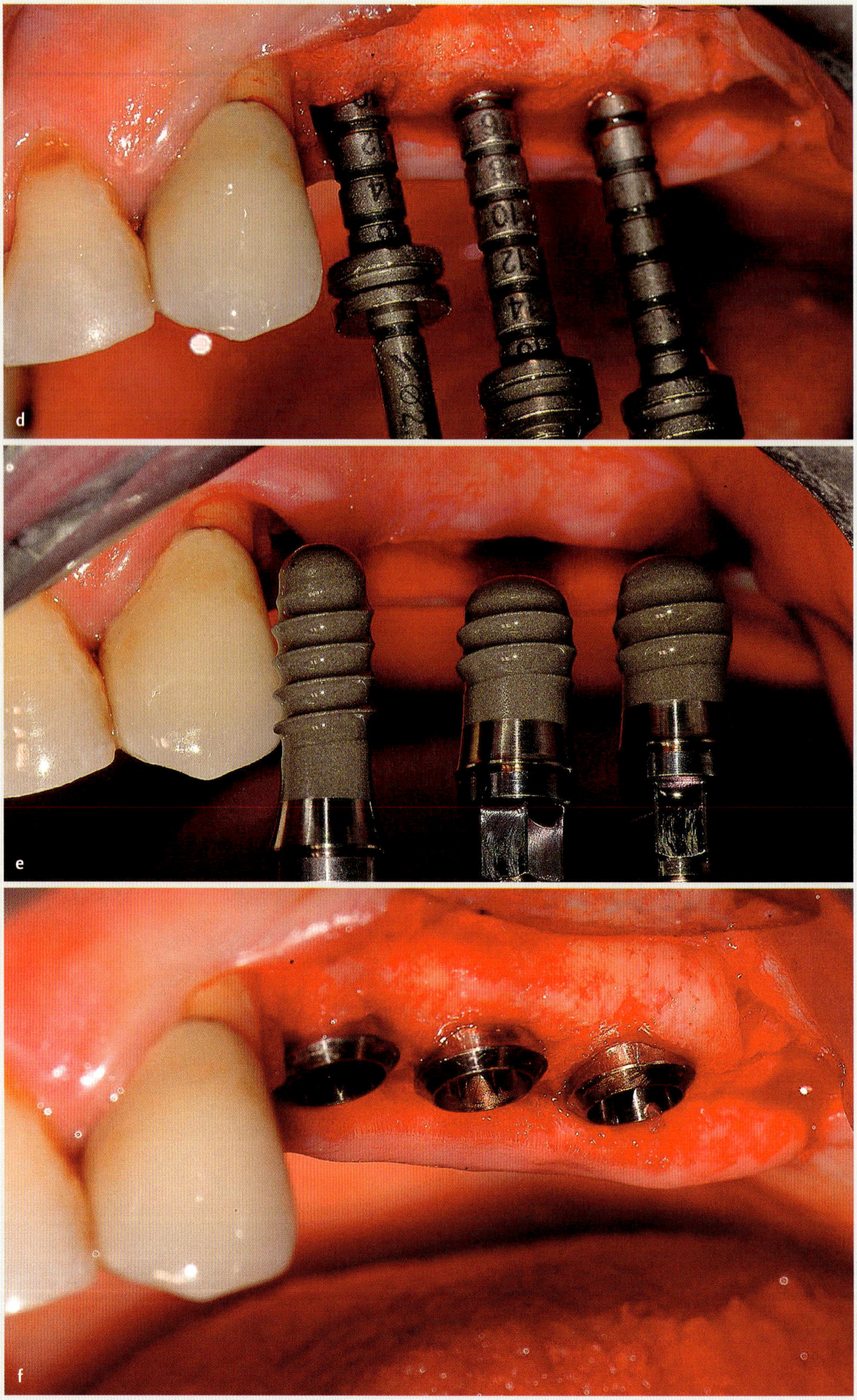

13.8 (*continued*)
d–e) preparation of the implant sites and placement of a 10 mm implant (standard length) and two 8 mm (short) implants. To compensate for the reduced length, a 5 mm diameter was chosen; **f)** implants placement completed: the use of one-piece implants may represent an ideal choice in the lateral-posterior areas of the jaws; (*continued*)

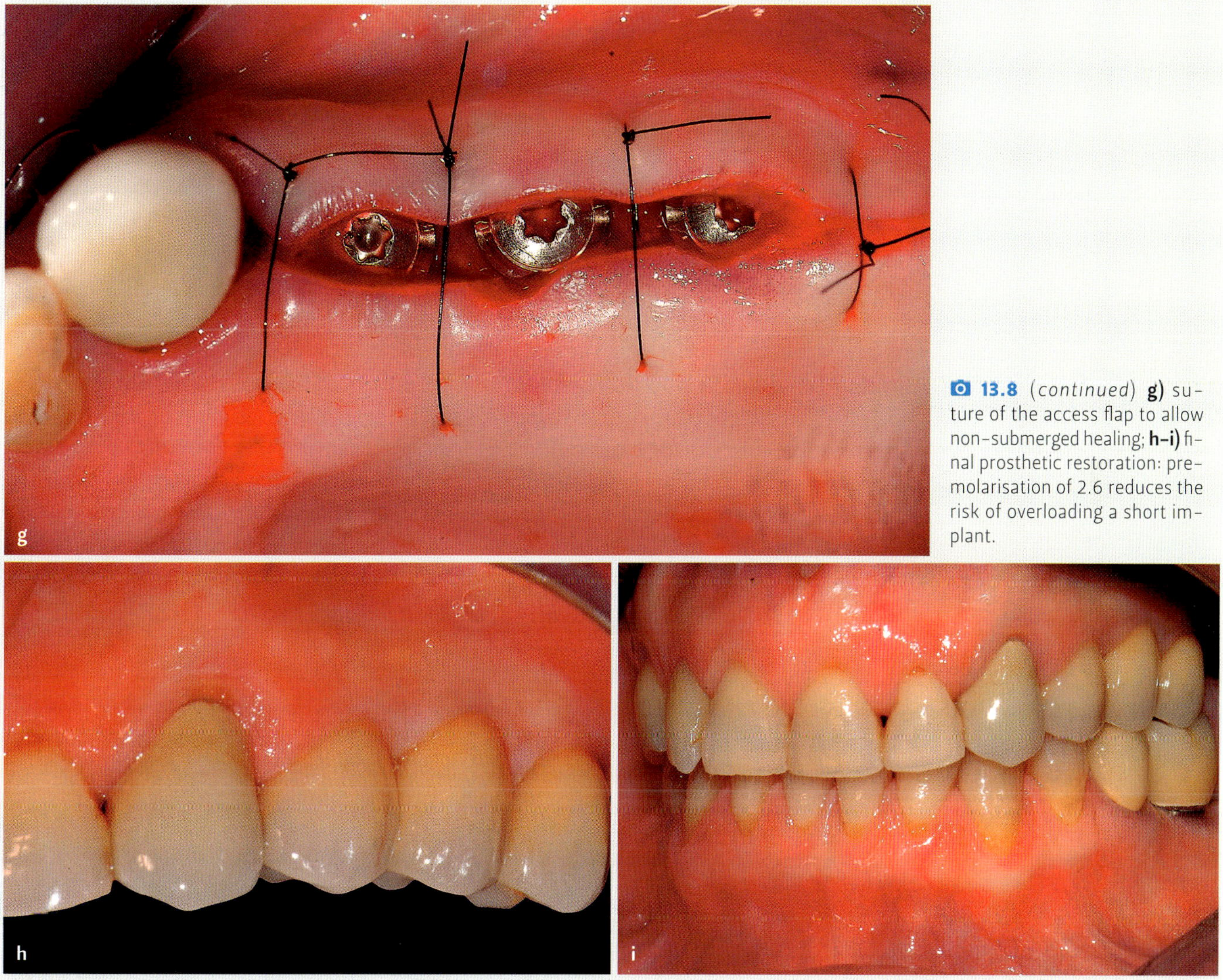

13.8 (*continued*) **g)** suture of the access flap to allow non-submerged healing; **h–i)** final prosthetic restoration: premolarisation of 2.6 reduces the risk of overloading a short implant.

dimension of the missing teeth in place; radiographic stents can be tooth-supported or mucosa-supported, according to the type of edentulism.

Implant planning software can directly import the digital files created by the CT scanner (identified by the ".dcm" extension), and have a built-in library containing tridimensional models of implants of different length and diameter, allowing the clinician to choose the ideal dimensions and position of the implants according to the aforementioned criteria.

Furthermore, the main advantage of computer-guided surgery is represented by the possibility of transforming the virtual planning made with the aid of the software into a surgical guide that is produced by means of a CAD-CAM (*Computer Aided Design - Computer Aided Manufacturing*) process.

It is possible to produce tooth-supported, mucosa-supported, and bone-supported surgical guides: calibrated metal sleeves allowing the guided preparation of the implant sites are embedded in the resin body of the surgical guide according to the positions established in the virtual planning. Specifically designed drills of increasing diameter are passed through the metal sleeves according to dedicated drilling sequences; the depth of the preparation is predetermined according to the implant length and is transferred to the surgical field either by means of drill stops or by a depth stop system integrated into the surgical guide.

The advantages of computer-guided surgery could be represented, theoretically, by a less invasive surgery and a precise implant positioning. When the available bone volume and morphology are adequate, and the preparation of the implant site can be achieved without the risk of creating bone dehiscences and fenestrations or damaging important anatomic structures, surgery can be performed without raising flaps. This "flapless" approach allows the preparation of the implant site through a small access created by removing a round portion of the mucosa with a tissue punch, thus reducing the postoperative discomfort.

However, it is worth noting that computer-guided implant surgery, like any other technique, requires specific training; moreover, even if CT scans are generally very precise, they are not immune to distortions that may expose planning errors, resulting in implant failures or damage to important anatomic structures. For a systematic review of the literature on this subject, see Jung et al. (2009).

A step-by-step clinical case is presented to illustrate the flapless computer-guided surgical protocol using a mucosa-supported guide, and the subsequent prosthetic rehabilitation (13.9a-l).

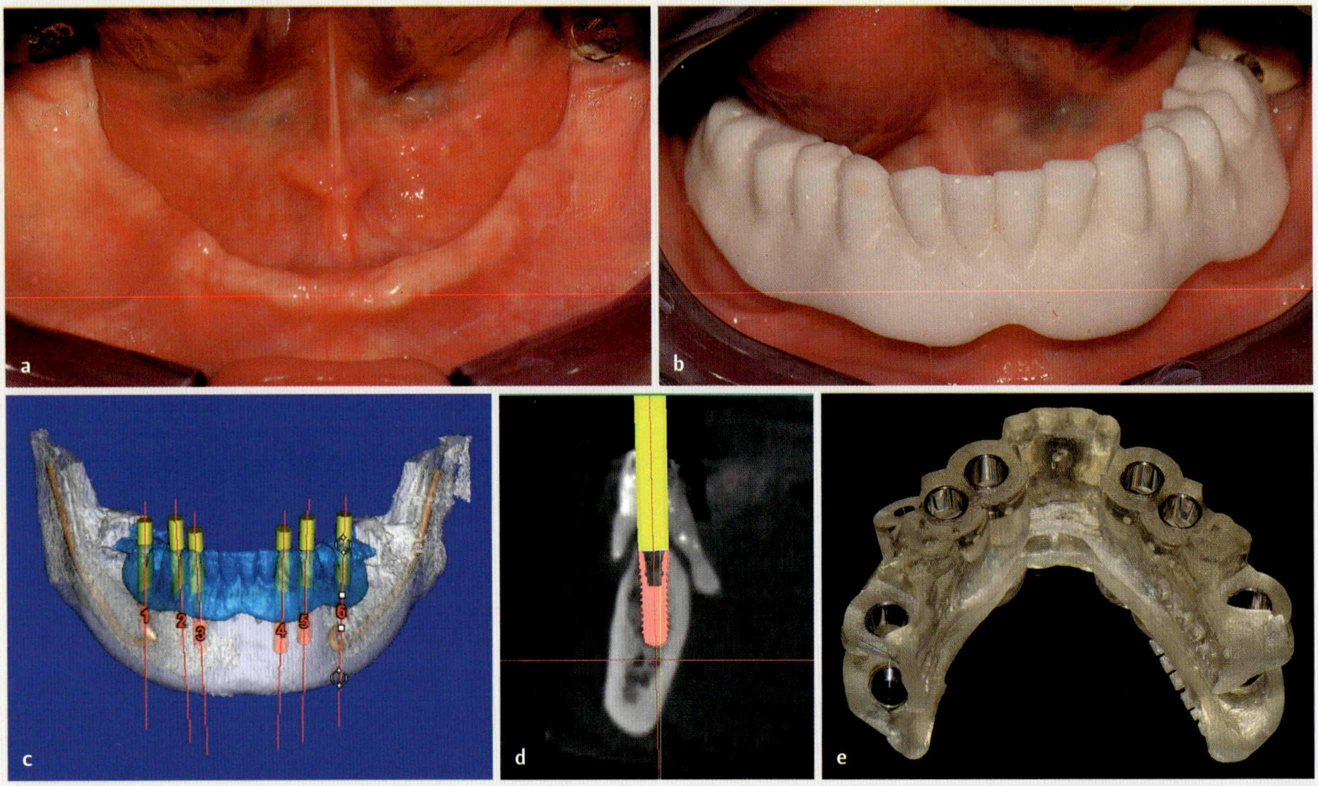

13.9 Computer-guided planning and surgery: **a)** initial clinical situation: complete mandibular edentulism; **b)** a radiographic stent is created; **c–d)** the CT scan is imported into a dedicated software (Simplant®) that makes it possible to plan the dimension, position, and inclination of 6 implants according to prosthetic considerations; **e)** a surgical guide that replicates the virtual plan is created; (*continued*)

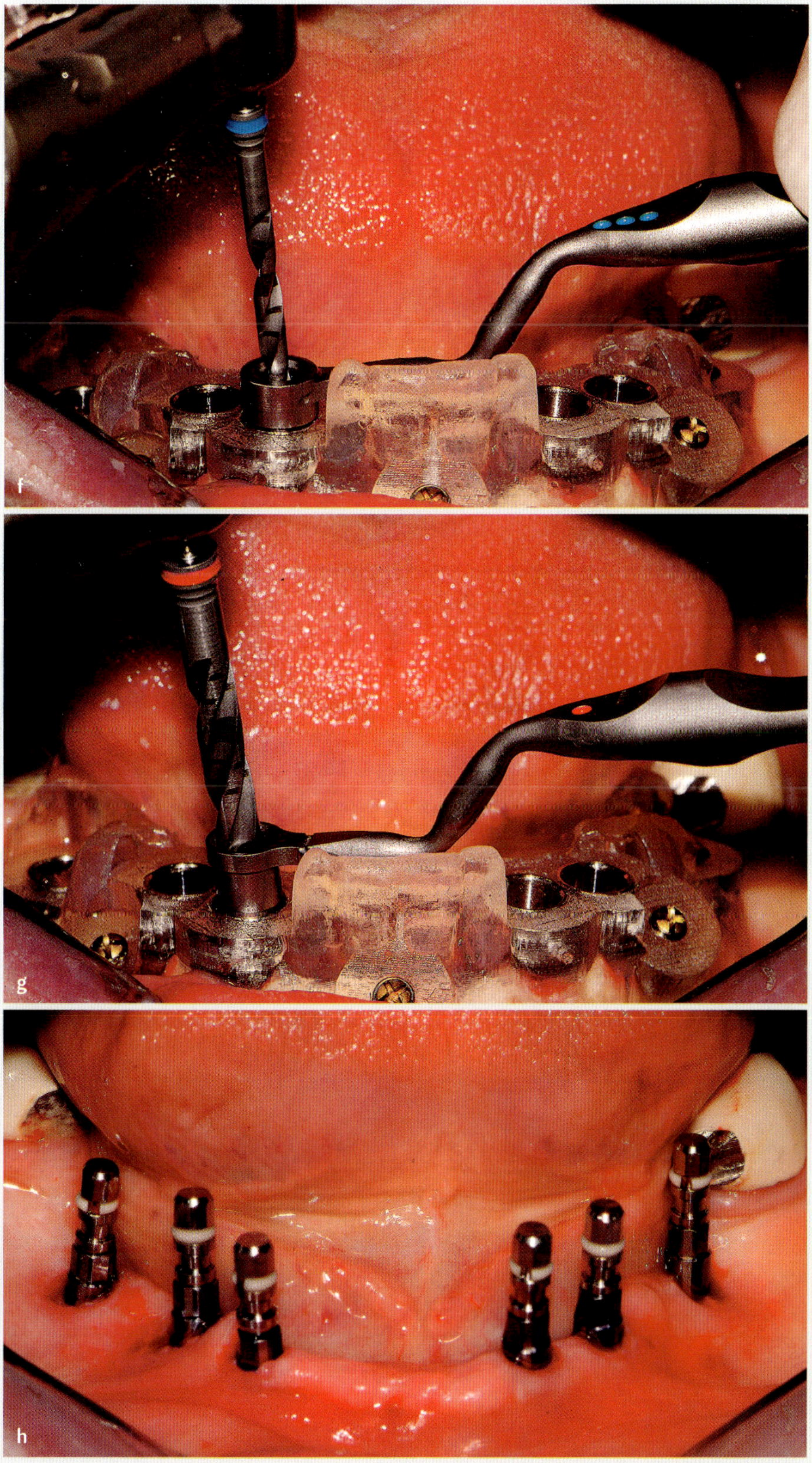

13.9 (*continued*) **f–g)** after fixation of the surgical guide in the correct position, implant sites are prepared with dedicated drilling sequences with the aid of specific cylinders calibrated according to the diameter of each drill; **h)** postoperative view after flapless implant placement and removal of the surgical guide; (*continued*)

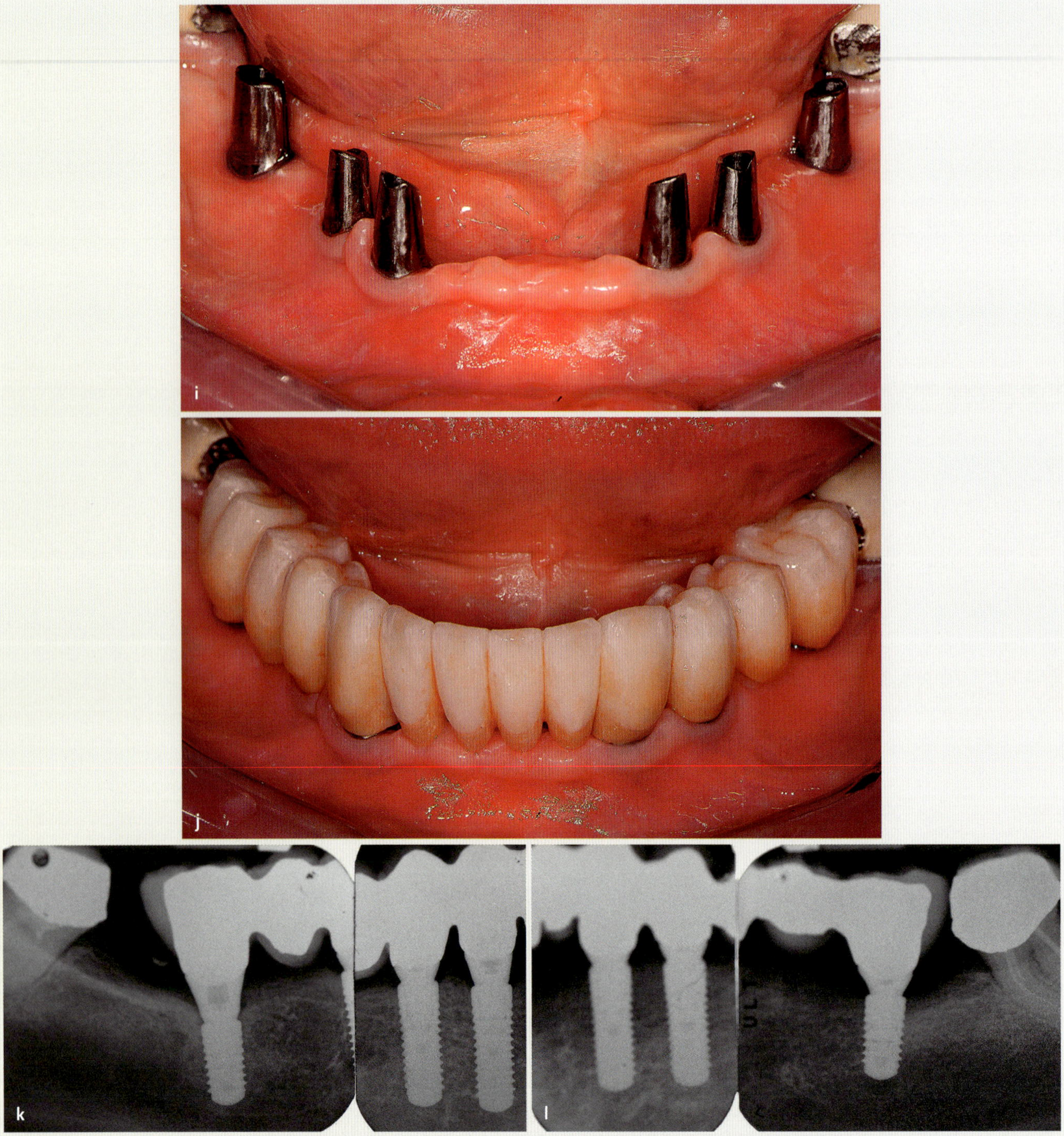

13.9 (*continued*) **i–j)** final prosthetic restoration completed after osseointegration of the implants is achieved; **k–l)** radiographic follow-up.

Implant surgery

Preparation of the surgical environment (operating room, operators, patient)

A surgical intervention for the placement of endosseous implants, like any other oral surgery intervention, implies the interruption of the mucosal barrier, thus creating a communication between the deep tissues and oral cavity, which is always colonised by different types of germs.

The penetration of pathogens may lead to a risk of local or systemic infection, and any possible contamination of the implant surface by oral bacteria prior to implant placement may lead to postoperative complications.

For these reasons, implant placement should always be performed in sterile conditions (see Chapter 3 for details).

Preoperative and postoperative medications

Oral cavity antisepsis with chlorhexidine mouthwashes

The use of 0.12% or 0.2% chlorhexidine mouthwashes prior to surgical intervention is recommended by the majority of authors. However, antibacterial control is even more effective if an antisepsis protocol with chlorhexidine mouthwash is started 2-3 days before surgery. The same protocol is then continued in the postoperative period until suture removal. Generally, the patient is instructed to rinse for sixty seconds three times per day, after meals.

Antibiotic prophylaxis in oral implantology

Type of procedure:	Prophylaxis
Basic implant surgery, when a limited number of implants are placed in native bone (adequate bone volume and morphology) with limited surgical access, and no reconstructive/regenerative procedures are performed	No antibiotic prophylaxis, or short-term prophylaxis consisting of a single dose (2 grams) of amoxicillin (or amoxicillin in association with clavulanate) one hour before surgery
More invasive procedures requiring ample access flaps for the placement of numerous implants	Short-term prophylaxis consisting of a single dose (2 grams) of amoxicillin (or amoxicillin in association with clavulanate) one hour before surgery. If deemed necessary, prophylaxis can be followed by antibiotic therapy in the 6 days following surgery (1 gram of amoxicillin every 8 hours, or 1 gram of amoxicillin+clavulanate every 12 hours)
Extensive treatments involving autologous bone harvesting, bone reconstruction/regeneration with autologous bone or biomaterials in association with barrier membranes; surgical interventions lasting more than 2 hours	Antibiotic prophylaxis consisting of a single dose (2 grams) of amoxicillin (or amoxicillin+clavulanate) one hour before surgery in association with antibiotic therapy in the 6 days following surgery (1 gram of amoxicillin every 8 hours, or 1 gram of amoxicillin+clavulanate every 12 hours) In patients with a history of adverse reactions or allergy to penicillins, amoxicillin can be substituted with claritromicin for short-term prophylaxis (500 mg 1 hour before surgery) and postoperative therapy (500 mg every 12 hours)

Antibiotic prophylaxis

Notwithstanding the lack of a general consensus regarding the recourse to antibiotic prophylaxis in systemically healthy patients, the majority of publications report the use of the prophylaxis protocol in all patients, even in cases of basic implant surgery.

However, the administration of antibiotics in the absence of specific indications does not seem to be justified as it may expose patients to potentially severe allergic reactions and to the development of antimicrobial resistance. In general, antibiotic prophylaxis is indicated in patients presenting risk factors for infective endocarditis, for immunocompromised patients, for invasive and prolonged procedures, and when grafting procedures with autogenous bone, biomaterials and barrier membranes are performed.

Types of anaesthesia

The techniques are the same used in all oral surgery procedures (see Chapter 3 for details), and choice is determined by the area in which the implants are to be placed. Preoperative assessment, particularly with regards to the duration and complexity of the procedure and the patient's compliance, may in some cases lead the clinician to consider the recourse to intravenous sedation or general anaesthesia.

Access flaps

The design of access flaps follows the principles described in Chapter 3: the objectives are the prevention of ischaemia, laceration, and dehiscence of the flap, while obtaining an optimal view in the operating field.

Partial edentulism

When the morphology of the alveolar crest is favourable, an envelope flap is created by means of an incision running along the centre of the edentulous alveolar ridge: the incision usually extends inside the sulcus of adjacent teeth both on the buccal and on the lingual/palatal side.

If a wider surgical access is needed during surgery, one or two releasing incisions can be added to transform the envelope flap into a three-corner or four-corner flap. (13.10a-c).

Distal edentulous ridge

Generally speaking, a three-corner flap is used in cases of distal edentulous ridges: a crestal incision is extended mesially inside the sulcus of the neighbouring tooth, while distally two divergent releasing incisions (forming a dovetail shape) are made to render the retraction and protection of the soft tissues easier (13.11a-b).

Totally edentulous mandible: placement of two implants in the interforaminal region to support an overdenture

A crestal incision connecting the areas of the left and right first premolar is made, in association with a median releasing incision. The limited distal extent of the incision avoids any interference with the emergence of the mental nerve that, in cases of mandibular atrophy, can be superficial. The median releasing incision allows an easier elevation of the flap and an adequate access to the surgical field (13.12a-b).

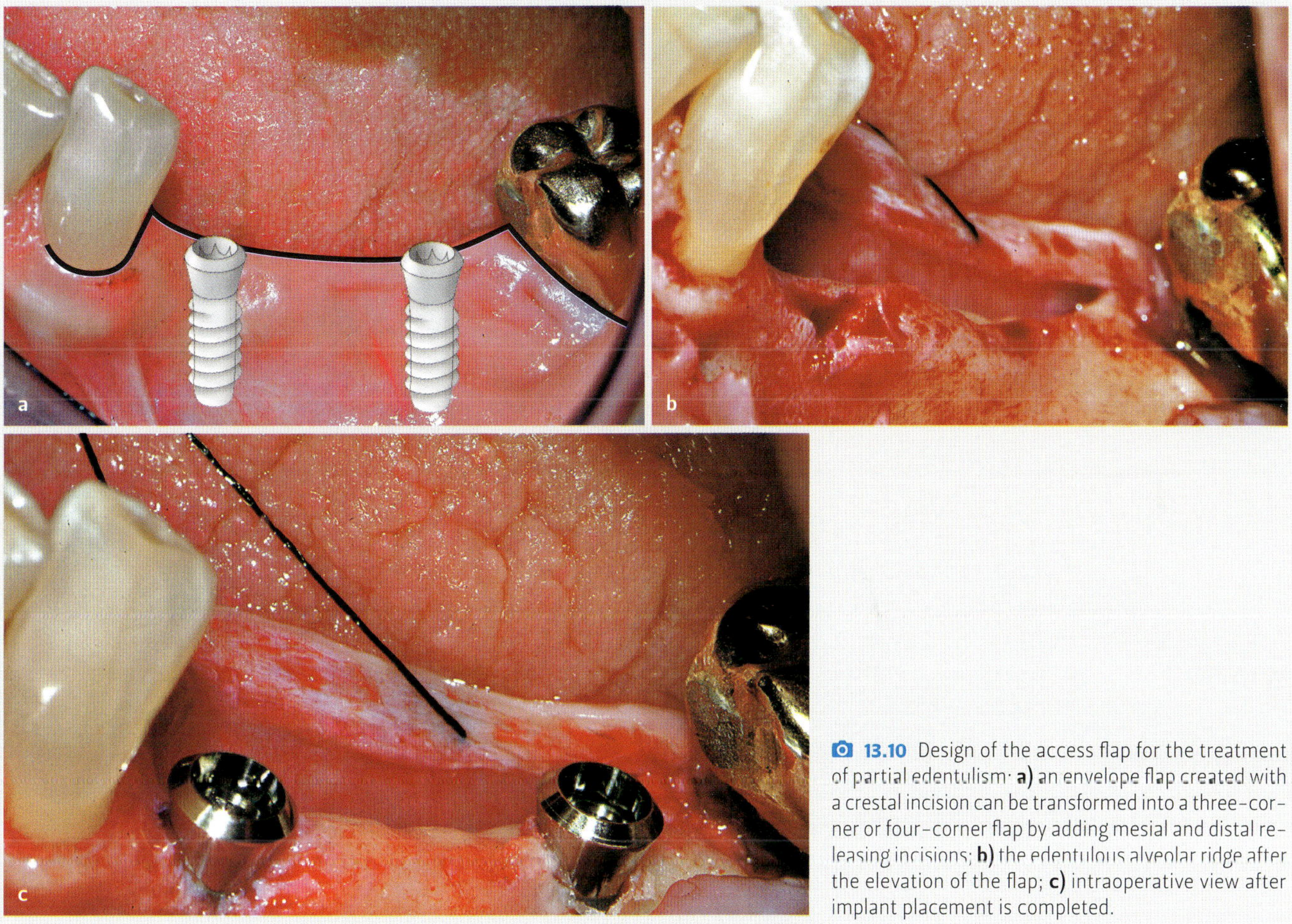

13.10 Design of the access flap for the treatment of partial edentulism: **a)** an envelope flap created with a crestal incision can be transformed into a three-corner or four-corner flap by adding mesial and distal releasing incisions; **b)** the edentulous alveolar ridge after the elevation of the flap; **c)** intraoperative view after implant placement is completed.

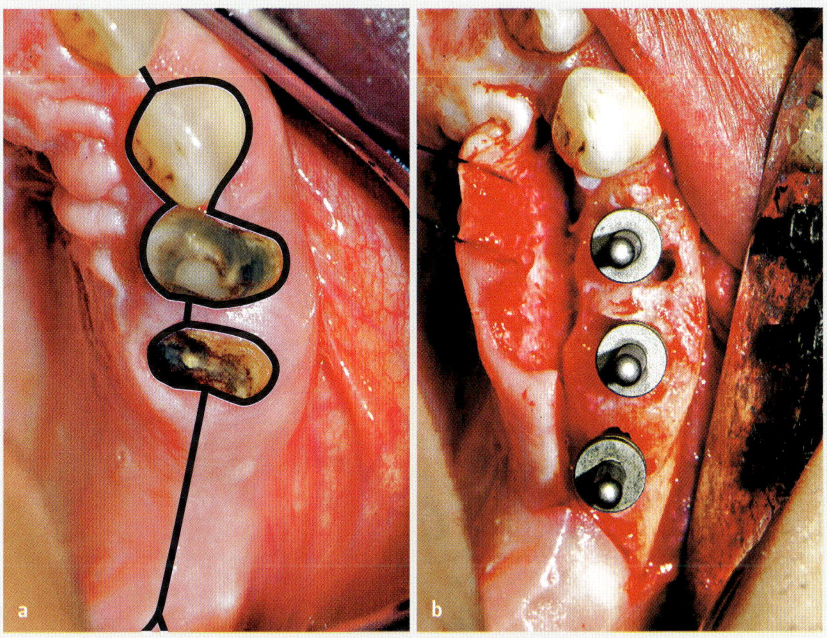

13.11 Design of the surgical flap for the treatment of distal edentulism: **a)** an intrasulcular incision is associated with a crestal incision and two divergent releasing incisions at the distal end of the flap; **b)** the alveolar ridge after flap elevation and implant placement.

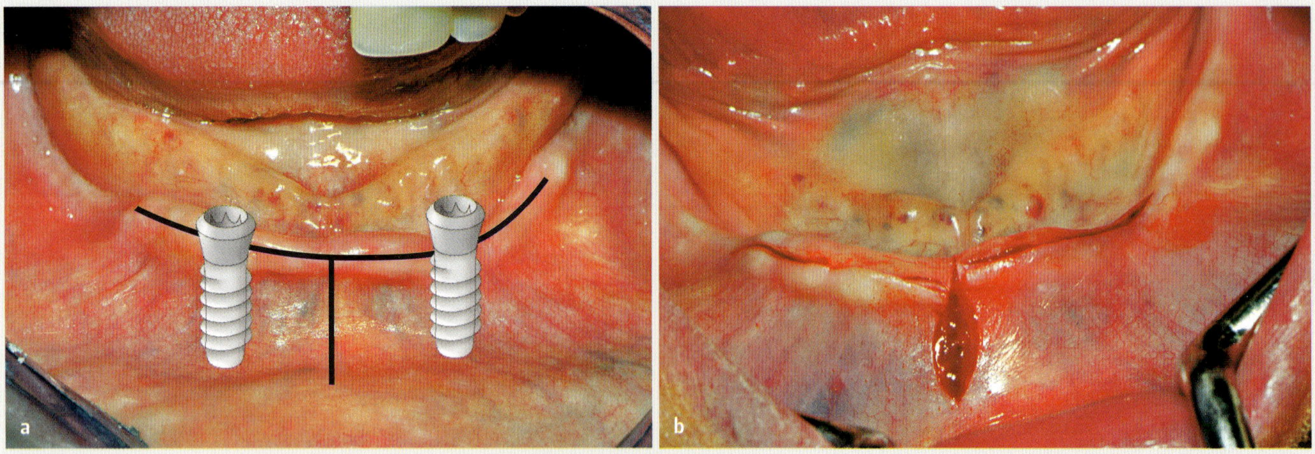

13.12 Design of the surgical flap for the treatment of complete mandibular edentulism with the placement of two implants in the interforaminal area: **a)** crestal incision associated with a median releasing incision; **b)** clinical view after the completion of the two incisions.

When transmucosal (soft tissue level) implants are used, the incision should divide the keratinised mucosa in half. This measure guarantees that, when the flap is sutured, the transmucosal portion of the implant is surrounded by keratinised tissue both on the buccal and on the lingual side.

Totally edentulous mandible: placement of four implants in the interforaminal region to support an overdenture

A crestal incision connecting the areas of the left and right first molar is made, in association with a median incision and, if necessary, with distal releasing incisions. Extending the incision up to the molar region and adding distal releasing incisions allows the elevation of a wider flap that guarantees an easier location of the mental foramina, which represent the fundamental reference points for the placement of the two most distal implants (13.13a-b).

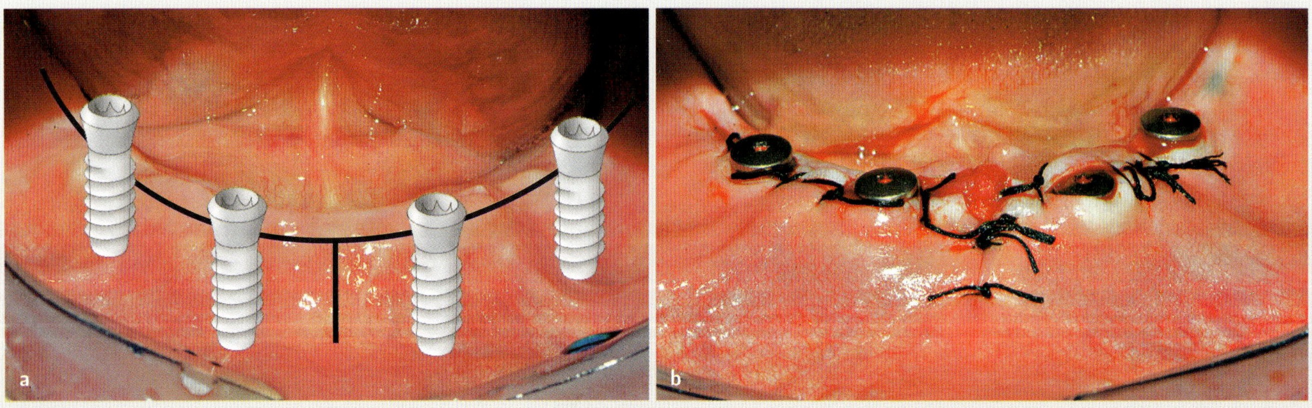

13.13 Design of the surgical flap for the treatment of complete mandibular edentulism with the placement of four implants in the interforaminal area: **a)** crestal incision associated with a median releasing incision; **b)** suture of the access flap after the completion of implant placement.

However, it is worth remembering that the crestal incision distally to the area of the first premolar should be conducted with great care in cases of severe mandibular atrophy, due to the risk of damaging the mental nerves. In fact, resorption of the alveolar ridge causes relative superficialisation of the mental foramina; in cases of extreme bone atrophy, the roof of the foramina can be absent and the mental nerve can emerge directly on top of the residual alveolar ridge.

Totally edentulous mandible: placement of five implants in the interforaminal region to support a full-arch Toronto bridge

A crestal incision connecting the areas of the left and right first molar is made, in association with distal releasing incisions. The difference between this flap and the previous one consists in the absence of the median releasing incision: this choice is determined by the need to place one of the five implants on the midline (13.14a–c).

Possible undercuts on the lingual side of the mandible should always be identified by palpation and, if necessary, confirmed by a CT scan. Should perforation of the lingual cortical plate occur, damage to the arterial vessels of the oral floor could result in severe haemorrhagic complications. To avoid any risk of damage to these blood vessels it is recommended that, particularly when lingual undercuts are present, the access flap on the lingual side be adequately elevated and protected with a retractor during the preparation of the implant sites.

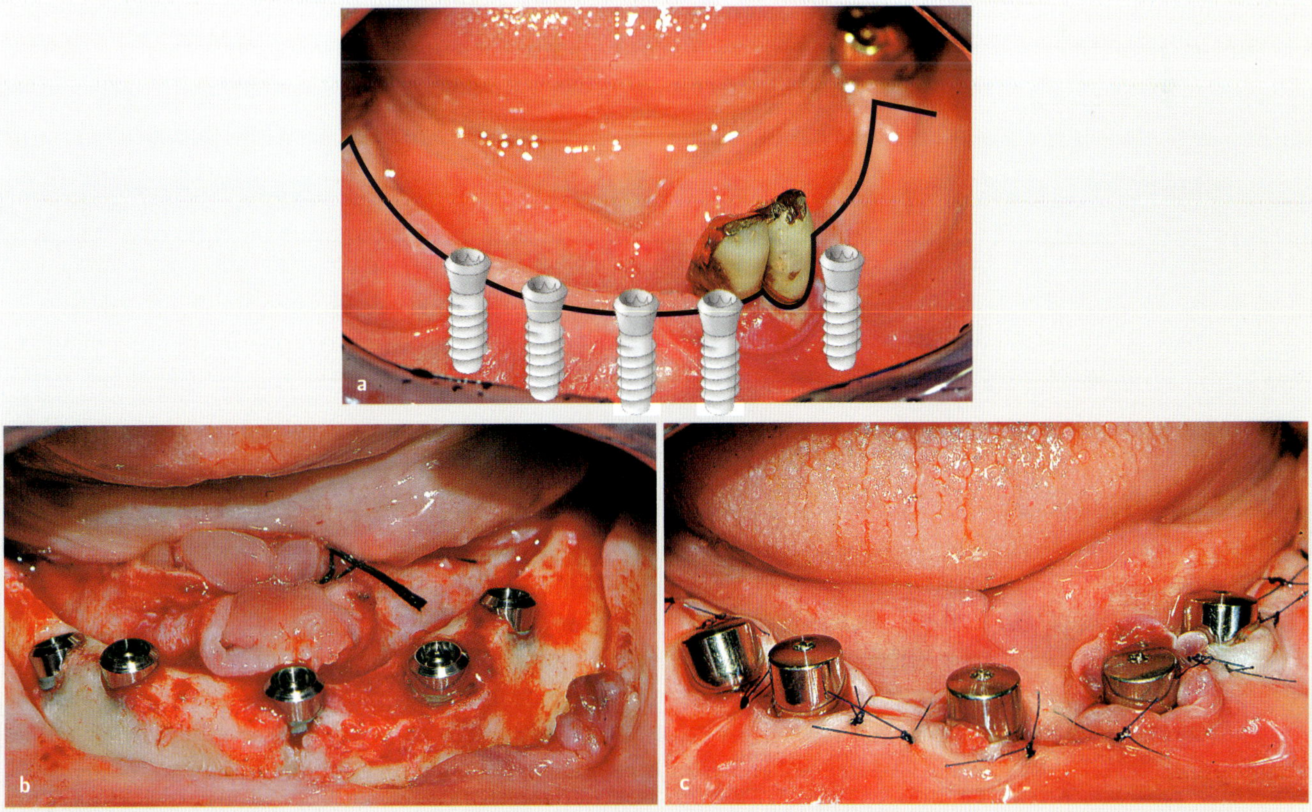

13.14 Design of the surgical flap for the treatment of complete mandibular edentulism with the placement of five implants in the interforaminal area: **a)** crestal incision associated with distal releasing incisions; **b)** intraoperative view after the completion of implant placement; **c)** suture.

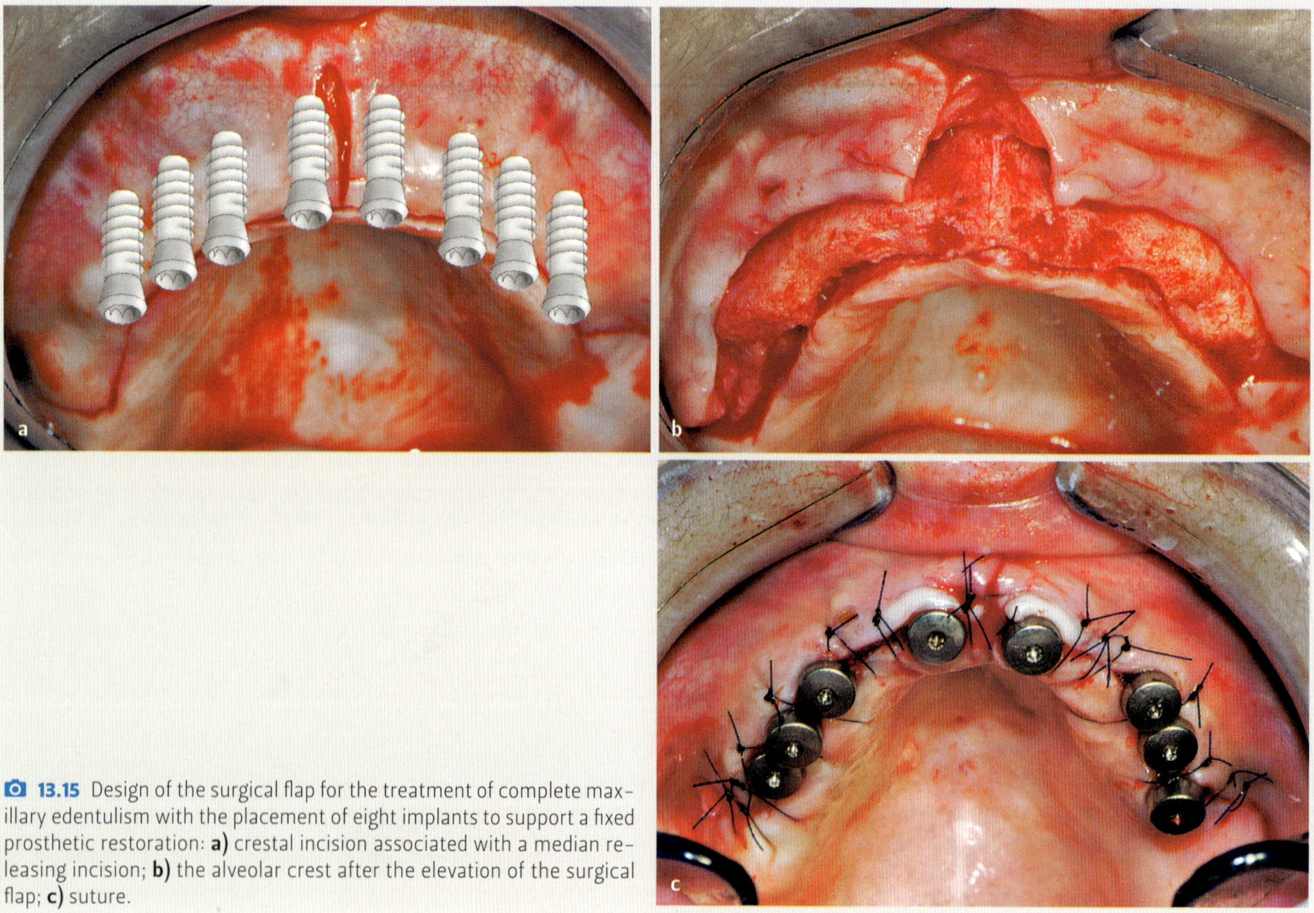

13.15 Design of the surgical flap for the treatment of complete maxillary edentulism with the placement of eight implants to support a fixed prosthetic restoration: **a)** crestal incision associated with a median releasing incision; **b)** the alveolar crest after the elevation of the surgical flap; **c)** suture.

Totally edentulous maxilla

As a rule, a crestal incision connecting the areas of the left and right second molar is made, in association with a median incision and with distal releasing incisions. However, the length of the crestal incision can be modified according to the planned number and positions of the implants (13.15a-c).

IMPLANT PLACEMENT WITHOUT FLAP ELEVATION: THE "FLAPLESS" APPROACH

In selected cases, the elevation of a full-thickness access flap can be avoided; this approach has been proposed both for the immediate placement of implants in post-extractive sockets and for implants placed in healed sites. The main advantages of flapless surgery are represented by the reduction of surgical trauma on the soft tissues, particularly in the case of immediate post-extractive implant placement or computer-guided placement of a significant number of implants. However, this approach also presents some drawbacks.

- For implant placement in healed sites, the technique is contraindicated if keratinised mucosa defects are present; in fact, the use of tissue punches to create access for the drilling of the implant site and for implant placement could result in the complete removal of the residual keratinised tissue that should surround the implant.

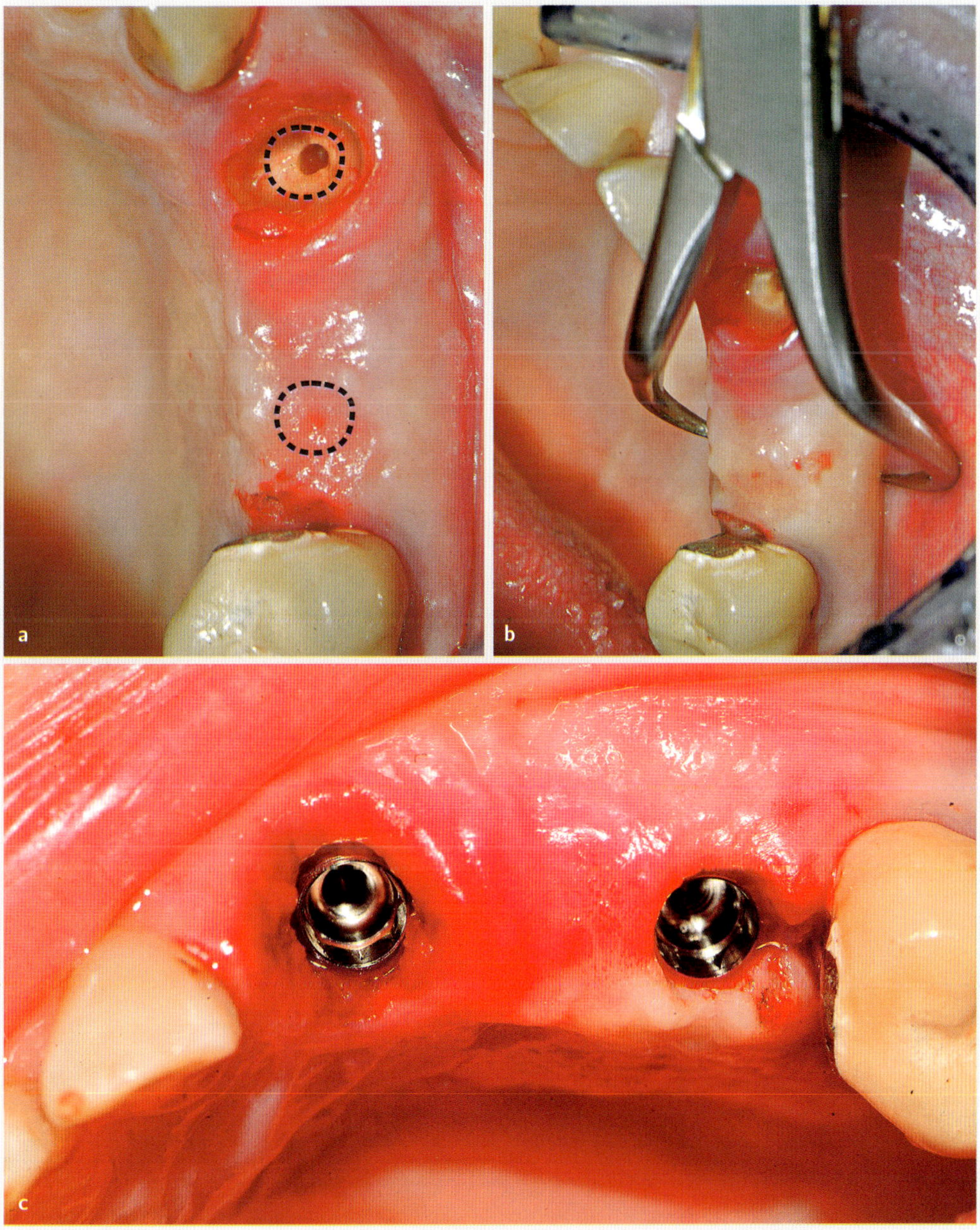

13.16 Flapless implant site preparation: **a)** the treatment plan includes the placement of an immediate post-extractive implant (2.3) and a second implant distally (2.5); **b)** the morphology of the alveolar ridge is particularly favourable, and is verified with the aid of a transmucosal calliper; **c)** occlusal view after implant placement is completed: the final prosthetic restoration is presented in 13.26a-b.

- The technique is also contraindicated when the morphology of the edentulous alveolar ridge is not favourable due to the presence of no bone defects or undercuts (13.16a-c).
- Some authors have demonstrated that a flapless approach may lead to errors in implant positioning, and differences between inexperienced and skilled operators are not statistically significant with respect to this subject.
- For immediate post-extractive implant placement, a flapless approach is more demanding because it is not possible to verify the integrity of the thin buccal cortical plate visually.

Preparation of the implant site

SELECTING THE IMPLANT POSITION

Notwithstanding the possible use of a surgical stent, the position of any implant should be planned according to specific criteria that include a minimum distance between the implant and the natural teeth, and between neighbouring implants (for multiple implant placement). More precisely, the minimum distance between the shoulders of two implants is 2 millimetres, while the minimum distance between a natural tooth and an implant is 1.5 millimetres. If minimum distances are not respected, the construction/customisation of prosthetic components can be difficult or impossible, the patient can experience difficulties in maintaining adequate oral hygiene in the area, the papillae can be lost due to the lack of space, and the risk of significant peri-implant bone resorption is higher. Using the cited minimum distances as a reference point, the first perforations needed to place two adjacent implants depend on the maximum diameter of the chosen implants, which is measured at the prosthetic platform. As an example, if two wide diameter (5 mm) implants are to be placed in a distal edentulous ridge, the distance between the first perforation and the last tooth should be 4-5 millimetres, while the distance between the first and the second perforation should be 7 millimetres (13.17).

If the diameter of the chosen implants is different, then the tooth-implant and implant-implant distances should be modified accordingly (13.18a-b). In general, implant manufacturers provide operative manuals with detailed instructions for recommended implant-tooth and implant-implant distances, as well as specific instruments that allow the reliable measurement of the exact distances during surgery.

The minimum distance between two implants is not only determined by biologic factors, but also by the type of prosthetic rehabilitation chosen by the clinician. As an example, for partial or total edentulous jaws to be rehabilitated with fixed implant-supported prostheses (with the exclusion of Toronto-type rehabilitations), the position of each implant is determined according to restorative criteria evaluated on casts with the aid of the diagnostic wax-up. The available space is measured, the implant diameters are chosen, and the most appropriate rehabilitation scheme is selected accordingly. Implant positioning is then guided by the surgical stent, which represents the means of transferring the original plan to the operating field. **Obviously, the surgical stent must respect the previously described minimum distances between teeth and implants, and between adjacent implants.**

When totally edentulous jaws are to be rehabilitated with implant-supported overdentures, only the minimum distance between adjacent implants can be considered, while the lack of natural teeth makes it possible to choose the position of each implant considering only specific technical requirements.

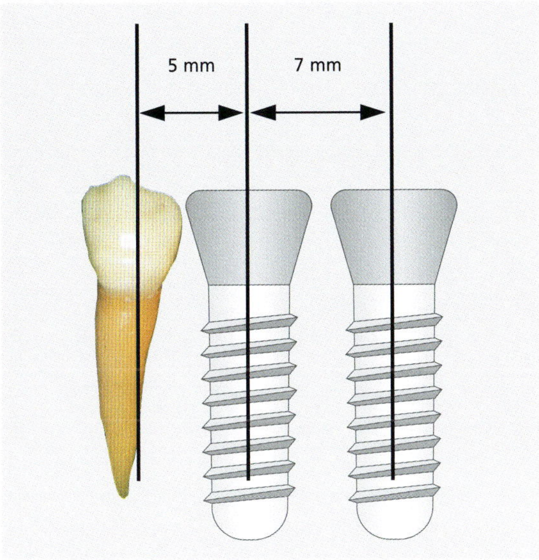

13.17 When choosing the implant position, minimum distances between teeth and implant, and between two adjacent implants, must be respected.

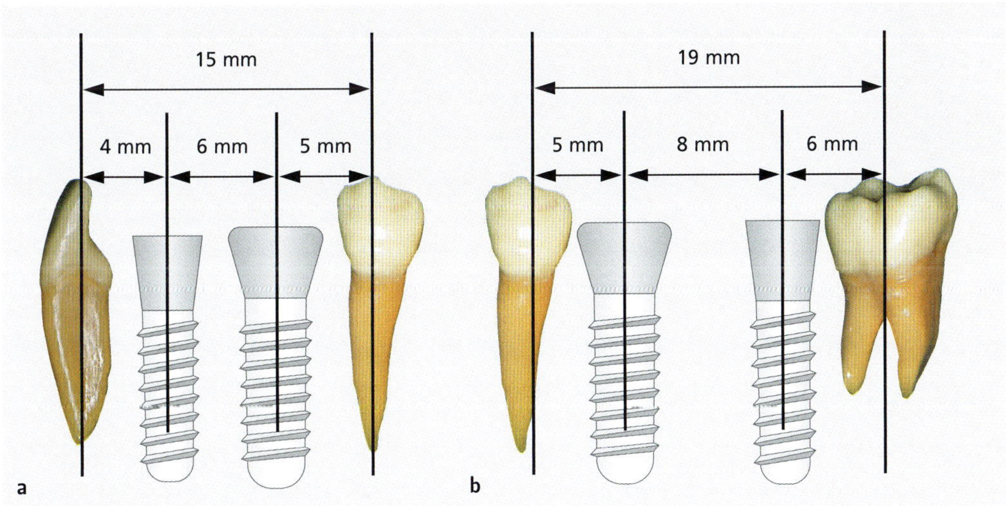

13.18 **a)** When narrow diameter implants are used, minimum distances are modified accordingly. **b)** When wide diameter implants are used, minimum distances must also be modified accordingly.

Surgical sequence for the preparation of the implant site

Every implant system has a specific drilling sequence for the atraumatic preparation of the implant site. After the access flap is elevated and possible connective tissue residuals are removed with a surgical curette, the main steps of the surgical sequence are as follows:

- preliminary regularisation of the alveolar ridge (if necessary);
- initial perforation to mark the mesial-distal and buccal-lingual/palatal position of the implant sites;
- preparation of the implant site with the dedicated drills;
- verification of the implant axis/implant site depth;
- bone tapping of the implant site (in cases of dense cortical bone);
- verification and irrigation of the implant site;
- implant placement;
- removal of the mounting device (if present);
- tightening of the cover screw (or healing abutment, in cases of non-submerged healing).

PREPARATION OF THE IMPLANT SITE ACCORDING TO BONE QUALITY

The technique for the preparation of the implant site should be adapted according to the local bone quality. Assessment of the latter is performed clinically, through analysis of CT scans that can give valuable information regarding the thickness of the cortical plates and the density of the cancellous bone. However, bone quality is chiefly evaluated during surgery, after the perforation of the cortical layer, and is based on the resistance offered by cancellous bone to drilling. However, in 1985 an empirical classification of bone density was proposed by Lekholm and Zarb, consisting of four classes.

Type I bone: highly corticalised dense bone, typically found in the interforaminal region of atrophic mandibles. In these cases, the resistance of the bone to the cutting action of the drills can be significant, leading to a higher risk of overheating. It is worth remembering that bone is very sensitive to temperature variations and, if it is heated to 47°-50° C, irreversible damage to the osteoblast can occur, potentially delaying or jeopardising bone healing around implants and, thus, osseointegration. Moreover, this type of bone presents a reduced blood supply compared to the other types, particularly in cases of severe mandibular atrophy where the endosteal vascularisation provided by the inferior alveolar artery is reduced. Therefore, sharp drills should always be used with an intermittent drilling technique, constantly removing bone particles and using cold sterile saline to irrigate while drilling. Use of a cortical drill or countersink at the end of the sequence and bone tapping are recommended.

Due to a reduced blood supply and higher risk of overheating, type I bone makes it possible to obtain high insertion torque and, thus, higher primary implant stability: this translates into the possibility of using shorter implants, if necessary.

Type II bone: it is characterised by a thick cortical layer and highly mineralised cancellous component, and it is typically found in the lateral-posterior areas of the mandible and in the anterior maxilla. The presence of type II bone represents an ideal clinical situation as the preparation of the implant site is easy, blood supply is excellent, and it is possible to obtain optimal primary implant stability by using the standard drilling sequence.

Type III and IV bone: the cortical layer is thin (type III) or absent (type IV), and the density of cancellous bone is acceptable (type III) to low (type IV). There is no correlation between bone density and anatomic region; however, these types of bone are usually found in the lateral-posterior areas of the maxilla, particularly in elderly patients. Obtaining adequate primary implant stability is critical: the survival rate of implants placed in type III and IV bone is generally lower compared to that of implants placed in type I and II bone. On the other hand, evolution of the macro- and micro-morphology of implants (design of the threads, active surfaces, etc.) has mitigated this difference.

Preparation of the implant site in type III and IV bone is modified to achieve sufficient primary implant stability:

- the last drill (or drills) included in the standard drilling sequence are not used: compression generated during implant placement increases the bone-to-implant contact surface, thus leading to a higher primary implant stability;
- bone tapping should always be avoided;
- countersink drills should not be used, to avoid unnecessary loss of cortical bone;

Technical tips to reduce surgical trauma and the risk of bone overheating

- Use of sharp drills (worn out or blunt drills require more pressure to be applied, with a higher risk of overheating)
- Removal of bone particles from the drills (bone particles reduce the cutting capacity of the drills)
- Implant site preparation with low speed (500-1500 rpm), high torque handpieces
- Intermittent (push-pull) movement under continuous irrigation with refrigerated sterile saline

- the use of wider diameter implants with a tapered profile makes it possible to increase the bone-to-implant contact surface, and to achieve better stability due to the proximity of the buccal and lingual/palatal cortical plates and the increased compression on the cancellous bone;
- the use of implants with a rough, active surface shortens the osseointegration process, leading to increased survival rates in type IV bone;
- preparing the implant site with osteotomes causes compression of the surrounding bone, thus leading to increased primary implant stability (13.19).

Suture

Submerged implants: soft tissues are sutured above the cover screw. Tension-free flap repositioning is mandatory to avoid spontaneous dehiscences and implant uncovering during the osseointegration period. If necessary, periosteal releasing incisions can be performed. Flaps can be closed with single interrupted sutures associated, if necessary, with U-sutures to obtain a watertight closure of the surgical access.

In general, whenever reconstructive/regenerative procedures are performed in conjunction with implant placement, a submerged healing protocol is recommended.

Transmucosal (soft tissue level) implants: the flap is sutured around the healing abutments; the recourse to periosteal releasing incisions is often unnecessary (13.20).

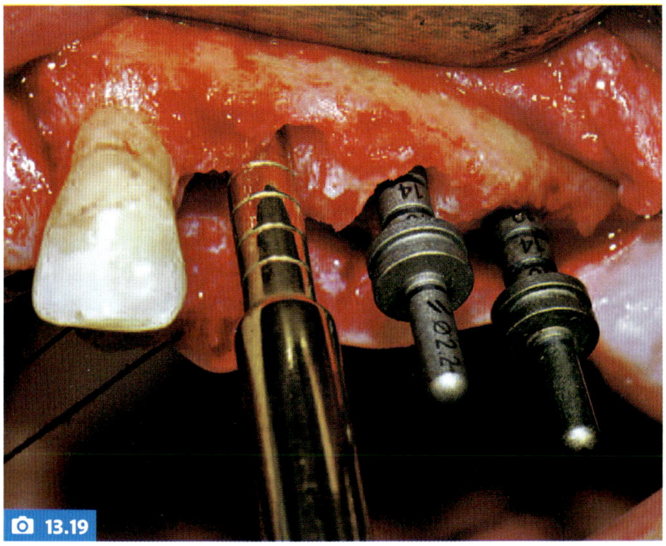

13.19

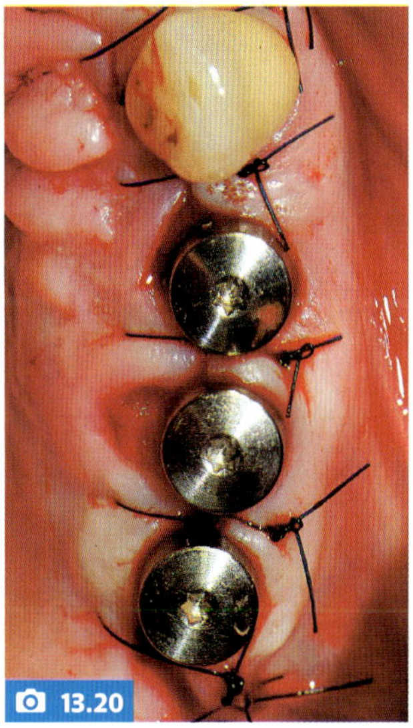

13.20

13.19 When bone quality is poor, implant site preparation can be performed with osteotomes to increase primary implant stability.

13.20 When a non-submerged healing protocol is used, the access flap is sutured around the healing abutments.

Peri-implant soft tissue management

Optimisation of soft tissue morphology and thickness around implants is particularly important in the aesthetic zone. When transmucosal implants are placed, thickening of the buccal mucosa can be performed in conjunction with implant placement by means of a connective tissue graft sutured under the buccal aspect of the flap. When submerged implants are used, the same surgical correction can be performed in conjunction with implant placement or at the time of implant uncovering (13.21a-c). For a critical review of the literature on techniques for the management of peri-implant soft tissues, see Esposito et al. (2012).

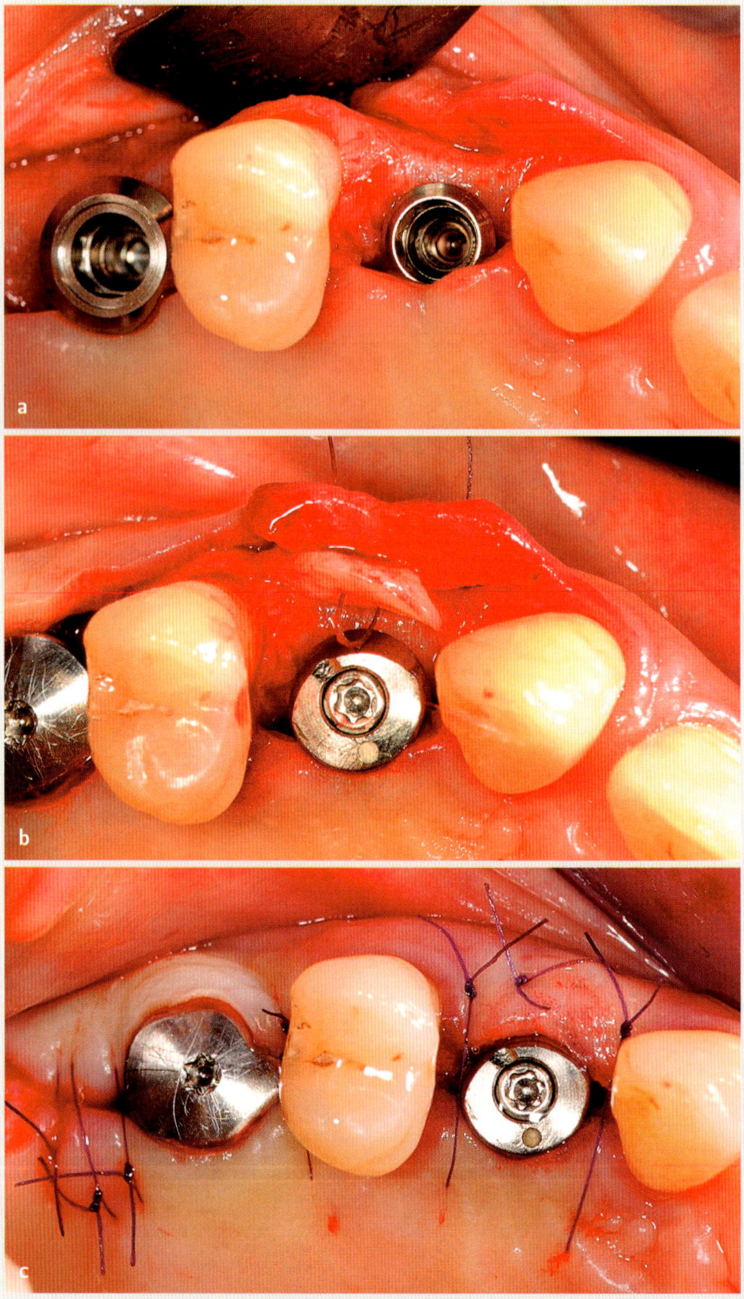

13.21 a–c) To improve the profile of the alveolar crest, and thus the emergence profile of the implant-supported prosthetic restoration, a connective tissue graft is sutured under the buccal aspect of the surgical flap.

Postoperative radiographic follow-up

The postoperative radiograph makes it possible to verify the correct positioning of implants, the safety distance between implants and important anatomic structures (e.g. inferior alveolar nerve, nasal cavities, maxillary sinus, etc.), and the correct placement of healing abutments. Moreover, it represents the reference point for evaluation of the following radiographs that will be taken annually to assess the behaviour and stability of peri-implant bone over time.

Postoperative treatment

For invasive or complex surgeries, antibiotics are administered together with analgesics. Oral antisepsis and plaque control are obtained with chlorhexidine mouthwashes: the patient is instructed to rinse three times per day for 10-15 days after surgery. A liquid/soft diet is prescribed for 2-3 days.

Sutures are removed 7-10 days after surgery: the use of mucosa-supported provisional prostheses on the operated area is proscribed until complete healing of the soft tissues, and relining with soft materials is recommended. Fixed provisional prostheses supported by neighbouring teeth can be cemented immediately after surgery, provided that the absence of any contact between the prosthesis and the soft tissues is verified.

After implant placement

The choice of a non submerged healing protocol allows the soft tissue to heal around specifically designed healing abutments. Once osseointegration is achieved, the healing abutments are removed and the appropriate prosthetic components are connected to the implants. The timing of implant loading is a critical factor: three loading protocols have been widely used in a large number of studies published in the literature, and validated by systematic reviews and consensus conferences (see Esposito et al., 2007, and Weber et al., 2009).

Conventional loading: the waiting time between implant placement and loading is equal to or greater than 2 months;

Early loading: the waiting time between implant placement and loading ranges from 1 week to 2 months;

Immediate loading: the waiting time between implant placement and loading is less than 1 week.

Basic techniques

Regularisation of the alveolar ridge

The alveolar ridge can be regularised with a 4–5 mm round bur mounted on a straight or contra-angle handpiece (13.22a). Whenever burs are used, irrigation with refrigerated sterile saline is recommended, to avoid bone overheating and necrosis, which may occur if bone temperature rises to 47°–50° C.

Initial perforation – marking the implant site

The drilling sequence generally begins with a small-diameter round bur used for the initial perforation of the cortical layer to mark the position of the planned implant site (13.22b). If the upper curvature of the alveolar ridge renders the use of a round bur difficult, a pointed bur can be used to avoid errors caused by bur swerving.

Preparation of the implant site with dedicated drills

Drills of increasing diameter are used to create an implant site that matches the implant diameter. Drills are used with an intermittent (push and pull) movement under constant irrigation to avoid bone overheating. Laser-marked bands on every drill allow the clinician to verify the depth of the preparation; however, it is worth remembering that these markings represent the length of the implant body, but they do not include the length of the point of each drill which in some cases may exceed 1 millimetre (13.22c–d).

The use of the last drill in the sequence is critical for primary implant stability: care must be taken to avoid inclination errors that may lead to drill vibration and deformation of the implant site.

The drilling sequence for some implant systems includes a countersink drill for the final preparation of the cortical layer, to allow a deeper positioning of the implant shoulder (particularly in the aesthetic zone).

Bone particles retrieved during drilling can prove useful in various clinical situations, such as the treatment of small dehiscences or fenestrations occurred during the preparation of the implant site. Bone particles can be easily retrieved from the flutes of each drill with the tip of a probe, and they are preserved in a small surgical bowl immersed in sterile saline.

An ideal rotation speed is recommended (expressed in rotations per minute or rpm) for different drills in the same sequence (and for drills from different implant systems). Typically, drills with a smaller diameter can be operated at higher speed (1000–1500 rpm), while for drills with a larger diameter the recommended speed is much lower.

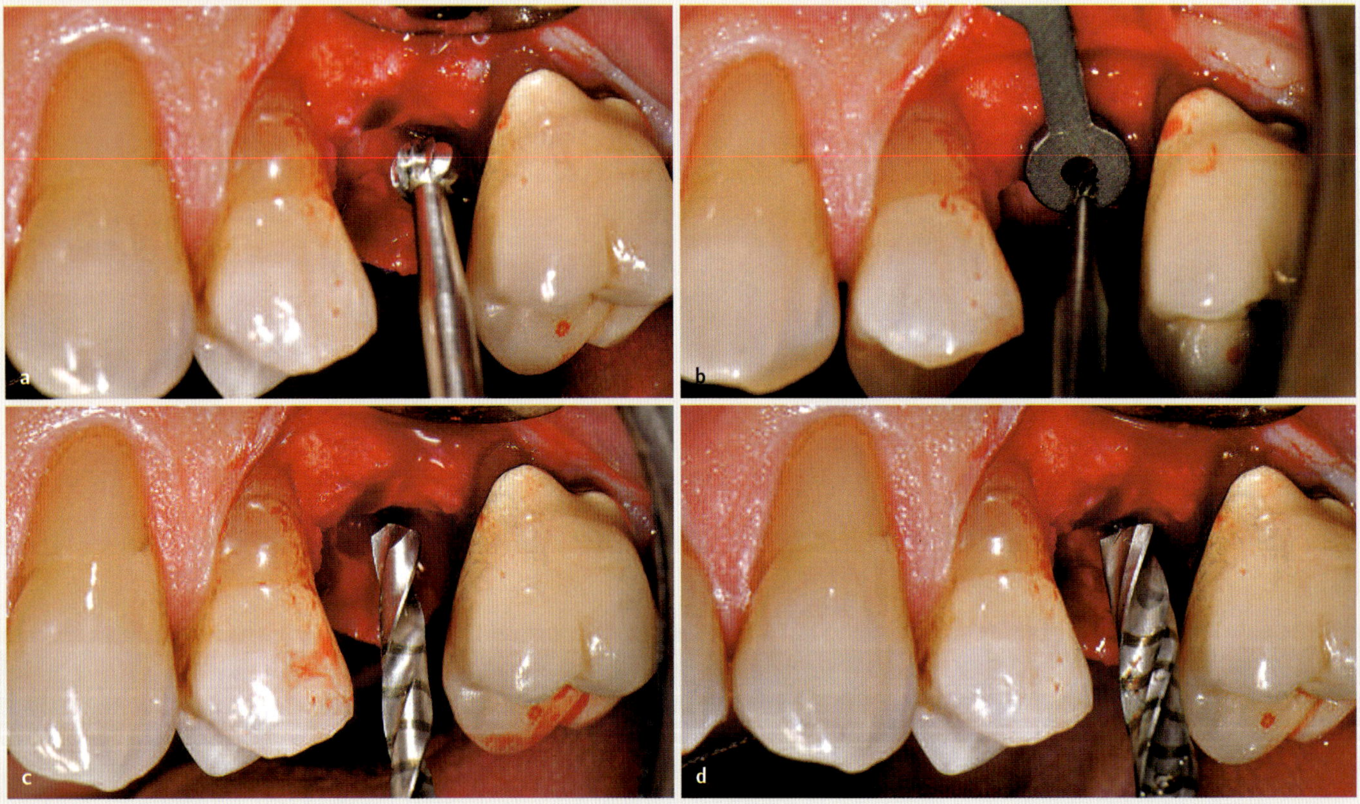

13.22 **a)** A round bur is used to level the profile of the alveolar ridge. **b)** The position of the implant site is marked with a small round bur: a surgical calliper replicating the diameter of the chosen implant is used to simplify the identification of the ideal position. **c–d)** The preparation of the implant site continues with dedicated drills and a specific drilling sequence: the depth marks on the drills allow easy verification of the drilling dept. (*continued*)

The use of a surgical unit is recommended, to provide complete control over speed, torque, and irrigation during the preparation of the implant site and implant placement.

Implant axis verification

After each drill is used, the axis of the implant bed should be verified with dedicated guide pins (13.22e). The following criteria should always be respected:

Parallelism between adjacent implants: an important prerequisite to simplify the prosthetic rehabilitation that follows (in cases where the use of tilted implants is not specifically planned);

Position of the implant according to the position of neighbouring teeth: in this case, the axis of the preparation must take into consideration the inclination and possible curves of the roots of neighbouring teeth, from which safety distances should always be maintained;

Correction: if a correction of the preparation axis is necessary, it can be performed with the bur that follows (larger diameter).

Implant site depth verification

Guide pins usually present depth marks as well, to allow verification of the implant site depth (13.22e).

Bone tapping (optional)

The recourse to bone tapping is rare, because the majority of implants are self-tapping. However, it can be performed with the dedicated instruments either by hand or with a handpiece at a very low speed (15–20 rpm), for implant placement in type I bone, to avoid excessive friction between the implant and the surrounding bone.

Implant site verification and irrigation

If the depth of the implant site exceeds the portion of the alveolar ridge that is visible after flap elevation, verification of the implant site with a probe allows verification of the presence of possible fenestrations on the cortical plates. Irrigation with sterile saline is performed to remove possible bone particles that may interfere with the correct placement of the implant.

Implant placement

Once the preparation of the implant site is completed, the implant can be inserted. The implant is picked up from its sterile box with a specific carrier, and it can be inserted either with manual instruments or with a low-speed contra-angle handpiece (13.22f).

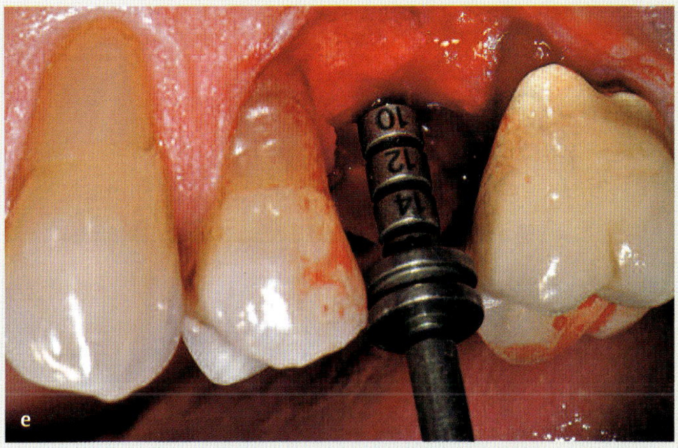

13.22 (*continued*) **e)** When two or more adjacent implants are placed, guide pins make it possible to verify the correct alignment, while depth marks are used to confirm that the planned depth is reached. (*continued*)

In both cases, insertion is performed slowly (15–30 rpm) while maintaining the correct axis created during preparation of the implant site. Before and during placement, the implant surface must never be contaminated by saliva or by direct contact with any other surface or instrument. Implant insertion by means of a controlled-torque device (torque wrench, contra-angle handpiece mounted on a surgical unit) makes it possible to evaluate the peak insertion torque, which is a fundamental parameter in the assessment of primary implant stability and, thus, in the choice of the loading protocol.

Cover screw and healing abutments

After the implant is placed, a cover screw is tightened at a low torque (5–10 Ncm) to protect the internal cavity of the implant from contamination and soft tissue ingrowth. Correct adaptation and tightening of the cover screws must be verified, to avoid possible unscrewing or bone formation on the implant shoulder.

Submerged healing: the cover screws, once in place, are level with the implant shoulder or present a reduced height, to avoid any interference with the closure of the access flap.

Non-submerged healing: the healing abutments are connected to the implants, and the access flap is sutured around them. The height of the healing abutment is chosen according to the thickness of the soft tissues (13.22g–j).

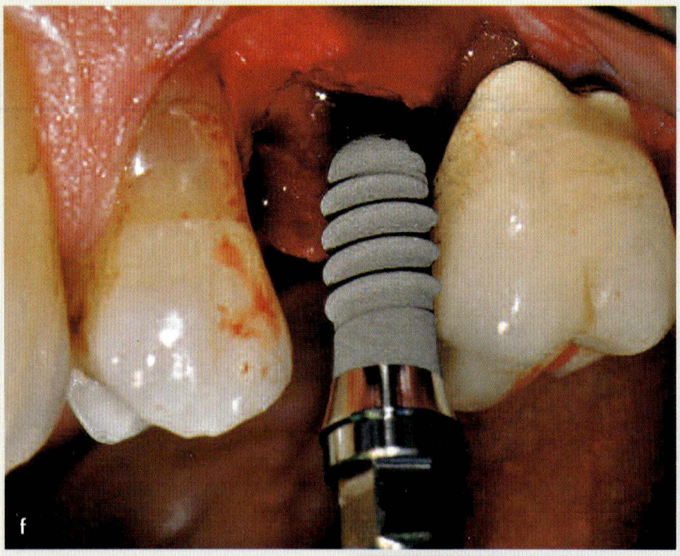

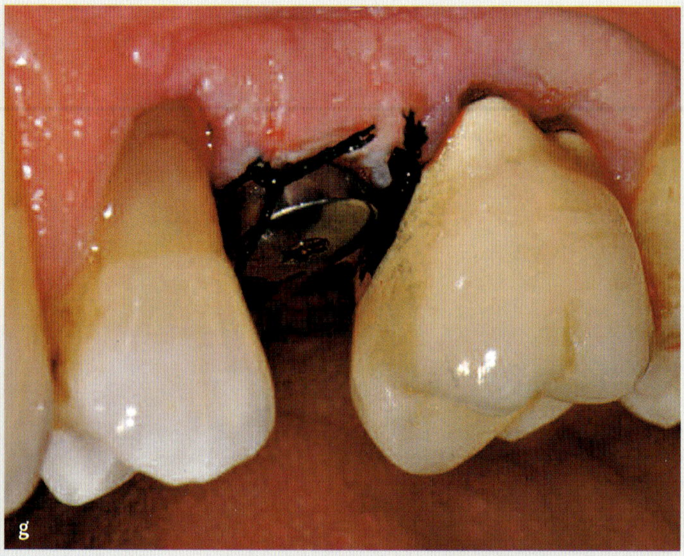

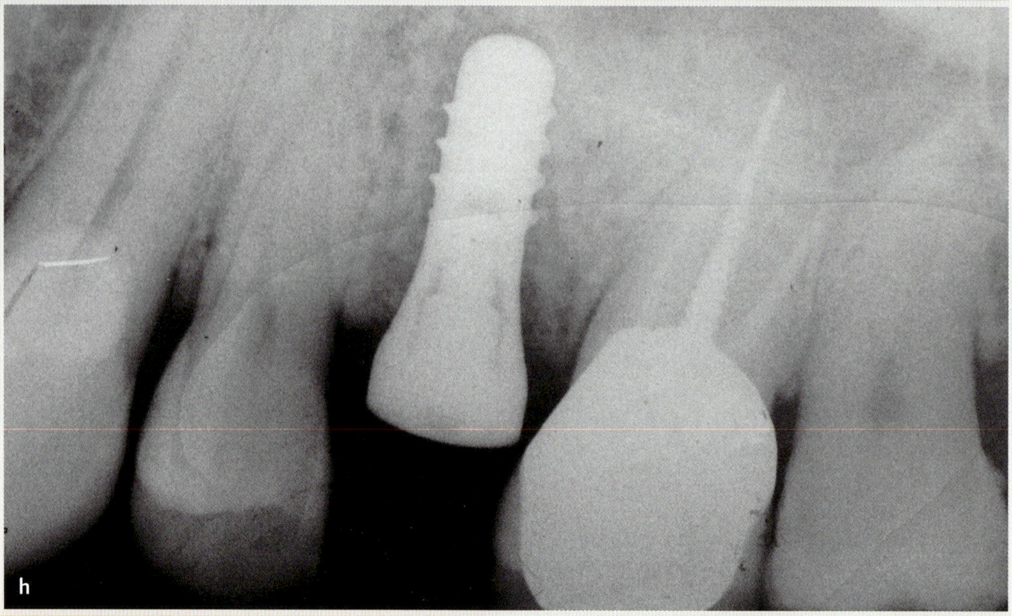

13.22 (*continued*) **f)** Placement of a one-piece implant. **g)** The healing abutment is screwed to the implant and the access flap is sutured around it to allow a non-submerged healing. **h)** Radiographic follow-up after implant placement. **i–j)** Final prosthetic restoration and radiographic follow-up.

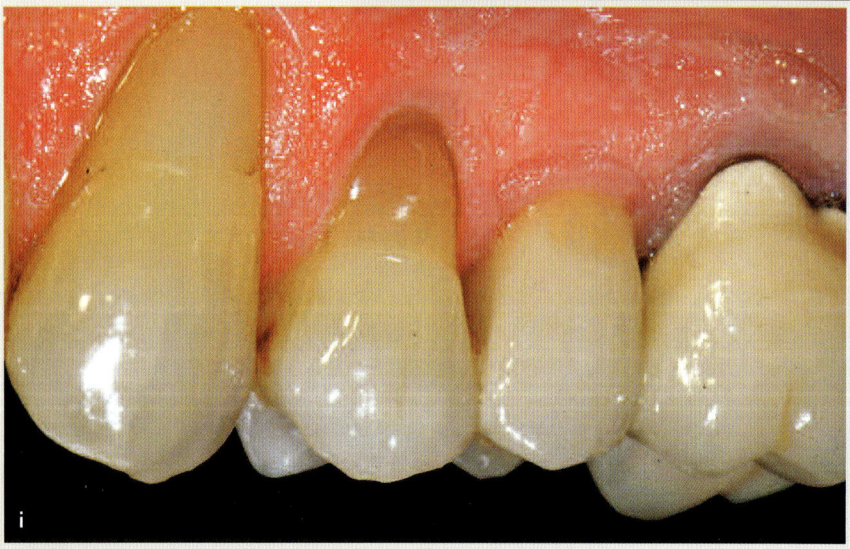

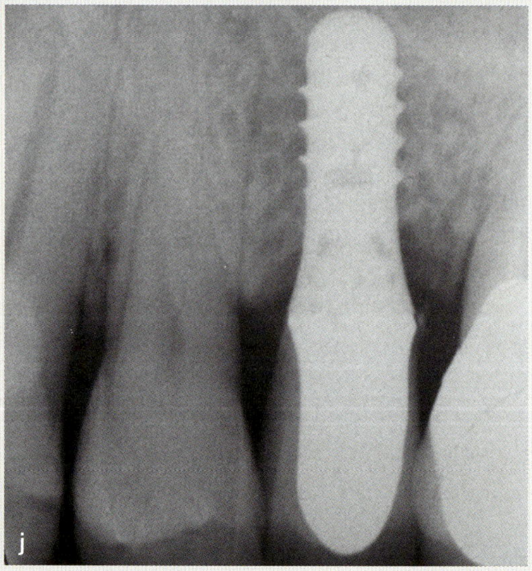

Two-piece (bone level) implants, if necessary, can be managed with a submerged healing protocol (e.g. when regenerative procedures are performed in conjunction with implant placement). In this case, a second surgical intervention to uncover the implants, remove the cover screw, and connect the healing abutments is required (13.23a–c). If necessary, ancillary procedures such as connective tissue grafting or keratinised mucosa grafting can be performed at the time of implant uncovering.

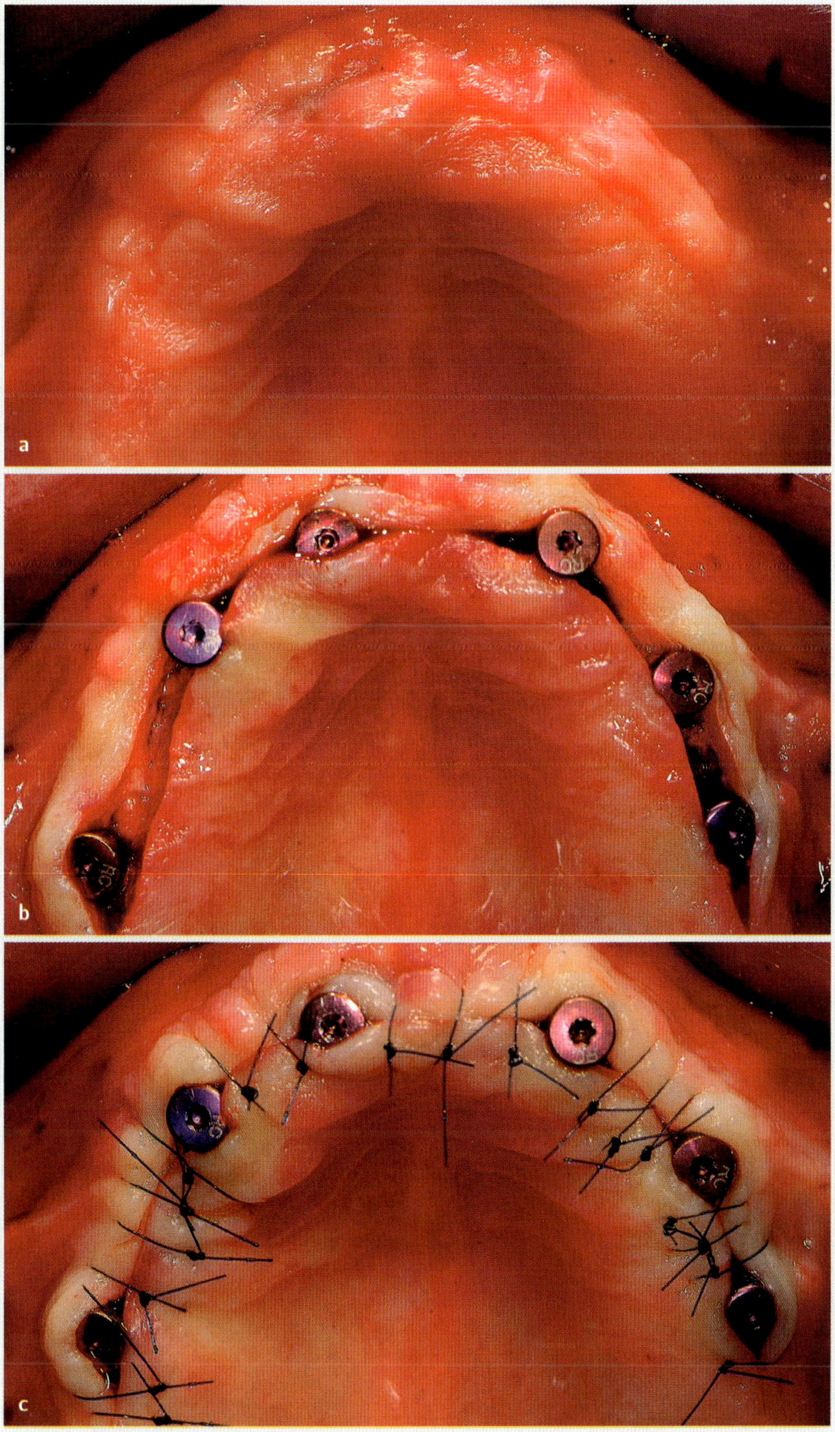

13.23 a–c) Uncovering of submerged implants in the maxilla.

The analysis of restorative options and the detailed description of prosthetic protocols are beyond scope of this manual. However, it is worth noting that if the initial planning follows the principle of prosthetic-driven implant placement, then the final result can meet high standards both in aesthetic and functional terms irrespective of the type of condition (partial edentulism, total edentulism) or prosthesis used (fixed, removable, screw-retained, cement-retained) (13.24a-b, 13.25a-d, 13.26a-c).

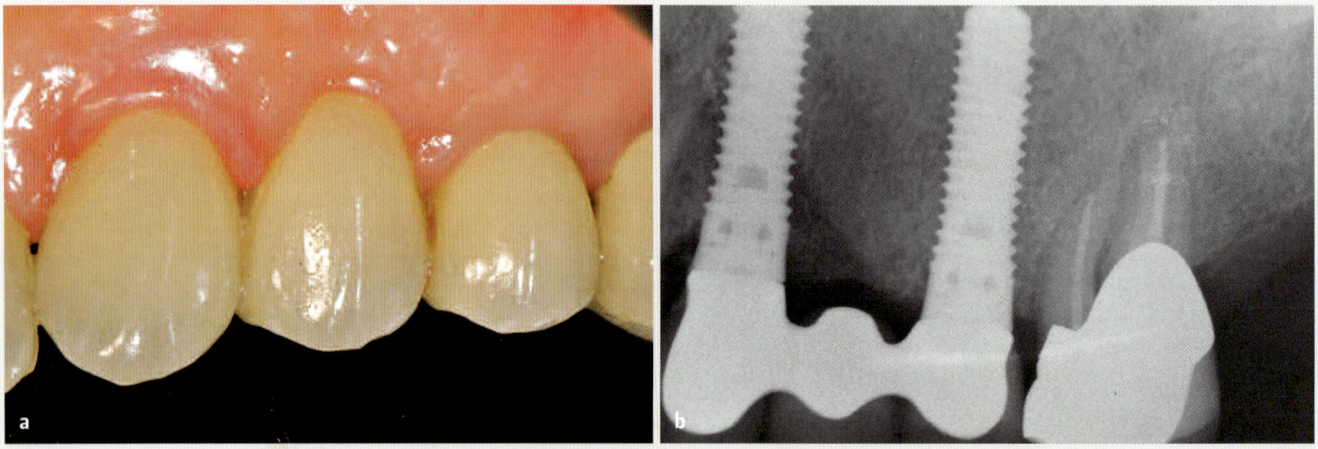

13.24 Implant-supported prosthetic rehabilitation of partially edentulous ridges: **a)** clinical follow-up; **b)** radiographic follow-up (case presented in 13.16a-c).

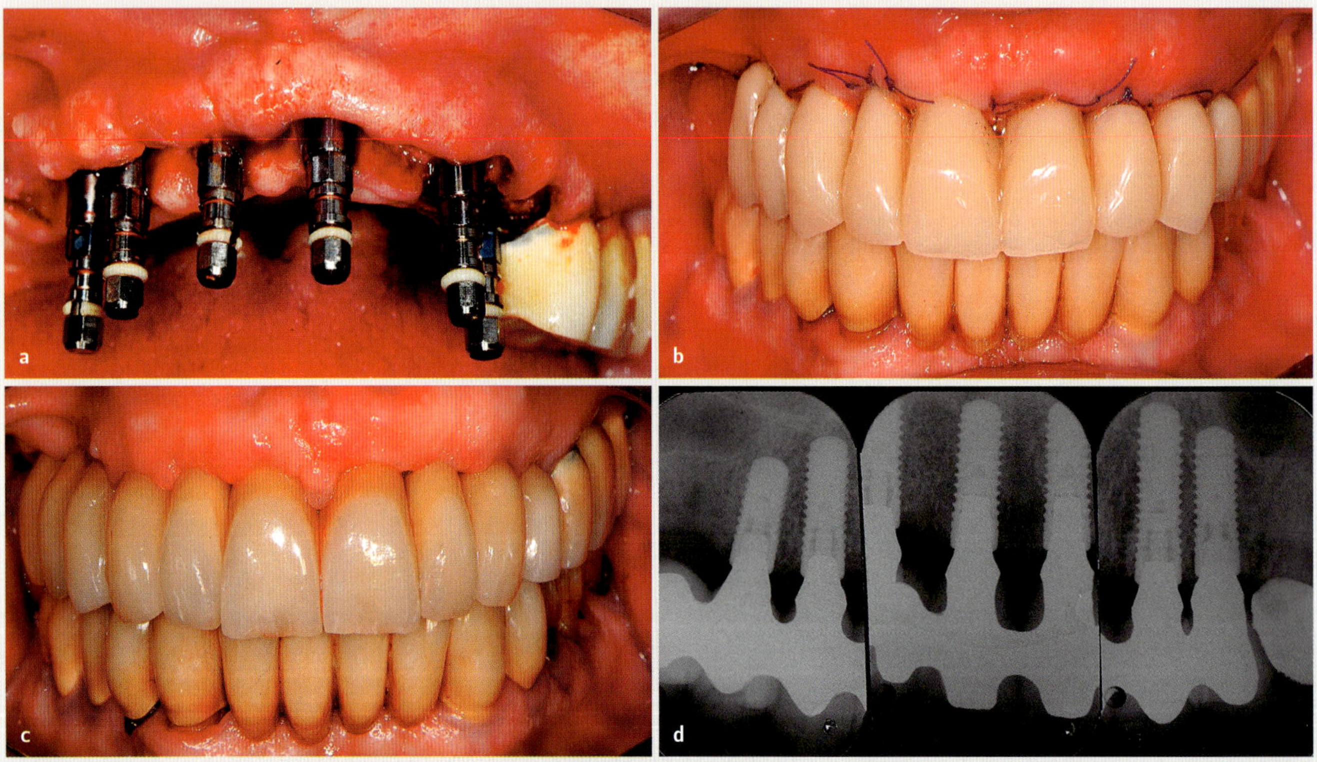

13.25 Implant-supported rehabilitation of partially edentulous maxilla: **a–b)** six implants are placed in the planned position: optimal primary stability is obtained, therefore an immediate loading protocol is chosen and provisional restorations are cemented 24 hours after implant placement; **c–d)** final clinical and radiographic follow-up.

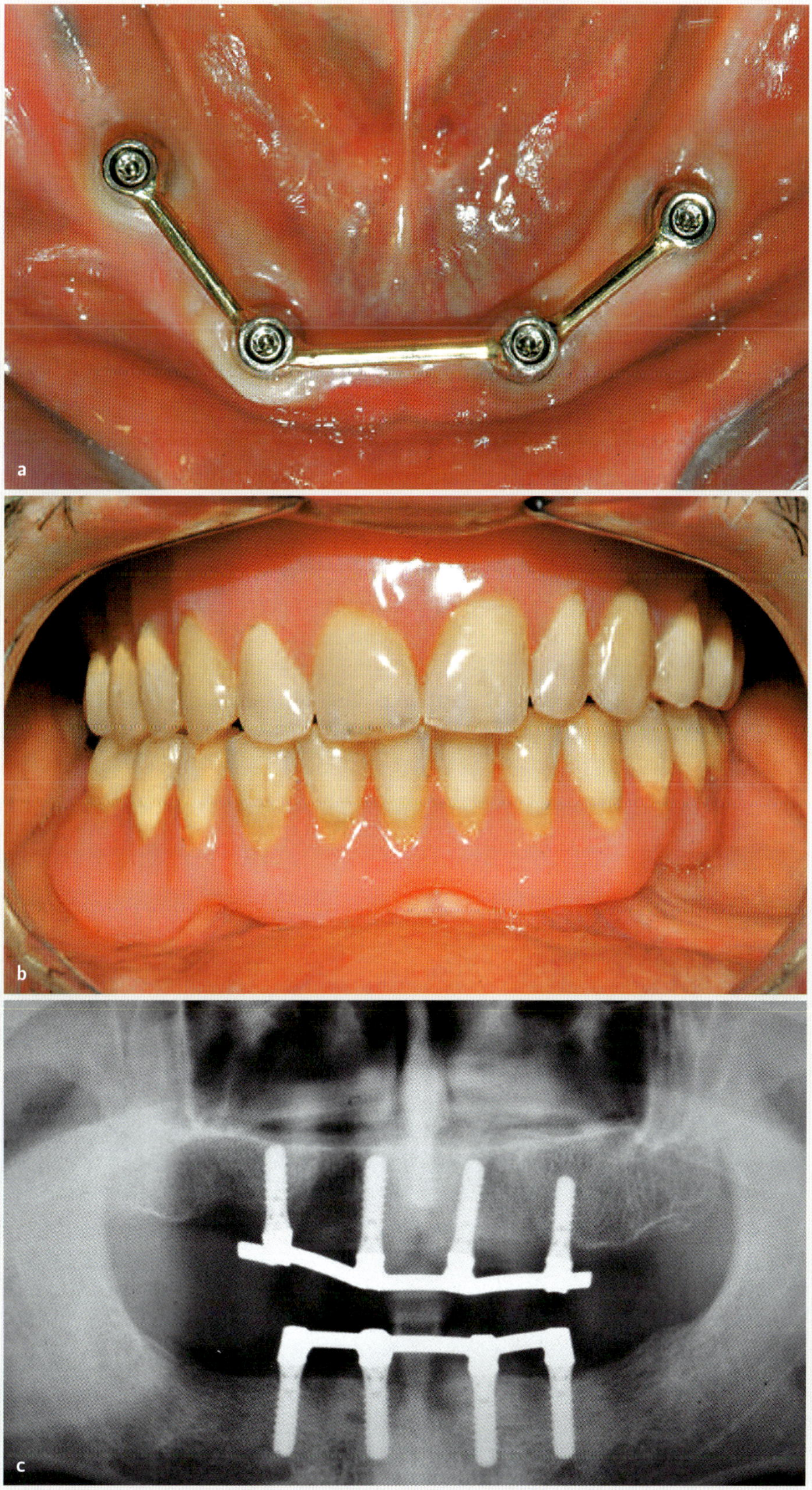

13.26 **a)** Implant-supported overdentures for the rehabilitation of totally edentulous jaws. **b)** Clinical follow-up. **c)** Radiographic follow-up.

Implant rehabilitation – Complex cases

The rehabilitation of partially or totally edentulous alveolar ridges with implant-supported prostheses should be planned according to the principles of prosthetic-driven implant placement. When bone volume and morphology are adequate, implants can be placed in the ideal position and good results can be obtained without additional procedures. However, the loss of teeth due to periodontal disease, trauma, tumour resection, as well as their absence due to agenesia associated with bone loss or atrophy which, in the lateral-posterior area of the maxilla, can be aggravated by maxillary sinus pneumatisation, bone loss and an unfavourable morphology of the edentulous ridge, may render the placement of implants in the ideal position impossible. In these cases, compromises in the positioning of implants to adapt to a less than ideal situation may result in functional and aesthetic complications, or even the failure of the rehabilitation. Instead, the same guidelines described for simple cases should be followed. The oral surgeon should plan the case in cooperation with the prosthodontist who, by studying the casts and diagnostic wax-up, is able to determine the correct form, dimension, and position of each implant-supported element. A radiographic/surgical stent is created and a CT scan is performed with the stent in place. With bone defects, discrepancies between the ideal implant position and the residual alveolar ridge can be evaluated and measured: this method makes it possible to assess the defect precisely and plan the procedures accurately to restore the lost bone volume and morphology.

A detailed description of all the alternatives to treat bone defects (guided bone regeneration, onlay bone grafts, inlay bone grafts, osteotomies, etc.) is beyond the scope of this manual, and can be found in specialist textbooks. However, it is worth noting that a single ideal solution to treat every possible condition does not exist: every technique and material presents peculiar advantages and disadvantages that the oral surgeon must evaluate according to the specific clinical situation. A fundamental parameter to consider when planning a complex rehabilitation is the optimal benefit-cost ratio, which should make it possible to obtain the best result with the least invasive approach. Once the optimal reconstructive procedure is chosen, the timing of implant placement can be planned. In the presence of small defects, particularly when the posterior areas of the jaws are involved and aesthetic considerations are not a predominant factor, the placement of implants in conjunction with the reconstructive procedure can represent a viable option. Conversely, for large defects or defects involving the aesthetic zone, delayed implant placement is indicated.

Generally, defects that can jeopardise an implant-supported prosthetic rehabilitation may involve both hard and soft tissues: in the latter case, the loss of keratinised mucosa is a critical factor.

Bone defects

Irrespective of the cause (atrophy, trauma, maxillary sinus pneumatisation, tumour ablation, congenital defect), alveolar bone may present the following types of defect that can render the placement of implants inadequate or impossible:

- horizontal defects (insufficient width of the alveolar ridge);
- vertical defects (insufficient height of the alveolar ridge);
- combined vertical/horizontal defects (tridimensional defects).

Horizontal defects: a moderate horizontal defect may result in the creation of dehiscences (coronal bone defects) or fenestrations (apical bone defects) while creating the implant site with the specific drilling sequence, and a portion of the implant surface is exposed and visible. If the initial defect is more ample, a greater portion of the implant surface is exposed and, thus, a lesser portion of the implant can osseointegrate. For extremely narrow ridges, creating an implant bed is impossible and may lead to the complete destruction of the alveolar ridge. Although in recent years, narrow diameter implants made with more resistant alloys (e.g. titanium-zirconium) or specially engineered surfaces have been introduced, it is undeniable that in some cases implant placement is not possible or, if technically possible, it is however contraindicated due to the impossibility of a prosthetic-driven placement with obvious consequences on aesthetics and function.

In these cases, different reconstructive and regenerative techniques are available to correct the initial defect and allow a delayed prosthetic-driven implant placement and subsequent satisfactory prosthetic rehabilitation.

Vertical defects: for vertical bone deficit, interarch distance is augmented proportionately to the extent of the defect. Moreover, vertical bone loss may reduce the bone height available for implant placement due to the relative proximity of important anatomic structures such as the inferior alveolar nerve, the maxillary sinus, and the nasal cavities. Although the introduction of short (<7-8 mm) implants with specifically engineered surfaces, designed to increase the bone-to-implant contact ratio, has made it possible to overcome some challenges, it is nonetheless undeniable that implant placement remains impossible under certain circumstances (e.g. when the mandibular nerve is just below the upper margin of the alveolar crest) or, despite being technically possible, it would result in less than ideal aesthetics and function of the implant-supported prosthetic rehabilitation.

It is worth noting that in the lateral-posterior areas of the edentulous maxilla the presence of a vertical bone defect is frequent, even when a normal interarch distance is preserved. This is due to the expansion (pneumatisation) of the maxillary sinus in the coronal direction, which normally occurs during adult life but is accelerated by the loss of the premolars and molars. In this case, the correction of the vertical defect (by means of a sinus floor elevation procedure) presents peculiarities that will be discussed in a dedicated section of this chapter.

Combined horizontal-vertical (tridimensional) defects: the disadvantages of both horizontal and vertical defects are present, determining more complex clinical situations that are more challenging to treat.

Soft tissue defects

Although it is still not widely accepted that the presence of an adequate band of keratinised mucosa around implants is fundamental for their long-term survival (Chen and Buser, 2009), its absence may cause a higher risk of gingival recession, difficulties in maintaining adequate oral hygiene, exposure of the prosthetic mesostructures (abutments), and finally a lack of aesthetic uniformity between natural teeth surrounded by keratinised tissue and implants.

Materials and surgical techniques for bone reconstruction/regeneration

Several techniques and grafting materials are currently available that allow predictable outcomes and long-term reliability in the reconstruction/regeneration of bone defects, with the aim of optimising implant placement and the final functional and aesthetic result of the implant-supported prosthetic rehabilitation.

Techniques:

- guided bone regeneration;
- onlay bone grafts;
- inlay bone grafts;
- sinus floor elevation;
- distraction osteogenesis;
- ridge expansion;
- revascularised free flaps.

Materials:

- autogenous bone (bone harvested from the patient);
- allogeneic bone (fresh frozen bone from the tissue bank);
- heterologous bone (bone derived from other animal species);
- synthetic biomaterials (e.g. tricalcium phosphate, bioglasses, hydroxylapatites);
- semi-permeable barriers/membranes (both synthetic and derived from animal tissues, resorbable and non-resorbable, primarily used for guided bone regeneration techniques).

These materials can be used separately, in conjunction one with the other, or mixed.

Despite the enormous development of research protocols on grafting materials, autogenous bone harvested from intraoral (mandibular body and ramus) and extraoral (iliac crest, calvarium) sites still represents the reference material for bone reconstruction due to its osteoconductive, osteoinductive, and osteogenic potential, and to the absence of any possible immune response.

Other grafting materials now available offer adequate osteoconductive characteristics, but lack osteoinductive and osteogenic potential. The latter could be obtained with the addition of bone morphogenetic proteins (BMPs) and cell cultures, but these methods are still in the experimental phase and cannot be introduced in the clinical routine, due to the high costs and complex management.

An analysis of all the characteristics of every grafting material is beyond the scope of this manual. Nonetheless, it is worth remembering that all grafting materials must be biocompatible, bio-inert, and present a calibrated porosity to allow the penetration of newly formed capillaries, which represent the basis for an adequate blood supply that conveys oxygen, cells, and growth factors in the area.

Detailed information on the biology of bone regeneration/repair, bone harvesting procedures, and grafting techniques can be found in specialty textbooks, but some basic information on these subjects is reported in the following sections.

Autogenous bone harvesting

Autogenous bone, as previously mentioned, can be harvested both from intraoral and extraoral sites.

The choice of the donor site depends on the extent of the defect and, as a consequence, the quantity of bone needed to restore an adequate bone volume in the area. Intraoral sites, such as the mental symphysis and the mandibular ramus, are characterised by the presence of a dense, cortical bone, which is an excellent grafting material. However, the quantity of bone available is relatively limited; therefore, bone harvesting from intraoral sites is indicated in the case of relevant defects with a limited extension.

Other intraoral areas, such as the maxillary tuberosity, have been proposed in the past as donor sites for bone harvesting, but the limited quantity and scarce quality of the available bone (which renders it more prone to resorption) represent a limit to its use.

Extraoral donor sites, such as the anterior iliac crest and the calvarium, offer a greater quantity of available bone to harvest, and extraoral harvesting procedures are therefore indicated for extended defects. With small defects, they rarely represent an alternative to intraoral donor sites, due to the higher technical complexity, postoperative morbidity, and the necessity of specific maxillofacial surgery skills to perform the intervention.

It is also worth noting that, while the anterior iliac crest can offer the greatest amount of bone to harvest, and the thin cortical layer and predominant cancellous component cause shorter revascularisation and integration times, they can also expose the grafted area to an augmented risk of bone resorption over time. Conversely, bone blocks harvested from the calvarium consist almost entirely of dense cortical bone: the quality is similar to that of bone harvested from intraoral sites, but the quantity is far superior. Revascularisation and integration of the graft is slower compared to iliac bone, but calvarial bone is significantly less prone to resorption over time.

Harvesting techniques and the surgical armamentarium are similar, and the latter includes:

- rotary instruments (round burs, fissure burs, disks), oscillating and reciprocating saws, and piezoelectric instruments are used to create osteotomies in cases where bone blocks are utilised;
- surgical chisels and hammers are used to detach the bone blocks.

More recently, bone scrapers have been introduced in the market: these instruments make it possible to harvest relevant quantities of bone particles with a less invasive and less traumatic procedure, as compared to bone block harvesting. However, these instruments are indicated only if the augmentation procedure of the deficient maxillary/mandibular bone will be performed not with blocks but with guided bone regeneration procedures (GBR) in which semi-permeable barriers are necessary.

Anaesthetic techniques and access flaps are obviously different and are briefly described in the following section.

BONE HARVESTING FROM THE MANDIBULAR SYMPHYSIS

Anaesthesia: local infiltration of anaesthetics in the interforaminal area in association with inferior alveolar nerve block is indicated.

Access flap: in dentate patients, an arched incision is made in the vestibular fornix, extending from one premolar region to the contralateral: care should be taken to avoid any damage to the branches of the mental nerves. The mental muscles are interrupted, and the separated portions will be reunited at the end of the harvesting procedure with resorbable sutures. Osteotomies depend on the quantity of bone to be harvested, but it is recommended that a safety distance be maintained: 0.5 cm mesially to the mental foramina, 0.5 cm apically to the root apexes of the anterior teeth, and 0.5 cm coronally to the inferior border of the mandible. Moreover, once the buccal cortical layer is perforated, osteotomies should not be extended to the underlying cancellous bone, due to the risk of damaging the incisive nerve.

BONE HARVESTING FROM THE MANDIBULAR RAMUS

Anaesthesia: inferior alveolar nerve block is performed in conjunction with buccal nerve block and infiltration anaesthesia in the area of the mandibular body and ramus to achieve adequate haemostasis. Lingual nerve block is not mandatory, and it usually occurs spontaneously when the inferior alveolar nerve block is performed.

Access flap: in dentate patients, a submarginal incision is made along the oblique line of the mandible towards. The distal extent of the incision is chosen according to surgical needs. Elevation of the buccal aspect of the flap is recommended, to allow better visibility, access, and protection of the soft tissues and to avoid possible damage to the facial artery. Osteotomies are performed according to the size of the bone block to be harvested, but once the buccal cortical layer is perforated, osteotomies should not extend too far in the underlying cancellous bone due to the risk of damaging the inferior alveolar nerve. Length of the incision as well as elevation of flaps can be significantly reduced if bone scrapers are used.

BONE HARVESTING FROM THE ANTERIOR ILIAC CREST

Anaesthesia: local infiltration of anaesthetic is performed on the superior, medial, and lateral face of the anterior iliac crest; however, these surgical interventions are frequently performed under general anaesthesia.

Access flap: a linear incision is made along the superior margin of the anterior iliac crest, keeping a 2 cm safety distance from the anterior iliac spine to avoid possible damage to the lateral femoral cutaneous nerve. Subperiosteal elevation of the surgical flap is performed to expose the superior margin and medial face of the iliac crest, while avoiding detachment of the tensor fasciae latae and gluteus medius muscles on the lateral face to limit postoperative discomfort and gait disturbances.

BONE HARVESTING FROM THE CALVARIUM

Anaesthesia: local infiltration of anaesthetic in the parietal region is performed; however, these surgical interventions are frequently performed under general anaesthesia.

Access flap: two different incisions can be used, a hemicoronal incision from the vertex of the cranial vault towards the auricular region or a parasagittal incision extending from the frontal region (distally to the hairline) to the distal limit of the parietal region. The incision of the skin, subcutaneous tissue, galea capitis, and pericranium, and their detachment from the cranial vault allow exposure of the parietal bone.

GUIDED BONE REGENERATION (GBR)

The principle underlying this group of reconstructive procedures is that using semi-permeable barriers as spacemakers over a bone defect, to create a chamber between residual bone and the overlying soft tissues, allows bone regeneration to occur. Barrier membranes can be either resorbable (collagen, polylactic-polyglycolic acid, pericardium etc.) or non-resorbable (PTFE, titanium, etc.).

Theoretically, the membrane alone should guarantee bone regeneration, due to the transformation of the blood clot that fills the void between the residual alveolar crest and the membrane itself into newly formed bone, particularly if the defect is surrounded by intact bony walls. However, the majority of, bone regeneration of horizontal and vertical defects are performed with the combined use of barrier membranes and different autogenous or non-autogenous grafting materials (allografts, xenografts, alloplastic materials), used as a support for the membrane and for their osteoconductive and/or osteoinductive properties. In summary, the grafting material is used to recreate adequate bone volume and morphology in the deficient area, and is then covered and stabilised for several months with the membrane. During the healing phase, the material undergoes organisation and consolidation that lead to new bone formation; the presence of newly formed bone allows the placement of implants in the edentulous area. This process requires a healing period of 4 to 12 months.

Guided bone regeneration allows correction of limited horizontal, vertical, and tridimensional defects. In fact, data reported in the literature generally refer to edentulous spaces ranging from one to 3-4 missing teeth (although in a minority of cases GBR procedures have been used also in fully edentulous patients). As far as horizontal GBR is concerned, resorbable membranes and alloplastic grafting materials may make it possible to obtain satisfactory results, while for vertical GBR the recourse to autologous bone (alone or mixed with alloplastic materials) and non-resorbable rigid membranes (such as titanium-reinforced PTFE membranes or titanium meshes) is indicated. When the initial situation is favourable, the defect is limited, and the implants can be inserted with a prosthetic-driven approach achieving adequate primary stability; implant placement can be performed in conjunction with the reconstructive procedure. If the initial situation does not allow immediate placement, implant insertion is performed months after the reconstructive procedure. The following prosthetic procedures follow the same protocol described for implants placed in native, non-reconstructed bone.

More precisely, the technique requires the elevation of a full-thickness flap and the exposure of the edentulous alveolar ridge; possible connective or periosteum remnants must be carefully eliminated from the recipient bed to avoid the interposition of soft tissues between the grafting material and the residual crest. The access flap should be wider than the defect, to allow adequate intraoperative visibility and simplify the reconstructive phase. The defect is filled with the chosen grafting material, which is then covered with the appropriate membrane to obtain adequate stabilisation. The membrane can be either simply laid onto the graft, in cases of small horizontal defects such as dehiscences and fenestrations, or fixed in place with pins and osteosynthesis screws, particularly in the case of vertical and tridimensional defects. Care must be taken in the choice of the membrane and fixation means to assure an adequate management of mechanical stress, in order to avoid any movement that could jeopardise bone regeneration and lead to soft tissue formation. Once the reconstructive phase is completed, periosteal releasing incisions are made to allow a tension-free, watertight suture of the access flap. The patients should not be allowed to wear any type of removable prostheses in the area due to the risk of soft tissues dehiscence and grafting material dislocation with subsequent failure of the reconstructive procedure.

Onlay bone grafts

Reconstruction by means of onlay grafts is the most documented technique to correct bone defects, both in terms of number of patients treated and follow-up.

Autogenous bone blocks harvested from intraoral or extraoral sites can be used, as well as homologous bone blocks and heterologous bone blocks. However, it is worth noting that autologous bone still represents the benchmark for the evaluation of other materials in terms of clinical results.

Onlay grafts share the same indications (treatment of horizontal, vertical, and tridimensional defects) of GBR techniques. However, while the recourse to these latter is generally used for the correction of relatively small defects, ample scientific documentation is available in the literature regarding the reconstruction of large (full-arch) defects and extreme bone atrophy with autologous onlay bone grafts.

The elevation of the access flap and preparation of the recipient site follow the same principles described for GBR techniques. The bone blocks are then modelled to obtain adequate adaptation to the residual alveolar ridge and stabilised by rigid fixation with titanium microscrews. The absence of empty spaces between the graft and the recipient bed is essential for avoiding connective tissue ingrowth that would jeopardise the integration process: particulated bone can be used to fill possible gaps. The closure of the access flap follows the same principles described for GBR techniques.

It is worth noting that, while immediate implant placement in conjunction with the reconstructive procedure may be possible when GBR techniques are used, delayed implant placement is mandatory when bone defects are reconstructed by means of onlay bone grafts. Graft integration can be obtained in 3-4 months when iliac bone is used, in 4 to 5 months when cortical bone harvested from intraoral sites is used, and in 5-6 months when calvarial bone is used. When homologous bone blocks are used, integration of the grafts may take up to 6-9 months to complete. Moreover, it is worth remembering that a bone block loses its vitality once harvested: when fixed to the recipient site, its integration depends on revascularisation supported by the formation of new capillaries from the endosteum of the residual crest and from the periosteum of the overlying soft tissues. The graft undergoes remodelling until the reconstructed volume is substituted by vital, newly formed bone (📷 13.27a-r).

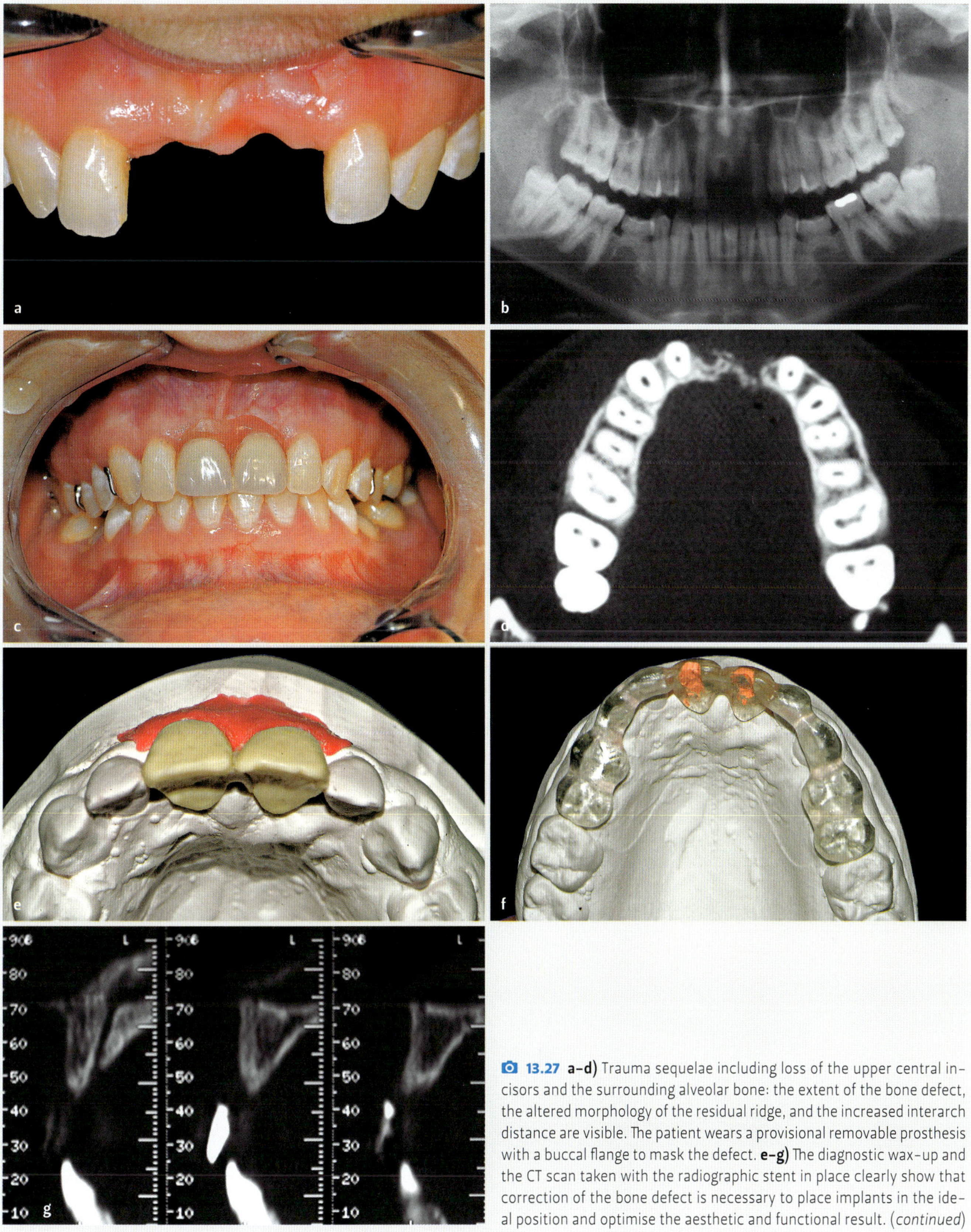

13.27 a–d) Trauma sequelae including loss of the upper central incisors and the surrounding alveolar bone: the extent of the bone defect, the altered morphology of the residual ridge, and the increased interarch distance are visible. The patient wears a provisional removable prosthesis with a buccal flange to mask the defect. **e–g)** The diagnostic wax-up and the CT scan taken with the radiographic stent in place clearly show that correction of the bone defect is necessary to place implants in the ideal position and optimise the aesthetic and functional result. (*continued*)

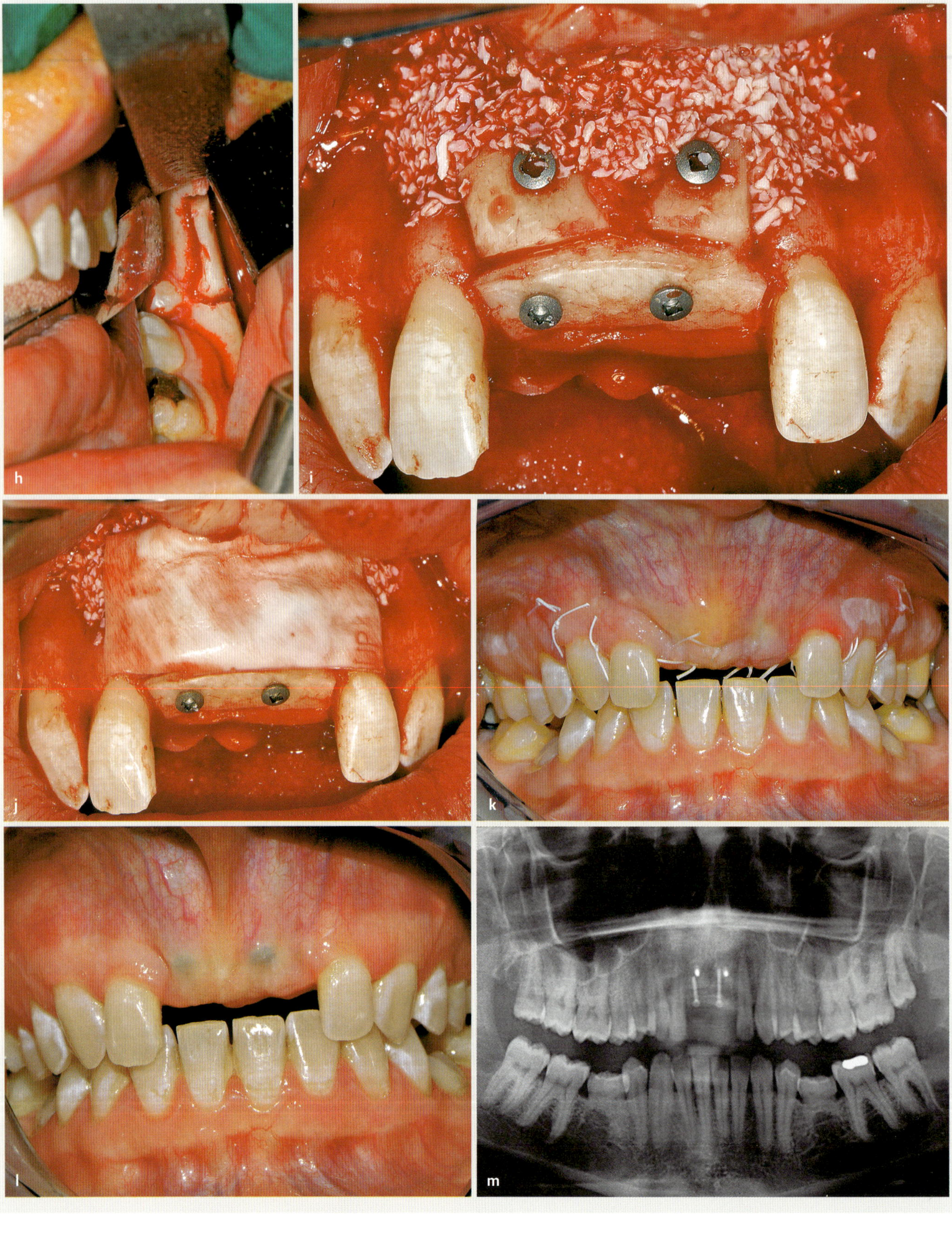
h
i
j
k
l
m

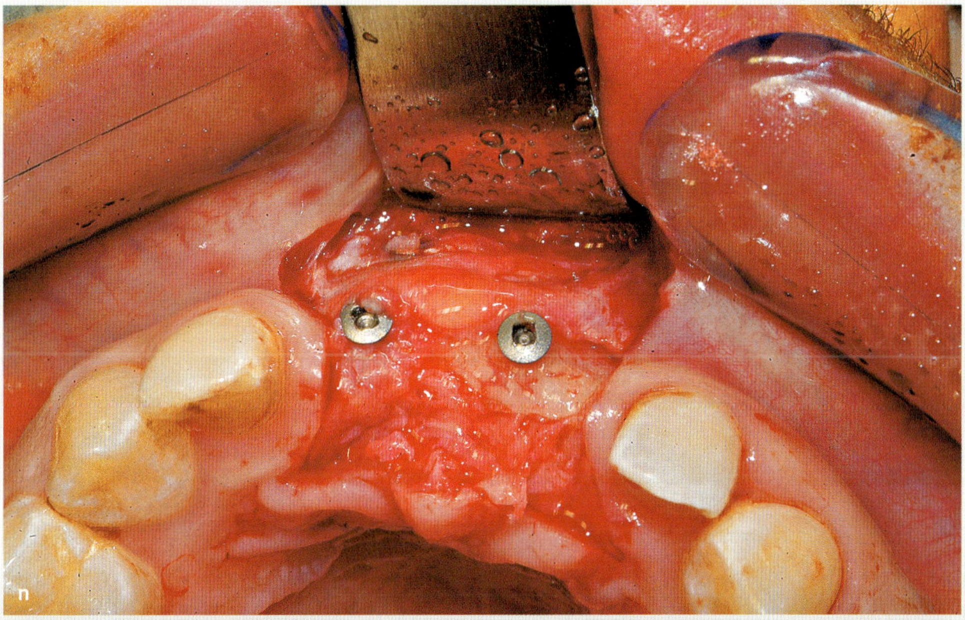

13.27 (*continued*) **h–k)** Reconstruction of the anterior maxilla with autologous onlay bone grafts harvested from the mandibular ramus, in association with particulated biomaterials and resorbable collagen membranes. **l–m)** Clinical and radiographic follow-up 4 months after the surgical procedure. **n)** A four-corner access flap is elevated and the reconstructed ridge is exposed. **o)** The radiographic/surgical stent is used to guide the correct positioning of the implants. **p)** Radiographic follow-up after implant placement. **q)** Final prosthetic restoration: a correct functional and aesthetic integration is obtained. **r)** Radiographic follow-up 6 months after prosthetic loading.

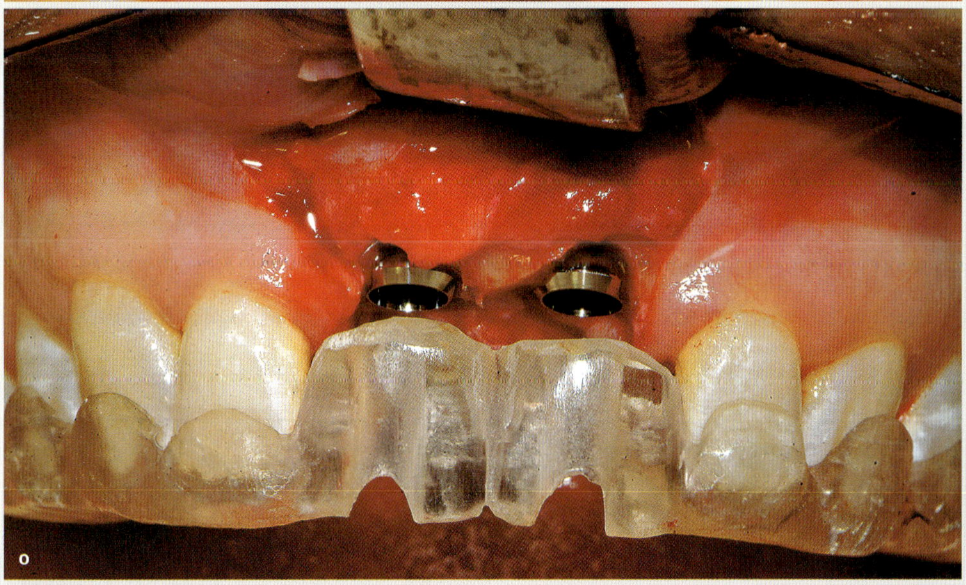

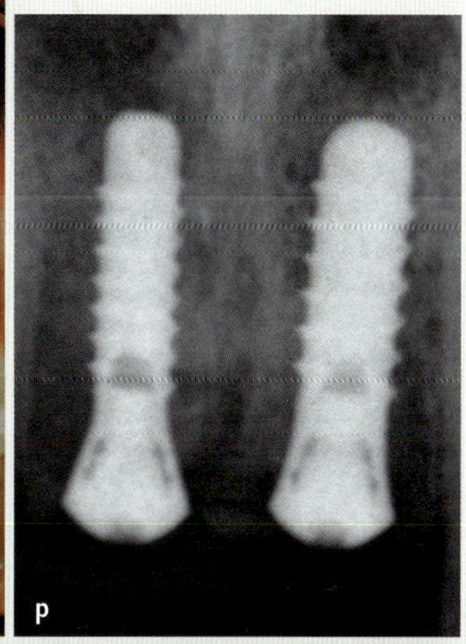

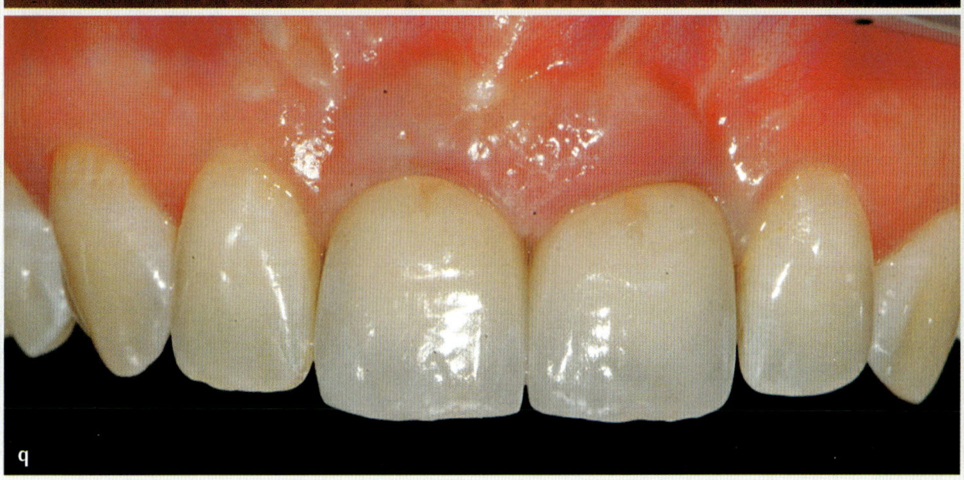

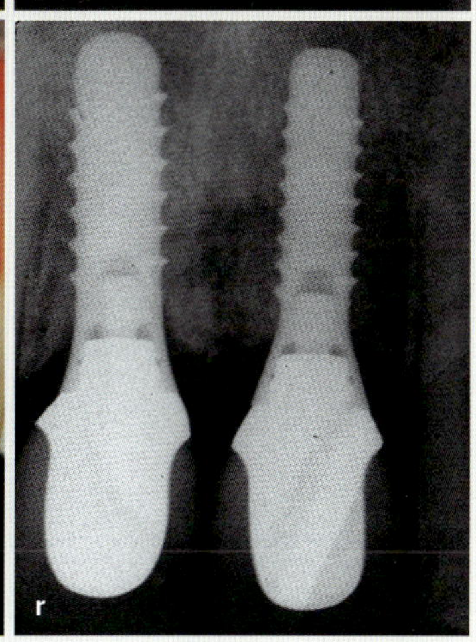

Inlay bone grafts

Reconstruction of bone defects by means of inlay grafts is rarely used due to its limited indications.

In summary, an osteotomy is made to separate the atrophic area of the alveolar crest from the basal bone, and to allow its repositioning: bone blocks are then used to fill the gap that is created between the basal bone and the osteotomised segment.

It is worth noting that there are some significant differences between the surgical technique used to perform inlay grafts and the technique used to perform onlay grafts and GBR procedures. With inlay grafts, the crestal incision must not be made on top of the alveolar ridge but rather along its base, on the buccal side; this fundamental precaution safeguards the vascularisation and, thus, the vitality of the mobilised segment. Failure to respect this principle may lead to necrosis of the mobilised segment and its total resorption.

Once the flap is elevated, three full-thickness osteotomies are made to separate the segment, which is then repositioned according to the preoperative plan. Generally, vertical increments are performed, but if complete maxillary osteotomy (Le Fort I osteotomy) is performed, it is also possible to modify the anterior-posterior position of the entire maxilla to correct sagittal intermaxillary discrepancies.

Bone blocks are positioned to fill the space created between the basal bone and the mobilised segment, and rigid fixation is achieved with the use of titanium microscrews or, if necessary, with titanium microplates and screws. Periosteal releasing incisions are made to allow a tension-free closure of the access flap; implant placement can be performed 4 to 6 months after the reconstructive procedure, to allow integration of the grafts.

Sinus floor elevation

Maxillary sinus expansion (pneumatisation), which normally occurs in the course of adult life, can be accelerated by the loss of teeth in the lateral-posterior areas of the maxilla, and cause a vertical bone loss incompatible with the placement of implants of adequate length (> 7-8 mm.)

To correct this condition, several techniques have been developed since the end of the 1970s associating the elevation of the Schneiderian membrane from the floor of the maxillary sinus (the so-called *sinus lifting procedure*) with the placement of different grafting materials in the space created under the membrane, to obtain adequate bone volume for the placement of endosseous implants.

Sinus floor elevation can be performed with two different approaches: the crestal approach and the lateral approach.

SINUS FLOOR ELEVATION WITH TRANS-CRESTAL APPROACH

Trans-crestal sinus floor elevation, which is generally associated with immediate implant placement, may be performed in situations where it is possible to obtain adequate primary implant stability: this is generally the case when bone quality is acceptable and at least 3-4 millimetres of residual bone are present.

Although many variants based on specifically designed devices have been proposed over the years, the basic technique involves the preparation of the implant site keeping a safety distance of 1 millimetre from the floor of the maxillary sinus. Once the standard drilling sequence is completed, specifically designed osteotomes are used to fracture the thin sinusal floor; then, the overlying Schneiderian membrane is gradually elevated by gently pushing the grafting material (alloplastic materials or xenografts are generally used) inside the implant bed with the aid of an osteotome. However, elevation of the sinus membrane should not exceed 4-5 millimetres to limit the risk of laceration and subsequent penetration of the implant apex and grafting material inside the sinus lumen, which may lead to local infection (sinusitis). Untreated sinusitis may cause the loss of the implant, or even extend to other paranasal cavities causing severe pansinusitis.

SINUS FLOOR ELEVATION WITH LATERAL APPROACH

The lateral approach consists in the creation of a bony window on the lateral wall of the maxillary sinus by means of rotary (round bur mounted on a straight surgical handpiece) or piezoelectric instruments. The Schneiderian membrane is then gently detached from the floor of the sinus with specifically designed elevators and folded upwards to allow the filling of the lower portion of the sinus with the grafting material.

Unlike the trans-crestal approach, this technique can be used even for severe vertical bone resorption (< 1 mm of residual bone), does not present limitations to the extent of the lifting, provides better control of the surgical field, and allows identification and repair of possible perforations of the sinus membrane. Implants can be placed in conjunction with this procedure if the quantity and quality of the residual bone can guarantee adequate primary implant stability; otherwise, the recourse to delayed implant placement is indicated to obtain complete integration of the grafted material (6-9 months). In fact, data reported in the literature demonstrates that immediate implant placement in the absence of favourable conditions providing adequate primary implant stability leads to lower implant survival rates (13.28a-k).

When vertical bone defects in the lateral-posterior areas of the maxilla are not caused solely by sinus pneumatisation but also by vertical resorption of the alveolar ridge, the association of onlay bone grafts (or GBR procedures) and sinus floor elevation techniques is indicated to correct both the defect and the alterations of interarch relationships (13.29a-n).

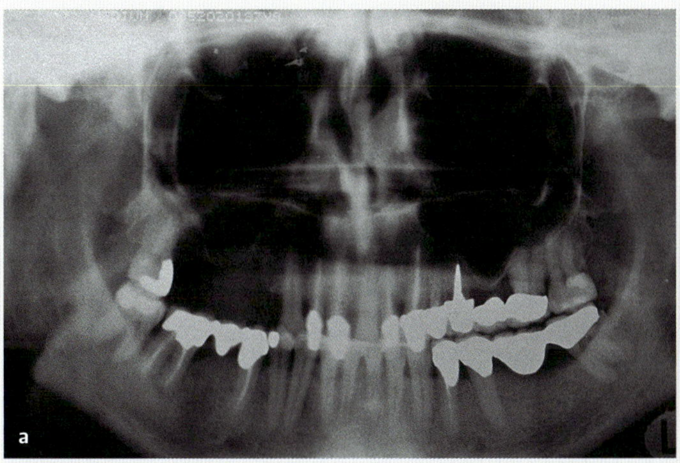

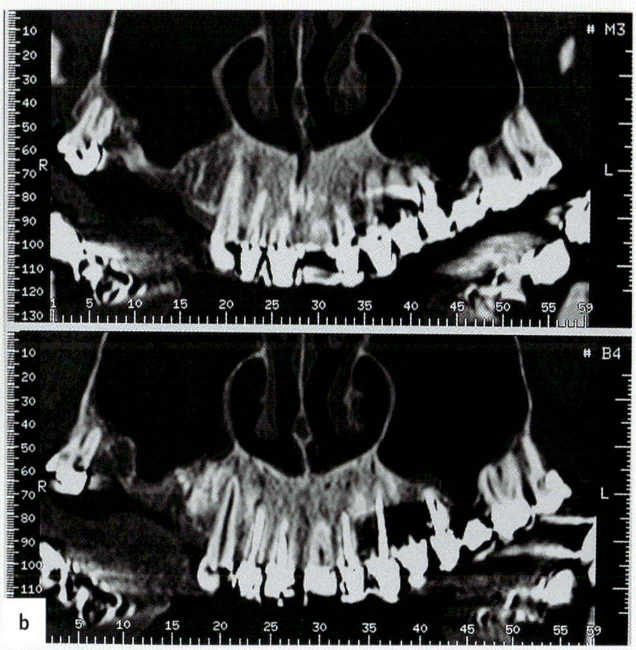

13.28 a-b) Preoperative panoramic radiograph and CT scan: partial edentulism in the lateral-posterior area of the maxilla is associated with maxillary sinus pneumatisation. (*continued*)

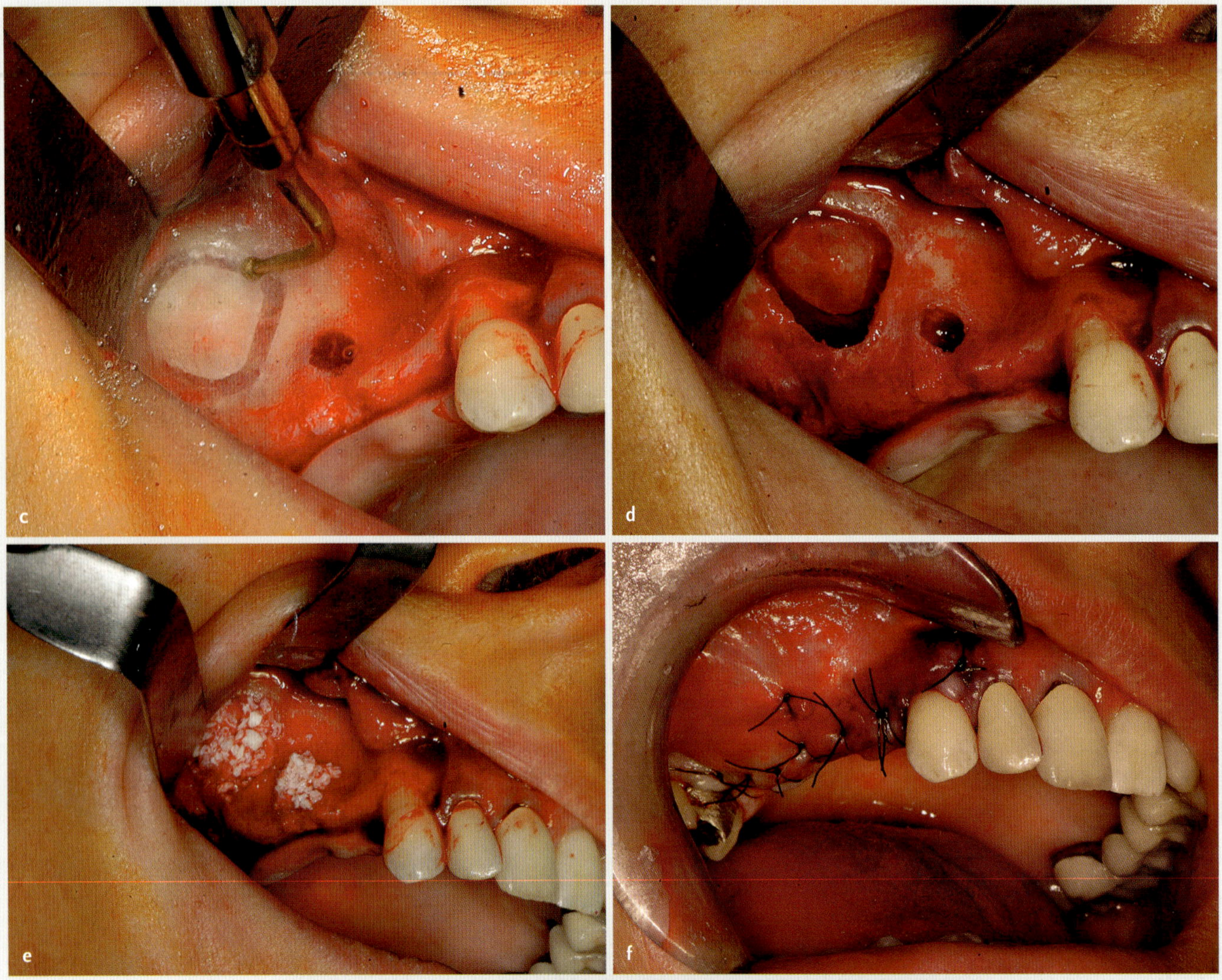

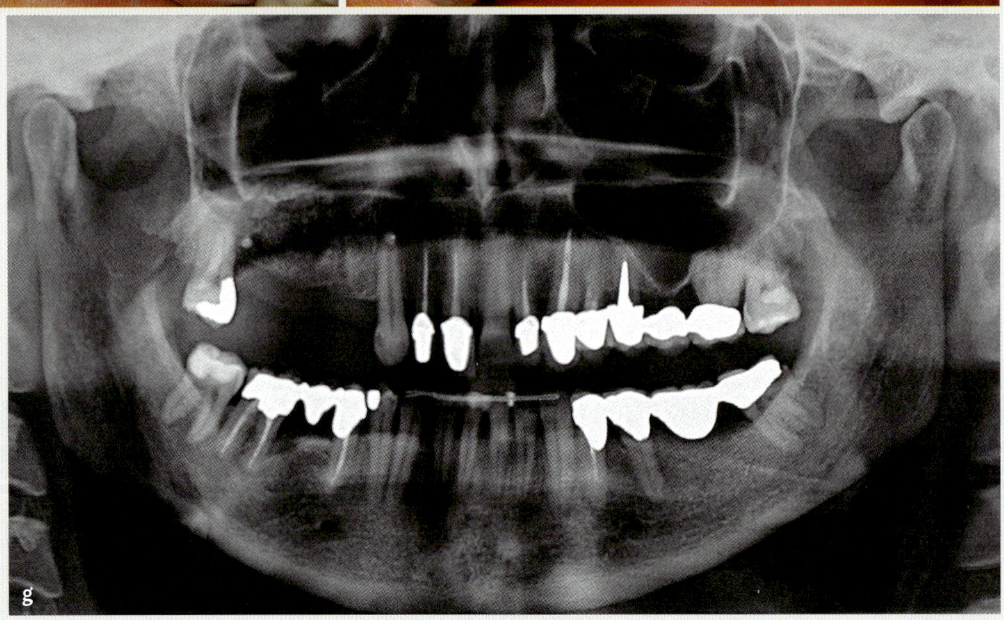

13.28 (*continued*) **c)** After elevation of the access flap, a window is created in the lateral wall of the maxillary sinus. **d)** The Schneiderian membrane is detached from the floor of the sinus and folded upwards. **e)** The space between the sinus floor and the lifted membrane is filled with alloplastic material (bovine bone mineral). **f)** Suture. **g)** Radiographic follow-up after sinus floor elevation and grafting is completed. (*continued*)

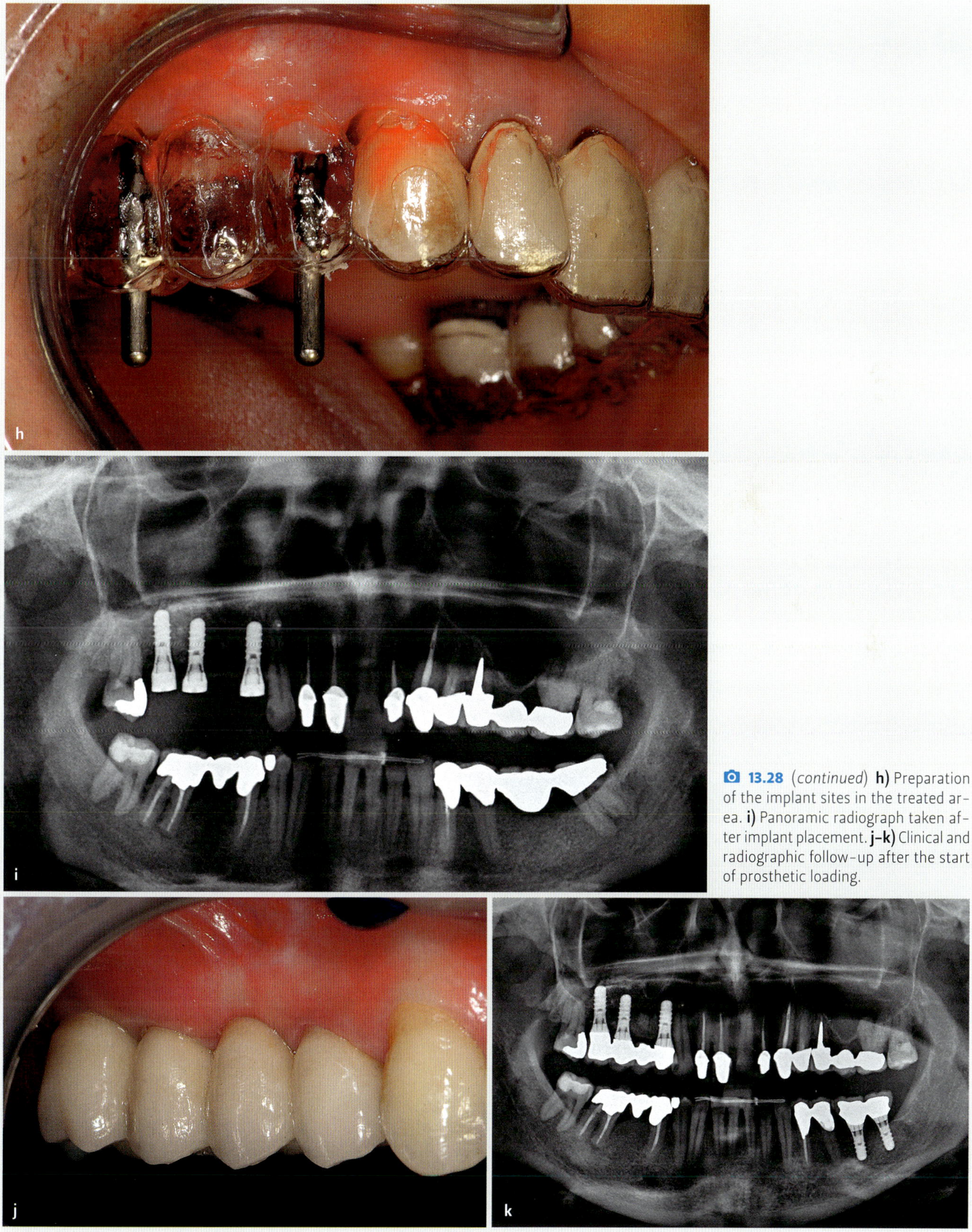

13.28 (*continued*) **h)** Preparation of the implant sites in the treated area. **i)** Panoramic radiograph taken after implant placement. **j–k)** Clinical and radiographic follow-up after the start of prosthetic loading.

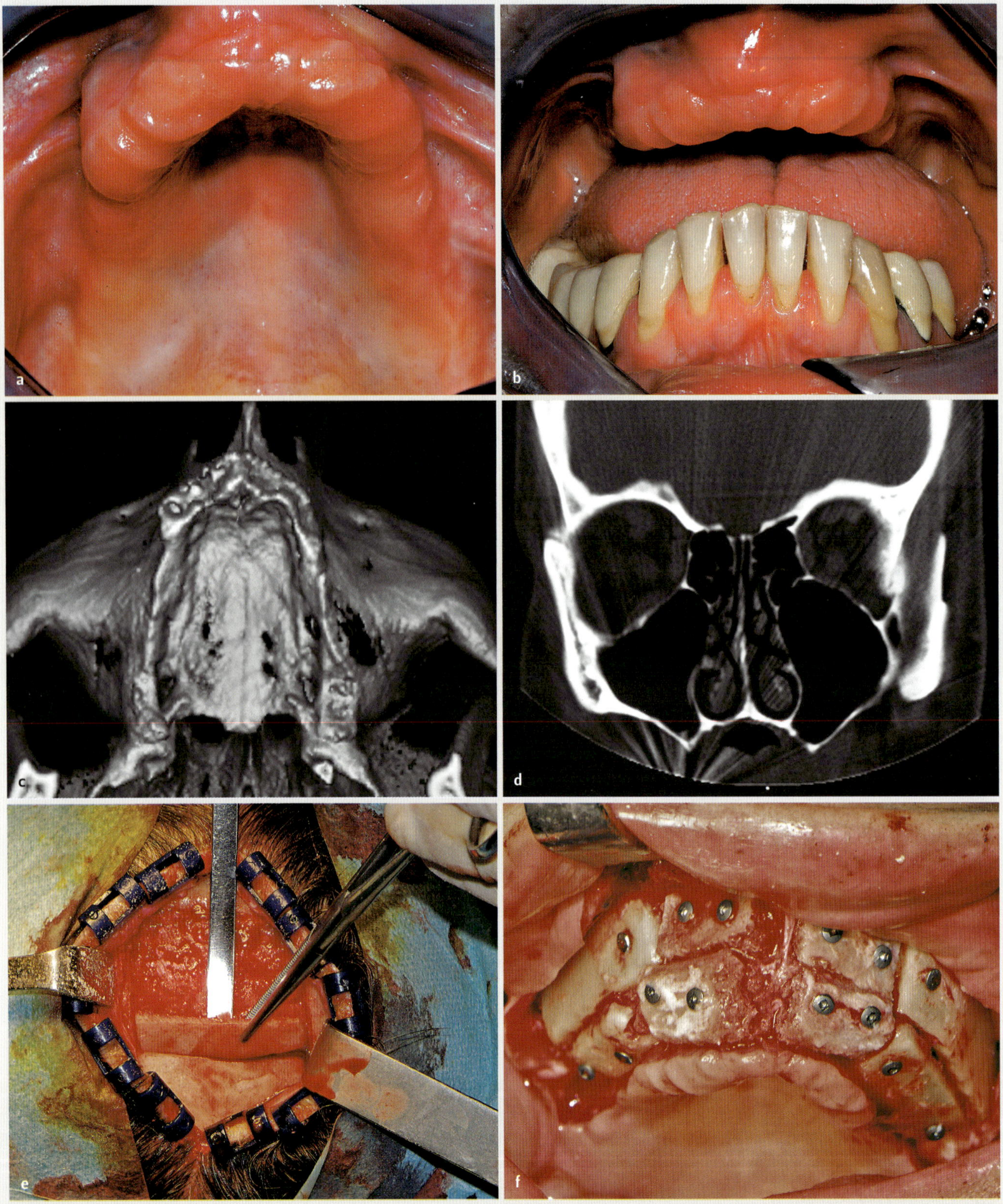

13.29 **a–d)** Preoperative clinical and radiographic situation: severe tridimensional atrophy of the maxilla with significant bilateral sinus pneumatisation preventing implant rehabilitation. **e–f)** Tridimensional reconstruction of the atrophic maxilla with autologous bone grafts harvested from the calvarium in association with bilateral sinus floor elevation. (*continued*)

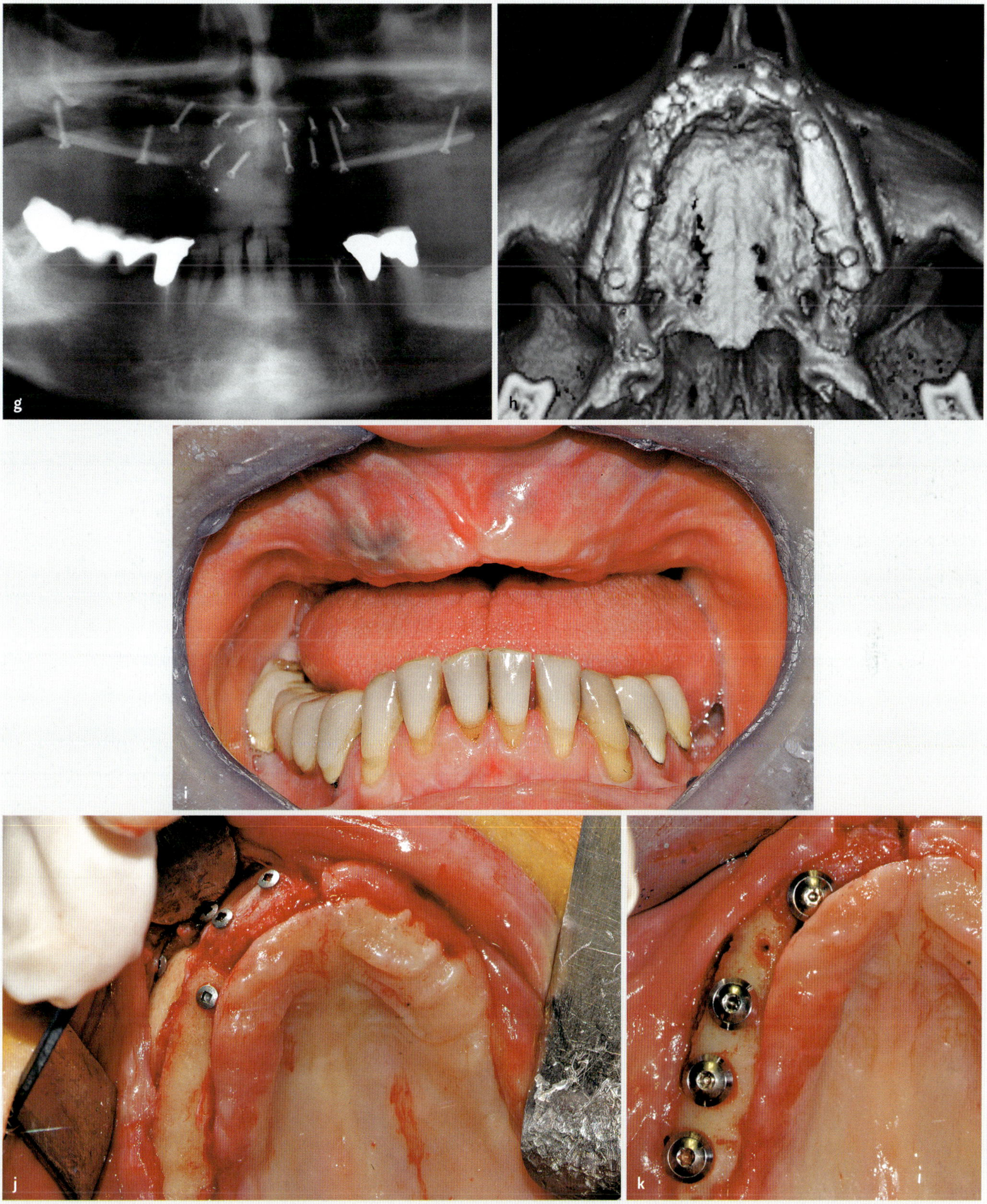

13.29 (*continued*) **g–i)** Radiographic and clinical follow-up months after the reconstructive procedure. **j–k)** After flap elevation, complete integration of the graft is observed and implants are placed according to the preoperative plan. (*continued*)

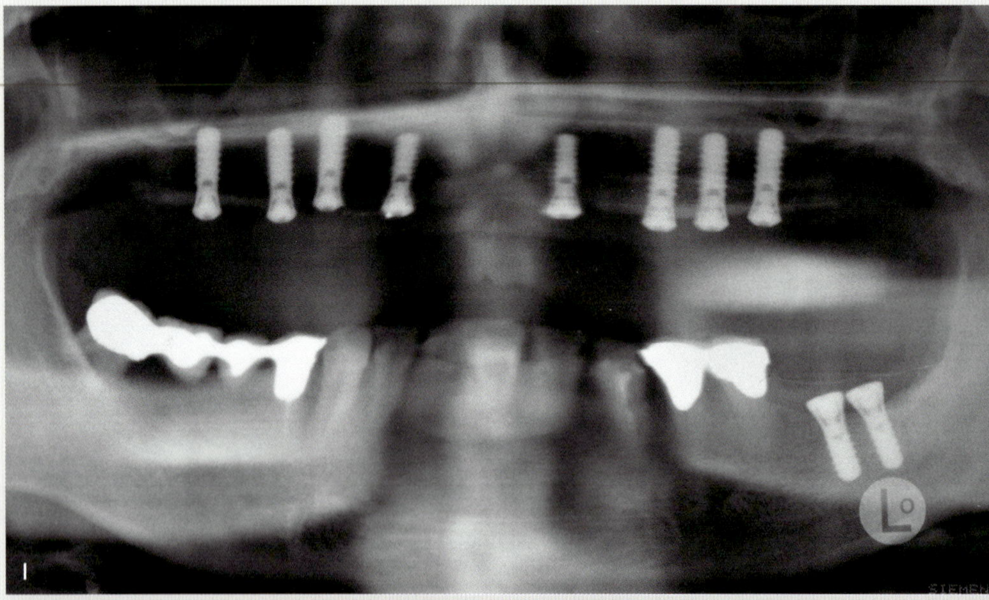

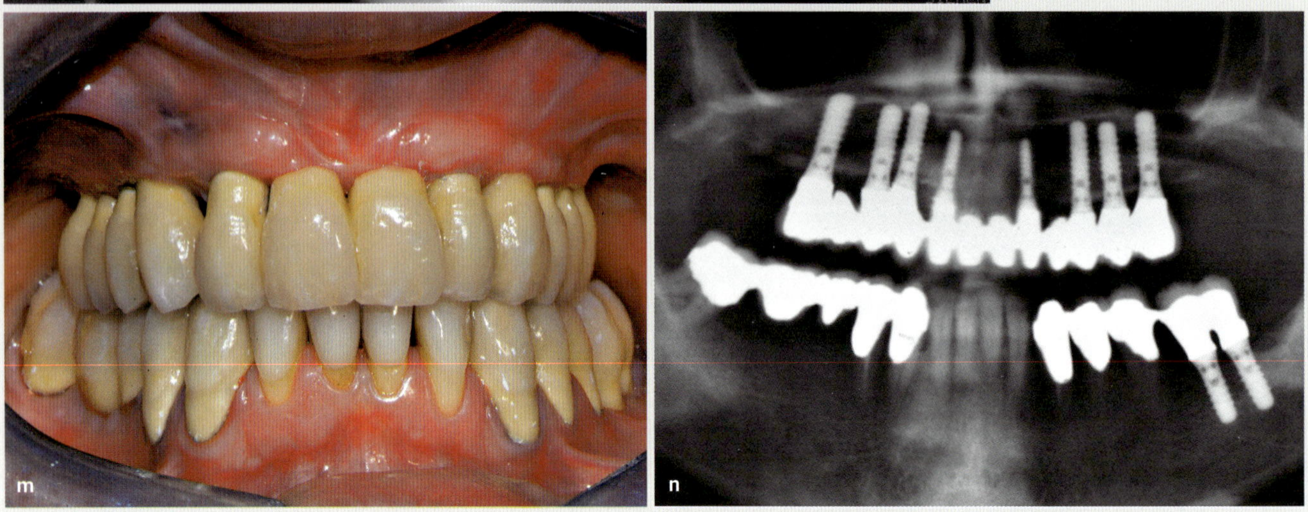

13.29 (*continued*) **l)** Radiographic follow-up after implant placement. **m–n)** Clinical and radiographic follow-up after c ompletion of the definitive implant-supported prosthetic rehabilitation.

Distraction osteogenesis

This technique, originally invented to correct the defects of long bones (femur, tibia, fibula, humerus, radius, ulna) in patients presenting congenital anomalies such as dwarfism, was then applied to the treatment of severe congenital defects of the cranio-maxillofacial complex associated with underdevelopment (craniosynostosis, first and second branchial arch syndromes, etc.), and was finally introduced in the field of oral surgery for the treatment of deficient edentulous ridges. The basic principle behind the process of distraction osteogenesis is that new bone formation will occur between two osteotomised bone segments when they are slowly and gradually separated (0.5-1 mm per day) by means of a specifically designed device (distractor).

The access flap and osteotomies are the same described for inlay grafts (see previous section for details); a distractor is then fixed to the osteotomised block and to the basal bone. When the access flap is sutured, care is taken to allow the activation screw of the distractor to protrude from the soft tissue. One week after surgery, the device is activated by rotating the activation screw to obtain a 0.5-1 millimetre distraction per day. The osteotomised segment follows the distraction vector, and new osteoid matrix forms in the gap created by the distraction that will develop into mature bone. Once the distraction phase is completed, a 4-month consolidation phase is allowed before the removal of the distractor and implant placement in the regenerated bone are performed.

However, it is worth noting that the remarkable results obtained in orthopaedics, as well as in maxillofacial surgery, cannot be entirely replicated in the field of oral surgery for numerous reasons such as limited indications, potential intraoperative (mandibular fracture) and postoperative complications (change of distraction vector, incomplete bone formation, scar formation), patient discomfort, etc. Therefore, the use of distraction osteogenesis to correct bone defects of the jaws has been limited, as is also apparent from the paucity of data reported in the literature.

Ridge expansion

This technique was introduced as an alternative to onlay grafts and GBR techniques to correct horizontal defects of the alveolar ridges.

In summary, the procedure consists of the separation of the buccal cortical plate from the lingual/palatal cortical plate by means of three osteotomies performed with rotary or piezoelectric instruments; the buccal cortical plate is then opened buccally with the aid of specifically designed devices, and a greenstick fracture leads to an increase in the width of the edentulous crest.

The access flap is peculiar: full-thickness elevation is performed on the lingual/palatal side, while a split-thickness elevation is performed on the buccal side to preserve the periosteal blood supply and avoid necrosis of the buccal cortical plate once it is fractured.

Once the crestal osteotomy and the mesial and distal releasing osteotomies are completed, progressive expansion of the crest is obtained in a few minutes with the aid of osteotomes, chisels, or wedges. The procedure is generally performed in conjunction with immediate implant placement, as the implants can act as expanders themselves. The gaps between the two cortical plates and between the implants can be left to heal by secondary intention (new bone formation occurs), or they can be filled with collagen sponges or biomaterials. A tension-free suture of the access flap concludes the procedure.

This technique presents precise indications and some limitations:

- it can be used only when the two cortical plates are separated by a layer of cancellous bone; fusion of the two cortical plates, which is typical for extremely narrow ridges, does not make it possible to find a cleavage plane and exposes to a high risk of fracturing the alveolar ridge;
- as the crestal expansion is greater at the coronal margin of the residual crest, while being negligible at the apical margin, a change occurs in the orientation of the edentulous crest which will be inclined buccally, thus determining a modification of the implant axis (the prosthetic implications of this factor must be carefully considered);
- only a limited amount of width-gain is possible due to the risk of complete fracture and subsequent necrosis of the buccal plate (associated with the loss of the implants placed) if excessive expansion is performed.

Revascularised free flaps

The technique consists in the harvesting of a bone segment (from the iliac crest or fibula), together with its vascular pedicle, which is then anastomosed with blood vessels of the neck (typically the facial artery and vein, but also lingual or superior thyroid vessels). Therefore, contrary to what happens when onlay bone blocks are used, the transplanted bone segment can immediately receive adequate blood supply and remain vital. The free flap may also include skin, subcutaneous tissues, and muscle that can be used to correct severe soft tissue defects.

The main advantage of free flaps is represented by the possibility of maintaining bone vitality even when the recipient site is unfavourable (severely atrophic, scarred, or irradiated areas). However, these procedures are very complex, present a relevant morbidity, and must be performed by maxillofacial surgeons specialised in reconstructive and microvascular surgery. Therefore, their use to correct bone defects of the jaws for preimplant purposes is limited to severely compromised situations, typically caused by tumour resection.

REFERENCES

Ahmad N, Saad N. Effects of antibiotics on dental implants: a review. *J Clin Med Res* 2012; 4(1):1-6.

Albrektsson T, Zarb G, Worthington P, Eriksson AR. The long-term efficacy of currently used dental implants: a review and proposed criteria of success. *Int J Oral Maxillofac Implants* 1986; 1:1-25.

Al-Nsour MM, Chan HL, Wang HL. Effect of the platform-switching technique on preservation of peri-implant marginal bone: a systematic review. *Int J Oral Maxillofac Implants* 2012; 27(1):138-45.

Annibali S, Cristalli MP, Dell'Aquila D, Bignozzi I, La Monaca G, Pilloni A. Short dental implants: a systematic review. *J Dent Res* 2012; 91(1):25-32.

Arvidson K, Bystedt H, Frykolm A, Won Konov L, Lothigius E. Five-year prospective follow-up report of Astra Tech Implant System in the treatment of edentulous mandible. *Clin Oral Impl Res* 1998; 9:225-34.

Atieh MA, Ibrahim HM, Atieh AH. Platform switching for marginal bone preservation around dental implants: a systematic review and meta-analysis. *J Periodontol* 2010; 81(10):1350-66.

Bianchi A, Sanfilippo F, Zaffe D. Implantologia e Implantoprotesi. Basi biologiche, Biomeccanica, Applicazioni Cliniche. Utet, Torino, 1999; pp. 150-3.

Brånemark PI, Adell R, Breine U, Hansson BO, Ohlsson A. Intra-osseous anchorage of dental prostheses. I. Experimental studies. *Scand Plastic Reconstructive Surg* 1969; 3:81-100.

Brånemark PI, Hansson BO, Adell R, Breine U, Lindström J, Hallen O, Öhman A. Osseointegrated implants in the treatment of the edentulus jaw: experience from a 10-year period. *Scand Plastic Reconstructive Surg* 1977; 16:1-132.

Brocard D, Barthet P, Baysse E, Duffort JF, Eller P, Justumus P, Marin P, Oscaby F, Simonet T, Benque E, Brunel G. A multicenter report on 1022 consecutively placed ITI implants: a 7-year longitudinal study. *Int Oral Maxillofac Implants* 2000 Sept-Oct; 15(5):691-700.

Buser D, Mericske-Stern R, Bernard JP, Behneke A, Behneke N, Hirt HP, Belser UC, Lang NP. Long-term evaluation of non-submerged ITI implants: 8-year life-table analysis of a prospective multi-center study with 2359 implants. *Clin Oral Impl Res* 1997; 8(3):161-72.

Buser D. Effects of various titanium surface configurations on osseointegration and clinical implant stability. In: Lang NP, Karring T, Linde J (eds). Implant Dentistry. Proceedings of the 3rd European Workshop on Periodontology. Quintessence, Berlin 1999; pp. 88-101.

Chen ST, Buser D. Clinical and *estetic outcome* of implants placed in postextraction sites. *Int J Oral Maxillofac Implants*, 2009; 24(suppl):186-217.

Chiapasco M, Romeo E. La riabilitazione implantoprotesica nei casi complessi. Utet, Torino 2003.

Chiapasco M, Lang NP, Bosshardt DD. Quality and quantity of bone following alveolar distraction osteogenesis in the human mandible. *Clin Oral Implants Res* 2006; 17(4):394-402.

Chiapasco M, Casentini P, Zaniboni M, Corsi E, Anello T. Titanium-zirconium alloy narrow-diameter implants (Straumann Roxolid(®)) for the rehabilitation of horizontally deficient edentulous ridges: prospective study on 18 consecutive patients. *Clin Oral Implants Res* 2012; 23(10):1136-41.

Chin M, Toth BA. Distraction osteogenesis in maxillo-facial surgery using internal devices: review of 5 cases. *J Oral Maxillofac Surg* 1996; 54(1):45-53.

Cochran DL, Buser D, Ten Bruggenkate C. The use of reduced healing times on ITI, implants with a sandblasted and acid-etched surface (SLA): early resuts from clinical trials on ITI, SLA implants. *Clin Oral Impl Res* 2002; 13:144-53.

Dominguez Campelo L, Dominguez Camara JR. Flapless implant surgery: a 10-year clinical retrospective analysis. *Int J Oral Maxillofac Implants* 2002; 17:271-6.

Ericsson I, Persson LG, Berglundh T, Marinello CP, Lindhe J, Klinge B. Different types of inflammatory reactions in peri-implant soft tissues. *J Clin Periodont* 1995; 22:255-61.

Ericsson I, Nilner K, Klinge B, Glantz PO. Radiographical and histological characteristics of submerged and non-submerged titanium implants. *Clin Oral Impl Res* 1996; 7:20-6.

Eriksson RA, Albrektsson T. Temperature Threshold levels for heat-induced bone tissue injury: a vital microscopic study in the rabbit. *J Prosthet Dent* 1983; 50:101.

Eriksson RA, Adell R. Temperatures during drilling for the placement of implants using the osseointegration technique. *J Oral Maxillofac Surg* 1986; 44:4-7.

Esposito M, Hirsch JM, Lekholm U, Thomsen P. Biological factors contributing to failures of osseointegrated oral implants. I. Success criteria and epidemiology. *Eur J Oral Sci* 1998a; 106(1):527-51.

Esposito M, Hirsch JM, Lekholm U, Thomsen P. Biological factors contributing to failures of osseointegrated oral implants. II. Success criteria and epidemiology. *Eur J Oral Sci* 1998b; 106(3):721-64.

Esposito M, Coulthard P, Oliver R, Thomsen P, Worthington HV. Antibiotics to prevent complications following dental implant treatment (Cochrane Rewiew). *Cochrane Database Syst Rev* 2003; (3):CD004152.

Esposito M, Coulthard P, Thomsen P, Worthington HV. The role of implant surface modifications, shape and material on the success of osseointegrated dental implants. A Cochrane systematic review. *Eur J Prosthodont Restor Dent* 2005; 13(1):15-31.

Esposito M, Grusovin MG, Coulthard P, Thomsen P, Worthington HV. A 5-year follow-up comparative analysis of the efficacy of various osseointegrated dental implant systems: a systematic review of randomized controlled clinical trials. *Int J Oral Maxillofac Implants* 2005; 20(4):557-68.

Esposito M, Grusovin MG, Willings M, Coulthard P, Worthington HV. The effectiveness of immediate, early, and conventional loading of dental implants: a Cochrane systematic review of randomized controlled clinical trials. *Int J Oral Maxillofac Implants* 2007; 22(6):893-904.

Esposito M, Grusovin MG, Chew YS, Coulthard P, Worthington HV. One-stage versus two-stage implant placement. A Cochrane systematic review of randomised controlled clinical trials. *Eur J Oral Implantol* 2009; 2(2):91-9.

Esposito M, Grusovin MG, Polyzos IP, Felice P, Worthington HV. Timing of implant placement after tooth extraction: immediate, immediate-delayed or delayed implants? A Cochrane systematic review. *Eur J Oral Implantol* 2010 Autumn; 3(3):189-205.

Esposito M, Maghaireh H, Grusovin MG, Ziounas I, Worthington HV. Soft tissue management for dental implants: what are the most effective techniques? A Cochrane systematic review. *Eur J Oral Implantol* 2012; 5(3): 221-238.

Garber DA, Belser UC. Restoration: driven implant placement with restoration-generated site development. *Compend Contin Educ Dent* 1995; 16:796-804.

Garber DA, Salama MA, Salama H. Immediate total tooth replacement. *Compend Contin Educ Dent* 2001; 22:210-18.

Gatti C, Chiapasco M, Casentini P, Procopio C. Manuale illustrato di implantologia orale: diagnosi, chirurgia e protesi. Elsevier, Milano 2007.

Gatti C, Chiapasco M, Casentini P, Procopio C. Manuale illustrato di implantologia orale. Diagnosi, chirurgia e protesi. Elsevier Masson, Milano 2009.

Ivanoff CJ, Widmark G, Hallgren C, Sennerby L, Wennerberg A. Histologic evaluation of the bone integration of TiO2 blasted and turned titanium microimplants in humans. *Clin Oral Impl Res* 2001; 12:128-34.

Jaffin O, Berman O. The excessive loss of Brånemark fixtures in type IV bone: a 5-year analysis. *J Periodontol* 1991; 62:2-4.

Jung RE, Schneider D, Ganeles J, Wismeijer D, Zwahlen M, Hämmerle CH, Tahmaseb A. Computer technology applications in surgical implant dentistry: a systematic review. *Int J Oral Maxillofac Implants* 2009; 24(Suppl):92-109.

Kalpidis CD, Setayesh RM. Hemorrhaging associated with endosseous implant placement in the anterior mandible: a review of the literature. *J Periodontol* 2004; 75(5):631-45.

Lang NP, Karring T, Lindhe J (eds). Implant Dentistry. Proceedings of the 3rd European Workshop on Periodontology. Quintessence, Berlin 1999.

Lazzara RJ, Siddiqui A, Binon P et al. Retrospective multicenter analysis of 3 I endosseous dental implants placed over a five-year period. *Clin Oral Impl Res* 1996; 7:73-83.

Lekholm U, Zarb GA. Patient selection and preparation. In: Tissue integrated prostheses: osseointegration in clinical dentistry. Quintessence, Chicago 1985; pp. 199-209.

Pavilkovà G, Foltàn R, Horkà M, Hanzelka T, Borunskà H, Sedy J. Piezosurgery in oral and maxillofacial surgery. *Int J Oral Maxillofac Surg* 2011 May; 40(5):451-7.

Persson LG, Lekholm U, Leonhardt A, Dahlen G, Lindhe J. Bacterial colonisation of internal surfaces of Brånemark system implant components. *Clin Oral Impl Res* 1996; 7:90-5.

Pjetursson BE, Tan WC, Zwahlen M, Lang NP. A systematic review of the success of sinus floor elevation and survival of implants inserted in combination with sinus floor elevation. *J Clin. Periodontol* 2009; 35(8 suppl):216-40.

Roberts E, Garetto L, Brezniak N. Bone physiology and metabolism. In: Misch C (ed). Contemporary implant dentistry. Mosby, St Louis, 1994; pp. 327-68.

Schroeder A, Pohler OM, Sutter F. Gewebsreaktion auf ein titan-hohlzylinderimplantat mit titan-Spritzschichoberflache. *Schweiz Monatsschr Zahnheilkd* 1976; 85:713.

Schroeder A, van der Zypen E, Stich H, Sutter F. The reactions of bone, connective tissue, and epithelium to endosteal implants with titanium- sprayed surfaces. *J Maxillofac Surg* 1981; 9:15-25.

Sennerby L, Thomsen P, Ericson LE. Early Bone tissue response to titanium implants inserted in rabit cortical bone. I. Light Microscopic Observations. *J Mater Sci Mater Med* 1993a; 4:240-50.

Sennerby L, Thomsen P, Ericson LE. Early Bone tissue response to titanium implants inserted in rabit cortical bone. II. Ultrastructural Observations. *J Mater Sci Mater Med* 1993b; 4:494-502.

Sennerby L, Roos J. Surgical determinants of clinical success of osseointegrated oral implants: a review of the literature. *Int J Prosthodont* 1998; 11(5):408-20.

Smith D, Zarb G. Criteria for success of osseointegrated endosseous implants. *J Prosthet Dent* 1989; 61:567-72.

Sohrabi K, Mushantat A, Esfandiari S, Feine J. How successful are small-diameter implants? A literature review. *Clin Oral Implants Res* 2012; 23(5):515-25.

Tarnow DP, Cho SC, Wallace SS. The effect of inter-implant distance on the height of inter-implant bone crest. *J Periodontol* 2000; 71:546-9.

Wennstrom JL, Palmer RM. Consensus of session C. In: Lang NP, Karring T, Linde J (eds). Implant Dentistry. Proceedings of the 3rd European Workshop on Periodontology. Quintessence, 1999; pp. 255-9.

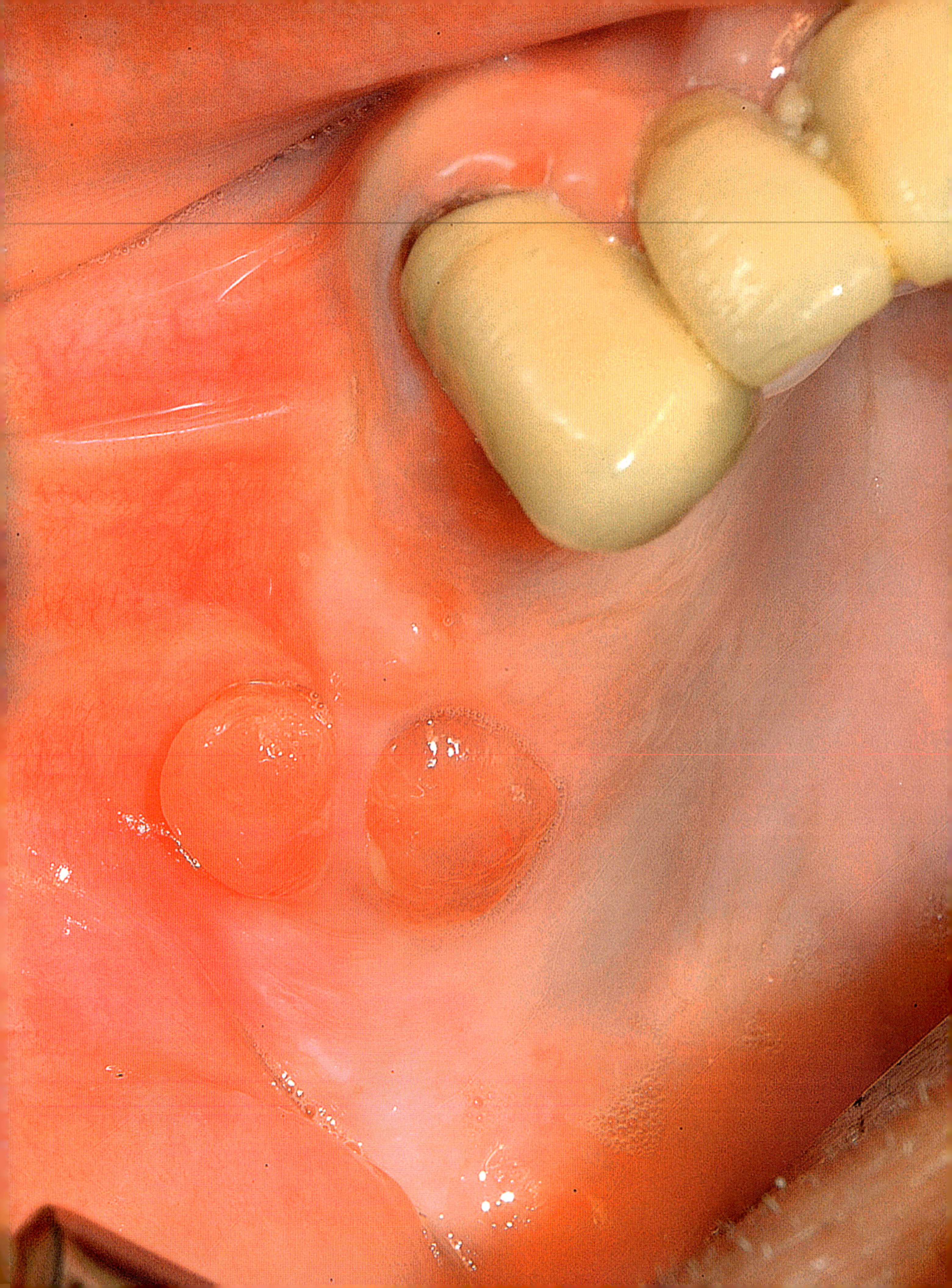

The most common complications in oral surgery: prevention and management

M. Chiapasco ▪ M. Zaniboni

Introduction

Any surgical intervention, even when performed by experienced operators, exposes the patient to a series of possible intraoperative and postoperative complications.

As a general rule, a surgeon should perform only those interventions whose specific complications he or she is able to manage.

The prerequisites for a significant reduction in potential accidents may be summarised as follows:

- thorough analysis of the patient's medical history;
- adequate knowledge of the local anatomy;
- accurate preoperative planning;
- proper surgical technique and reduced trauma.

Complications can be intraoperative or postoperative.

Common complications in oral surgery

Intraoperative
- Relevant haemorrhage
- Nerve lesions
- Soft tissue lacerations
- Root fractures
- Cortical fractures
- Mandibular fractures
- Temporomandibular joint dislocation
- Tooth dislocation inside the soft tissues
- Buccal fat pad herniation
- Oroantral communications
- Migration of foreign bodies inside the maxillary sinus

Postoperative
- Delayed haemorrhage
- Wound dehiscence
- Postoperative infections (alveolar osteitis and subperiosteal abscess)
- Oroantral communications and fistulas
- Nerve lesion sequelae
- Bone sequestra

Intraoperative complications

Relevant haemorrhage

Intraoperative bleeding is inherently inevitable when a surgical procedure is performed, but it is generally limited. In fact, it is relatively rare for blood vessels with a significant diameter to be involved in oral surgery procedures; therefore, the risk of profuse bleeding and subsequent hypovolaemia is negligible. However, significant intraoperative bleeding may represent an obstacle, as it reduces visibility in the operating field, and produces psychological stress in the patient and surgeon in addition to augmenting the risk of postoperative haematoma.

Prevention

Among the first indicators to check when gathering the patient's medical history are the results of coagulation tests, which include factor V assay, fibrinogen level, prothrombin time, platelet count, thrombin time, and bleeding time. It is important to exclude the presence of congenital as well as acquired coagulopathies (e.g. caused by antiaggregant medications) and serious liver or renal diseases (see Chapter 1). If severe coagulopathies are present or suspected, the patient should be referred to the haematologist for a specialist examination, and any surgical treatment should be performed in a protected environment (hospital). For on-going antiaggregant therapy, if surgery is to be performed in a private practice environment it is important that coagulation values are brought back inside the range of normality; cooperation with the specialist (cardiologist, haematologist) or family physician is essential.

The second requisite to avoid relevant intraoperative bleeding is a thorough knowledge of the local anatomy (see Chapter 2 for details); incision of the soft tissues in safe areas and elevation of access flaps along the correct cleavage plane prevents damage to major blood vessels.

The third requisite is represented by the identification and adequate protection of major blood vessels, particularly when rotary instruments are used.

Management

The choice of the best method to halt intraoperative bleeding depends on the following factors:

- type of bleeding (venous or arterial);
- location (soft tissues, intraosseous);
- relationship of the damaged vessel with neighbouring anatomic structures such as nerves.

All available methods (compression, haemostatic materials, bipolar coagulation, and ligature) have already been described in Chapter 3 (see Haemostasis section).

As a rule, haemostasis can be obtained quickly and effectively when the origin of the bleeding is precisely located.

Nerve lesions

Nerve lesions can involve both sensory and motor fibres. In oral surgery, the vast majority of these complications are represented by damage to the sensory branches of the 5th cranial nerve, particularly the inferior alveolar nerve, lingual nerve and, less often, the major palatine, nasopalatine, and infraorbital nerve.

Nerve lesions can be subdivided into three degrees, based on the severity of the damage.

Neurapraxia: it is characterised by a transient functional interruption of electrical conduction, caused by compression or stretching of the involved nerve due to surgical manoeuvres or postoperative swelling. The integrity of the axons and nerve sheath is preserved, and complete functional recovery is usually achieved in a few days.

Axonotmesis: it is characterised by the anatomical interruption of the axons, while the integrity of the nerve sheath is preserved. The distal nerve stump undergoes degeneration, and the proximal stump undergoes degeneration up to the first node of Ranvier. Nerve regeneration is possible and proceeds from the proximal stump at a 1 millimetre per day rate, following the guide represented by the intact nerve sheath. Functional recovery can be achieved if regeneration of the interrupted fibres is complete, but the entire process may take several months.

Neurotmesis: it is characterised by the anatomical interruption of both axons and nerve sheath. Degeneration follows the same scheme described for axonotmesis, while regeneration may occur but the lack of integrity of the nerve sheath implies the loss of its function as a guide. Therefore, disorganised proliferation of the nervous tissue occurs, which leads to traumatic neuroma formation. Spontaneous functional recovery is infrequent, and even more rarely complete, and it may occur only in cases of incomplete amputation of the nerve. It is worth noting that 12 months after the trauma has occurred, no further improvements are likely to occur as far as functional recovery is concerned.

SYMPTOMS

Symptoms caused by nerve lesions are:

- paraesthesia: sensory alteration;
- dysaesthesia: sensory alteration associated with pain;
- anaesthesia: absence of any sensory response;
- hyperaesthesia: accentuated sensory response.

Prevention

To minimise the risk of nerve lesions, it is essential to plan any surgical intervention thoroughly and know the local anatomy comprehensively.

During surgery, the nerve at risk must be identified and protected from any trauma, particularly those produced by sharp and rotary instruments.

In the case of neurovascular bundles, the use of bipolar coagulation should be averted even with profuse bleeding due to a high risk of direct (through any contact with the tips of the forceps) and indirect (through the heat irradiated by the tips of the forceps) damage to the nerve. It is worth noting that the risk of direct and indirect nerve damage is even higher for intrabony bundles, such as the inferior alveolar neurovascular bundle.

If the aforementioned criteria are respected, the incidence of unjustified nerve lesions is very low. Further details on the prevention of intraoperative complications are reported in Chapter 3 and other chapters (particularly Chapter 5, where technical tips are given on how to avoid lesions of the lingual nerve and the inferior alveolar nerve during surgery for the removal of impacted lower third molars).

Management

Neurapraxia does not require treatment: functional recovery occurs spontaneously. Anti-inflammatory and anti-edematous medications may help recovery only when inflammation and swelling are the primary causes of neurapraxia, while neurotrophic medications (B vitamins) may shorten recovery time.

Axonotmesis is generally managed with a wait-and-see approach. Neurotrophic medications can be administered to help recovery, and signs of improvement should be regularly assessed to evaluate different treatment options; it is worth remembering that 12 months is the time limit after which no spontaneous improvements can occur.

Nerve lesions

Type of lesion	Complications	Functional recovery
Neurapraxia	Transient functional interruption	Within days
Axonotmesis	Anatomical interruption of the axons with preservation of the nerve sheath	Within months
Neurotmesis	Anatomical interruption of both the axons and the nerve sheath	Rare: after 12 months, spontaneous recovery is almost impossible

Neurotmesis requires microsurgical suturing of the damaged nerve (neurorrhaphy); in cases of neural tissue loss, an autologous nerve graft should be associated to nerve suturing in order to recreate nerve continuity. Unfortunately, to this day, results of nerve reconstruction procedures are not always encouraging; in some cases, surgical reconstruction may even be followed by exacerbation of symptoms. Therefore, the recourse to this treatment option is indicated only for severe dysaesthesia or anaesthesia.

Monitoring nerve lesions

The patient must be followed regularly to evaluate any variation in the involved area, and in the intensity of symptoms. Possible variations should be reported on a dedicated medical record.

To evaluate sensory response, three different tests are used:

- pinprick is tested with the sharp tip of a dental probe;
- light touch is tested with a cotton wisp or the tip of a small brush;
- temperature is tested using cold and warm stimuli;
- discrimination ability is tested by simultaneous stimulation of two different areas.

Soft tissue laceration

Soft tissue laceration can be the result of improper use of forceps or elevators during tooth extraction, excessive flap retraction, and lack of adequate protection of the soft tissues when sharp or rotary instruments are used.

Prevention

The controlled use of forceps and elevators during tooth extraction, adequate protection of the surrounding soft tissues when sharp or rotary instruments are used, and the elevation of access flaps wide enough to allow sufficient visibility and operative freedom represent the basis to avoid lacerations. As far as rotary instruments are concerned, the use of diamond burs instead of carbide blade burs is preferable when working in close proximity to relevant anatomic structures such as neurovascular bundles, as these tools are less aggressive.

Management

After a laceration is produced, care should be taken to avoid that it extends further; if it is necessary to obtain a wider access to the surgical field, the flap can be enlarged. Once surgery is completed, the laceration must be sutured. It is important to obtain a tension-free closure and avoid applying an excessive number of sutures to reduce stress on the traumatised soft tissues.

Rotary instruments may cause not only lacerations, but also burns by possible overheating of the handpiece, or by friction exerted by the bur shank during contact with the soft tissues. In these events, the treatment is represented solely by the application of a chlorhexidine gel in the area 2-3 times a day to prevent bacterial infection.

Root fractures

As previously mentioned, the most important factor in the prevention of root fractures is the preoperative evaluation of the root anatomy; if it is unfavourable, the recourse to open surgery (elevation of an access flap, ostectomy, odontotomy) is recommended. Details on the techniques used for the extraction of fractured roots are reported in Chapter 4.

Cortical fractures

The application of excessive force during tooth luxation, particularly if extraction forceps are used, may cause the fracture of portions of the alveolar ridge. The incidence of this complication is higher in the maxilla, due to the thinness of the buccal cortical plate; the area of the maxillary tuberosity is particularly at risk during extraction of the upper third molars (14.1a-b).

Prevention

As for all surgical procedures, delicate and precise manipulation of the involved tissues is essential to reducing the risk of complications and postoperative discomfort. When preoperative radiographs demonstrate the presence of long, curved, or divergent roots, or the absence of the periodontal space (sign of tooth ankylosis), the recourse to open surgery, ostectomy and root separation is indicated to prevent cortical fractures.

Management

If the fractured segment is still attached to the periosteum, spontaneous healing may occur; as with any bone fracture, stabilisation leads to callus formation and consolidation. If connection with the periosteum is lost or severely compromised, the fractured segment must be removed. When the maxillary tuberosity is fractured, a further evaluation must be made regarding the possible formation of an oroantral communication that, if present, must be immediately treated (see further for details).

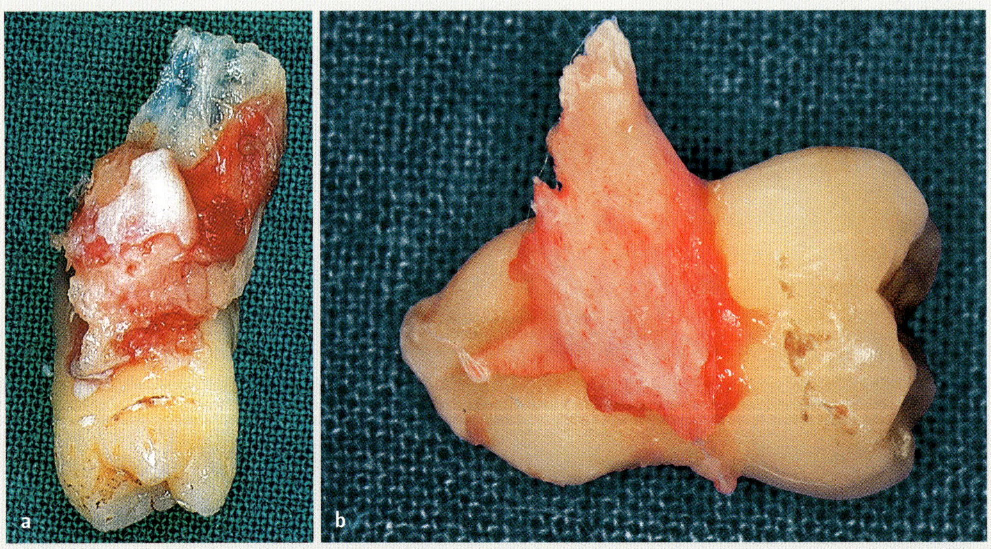

14.1 a) Alveolar ridge fracture. **b)** Fracture of the maxillary tuberosity, which is extracted together with 1.8.

Mandibular fracture

Mandibular fracture is a serious complication that may typically occur during the surgical removal of impacted inferior third molars. Specific risk factors are deep impaction, ankylosis, and the presence of large dentigerous cysts associated with an impacted third molar.

Prevention

A thorough preoperative evaluation, and the application of controlled force previously mentioned as recommendations to avoid cortical fractures also apply to mandibular fractures. In the presence of large dentigerous cysts associated with impacted lower third molars, marsupialisation is indicated to reduce the cyst dimension and stimulate peripheral bone regeneration prior to enucleation.

Management

Generally, the treatment of a complete fracture of the mandibular body falls out of the duties of the oral surgeon. However, all the standard criteria for fracture management apply, including reduction of the fracture (with restoration of the natural occlusion) and rigid fixation with osteosynthesis plates and screws; intermaxillary fixation is used to prevent movements that may jeopardise callus formation (14.2a-c) (see Chapter 12 for further details).

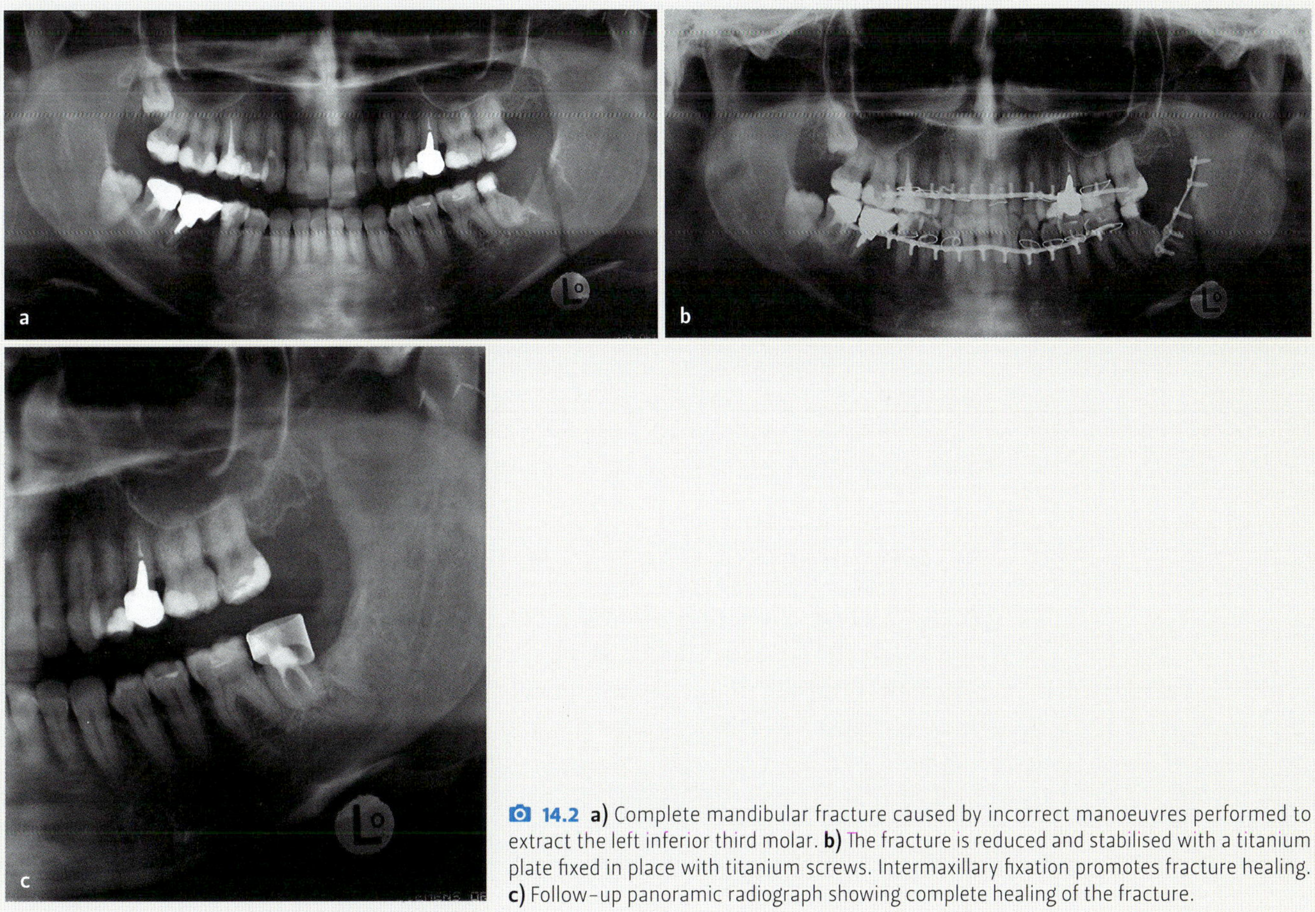

14.2 a) Complete mandibular fracture caused by incorrect manoeuvres performed to extract the left inferior third molar. **b)** The fracture is reduced and stabilised with a titanium plate fixed in place with titanium screws. Intermaxillary fixation promotes fracture healing. **c)** Follow-up panoramic radiograph showing complete healing of the fracture.

Temporomandibular joint (TMJ) dislocation

Temporomandibular joint dislocation typically occurs in predisposed patients, particularly when maximum mouth opening is attempted, or when excessive force is exerted on the mandible during surgery. Generally, the mandibular condyle is dislocated anteriorly to the articular eminence.

Prevention

A thorough preoperative evaluation of the TMJ function, in association with the application of controlled force during surgery, reduces the risk of TMJ dislocation. A mouth prop may help the patient to stabilise the mandible when the mouth must be kept open for prolonged periods, or when controlled force need to be exerted.

Management

Dislocation must be manually reduced as soon as possible to avoid spontaneous muscle contraction, which occurs as a reaction and renders reduction more difficult.

Generally, reduction of a temporomandibular joint dislocation is performed with an intraoral approach: with the patient seated in an upright position, thumbs are placed on the occlusal face of the molars, as far back as possible, while the other fingers are wrapped externally around the mandible. A firm, slow, and steady pressure is applied in a downward and posterior direction until the condyles are back in place. If bilateral reduction is difficult or impossible, the manoeuvre can be completed one side at a time. The patient should be instructed to avoid excessive mandibular excursions during the postoperative period to prevent further dislocations.

Tooth dislocation inside the soft tissues

It is a rare complication that is always caused by incorrect and traumatic manoeuvres during tooth extraction. Typically, tooth dislocation can occur in the maxillary retromolar area (cases of upper third molars dislocated in the infratemporal fossa have been reported in the literature) or on the lingual side in the mandibular retromolar area (📷 14.3).

To prevent tooth (or root) dislocation inside the soft tissues, adequate visibility and controlled application of any force during tooth luxation are fundamental.

Management

Immediate retrieval of the tooth (or tooth fragments, or root) is necessary. However, in some cases the lack of visibility or the proximity of important anatomic structures may determine the need for specific instruments, specific skills, and even the recourse to sedation or general anaesthesia.

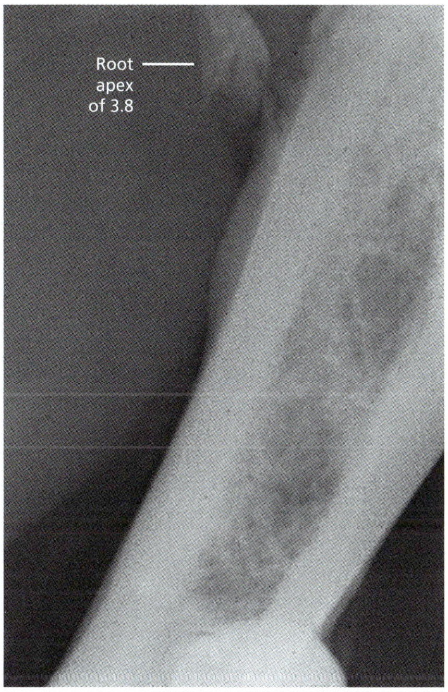

14.3 Mandibular third molar extraction: dislocation of a root apex inside the floor of the oral cavity.

Buccal fat pad herniation

Buccal fat pad herniation may occur, accidentally or intentionally, during elevation of buccal flaps in the posterior areas of the maxilla when the periosteum is interrupted (e.g. periosteal releasing incisions).

Subperiosteal elevation of the access flap and its protection during surgery are key factors in preventing this complication.

Management

If only a small portion of the fat pad is herniated, it can be repositioned under the access flap prior to suturing. If a larger portion is herniated, which renders the completion of the surgical procedure difficult, it can be removed via cut or bipolar coagulation (14.4a-b).

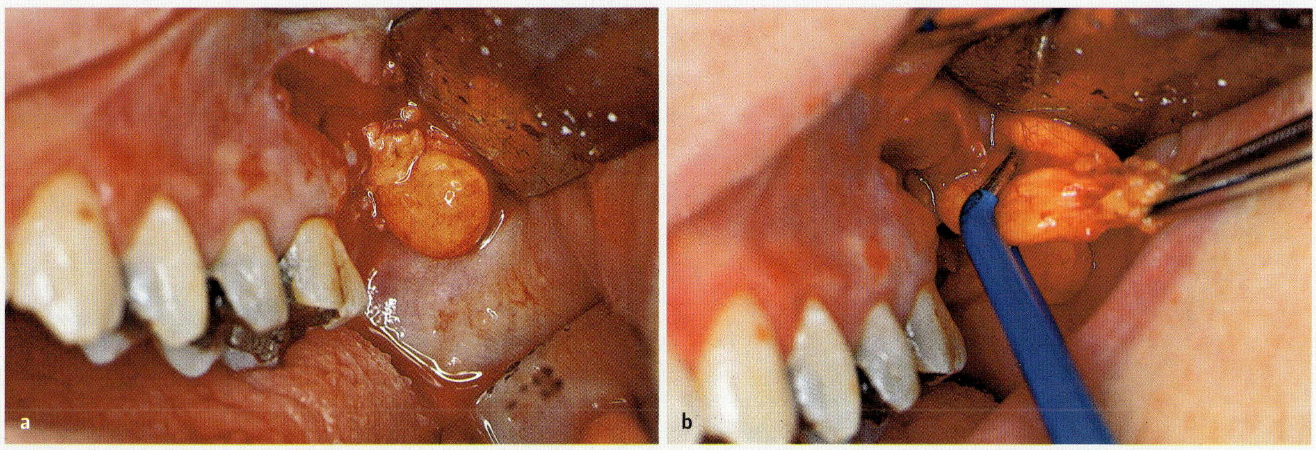

14.4 **a)** Herniation of the buccal fat pad during extraction of impacted 2.8. **b)** The herniated portion is removed by means of bipolar coagulation.

Oroantral communications

The maxillary sinus is the largest paranasal cavity and it usually occupies the entire body of the maxillary bone, and its walls are lined with a thin respiratory mucosa. At birth, it is only a small "pneumatised cell" under the orbital floor, but it undergoes an expansion process during the entire lifespan. In particular, although with a significant interindividual variability, the maxillary sinus tends to expand downwards, towards the alveolar ridge.

This particular anatomic situation may increase the risk of creating a communication between the oral cavity and the sinus during oral surgery procedures (e.g. extraction of maxillary molars). If oroantral communications are not immediately treated, signs and symptoms of inflammation prelude to the onset of sinus infection.

The formation of an oroantral communication is sometimes inevitable (eg, extraction of a tooth with roots protruding inside the maxillary sinus), but in the majority of cases it is the result of incorrect maneuvers such as the application of excessive force during tooth extraction or contamination of the surgical field during sinus surgery.

Based on histologic criteria, three different clinical entities can be identified:

- oroantral communications;
- oroantral fistulas;
- pseudopolyps.

Oroantral communications: are characterised by the presence of a passage between the oral cavity and the maxillary sinus that lacks an epithelial lining. It represents the initial phase of the pathologic process and spontaneous healing is possible on occasion.

Oroantral fistulas: represent the evolution of the former: the passage between the oral cavity and the maxillary sinus is lined with an epithelial layer that prevents spontaneous healing. It represents the advanced phase of the pathologic process (14.5).

Pseudopolyps: form due to the evagination of the Schneiderian membrane through the communication between the oral cavity and the maxillary sinus. Typically, they are observed when the communication is relatively large, and associated with chronic sinus infection (14.6).

Causes of oroantral communication

- Extraction of erupted teeth in the lateral-posterior areas of the maxilla
- Surgical extraction of impacted upper third molars
- Migration of teeth or roots inside the maxillary sinus
- Enucleation of periapical or cystic lesions involving the maxillary canines, premolars, and molars
- Enucleation of benign lesion in the lateral-posterior area of the maxilla
- Preparation of implant sites in the lateral-posterior maxilla

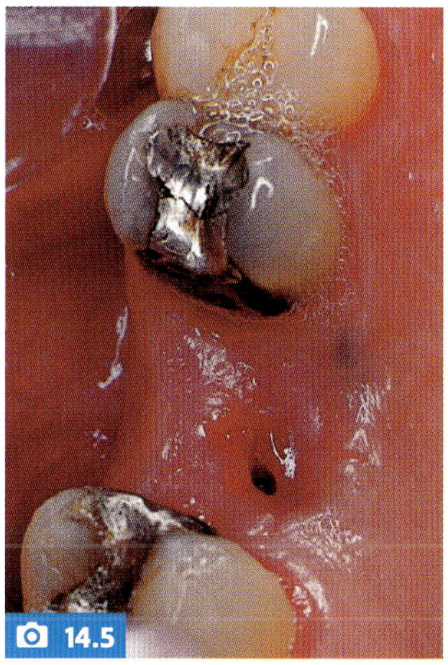

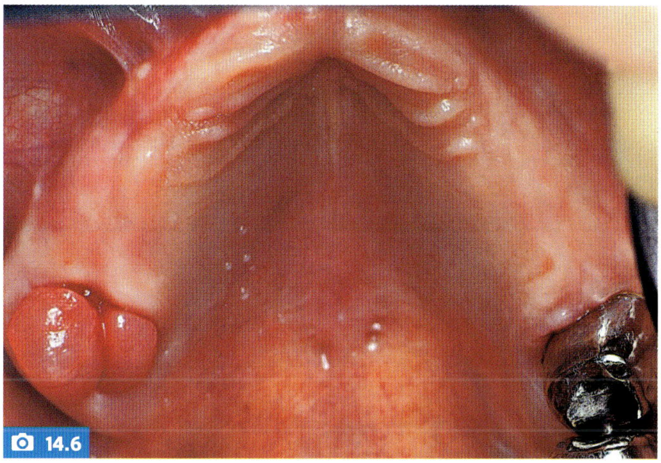

14.5 Oroantral fistula following the extraction of 1.7.

14.6 Pseudopolyp resulting from the herniation of the sinus mucosa through an oroantral communication caused during the extraction of 1.7.

Oroantral communications, if not treated, can develop in different ways according to their extent, and to the degree of sinus infection. As a rule, small traumatic communications (< 5 mm) may spontaneously heal after the formation and organisation of the blood clot. For larger communications, the chances of spontaneous healing decrease, while the risk of sinus infection from contamination by oral bacterial flora increases.

Clinical examination: analysis of signs and symptoms

Clinical examination should be conducted according to the principles of classic semiology, particularly regarding inspection and auscultation.

Intraoral examination

Inspection: small oroantral communications may not be evident upon inspection. Therefore, the use of a mirror and blunt-pointed probe can help to detect passages that may be covered by mucosal folds (14.7a).

Aspiration: placing the tip of a suction cannula on the intraoral opening of the communication makes it possible to hear a dull, amplified sound caused by airflow inside the maxillary sinus.

Oroantral communications

Signs
- Dull or amplified sound inside the maxillary sinus while suctioning
- Small bubbles at the intraoral opening of the passage
- Rare bloody discharge from the nose
- Discharge of serous fluid or purulent material

Symptoms
- Feeling of air or fluids flowing from the oral cavity to the sinus and vice versa
- Feeling of tension in the area of the sinus with possible irradiation to the orbital region

Irrigation: when irrigation of the operating field at the end of the surgical procedure is performed, a feeling of liquid passing to the nose may be reported by the patient.

Valsalva manoeuvre: by increasing air pressure inside the maxillary sinus, in cases of oroantral communication, this manoeuvre causes the formation of small bubbles at its intraoral opening. Less often, clear fluid or blood may leak from the communication (14.7b).

When the communication is left untreated for weeks or months, two clinical pictures may be observed: the first is characterised by the presence of a purulent discharge, while the second is characterised by the presence of a polypoid herniation of the Schneiderian membrane through the intraoral opening of the communication, occasionally associated with purulent discharge (14.6).

Extraoral examination

In the absence of full-blown sinus infection, extraoral examination may prove ineffective, while in cases of sinusitis a variable swelling involving the paranasal and malar regions can be observed, in association with reddening and pain.

SYMPTOMS

Oroantral communications cause a variable symptomatology depending on the duration of the infectious process, and the extent of the communication itself. Symptoms may arise immediately, or they can arise some time after the lesion is created; typically, these include the feeling of air and fluids passing from the oral cavity to the nasal cavity and vice versa. Absence of pain is the norm, provided that no concomitant acute inflammation of the sinus mucosa is present. In the latter case, pain can be exacerbated by palpation in the area of the anterior wall of the maxillary sinus. The patient may also report a sense of tension in the malar region with possible irradiation to the orbital region, or a sense of stretch or tension to the canine, premolars, and molars.

Instrumental screening

On radiographic exams, oroantral communications may appear as discontinuities of the bony floor of the sinus associated with a reduction of the sinus radiolucency when inflammation of the sinus mucosa or a purulent collection are present. A periapical radiograph taken with a probe or a gutta percha cone introduced in the intraoral opening makes it possible to verify the presence of a complete communication (14.7c). Occasionally, oroantral communications are complicated by the migration of root fragments or fractured instruments inside the maxillary sinus due to incorrect surgical manoeuvres, determining a higher risk of inflammatory reaction of the sinus mucosa that may lead to full-blown sinusitis. *Periapical radiographs* are widely used to evaluate possible post-extractive oroantral communications, but the field of view is limited; conversely, *panoramic radiographs* can give an overall, albeit less detailed, view of the jaws. Finally, *CT scans* can give a detailed tridimensional view of the area of interest, thus representing the ideal radiographic exam particularly for oroantral communications associated with sinus infection (14.7d). Today, due to the numerous advantages and reduced radiation doses, digital CT scans have supplanted exams such as stratigraphies and occipitomental radiographs (Waters' view).

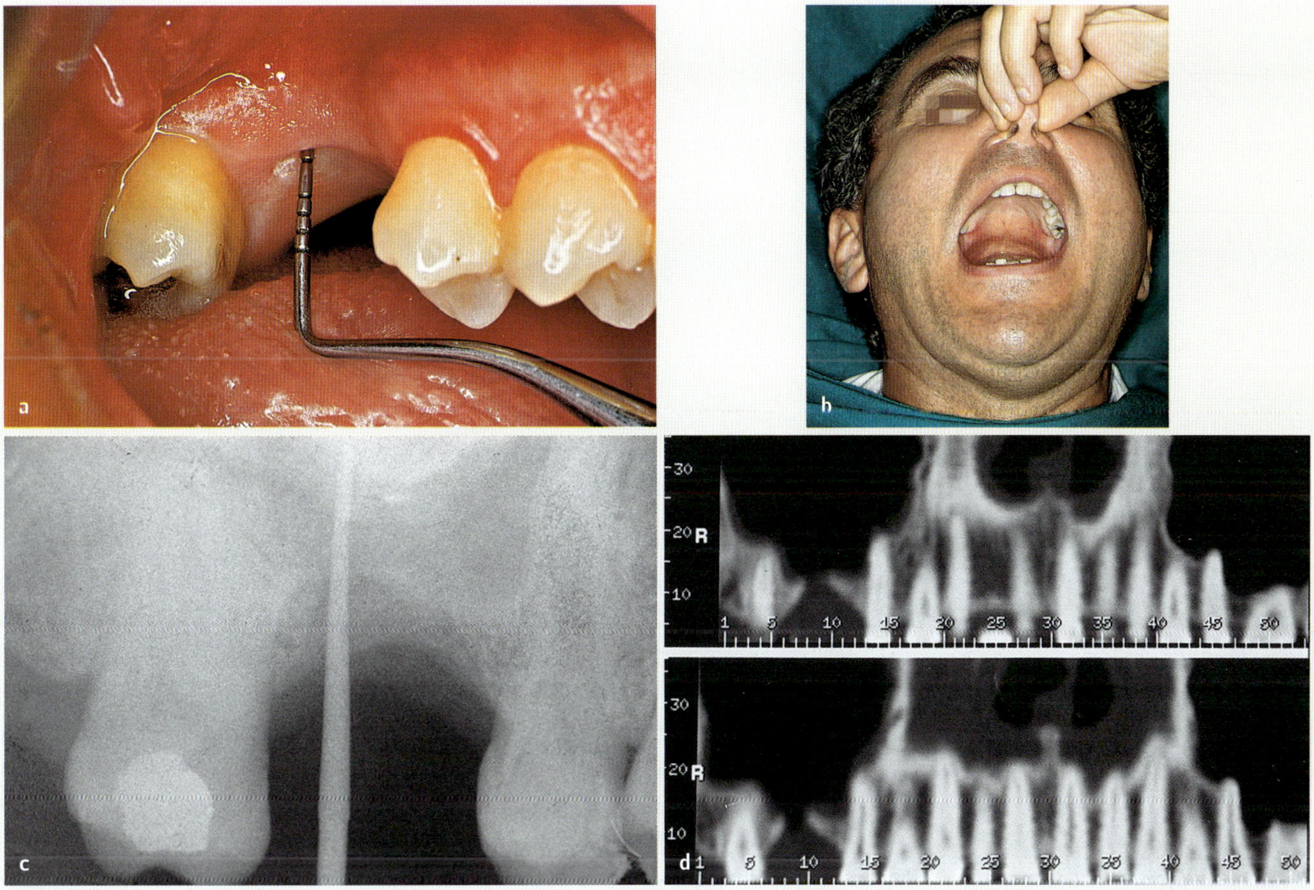

14.7 **a)** Intraoral probing of an oroantral communication caused during the extraction of 1.6. **b)** Valsalva manoeuvre. **c)** The gutta percha cone shows the interruption of the alveolar crest, and the penetration inside the maxillary sinus. **d)** CT scan showing interruption of the floor of the sinus.

Management

Choice of the appropriate treatment modality depends on the following:

- extent of the oroantral communication;
- epithelisation of the communication;
- presence of sinus infection.

For small (< 5 mm) communications without sinus infection, spontaneous healing may occur following the formation and organisation of the blood clot. This process may be facilitated by the use of haemostatic materials such as oxidised regenerated cellulose and collagen sponge, and by instructing the patient to avoid any air pressure surge inside the nasal and oral cavities. In the presence of large communications without sinus infection, notwithstanding the possible epithelisation of the passage (fistula), surgical closure with local advancement or rotational flaps is necessary. Conversely, in cases of concomitant infection, the latter must be treated before attempting any procedure to close the communication, as the elimination of this drainage way may cause sinus empyema.

Sinusitis can be treated by irrigating the maxillary sinus with antibiotic solutions through the intraoral opening of the communication for one week. Systemic antibiotic therapy is necessary only for severe sinus infection.

The most frequently used flaps for the closure of oroantral communications are:

- buccal flap;
- palatal flap;
- buccal flap associated with palatal flap;
- buccal fat pad flap;
- lingual flap (rarely used).

These flaps have two fundamental characteristics in common: good vascularisation and the possibility of obtaining a tension-free suture and an airtight closure of the communication.

BUCCAL FLAP

The buccal flap is a four-corner, full-thickness flap also known as Rehrmann flap. An incision is made around the communication, in association with two (mesial and distal) vertical releasing incisions delimiting a flap of adequate proportions; care must be taken to limit the extension of the releasing incisions to avoid any damage to the parotid duct (14.8a-f). For simple communication, flap preparation is sufficient, while for epithelisation of the passage, the fistula must be surgically removed. Once the flap is elevated, the extent and morphology of the communication, as well as the conditions of the sinus, are assessed. Remodelling of the alveolar crest may be necessary should morphologic anomalies be present that may interfere with the healing process, such as the sharp margins of post-extractive sockets.

To close the communication, the flap should be adequately mobilised by performing a periosteal releasing incision at the base of the flap itself. Once the absence of any tension is verified, the flap can be sutured in place. The mucosa on the palatal side of the flap can be disepithelialised prior to suturing to improve peripheral support and seal (14.9a-g).

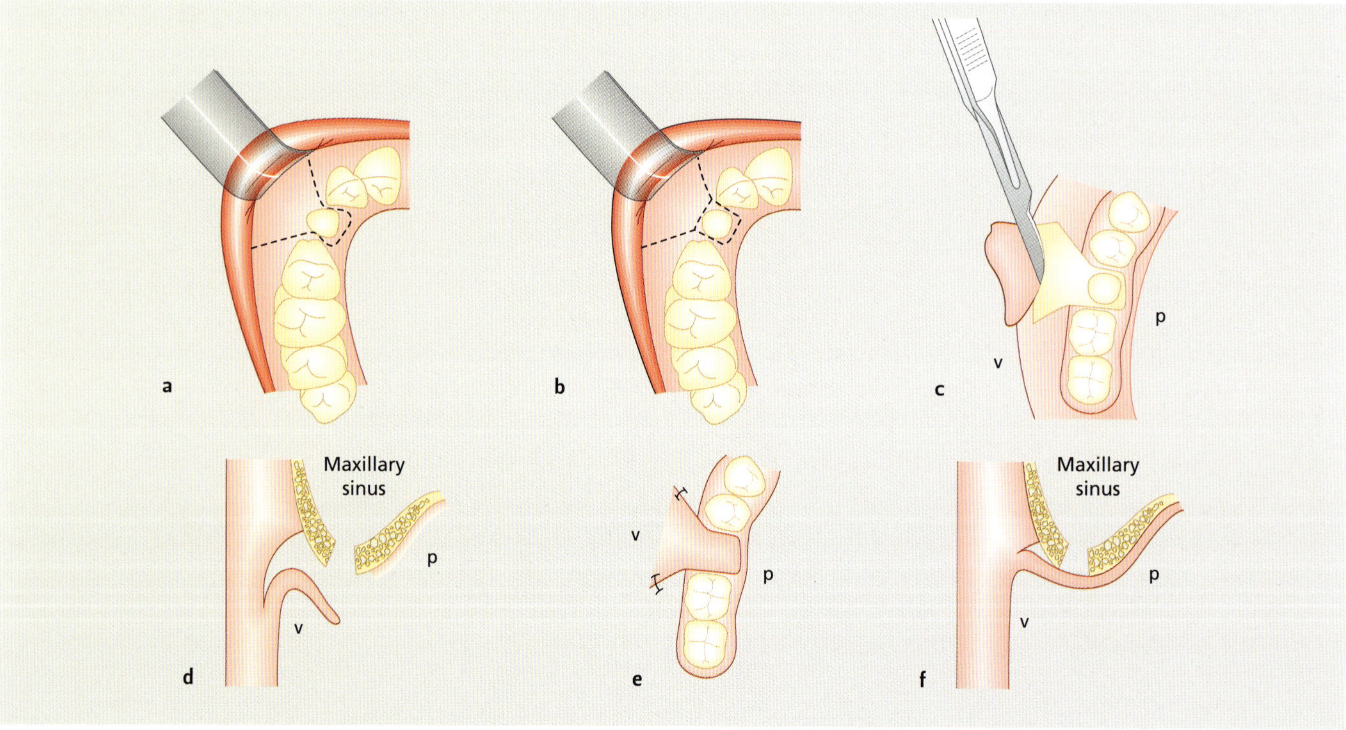

14.8 a–f) Buccal flap for the closure of an oroantral communication.

Local flaps for the closure of oroantral communications

	Advantages	Disadvantages
Buccal flap	+ Easy to prepare + Can be used to treat large communications	+ Possible reduction of the buccal vestibule depth
Palatal flap	+ Good vascularisation + Thickness of the soft tissues	+ Secondary intention healing of the palatine surface + Limited rotation
Buccal fat pad flap	+ Easy to prepare + Large quantity of soft tissues available	+ None + Must be performed under general anaesthesia
Lingual flap	+ Excellent vascularisation	+ Prolonged functional impairment

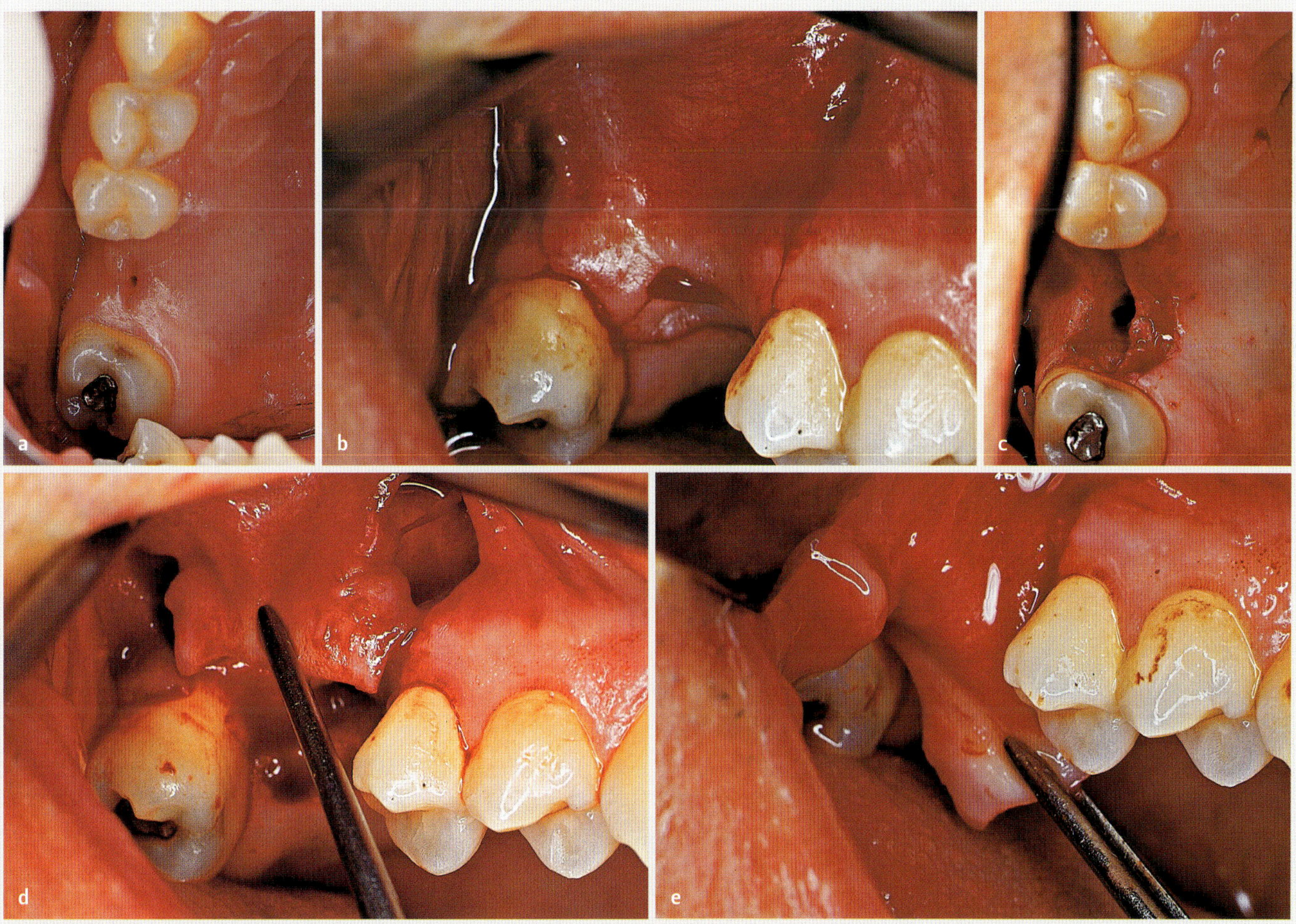

14.9 **a)** Oroantral fistula following the extraction of 1.6 (radiographs are shown in 14.7c–d). **b)** A buccal, four-corner flap is prepared (Rehrmann flap). **c)** Surgical removal of the fistula. **d)** The mobility of the access flap is insufficient to allow the closure of the communication. **e)** Periosteal releasing incisions allow adequate advancement of the flap. (*continued*)

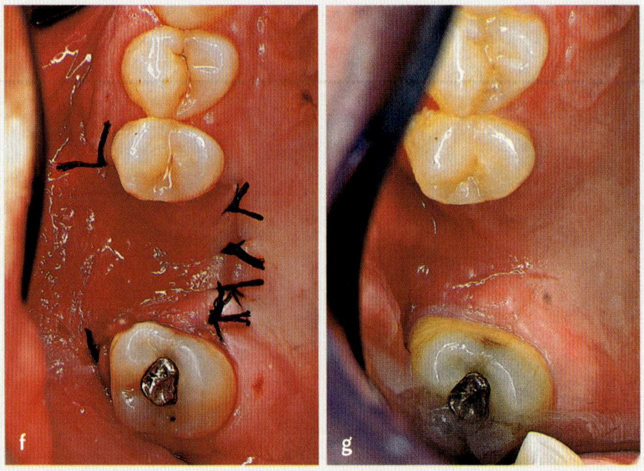

14.9 (*continued*) **f)** Suture. **g)** Complete healing some time after surgery.

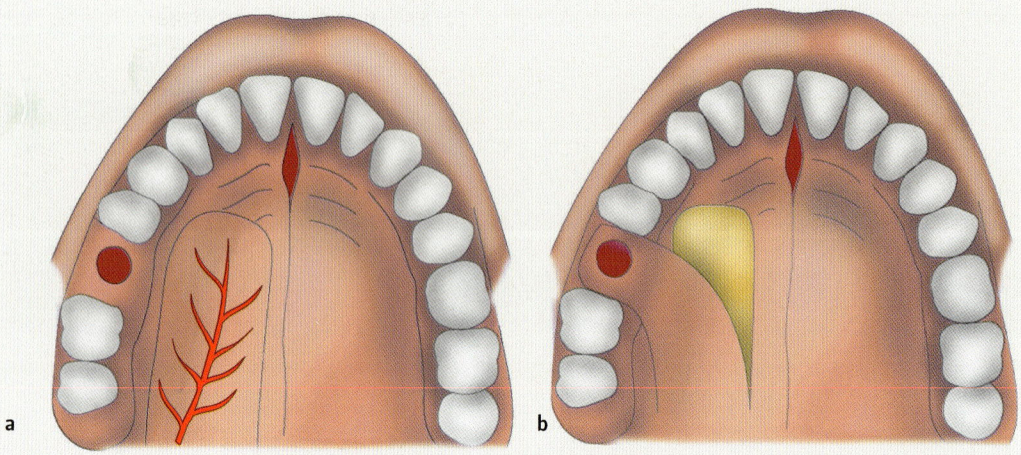

14.10 **a–b)** Palatal flap.

PALATAL FLAP

This flap is obtained by means of a full-thickness incision of the palatine mucosa aimed at creating an axial pedicle flap with a posterior base vascularised by the major palatine artery. The flap is elevated, rotated, and positioned over the communication to obtain its complete closure. Secondary intention healing will then occur on the exposed palatine surface (14.10a-b). This flap is particularly indicated for communications occurring in the premolar region. Conversely, if the communication occurs in the molar region, excessive rotation of the flap may be necessary to obtain adequate closure; this can cause occlusion of the major palatine artery with subsequent ischaemia and necrosis of the flap. A technical variation of this flap, the split-thickness palatal flap, can help avoid arterial occlusion: the superficial (epithelial) and deep (connective) portions of the flap are separated, and while the deep portion containing the artery is sutured over the communication, the superficial portion is sutured back in place. Separation from the epithelial layer renders the connective portion of the flap more flexible, allowing a tension-free adaptation even in cases of sharper rotation angles (14.11a-i).

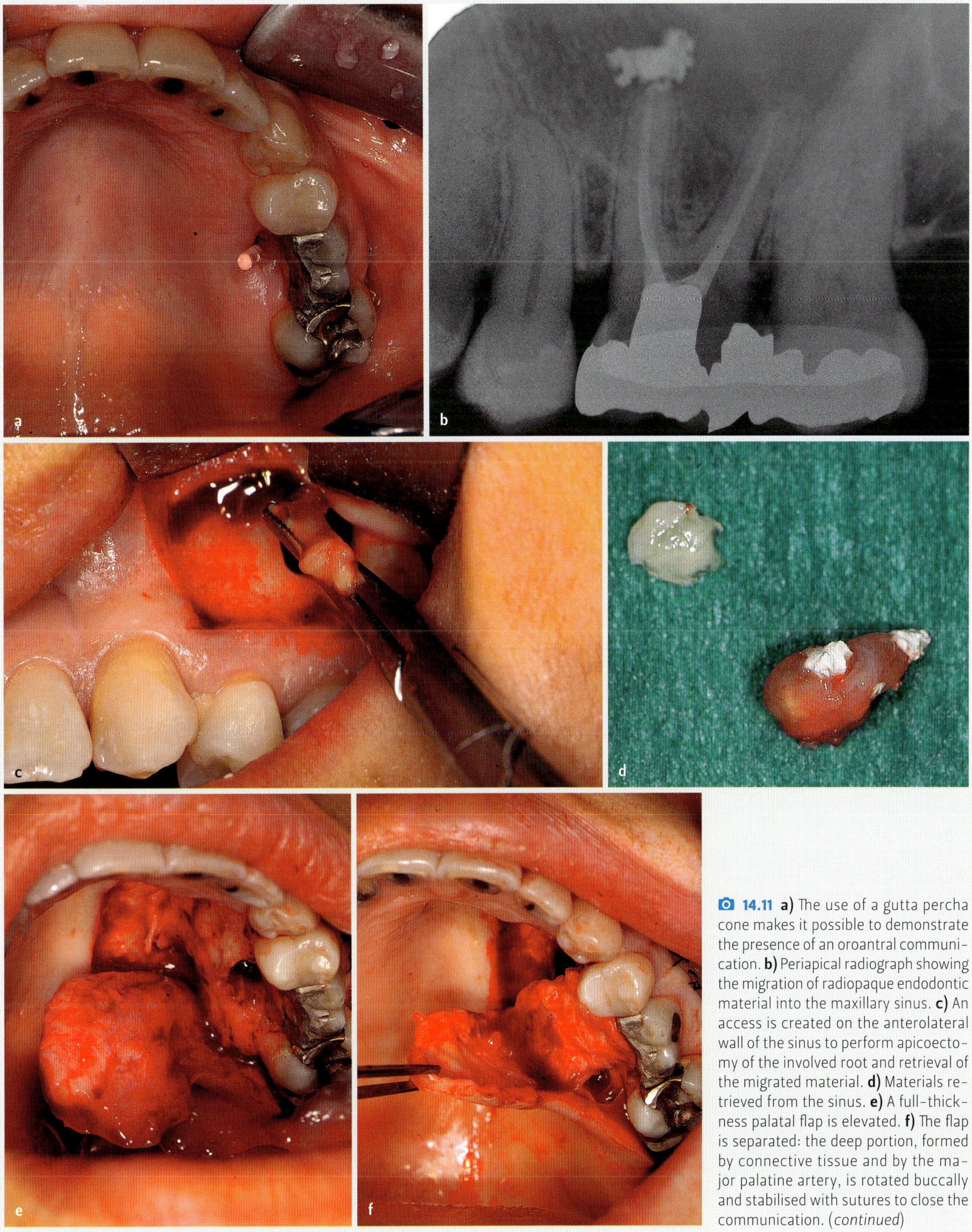

14.11 **a)** The use of a gutta percha cone makes it possible to demonstrate the presence of an oroantral communication. **b)** Periapical radiograph showing the migration of radiopaque endodontic material into the maxillary sinus. **c)** An access is created on the anterolateral wall of the sinus to perform apicoectomy of the involved root and retrieval of the migrated material. **d)** Materials retrieved from the sinus. **e)** A full-thickness palatal flap is elevated. **f)** The flap is separated: the deep portion, formed by connective tissue and by the major palatine artery, is rotated buccally and stabilised with sutures to close the communication. (*continued*)

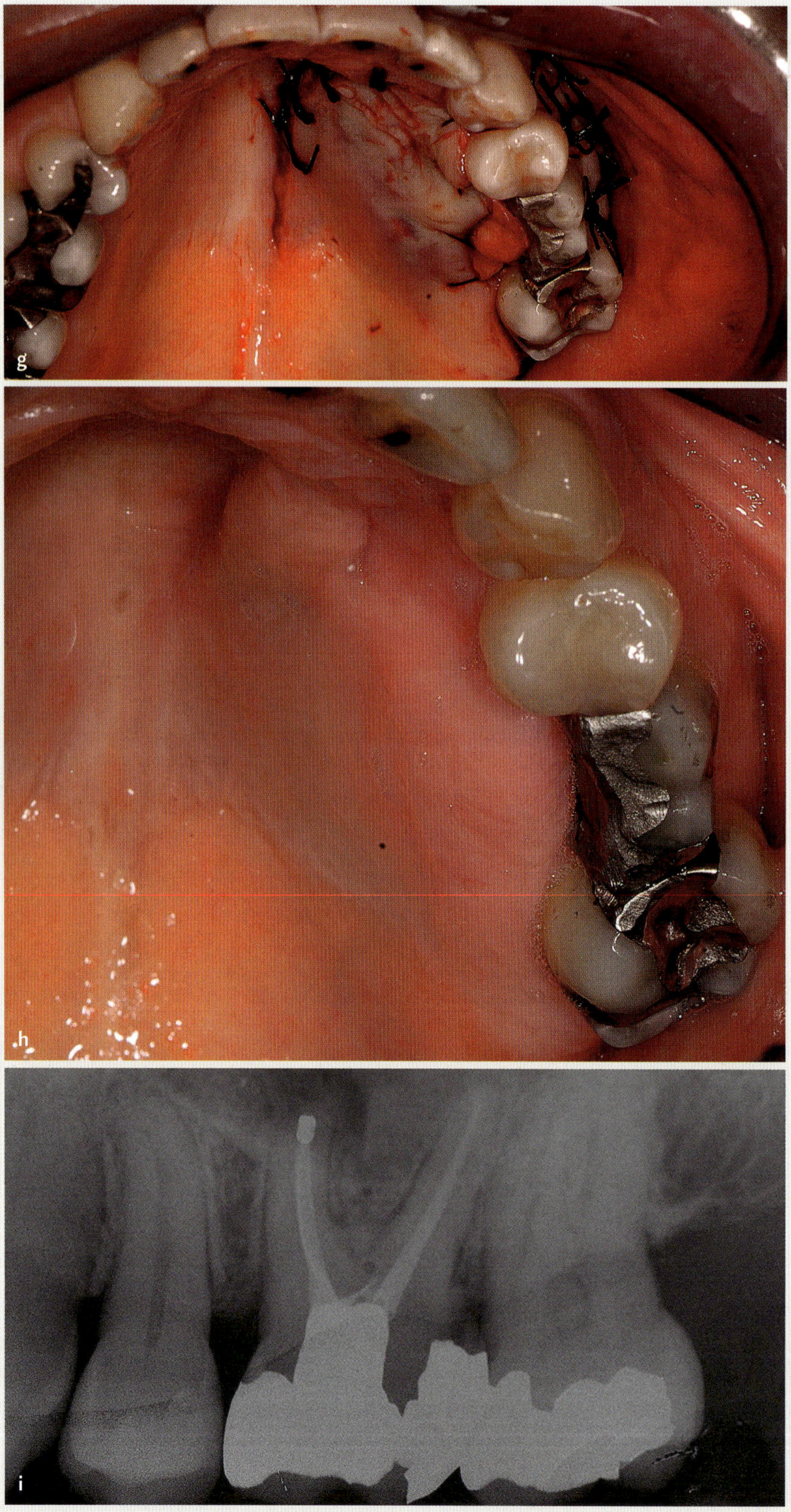

14.11 (*continued*) **g)** The superficial portion of the flap, represented by the palatine mucosa, is sutured in its original position. **h)** Complete healing some time after surgery. **i)** Periapical radiograph showing the positive outcome of the retrograde endodontic treatment.

BUCCAL FLAP ASSOCIATED WITH PALATAL FLAP

In cases of large oroantral communications, it is possible to associate the two types of flap to increase the quantity of soft tissues available for the closure.

BUCCAL FAT PAD FLAP

Typically, the buccal fat pad flap is used for the closure of oroantral communications in the area of the second and third maxillary molars, where the use of the palatal flap may result in ischaemic complications, and recourse to the buccal flap alone can cause alterations of the buccal vestibule depth. By virtue of the large quantity of tissue available, this flap allows the closure of even wide communications, and it may also be associated with the buccal flap to increase the quantity of tissue even more.

A buccal, four-corner flap is elevated around the margins of the communication, and the periosteum is incised to expose the buccal fat pad, which is then freed by blunt dissection. Care must be taken to extract the anterior portion without separating it from the posterior portion, to avoid interruption of its blood support. The fat pad is then sutured to the palatal mucosa and the mucosal flap is repositioned to restore the original anatomy of the buccal vestibule. The portion of the fat pad covering the communication rapidly undergoes spontaneous epithelisation (14.12a-j).

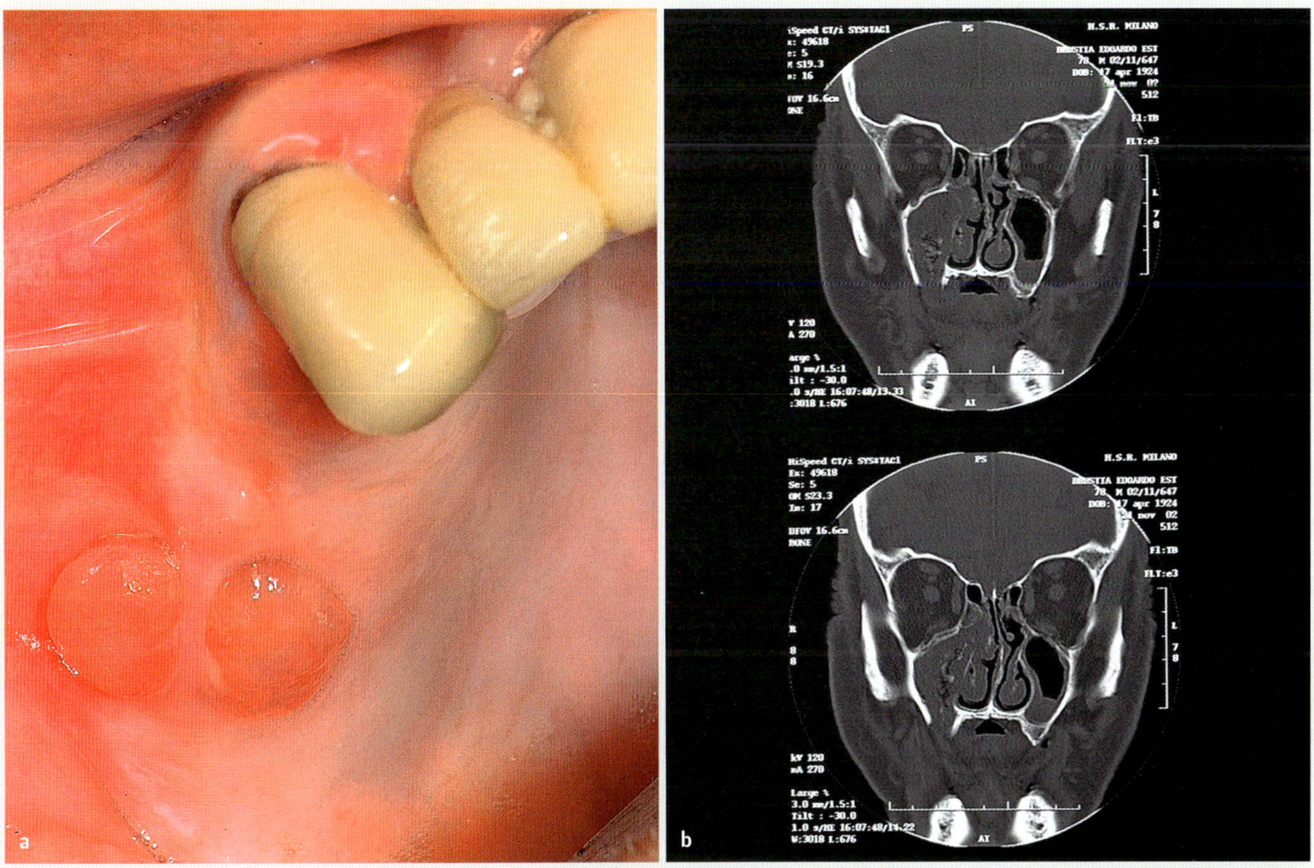

14.12 a) Pseudopolyp resulting from the herniation of the sinus mucosa through an oroantral communication caused during the extraction of 1.7. **b)** CT scan showing a wide oroantral communication associated with opacification of the maxillary sinus and involvement of the ethmoidal cells. (*continued*)

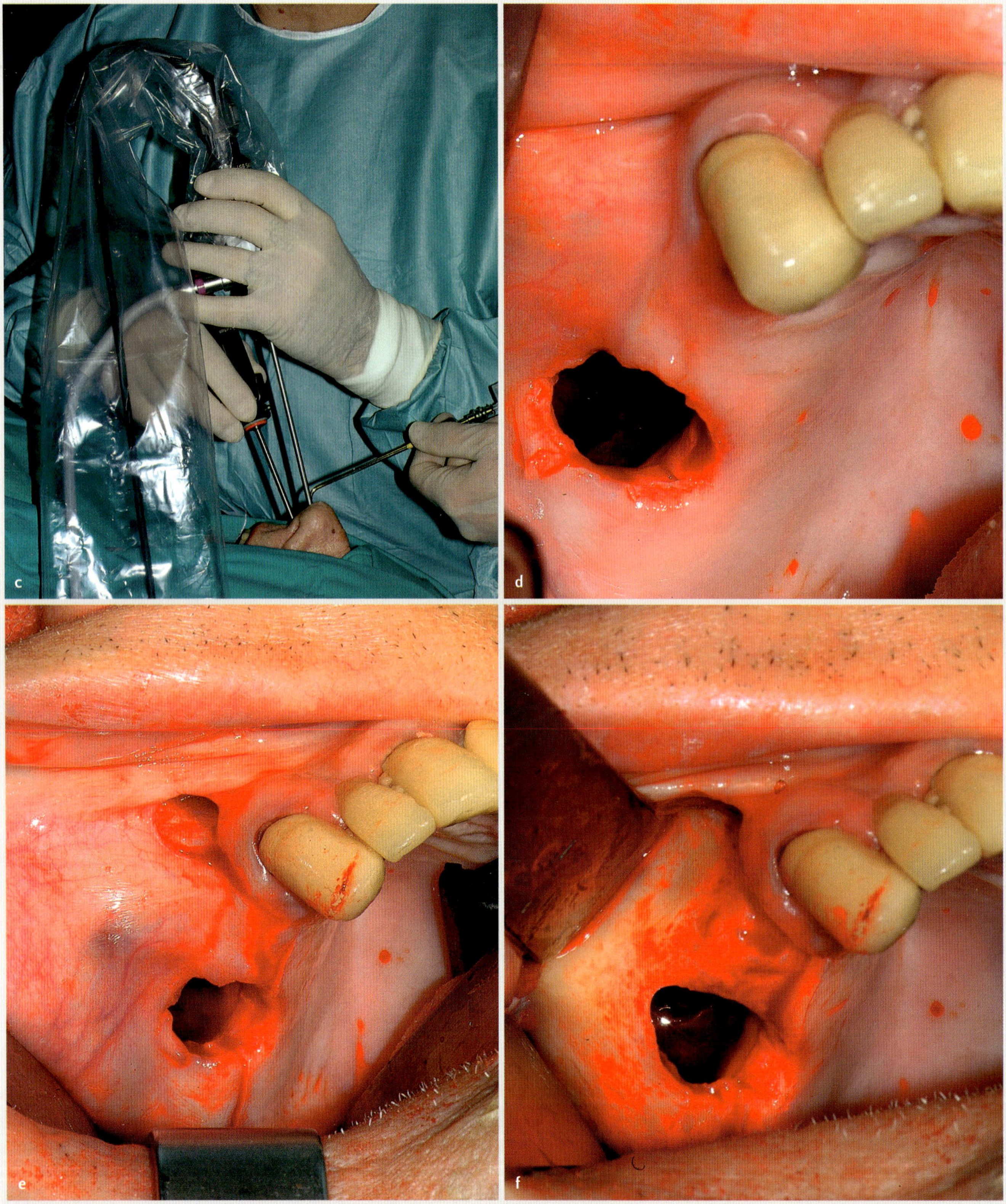

14.12 (*continued*) **c)** FESS (Functional Endoscopic Sinus Surgery) to treat infection of the paranasal cavities (endoscopic phase performed by Dr. Mario Mantovani - Milan). **d)** The oroantral communication after removal of the pseudopolyp is completed. **e)** A buccal, four-corner flap is prepared. **f)** Full-thickness elevation of the flap. (*continued*)

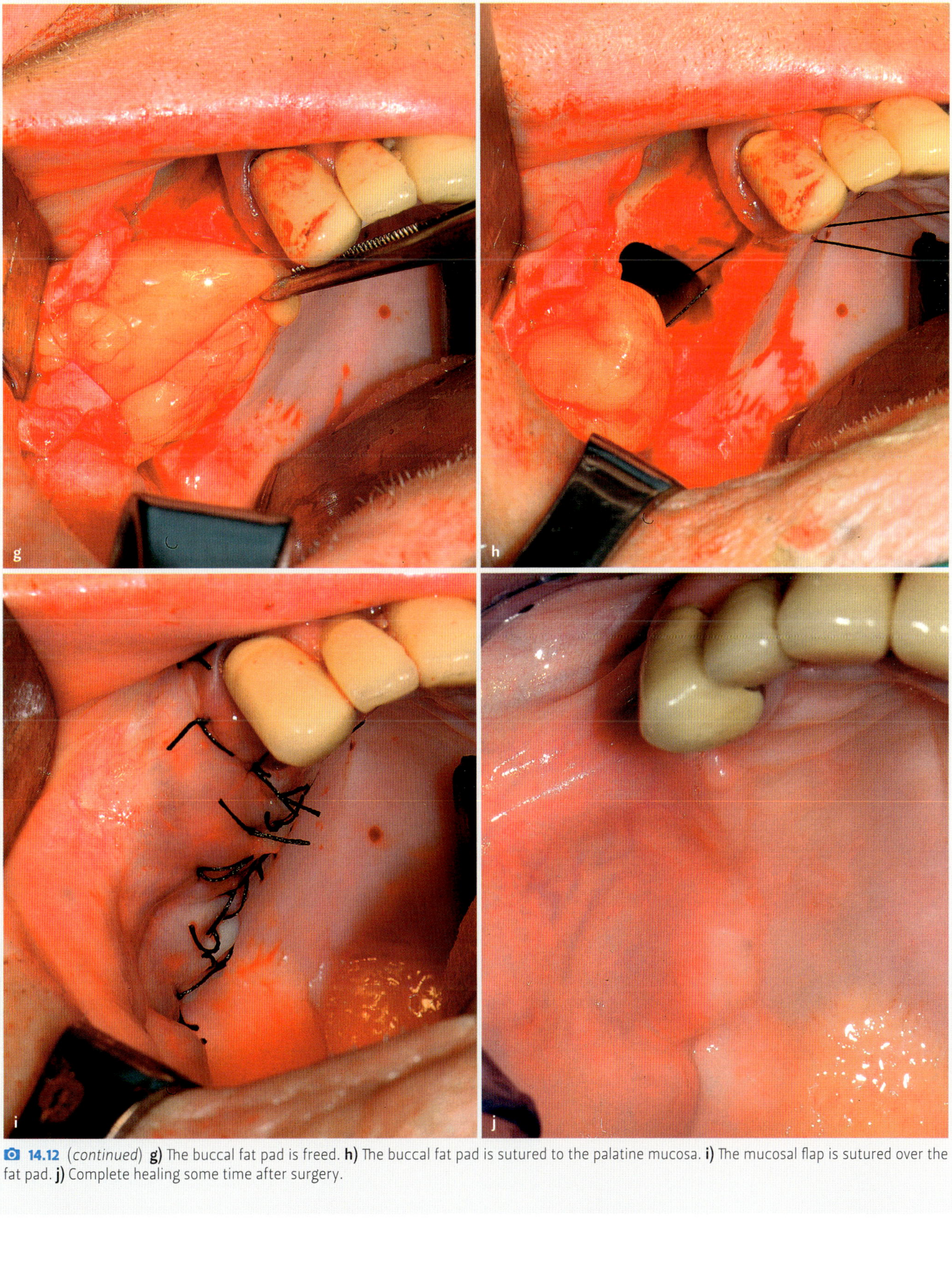

14.12 (*continued*) **g)** The buccal fat pad is freed. **h)** The buccal fat pad is sutured to the palatine mucosa. **i)** The mucosal flap is sutured over the fat pad. **j)** Complete healing some time after surgery.

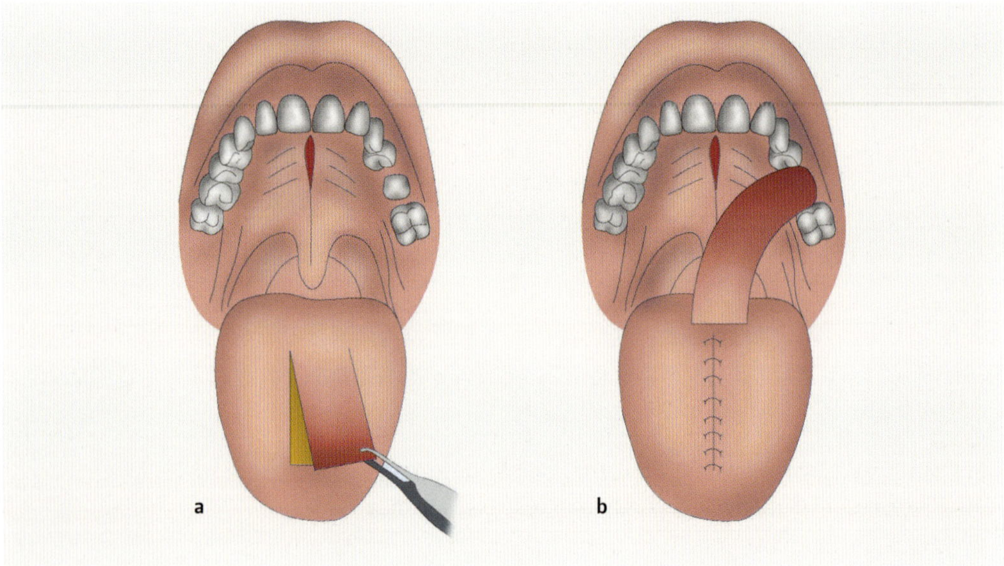

14.13 a–b) Lingual flap.

LINGUAL FLAP

Lingual pedicle flaps are divided into two categories: dorsal flaps and lateral flaps (14.13a-b). In light of the relevant disadvantages that these flaps entail, they are rarely used today. Since the procedure should be performed under sedation or general anaesthesia in a protected environment (hospital), their description is beyond the scope of this manual.

Communications and fistulae associated with sinus infection

As previously noted, for chronic sinus infection refractory to medical treatment (irrigation with antibiotic solutions and systemic antibiotic therapy), the closure of an oroantral communication is contraindicated due to the risk of sinus empyema, which could eventually spread also to other paranasal cavities. In these cases, the treatment of choice is the removal of infectious material from the sinus. It is performed with the Caldwell-Luc technique or with an endoscopic approach (FESS - Functional Endoscopic Sinus Surgery), associated with the closure of the oroantral communication with local flaps.

This treatment modality is also indicated for migration of foreign bodies such as dental roots, implants, and biomaterials inside the maxillary sinus.

The Caldwell-Luc technique is performed by elevating a full-thickness flap to expose the anterolateral wall of the maxillary sinus, on which a window is opened with rotary or piezoelectric instruments to access the sinus and remove the infected, hyperplastic mucosa. The medial wall of the sinus is then identified and an opening is created at its base (antrostomy), from which a surgical drain is passed to the inferior meatus of the ipsilateral nasal cavity to allow spontaneous discharge of fluids from the sinus: the drain is kept in place for 5-7 days postoperatively.

Finally, the access flap is sutured; irrigation with sterile saline or antibiotic solutions is possible through the surgical drain. Once removed, communication between the sinus and the nasal cavity will remain pervious, allowing fluids to drain from the sinus to the nasal cavity even when the natural ostium of the sinus is obliterated and the mucociliary clearance of the sinus mucosa is impaired, as occurs in the case of chronic sinusitis.

The Caldwell-Luc technique, which was widely used in the past, has today fallen into disuse and has been replaced by the transnasal endoscopic approach known as FESS.

The rationale for this procedure is the reduced invasivity and the respect of the sinus physiology. In fact, performing the procedure with the endoscope makes it possible to access the maxillary sinus from its natural ostium that is surgically enlarged to facilitate spontaneous sinus drainage. Therefore, antrostomy and the placement of a surgical drain are no longer necessary and the approach makes it possible to manage the possible involvement of other paranasal cavities in the infectious process in a single surgical procedure (14.14a-g).

Migration of foreign bodies inside the maxillary sinus

During oral surgery procedures, due to technical errors, foreign bodies such as teeth, roots, fractured instruments, implants, or biomaterials can migrate inside the maxillary sinus. The presence of a foreign body inside the sinus may cause:

- the presence of an oroantral communication;
- a chronic, irritative stimulus that may cause the onset of sinusitis.

As far as prevention of this complication is concerned, the correct application of surgical techniques is the only means to avoid such an adverse event.

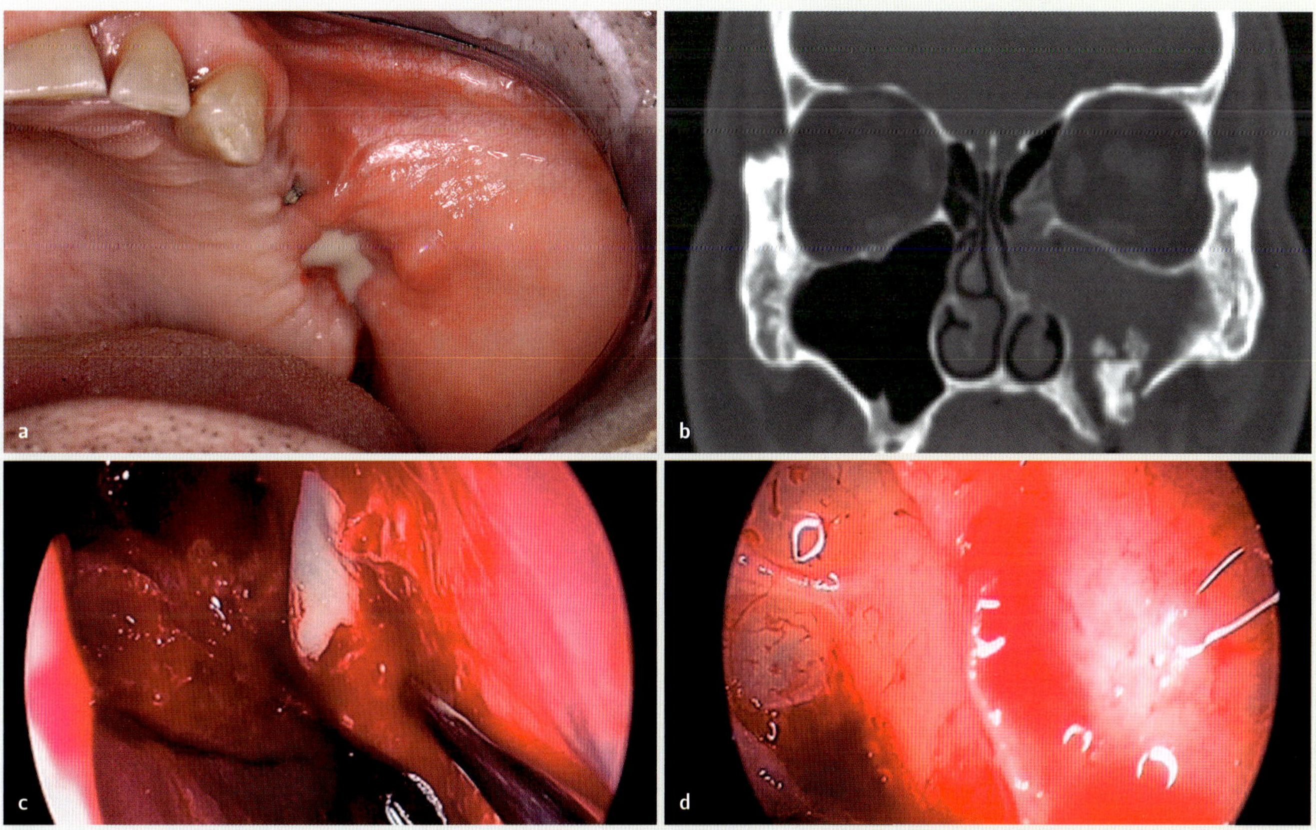

14.14 a-b) Oroantral communication associated with purulent discharge caused by sinus infection (involving the ethmoidal cells) following an attempted sinus lifting procedure: penetration of the grafting material inside the sinus is visible. **c-d)** Infectious material is removed from the maxillary sinus and the ethmoidal cells via an endoscopic approach (FESS performed by Prof. Giovanni Felisati - Milan). (*continued*)

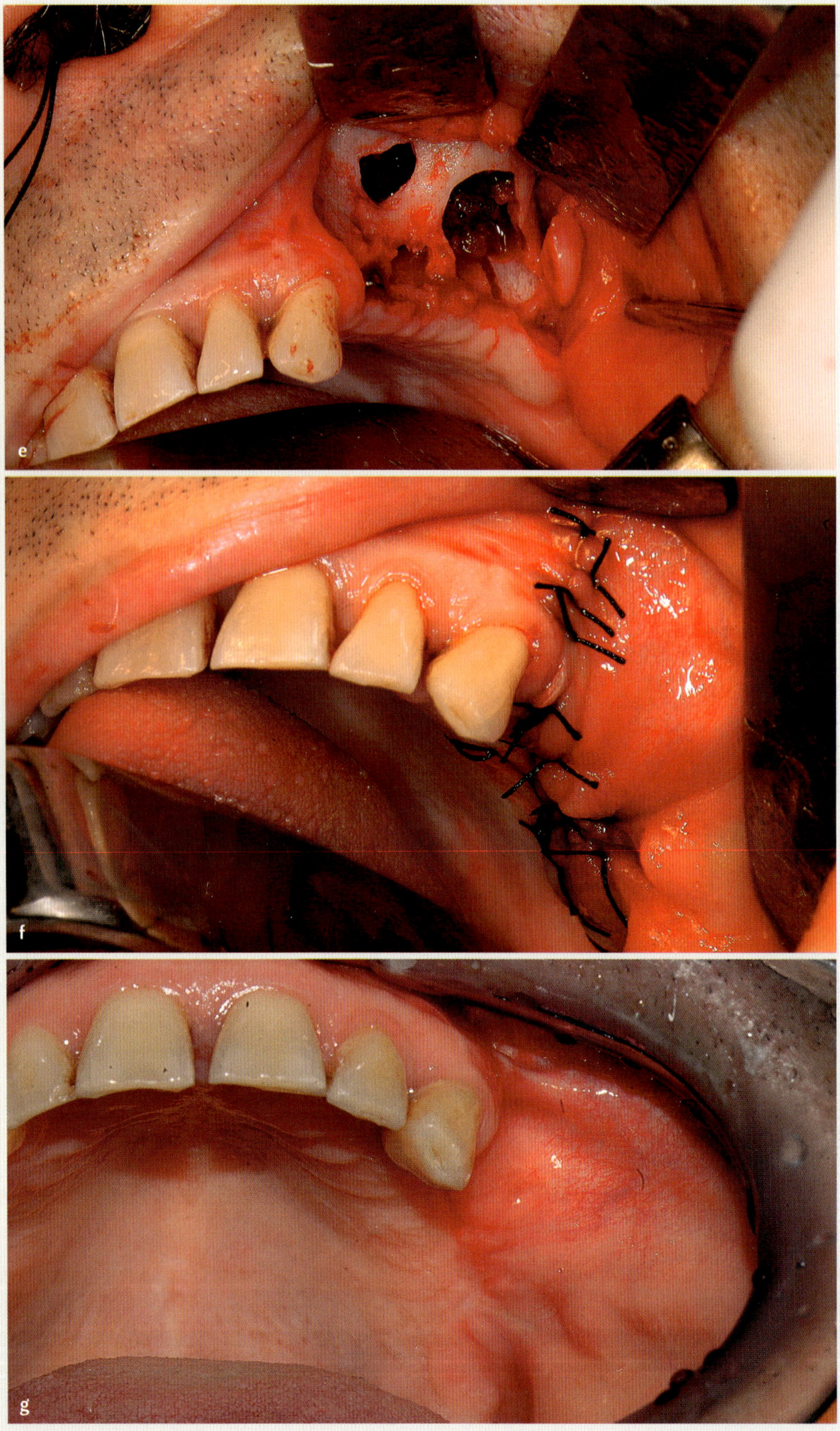

14.14 (*continued*) **e–f)** The migrated alloplastic material is removed, and the oroantral communications are closed with a Rehrmann flap. **g)** Complete healing some time after surgery.

Management

Foreign bodies must be removed from the maxillary sinus as soon as possible, and the oroantral communication immediately closed.

A first attempt at retrieving the migrated foreign body should be made immediately after the complication occurs, using the breach through which it has penetrated into the sinus. Periapical radiographs may help to assess its position and suction cannulas, as well as surgical curettes, can be used to extract it.

Should this first attempt fail, the retrieval must be performed by creating a window on the anterolateral wall of the sinus as detailed in the description of the Caldwell-Luc technique. Another technique involves creating a pedicle bone lid that can be repositioned with resorbable sutures after the foreign body is retrieved.

After sinus irrigation with sterile saline, the oroantral communication should be closed by repositioning the access flap with an airtight suture (14.15a–k).

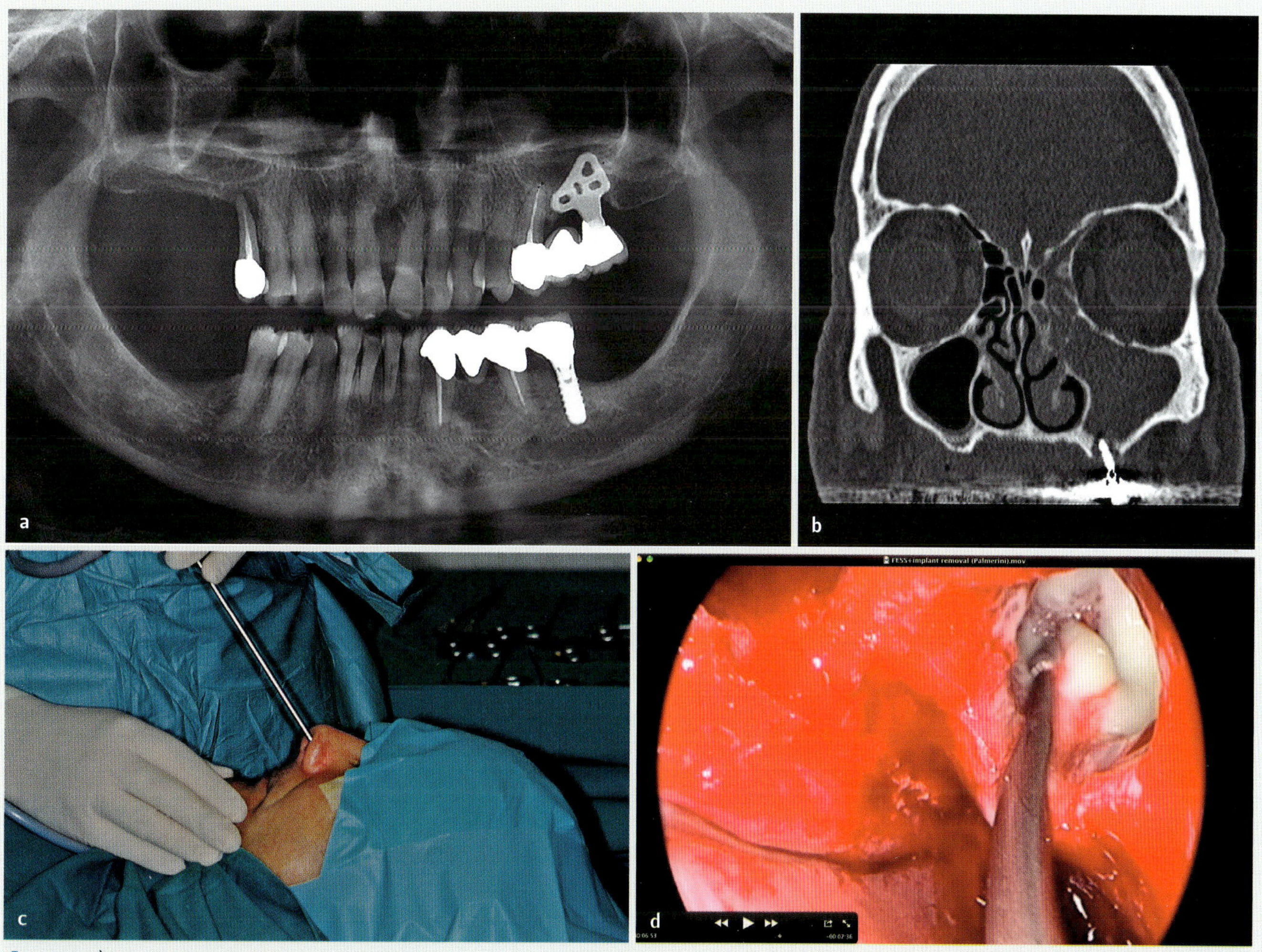

14.15 **a)** Panoramic radiograph showing the penetration of a blade implant inside the maxillary sinus. **b)** CT scan demonstrating the presence of an oroantral communication associated with complete opacification of the right maxillary sinus and involvement of the ipsilateral ethmoidal cells. **c)** FESS procedure: the endoscopic approach is used to remove the infectious material from the maxillary sinus and from the ethmoidal cells, while the following intraoral phase is aimed at closing the intraoral communication. **d)** During the endoscopic phase, inflammation and hyperaemia of the sinus mucosa, as well as the presence of purulent material, are clearly visible. (*continued*)

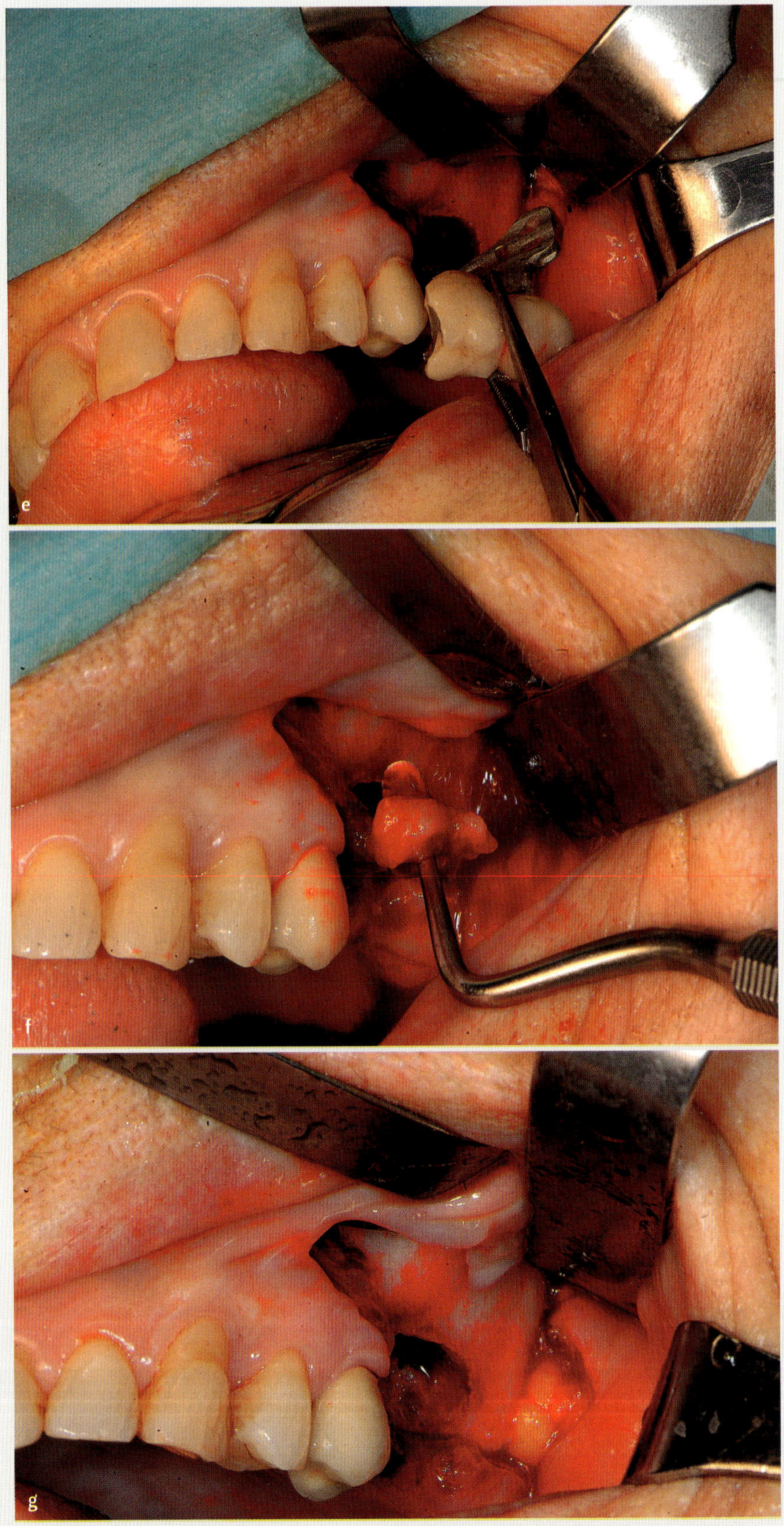

14.15 (*continued*) **e)** Intraoral phase: removal of the blade implant after elevation of a full-thickness flap. **f)** Removal of the inflamed tissue from the alveolar recess of the maxillary sinus. **g)** The buccal fat pad is exposed after the periosteum is interrupted. (*continued*)

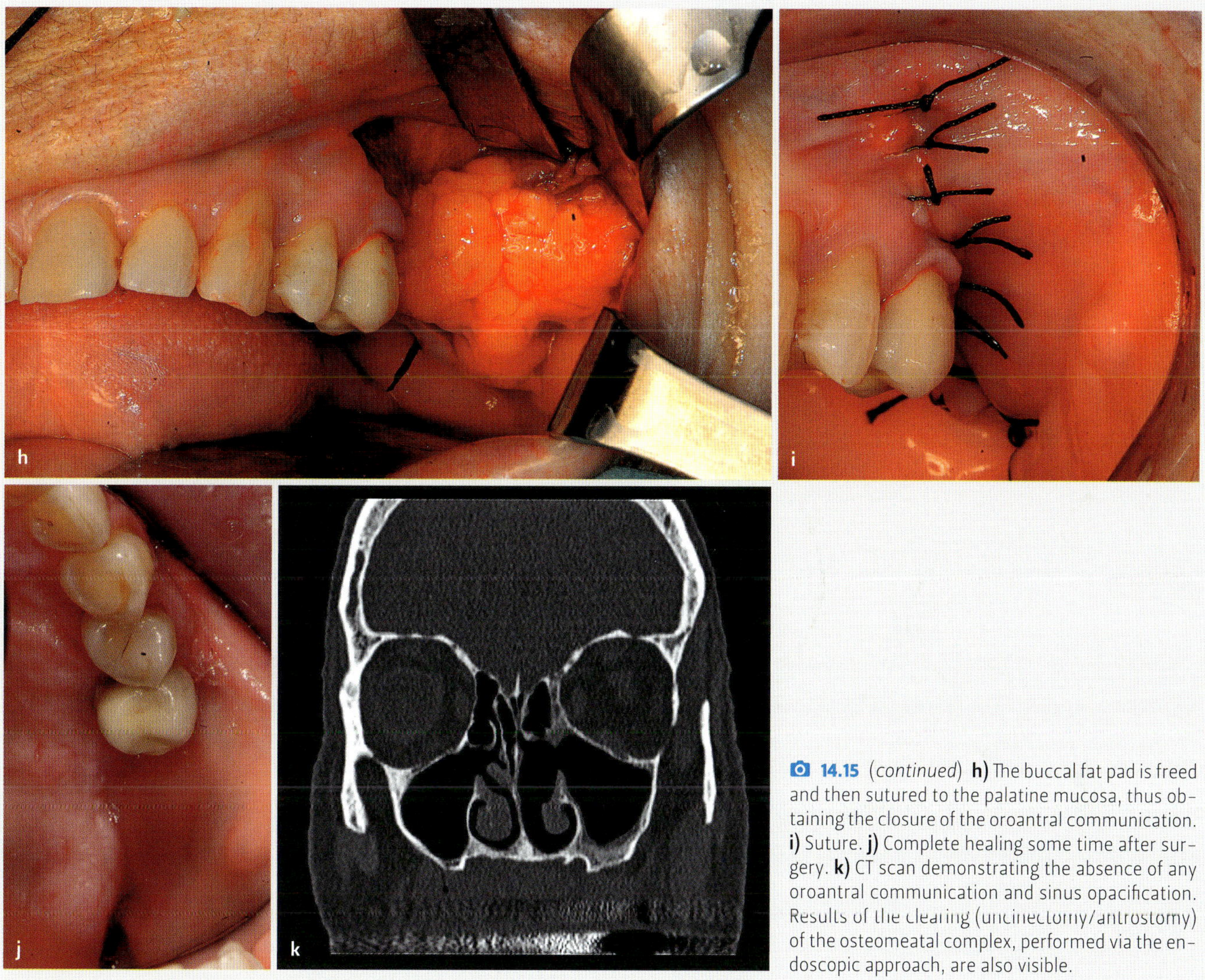

14.15 (*continued*) **h)** The buccal fat pad is freed and then sutured to the palatine mucosa, thus obtaining the closure of the oroantral communication. **i)** Suture. **j)** Complete healing some time after surgery. **k)** CT scan demonstrating the absence of any oroantral communication and sinus opacification. Results of the clearing (uncinectomy/antrostomy) of the osteomeatal complex, performed via the endoscopic approach, are also visible.

Postoperative complications

Delayed haemorrhage

Delayed bleeding may occur even after an apparently adequate haemostasis is obtained. This may be partially justified by the end of the vasoconstriction caused by the adrenaline (epinephrine) contained in the local anaesthetics used before and during the surgical procedure.

As far as prevention of this complication is concerned, the same criteria described in the section regarding intraoperative bleeding apply.

Management

Compressing the surgical wound with a damp gauze swab for 10-15 minutes may promote coagulation. In cases of protracted haemorrhage, the access flap must be reopened and the bleeding vessels identified before proceeding to enact the most appropriate manoeuvres to obtain adequate haemostasis. Bleeding control is important not only for the patients' comfort, but also to avoid haematoma formation that may cause any of the following:

- swelling that, in some cases, may be relevant or involve areas such as the floor of the mouth, where it can cause partial or total obstruction of the upper aerodigestive tract;
- formation of a particularly favourable medium for bacterial growth leading to secondary infections.

Wound dehiscence

Wound dehiscence can occur both before and after suture removal, and it can be caused by:

- infection;
- excessive suture tension;
- suture of the flap over an inadequately vascularised area;
- excessive trauma on the tissues during surgery.

Prevention

The risk of wound dehiscence can be significantly reduced if an atraumatic surgical technique is used, good oral hygiene is maintained in the postoperative period, and a tension-free suture of the access flap over an adequately vascularised area is performed. If excessive tension is felt while suturing, it must never be dealt with by placing more sutures or over-tightening the knots, as this may cause ischaemia of the soft tissues. The recourse to periosteal releasing incision, however, makes it possible to obtain adequate flap advancement and proceed with a tension-free suture of the access flap.

Management

In cases of early wound dehiscence, the access flap must be inspected and, in the absence of infection, can be sutured anew.

In cases of late dehiscence, epithelisation of the wound edges occurs: if no signs of infection are observed, refreshing of the wound edges and suturing can be performed. Alternatively, the wound can be left to heal by secondary intention.

Post-extractive infections: alveolar osteitis

Alveolar osteitis (also known as alveolitis sicca dolorosa or dry socket) is a post-extractive infection of the alveolar bone: its incidence ranges from 1% to 5%, and is generally higher in female patients. Symptoms of alveolar osteitis include pain (with a flare-up typically occurring 3-4 days after the extraction), halitosis, and regional lymph node involvement. The socket appears empty and greyish, occasionally filled with food debris. Alveolar osteitis seems to be caused by the early lysis of the blood clot, probably caused by bacterial contamination; several factors have been positively correlated with its onset, such as age, the use of oral contraceptives, the menstrual cycle, cigarette smoke, poor oral hygiene, and the intraligamentary infiltration of local anaesthetic containing adrenaline.

Prevention

To reduce the risk of alveolar osteitis, it is important to:

- eliminate bacterial plaque by means of a professional teeth cleaning session and a chlorhexidine mouthrinse protocol prior to the extraction;
- eliminate or reduce cigarette smoking habits in the postoperative period;
- perform the extraction between the 23rd and 28th day of the menstrual cycle in female patients who are taking oral contraceptives;
- choose a flap design that guarantees adequate blood supply to the area involved in the extraction;
- use refrigerated sterile saline as a cooling agent when rotary or piezoelectric instruments are used to perform ostectomy and odontotomy;
- irrigate the socket with sterile saline before suturing;
- eliminate contamination of the socket by oral fluids while suturing;
- instruct the patient to follow a protocol of chlorhexidine mouthrinse 3 times per day until suture removal;
- administer antibiotic prophylaxis (single dose, 1 hour before surgery).

Management

Irrigation of the empty socket allows the removal of possible food debris colonised by bacteria. In some cases, particularly when severe pain is present, curettage of the empty socket under local anaesthesia is indicated. The socket is then packed with an iodoform gauze, or with vegetable fibres impregnated with eugenol. Furthermore, it may be necessary to repeat this operation during the postoperative period. Vegetable fibres impregnated with eugenol present the advantage of being spontaneously expulsed from the socket during the healing phase (📷 14.16a-f).

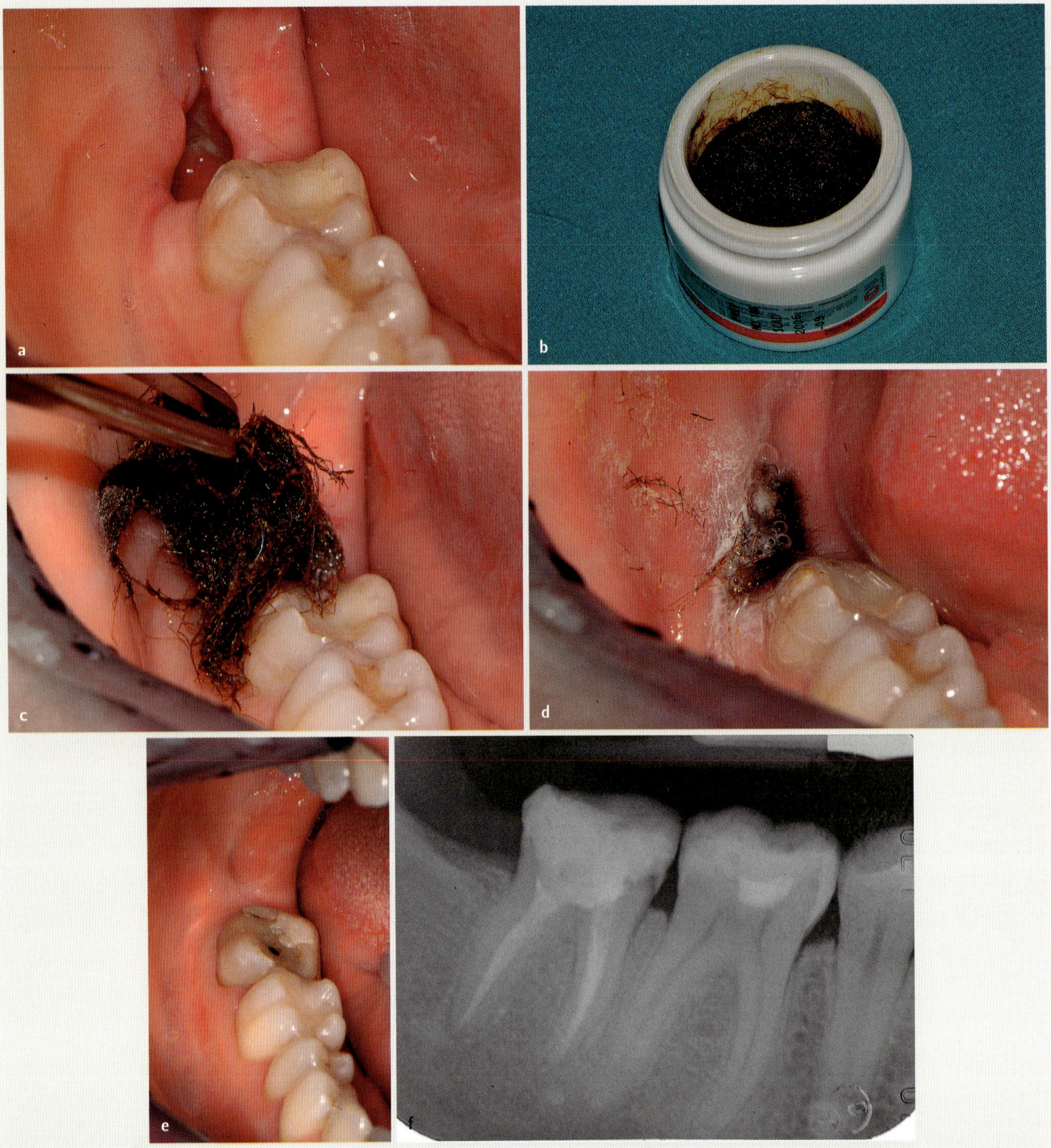

14.16 **a)** Clinical presentation of alveolar osteitis. **b)** Vegetable fibres impregnated with eugenol for the treatment of alveolar osteitis. **c–d)** Application of the impregnated vegetable fibres inside the empty socket. **e–f)** Radiographic and clinical follow-up showing complete healing.

Post-extractive infections: subperiosteal abscess

The subperiosteal abscess is caused by colonisation of the surgical wound by bacteria during the healing process and is characterised by the collection of purulent material under the soft tissues. The risk is higher in immunosuppressed patients. In some cases, a root fragment or foreign materials abandoned inside the socket can cause the formation of a subperiosteal abscess. The clinical picture can become evident days after surgery and includes swelling, pain, and in some cases also fever. The appearance of the superficial tissues may be normal; typically, subperiosteal abscesses develop when impacted teeth are extracted and complete closure of the soft tissues over the empty socket is achieved. No specific precautions have been identified to prevent suppurative complications. However, the same criteria described to prevent alveolar osteitis may apply.

Management

The treatment consists in the incision and drainage of the abscess, in association with antibiotic therapy (see Chapter 6). The incision is performed under local anesthesia, and allows the drainage of the purulent material. The wound is then irrigated with sterile saline, and a surgical drainage (iodoform gauze or rubber tube) is fixed in place. The drainage allows to expose the anaerobic bacteria inside the lesion to the external environment. Dressings should be removed, or substituted, within two days (14.17a–g).

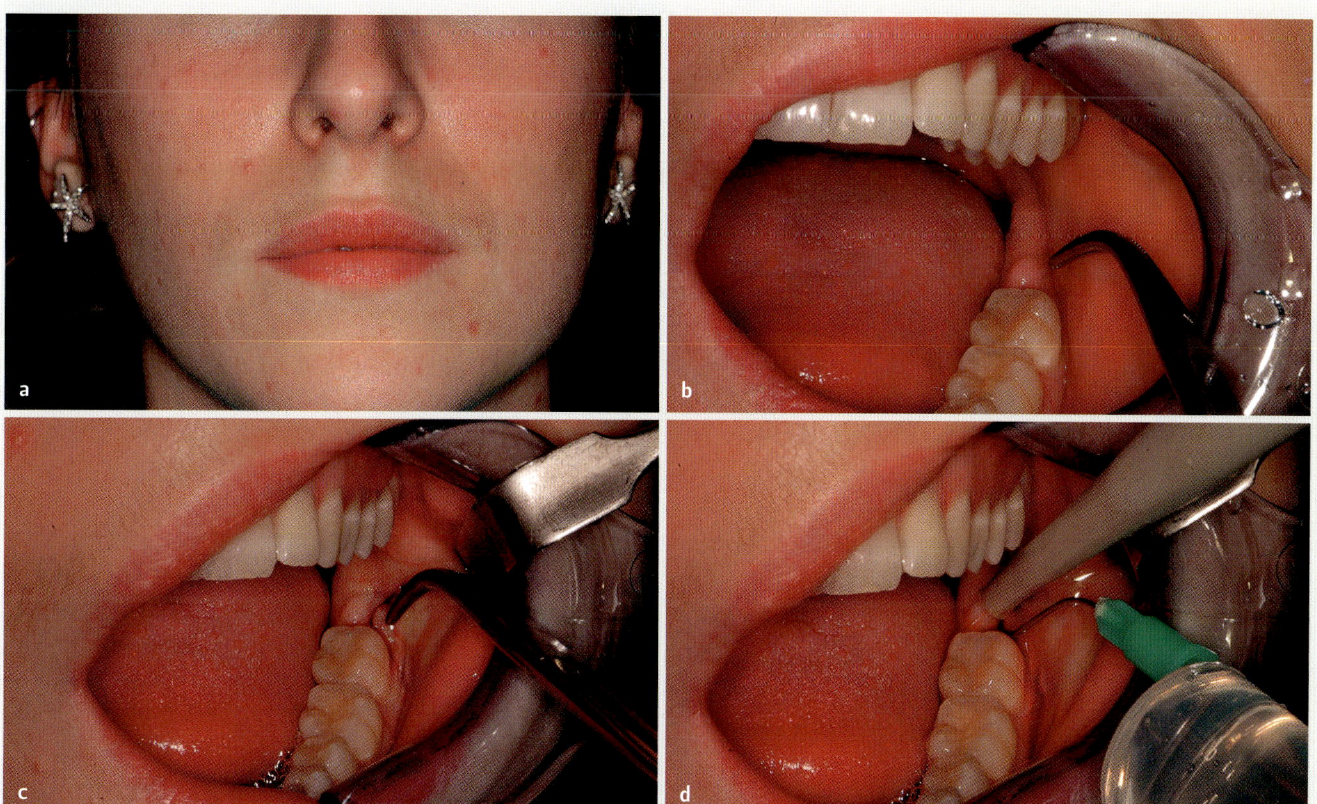

14.17 **a)** Upon extraoral examination, moderate swelling in the area of the left mandibular third molar is visible. **b)** Intraoral examination: the patient underwent surgical extraction of 3.8, and swelling of the soft tissues in the area is visible. **c)** An incision is made to facilitate the drainage of the subperiosteal abscess. **d)** Irrigation with sterile saline helps eliminate the purulent collection. (*continued*)

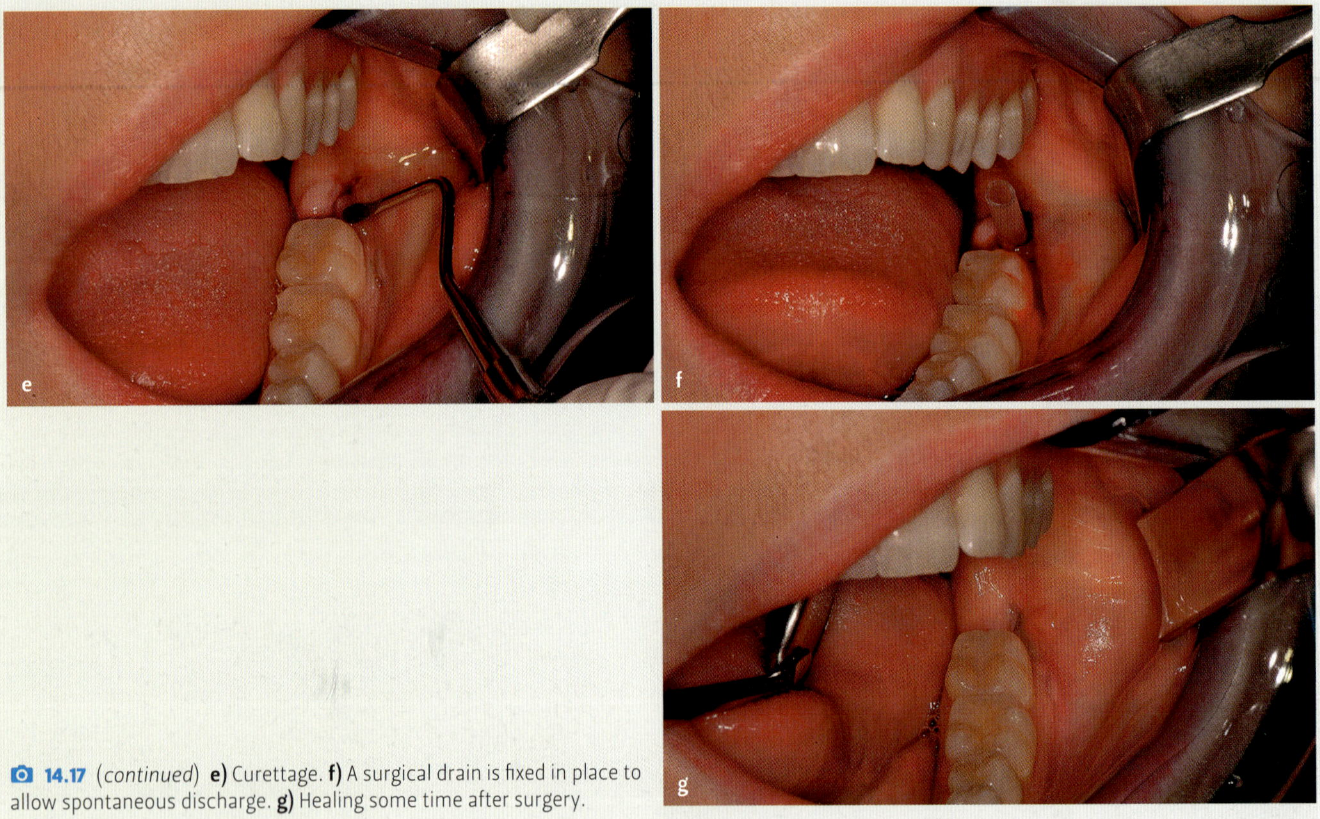

14.17 (*continued*) **e)** Curettage. **f)** A surgical drain is fixed in place to allow spontaneous discharge. **g)** Healing some time after surgery.

Bone sequestra

Bone sequestra represent the evolution of a localised bone infection that has a self-delimiting tendency: the infectious, non-viable bone segment is expelled. They are usually caused by traumatic injuries determining the presence of mobile or infected bone fragments that are not adequately vascularised, or by traumatic surgical manoeuvres determining alveolar fractures, laceration of the soft tissues, or bone overheating.

Radiographically, bone sequestra appear as bone segments surrounded by a radiolucent border; symptoms may include pain, which, however, is not always present, and the infected segment can be exposed and mobile.

Prevention

In cases of trauma, prevention of bone sequestrum is obtained by adequate stabilisation of bone fragments and coverage by well-vascularised soft tissues. Prevention of iatrogenic damage is obtained by respecting the principles of correct surgical techniques.

Management

Sequestra must be surgically removed and the surrounding bone vigorously curetted until vital tissue is found and bleeding is induced (14.18a–j).

Clinical case 1 – Surgical removal of mandibular bone sequestrum

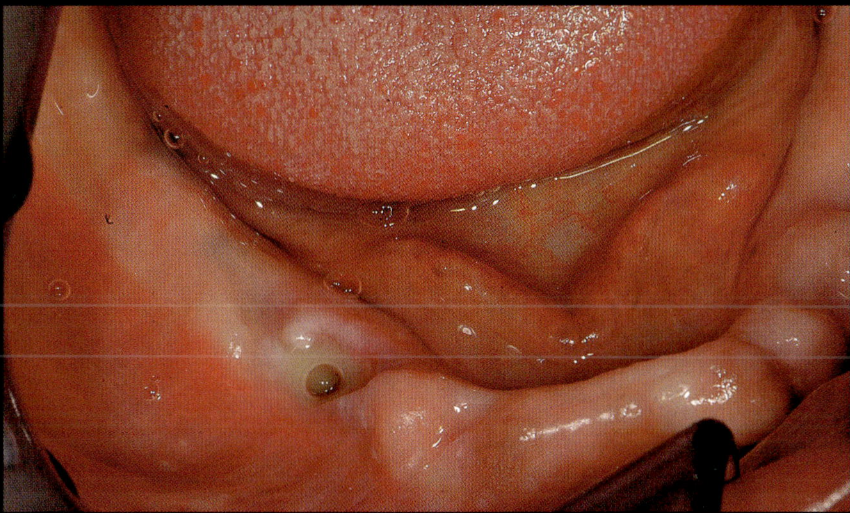

14.18a Intraoral view: purulent discharge is visible in the right hemimandible.

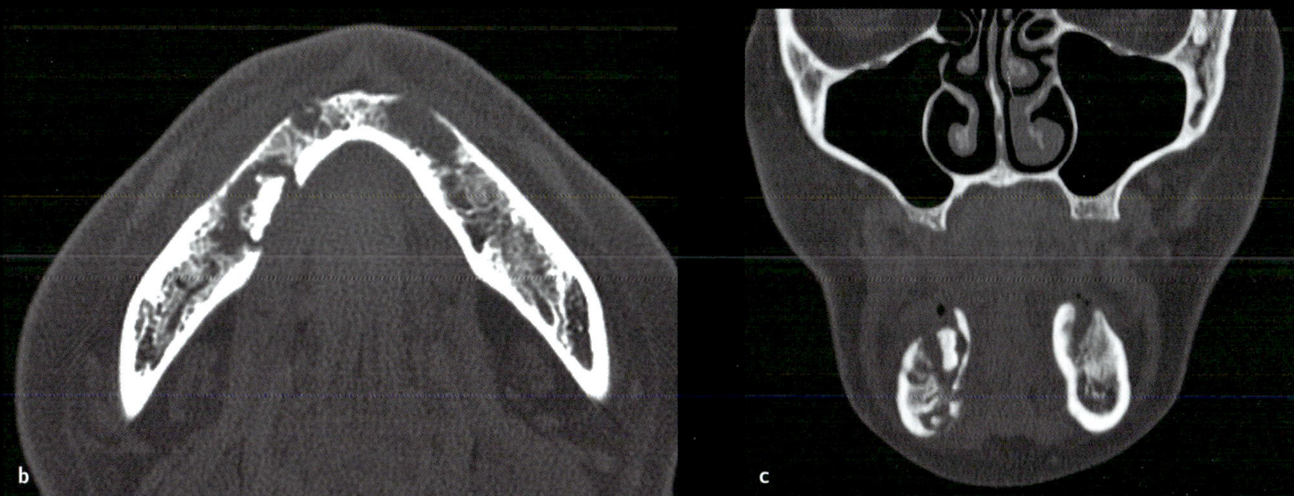

14.18b–c CT scan showing the presence of a bone sequestrum.

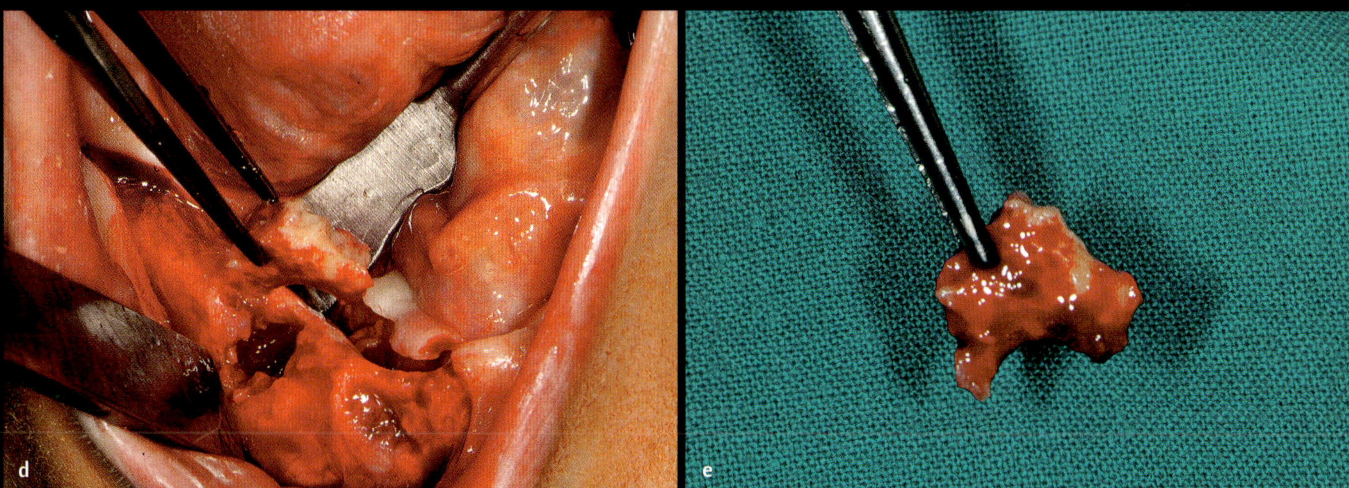

14.18d–e Surgical removal of the bone sequestrum.

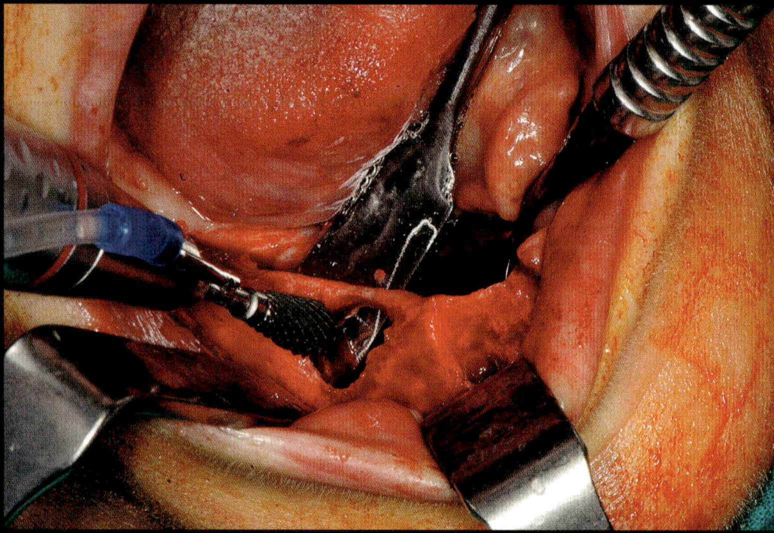

14.18f Vigorous curettage of the surrounding bone performed with rotary instruments to remove all traces of infected, non-vital tissue.

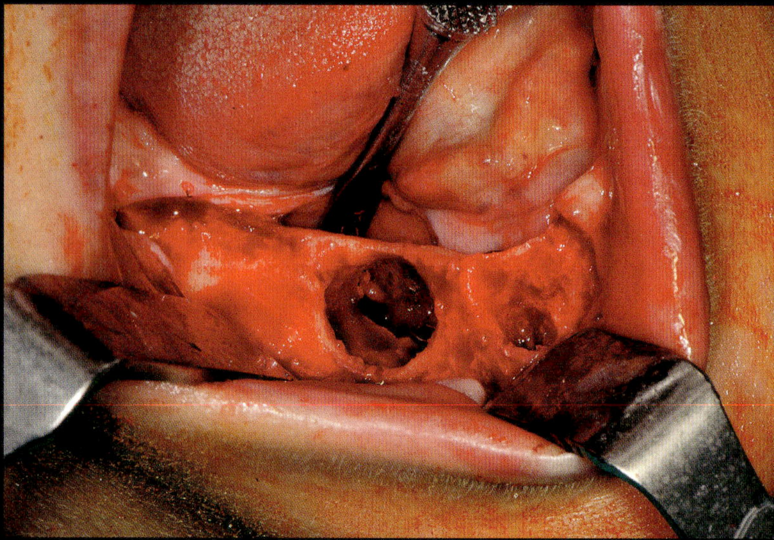

14.18g Curettage is completed.

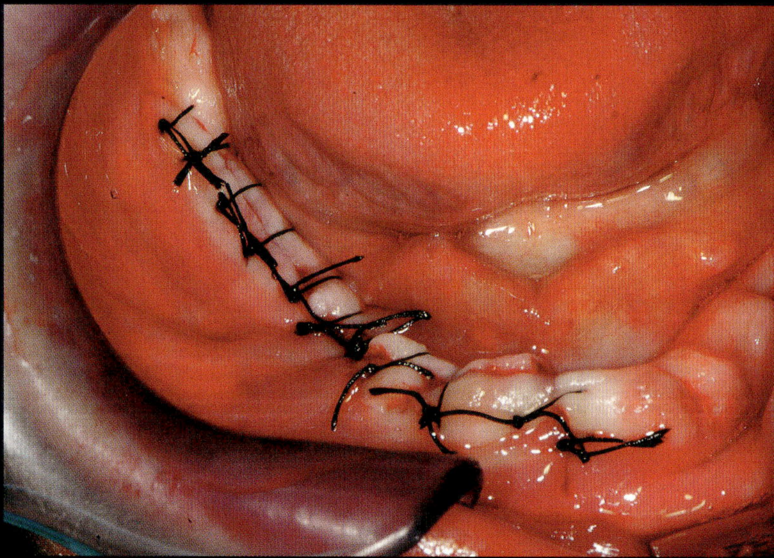

14.18h Suture.

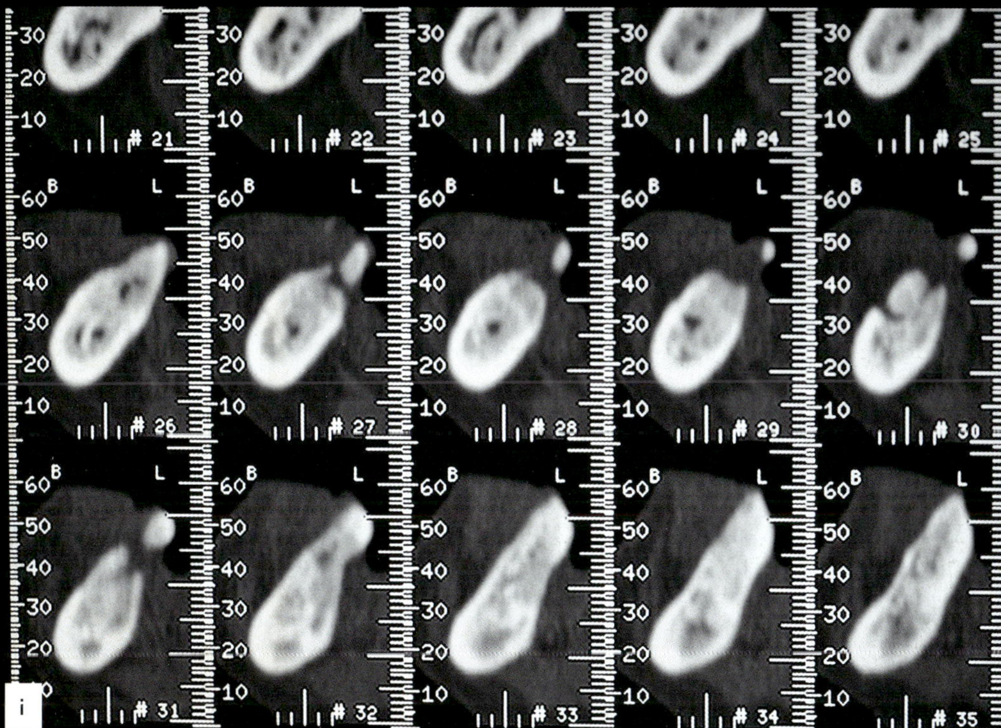

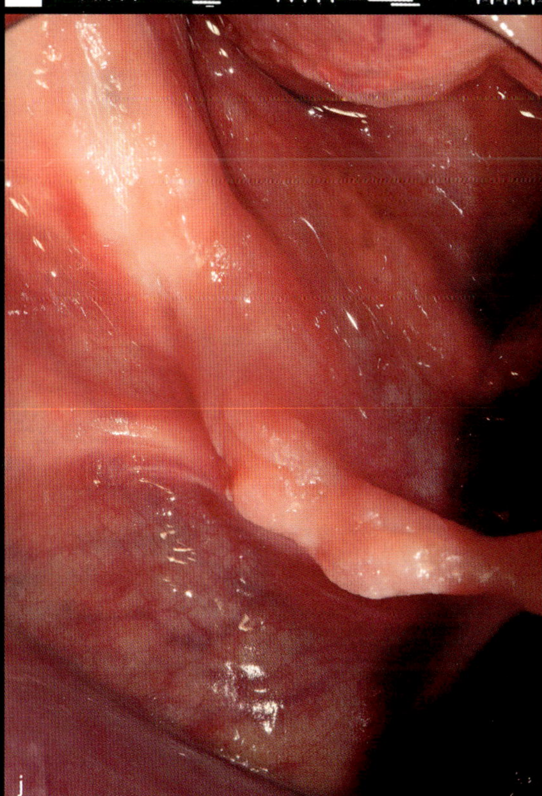

14.18i–j Radiographic and clini cal follow-up demonstrating complete healing.

REFERENCES

Almazrooa SA, Woo SB. Bisphosphonate and nonbisphosphonate-associated osteonecrosis of the jaw: a review. *J Am Dent Assoc.* 2009 Jul; 140(7):864-75.

Auyong TG, Le A. Dentoalveolar nerve injury. *Oral Maxillofac Surg Clin North Am* 2011 Aug; 23(3):395-400.

Bodner L, Brennan PA, McLeod NM. Characteristics of iatrogenic mandibular fractures associated with tooth removal: review and analysis of 189 cases. *Br J Oral Maxillofac Surg* 2011 Oct; 49(7):567-72.

Bowe DC, Rogers S, Stassen LF. The management of dry socket/alveolar osteitis. *J Ir Dent Assoc.* 2011 Dec-2012 Jan; 57(6):305-10.

Brauer HU. Unusual complications associated with third molar surgery: a systematic review. *Quintessence Int* 2009 Jul-Aug; 40(7):565-72.

Brook I. Sinusitis of odontogenic origin. Review. *Otolaryngology-Head and Neck Surgery* 2006; 136:349-55.

Bui CH, Seldin EB, Dodson TB. Types, frequencies, and risk factors for complications after third molar extraction. *J Oral Maxillofac Surg* 2003 Dec; 61(12):1379-89.

Cankaya AB, Erdem MA, Cakarer S, Cifter M, Oral CK. Iatrogenic mandibular fracture associated with third molar removal. *Int J Med Sci* 2011; 8(7):547-53.

Chiapasco M, De Cicco L, Marrone G. Side effects and complications associated with third molar surgery. *Oral Surg Oral Med Oral Pathol* 1993; 412-20.

Chrcanovic BR, Freire-Maia B. Considerations of maxillary tuberosity fractures during extraction of upper molars: a literature review. *Dent Traumatol* 2011 Oct; 27(5):393-8.

Clavero J, Lundgren S. Ramus or chin grafts for maxillary sinus inlay and local onlay augmentation: comparison of donor site morbidity and complications. *Clin Impl Dent Rel Res* 2003; 5:154-60.

Flanagan D. Important arterial supply of the mandible, control of an arterial hemorrage, and report of hemorrhagic incident. *J Oral Implantol* 2003; 29:165-73.

Giltay GB, Malvoz RE. Responsability and legal aspect of implantology. *Rev Belge Med Dent* 2001; 56:85-106.

Givol N, Chaushu G, Halamish-Shani T. Emergency tracheostomy following life threatening hemorrage in the floor of the mouth during immediaty implant placemen in the mandibular canine region. *J Periodontol* 2000; 71:1893-5.

Graff-Radford SB, Evans RW. Lingual nerve injury. *Headache*, 2003 Oct; 43(9):975-83.

Kalpidis CD, Setayesh RM. Haemorrhaging associated with endosseous implant placement in the anterior mandible: a review of the literature. *J Periodontol* 2004 May; 75(5):631-45.

Kalpidis CD, Konstantinidis AB. Critical hemorrage in the floor of the mouth during implant placement in the first mandibular premolar position: a case report. *Implant Dent* 2005; 14:117-24.

Laboda G. Life-threatening hemorrhage after placement of an endosseous implant: report of case. *J Am Dent Ass* 1990; 121(5):599-600.

Mason ME, Triplett RG, Alfonso WF. Life-threatening hemorrhage from placement of a dental implant. *J Oral Maxillofac Surg* 1990; 48:201-4.

Moore UJ. Principles of oral and maxillofacial surgery. 5th ed. Blackwell, Oxford 2001.

Mordenfeld A, Andersson L, Bergstrom B. Hemorrage in the floor of the mouth during implant placement in the edentolous mandible: a case report. *Int J Oral Maxillofac Impl* 1997; 12:558-61.

Nabil S, Samman N. Incidence and prevention of osteoradionecrosis after dental extraction in irradiated patients: a systematic review. *Int J Oral Maxillofac Surg* 2011 Mar; 40(3):229-43.

Niamtu. Near-fatal airway obstruction after routine implant placement. *Oral Surg Oral Med Oral Pathol Oral Radiol Endod* 2001; 92:597-600.

Pogrel MA, Perrott DH, Kaban LB. Complications in oral and maxillofacial surgery. WB Saunders, Philadelphia 1997.

Pogrel MA, Goldman KE. Lingual flap retraction for third molary surgery. *J Oral Maxillofac Surg* 2004; 62:1125-30.

Reich W, Kriwalsky MS, Wolf HH, Schubert J. Bleeding complications after oral surgery in outpatients with compromised haemostasis: incidence and management. *Oral Maxillofac Surg* 2009; 13:73-7.

Robert RC, Bacchetti P, Pogrel MA. Frequency of trigeminal nerve injuries following third molar removal. *J Oral Maxillofac Surg* 2005; 63:732-6.

Rothamed D, Wahl G, d'Hoedt B, Nentwig GH, Schwarz F, Becker J. Incidence and predictive factors for perforation of the maxillary antrum in operations to remove upper wisdom teeth: Prospective multicentre study. *British J Oral Maxillofac Surg* 2007; 45:387-91.

Scribano E, Ascenti G, Mazziotti S, Blandino A, Racchiusa S, Gualniera P. Computed tomography in dental implantology: medico-legal implications. *Radiol Med* 2003; 105:92-9.

Singh H, Lee K, Ayoub AF. Management of asymptomatic impacted wisdom teeth: a multicentre comparison. *Br J Oral Maxillofac Surg* 1996; 34:389-93.

Index